A LANGE Medical Book

Behavioral Medicine in Primary Care

A Practical Guide

Second Edition

Edited by

Mitchell D. Feldman, MD, MPhil
Associate Professor of Medicine
Division of General Internal Medicine
Department of Medicine
University of California, San Francisco

John F. Christensen, PhD
Department of Medicine
Legacy Portland Hospitals
Portland, Oregon

Lange Medical Books/McGraw-Hill
Medical Publishing Division

New York   Chicago   San Francisco   Lisbon   London   Madrid   Mexico City
Milan   New Delhi   San Juan   Seoul   Singapore   Sydney   Toronto

This book was set in Adobe Garamond by Circle Graphics.
The editors were Shelley Reinhardt, Harriet Lebowitz, and Regina Y. Brown.
The production supervisor was Lisa Mendez.
The illustration manager was Charissa Baker.
The cover designer was Mary McKeon.
RR Donnelley was the printer and binder.

This book is printed on acid-free paper.

Contents

Authors

Robert B. Baron, MD, MS
Professor of Medicine; Associate Dean for Continuing
Medical Education; Vice Chief and Director,
Educational Programs, Division of General Internal
Medicine; Director, Primary Care Internal Medicine
Residency Program, University of California,
San Francisco
baron@medicine.ucsf.edu
Obesity

Howard B. Beckman, MD, FACP
Clinical Professor of Medicine and Family Medicine,
University of Rochester School of Medicine and
Dentistry; Medical Director, Rochester Individual
Practice Association, Rochester, New York
hbeckman@ripa.org
Difficult Patients

Douglas Beers, MD
Assistant Chief of Medicine, Legacy Portland
Hospitals, Portland, Oregon
dbeers@lhs.org
Pain

Jeffrey L. Boone, MD, MS
Assistant Clinical Professor of Medicine, University
of Colorado College of Medicine, Denver; Preventive
Cardiology Consultant, Denver Broncos National
Football League Club, Colorado
Stress & Disease

Gail F. Brenner, PhD
Assistant Clinical Professor, Department of
Psychiatry, University of California, San Francisco
brenner@itsa.ucsf.edu
Chronic Illness

David G. Bullard, PhD
Clinical Professor of Medicine and Medical
Psychology (Psychiatry), University of California,
San Francisco; Psychotherapist in Private Practice,
San Francisco, California
dgbullard@yahoo.com
Sexual Problems

Jeffrey H. Burack, MD, MPP, BPhil
Assistant Adjunct Professor of Bioethics and Medical
Humanities, University of California, Berkeley;
Assistant Clinical Professor of Medicine, University of
California, San Francisco; Attending Physician,
East Bay AIDS Center, Berkeley, California
jburack@socrates.berkeley.edu
HIV/AIDS

Lisa Capaldini, MD, MPH
Assistant Clinical Professor of Medicine, University of
California, San Francisco; Director, Castro Medical
Clinic, San Francisco, California
lcapaldini@earthlink.net
HIV/AIDS

Harvey Caplan, MD
Former Co-Director of Clinical Training, Human
Sexuality Program, University of California,
San Francisco
hcaplan@ix.netcom.com
Sexual Problems

John R. Chamberlain, MD
Clinical Instructor, Department of Psychiatry,
University of California, San Francisco
johncmd@hotmail.com
Somatization

John F. Christensen, PhD
Director of Behavioral Medicine Training, Department
of Medicine, Legacy Portland Hospitals, Portland,
Oregon
jchriste@lhs.org
*Suggestion & Hypnosis; Depression; Stress & Disease;
Mistakes in Medical Practice*

William D. Clark, MD
Lecturer in Medicine, Harvard Medical School,
Boston, Massachusetts; Addiction Resource
Center, Brunswick, Maine
wclark@midcoasthealth.com
Alcohol & Substance Use

Thomas J. Coates, PhD
Professor of Medicine and Epidemiology, University of California, San Francisco; Director, Center for AIDS Prevention Studies; Director, University of California, San Francisco, AIDS Research Institute, tcoates@psg.ucsf.edu
HIV/AIDS

Mary Raju Cole, RN, MSN, FNP
Formerly Director, Northport VA Primary Care Depression Project; Currently, Contributing Editor, The Nursing Spectrum, Huntington, New York
mrajucole@aol.com
Depression

Steven A. Cole, MD
Professor of Psychiatry and Co-Director, Center for Health Policy, University of Connecticut Health Center, Farmington
scole@psychiatry.uchc.edu
Depression

Thomas Denberg, MD, PhD
Instructor of Medicine, Division of General Internal Medicine, Department of Medicine, University of California, San Francisco
tdenberg@medicine.ucsf.edu
Cross-Cultural Communication

M. Robin DiMatteo, PhD
Professor, Department of Psychology, University of California, Riverside
robin@citrus.ucr.edu
Patient Adherence

Elizabeth A. Edwardsen, MD
Associate Professor, Department of Emergency Medicine, University of Rochester Medical Center
elizabeth_edwardsen@urmc.rochester.edu
Sexual Issues and Professional Development: A Challenge for Medical Education

Barry Egener, MD
Medical Director, The Foundation for Medical Excellence; Faculty, Portland Program in Internal Medicine, Portland, Oregon
begener@lhs.org
Empathy

Stuart J. Eisendrath, MD
Professor of Clinical Psychiatry, University of California, San Francisco; Director, Ambulatory Services, Langley Porter Psychiatric Hospital and Clinics, San Francisco, California
eisen@itsa.ucsf.edu
Somatization

Michael Eisman, MD
Medical Director, Seneca View Nursing Facility, Montour Falls, New York
Death & Dying

Adriana Feder, MD
Assistant Clinical Professor of Psychiatry (in Medicine), Department of Psychiatry, Columbia University College of Physicians and Surgeons, New York, New York
af286@columbia.edu
Personality Disorders

Mitchell D. Feldman, MD, MPhil
Associate Professor of Medicine, Division of General Internal Medicine, Department of Medicine, University of California, San Francisco
mfeldman@medicine.ucsf.edu
Cross-Cultural Communication; Depression; HIV/AIDS; Domestic Violence

Susan Folkman, PhD
Director, Osher Center for Integrative Medicine; Professor of Medicine, Osher Foundation Distinguished Professor in Integrative Medicine, University of California, San Francisco
folkman@ocim.ucsf.edu
Complementary & Alternative Medicine

Richard M. Frankel, PhD
Professor of Medicine, Indiana University School of Medicine; Senior Scientist, The Regenstrief Institute for Health Care, Indianapolis, Indiana
rfrankel@iupui.edu
Sexual Issues and Professional Development: A Challenge for Medical Education

Lawrence S. Friedman, MD
Professor of Pediatrics and Chief, Division of General Pediatrics and Adolescent Medicine, University of California, San Diego
lsfriedman@ucsd.edu
Adolescents

Linda Ganzini, MD
Professor of Psychiatry, Oregon Health and Science University, Portland; Director, Geriatric Psychiatry Fellowship Training, Portland Veterans Affairs Medical Center, Oregon
ganzinil@ohsu.edu
Older Patients

Geoffrey H. Gordon, MD
Adjunct Professor of Medicine, Division of General Medicine & Geriatrics, Oregon Health and Science University, Portland, Oregon
gordong@ohsu.edu
Giving Bad News

Steven R. Hahn, MD
Professor of Clinical Medicine and Instructor in Psychiatry, Albert Einstein College of Medicine; Director, Primary Care Internal Medicine Residency Program of the Albert Einstein College of Medicine at Jacobi Medical Center, Bronx, New York
shahn@aecom.yu.edu
Families

Katherine A. Halmi, MD
Professor of Psychiatry; Director, Eating Disorder Program, Weill-Cornell Medical Center-Westchester Division, White Plains, New York
kah29@cornell.edu
Eating Disorders

Ellen Hughes, MD, PhD
Clinical Professor of Medicine, University of California, San Francisco, Director for Education, Osher Center for Integrative Medicine, San Francisco, California
ehughes@medicine.ucsf.edu
Complementary & Alternative Medicine

Martina J. Jelley, MD, MSPH
Associate Professor, Department of Internal Medicine, University of Oklahoma College of Medicine, Tulsa
martina-jelley@ouhsc.edu
Women

Stephen R. Jones, MD
Chief, Department of Medicine, Legacy Portland Hospitals; Professor of Medicine, Oregon Health Sciences University, Portland, Oregon
sjones@lhs.org
Older Patients

Wendy Levinson, MD
Vice Chairman, Department of Medicine, The University of Toronto; Associate Director of Research Administration, St. Michael's Hospital, Toronto, Ontario, Canada
wendy.levinson@utoronto.ca
Anxiety

Mack Lipkin, Jr., MD
Professor of Medicine; Director, Division of Primary Care, New York University School of Medicine; Founding President, American Academy on Physician and Patient, New York, New York
lipkim01@popmail.med.nyu.edu
The Medical Interview

William L. Lyons, MD
Medical Director, Geropsychiatric Nursing Home Care Unit, Department of Veterans Affairs, Palo Alto Health Care System, Menlo Park, California
william.lyons@med.va.gov
Dementia

Stephen J. McPhee, MD
Professor of Medicine, Division of General Internal Medicine, Department of Medicine, University of California, San Francisco
smcphee@medicine.ucsf.edu
Mistakes in Medical Practice

E. Montez Mutzig, MD, MPH, FACP
Former Associate Professor, Department of Internal Medicine & Obstetrics/Gynecology, University of Oklahoma College of Medicine, Tulsa; Present Internist in Private Practice, Tulsa, Oklahoma
Women

Daniel O'Connell, PhD
Private Practice in Coaching, Consulting and Counseling, Seattle, Washington; Clinical Instructor, Department of Psychiatry and Human Behavior, University of Washington School of Medicine, Seattle
danoconn@mindspring.com
Behavior Change

Britta Ostermeyer, MD
Fellow, Department of Forensic Psychiatry, Case
Western Reserve University, Cleveland, Ohio
brittamd@aol.com
Personality Disorders

Timothy E. Quill, MD
Professor of Medicine, Psychiatry and Medical
Humanities, University of Rochester School of
Medicine and Dentistry; Director, Primary Care
Internist, University of Rochester Medical Center,
Rochester, New York
Death & Dying

Gita Ramamurthy, MD
Clinical Assistant Professor, State University of
New York, Syracuse; Cayuga Medical Center, Ithaca,
New York
murthg@aol.com
Physician Well-Being

Nancy A. Rigotti, MD
Associate Professor of Medicine, Harvard Medical
School; Director, Tobacco Research & Treatment
Center, Massachusetts General Hospital, Boston
nrigotti@partners.org
Smoking

Seth Wigdor Robbins, MD, MPH
Private Practice, San Francisco and Berkeley,
California
swrobbins@earthlink.net
Personality Disorders

Steven J. Romano, MD
Senior Medical Director/Neuroscience, Pfizer Inc.,
New York, New York
steve.romano@pfizer.com
Eating Disorders

Robert Sack, MD
Professor of Psychiatry, Oregon Health and Sciences
University, Portland, Oregon
sackr@ohsu.edu
Sleep Disorders

Jason M. Satterfield, PhD
Assistant Clinical Professor, Department of
Medicine, University of California,
San Francisco
jsatter@medicine.ucsf.edu
Anxiety

Clifford Milo Singer, MD
Associate Professor of Psychiatry and Neurology;
Clinical Director of Geriatric Psychiatry;
Attending Physician and Investigator, Alzheimer's
Disease Research Center; Medical Director of the
Oregon Geriatric Education Center, Oregon Health
and Science University, Portland, Oregon
singerc@ohsu.edu
Older Patients; Sleep Disorders

Gregory T. Smith, PhD
Clinical Psychologist and Director, Progressive
Rehabilitation Associates, Portland, Oregon
greg@progrehab.com
Pain

Anthony L. Suchman, MD, MA
Senior Consultant, Relationship Centered Health
Care, Rochester, New York; Clinical Professor
of Medicine and Psychiatry, University of Rochester
School of Medicine and Dentistry, New York
asuchman@rochester.rr.com
Physician Well-Being

Howard L. Taras, MD
Professor, University of California, San Diego,
La Jolla, California
Children

Judith Walsh, MD, MPH
Associate Professor of Clinical Medicine, Women's
Health Clinical Research Center, Department of
Medicine, University of California,
San Francisco
jwalsh@medicine.ucsf.edu
Women

Melissa Welch, MD, MPH
Associate Clinical Professor of Medicine, University
of California, San Francisco; Medical Director,
Health Plan of San Mateo, South San Francisco,
California
podsdt@aol.com
Cross-Cultural Communication

Jocelyn C. White, MD, FACP
Assistant Professor of Medicine, Oregon Health and
Science University, Faculty, Legacy
Portland Hospitals, Portland, Oregon
jwhite@lhs.org
Lesbian & Gay Patients

Sarah Williams, MD
Instructor, Department of Psychiatry, New York
University Medical Center; Private Practice,
New York, New York
*Sexual Issues and Professional Development:
A Challenge for Medical Education*

Albert W. Wu, MD, MPH
Associate Professor of Health Policy and
Management and Epidemiology, Bloomberg School
of Public Health and Medicine, School of Medicine,
Johns Hopkins University, Baltimore, Maryland
awu@jhsph.edu
Mistakes in Medical Practice

Kristine Yaffe, MD
Assistant Professor in Residency, Department of
Psychiatry, Neurology, Epidemiology &
Biostatistics, University of California,
San Francisco; Chief, Geriatric Psychiatry,
San Francisco Veterans Affairs Medical Center,
San Francisco, California
kyaffe@itsa.ucsf.edu
Dementia

Foreword

Not the least of the many important changes that have occurred in medical care over the past 10 years is the heightened emphasis on primary care and its practitioners. The resulting new prominence has been accompanied by high expectations and expanded responsibilities—for greater productivity, for increased cost-effectiveness, for gatekeeping, and for integrating all aspects of patient care. In a sense, primary care has come to be seen as a solution for many of the problems in our medical system.

High expectations are of course burdensome. But in this setting they are more so because of the ways in which many primary care practitioners view themselves—as victims rather than beneficiaries of all this attention, expected to do more with less, with greater responsibility but no greater resources, and with a scope that is broader than what their expertise may permit.

Behavioral medicine offers help. While not a panacea, behavioral medicine can enrich primary care practice by providing a new perspective and the tools to implement it. For behavioral medicine holds the promise that greater attention to the mind/body connection—and to the effect of emotions on physical health and on the way patients seek medical care—can enhance physician and patient satisfaction, produce better treatment outcomes, and reduce inappropriate use of medical care. A behavioral medicine orientation can also help physicians look at themselves and better understand the ways in which their own behavior affects the patient. The ways physicians relate to their patients—what they say, how they say it, and nonverbal messages—have an important effect on the course and outcome of treatment and on compliance. Skillful communication is, of course, not a substitute for biomedical competence; both are necessary.

Behavioral medicine is both simple and profound, traditional and new, commonsensical and scientific. New research in psychoneuroimmunology, for example, suggests that the way people feel can affect, perhaps significantly, the immune system. Also, researchers using new brain scanning techniques, such as positron emission tomography (PET), are demonstrating the plasticity of the brain, the susceptibility to changes in its physical properties as a result of life experiences. Less esoteric is the good evidence that supportive group counseling with cancer patients can enhance compliance with treatment.

Above all, a behavioral medicine orientation instructs but also reminds physicians of much of what they already know but often fail to incorporate into practice—the symbiosis between psyche and soma, the inseparability of psychological well-being from general physical health, and the importance of being alert to signs of psychological distress, such as depression.

Doctors Feldman and Christensen have done primary care practice a good and important service with the publication of their book. It remains for clinicians and teachers to open their minds and practices to the ideas within it.

Steven A. Schroeder, MD
Distinguished Professor of Health and Health Care
Department of Medicine
Director
Center for Health Professions Leadership on Tobacco Cessation
University of California, San Francisco

Preface

Behavioral Medicine in Primary Care is a comprehensive text for clinicians, students, and teachers. The second edition builds on the contributions of the first by addressing the broad spectrum of psychosocial problems commonly seen in the practice of primary care medicine and providing practical, clinically relevant solutions. This edition retains the core concepts and principles of behavioral medicine that informed the first edition while incorporating many of the new developments in medical practice over the past five years. Every chapter has been significantly revised to reflect these developments as well as to provide updates on new approaches to diagnosis and treatment. For example, greater emphasis has been placed on evidence-based medicine and its influence on the content and practice of medicine. It is our belief that the incorporation of behavioral medicine principles and techniques into practice can help clinicians work more effectively and derive more satisfaction from their work. We have also added a chapter on complementary and alternative medicine, as the rise of CAM has created new challenges and opportunities in the behavioral arena for both patients and practitioners.

Although the term "behavioral medicine" is used widely in both medical and social science literature, there is little agreement as to its exact definition. We broadly define it as an interdisciplinary field that aims to integrate the biological and psychosocial perspectives on human behavior and apply them to the practice of medicine. Our perspective includes a behavioral approach to somatic disease, the mental disorders as they commonly appear in medical practice, issues in the relationship between physician and patient, and other important topics that affect the delivery of medical care, such as adherence to medical treatment, complementary and alternative medicine, and care of the dying.

It is our hope that general internists, family practitioners, nurse practitioners, and other primary care providers will find that this book helps them better understand and care for persons with a wide variety of mental and behavioral problems. For residents and students in primary care settings, *Behavioral Medicine in Primary Care* can function as a valuable resource for understanding the psychosocial dimensions of medicine in much the same way that *Current Medical Diagnosis & Treatment* (42nd edition, Lange, 2003) helps them to understand the biomedical domain.

We also hope that this book will serve as a clinically relevant text for the increasing number of primary care residency programs, schools of nursing, and medical schools that are adding behavioral medicine to their required curricula. As medical educators and policy-makers seek to define the core competencies in medical education, we expect that this book will help them better describe the behavioral and psychosocial domains that are key to developing competency in doctor-patient communication, professionalism, cultural competence, and other areas. For faculty and students who wish to explore a topic in greater depth, the suggestions for further reading and web based resources provided at the end of each chapter will be helpful.

Most chapters include case illustrations of behavioral strategies that can be used in the context of primary care. Many of these cases include sample dialogues to help illustrate—and, it is hoped, enhance—clinician-patient communication. Behavioral approaches can also help clinicians obtain greater satisfaction from patient care.

This second edition of *Behavioral Medicine in Primary Care* is divided into five sections. Section I, "The Doctor & Patient," focuses on topics that influence the development and maintenance of the doctor-patient relationship. Chapter 1, "The Medical Interview," lays the groundwork for how to communicate with patients effectively and efficiently. Chapter 2 explores a key element in doctor-patient communication, empathy, and suggests ways in which primary care clinicians can use empathy therapeutically. Chapters 3 and 4 focus on some specific challenges to doctor-patient communication, such as giving bad news and dealing with "difficult" patients. In Chapter 5, "Sexual Issues and Professional Development: A Challenge for Medical Education," the authors draw on material gathered from primary care providers at numerous workshops to explore the important but rarely acknowledged issue of how sexuality affects interactions with both patients and colleagues. Chapter 6 reviews ways in which busy primary care clinicians can use suggestion and hypnosis as part of their ongoing care of patients. The final chapter in this section focuses on physician well-being. Effective doctor-patient communication requires that physicians (and all clinicians) learn ways to enhance their own well-being and remain professionally and personally fulfilled.

Section II, "Working With Specific Populations," takes a broader perspective yet provides an in-depth review of some specific groups of patients cared for in the primary care setting. In Chapter 8, "Families," the author draws on an extensive case discussion to illustrate the importance of a family systems approach in caring for patients. Chapters 9, 10, and 11 focus on the developmental cycle from childhood to adolescence to old age, touching on the key developmental and emotional problems the primary care provider is likely to encounter in each patient group. The emphasis in these chapters, as it is throughout the book, is on both recognition and treatment of common disorders. The next three chapters, "Cross-Cultural Communication," "Lesbian & Gay Patients," and "Women," offer suggestions for enhancing the diagnosis and treatment of primary care patients who often have specific needs and concerns.

Section III focuses on health-related behavior in the primary care context. The framework for this section is provided in Chapter 15, "Behavior Change," in which the theory of stages of change is applied to the primary care setting, and in Chapter 16, "Patient Adherence." Chapters 17, 18, 19, and 20 address specific health-related behaviors most commonly encountered in the primary care setting—smoking, obesity, eating disorders, and alcohol and substance use.

Section IV, "Mental & Behavioral Disorders," is a guide to diagnosis and treatment of several problems often seen in primary care. The chapters on depression and anxiety offer clinical guidelines for patient management, in which both pharmacotherapy and counseling are provided by the primary care practitioner. Chapters 23 and 24 address the challenges of working with patients with somatization and personality disorders; included are practical, clinically relevant suggestions to aid clinicians in the management of these patients. Primary care approaches to working with patients with dementia, sleep disorders, and sexual problems (Chapters 25, 26, and 27, respectively) are also covered in this section. Guidelines for when to refer patients to a mental health specialist are included.

Section V, "Special Topics," examines a variety of additional behavioral issues seen in primary care medicine. Chapter 28 provides practical suggestions for communicating with patients about their use of complementary and alternative medicine, including herbal medicines and dietary supplements. The authors provide a collaborative model to help patients make informed decisions and help clinicians better understand their patients' beliefs and health practices. Chapter 29, "Stress & Disease," presents a model of the complex interaction between stress and somatic illness that can guide clinicians in diagnosis, prevention, and treatment. Chapters on pain (30) and HIV/AIDS (31) offer a behavioral perspective on managing patients with these problems. Mistakes in medical practice can be devastating for both clinicians and patients; Chapter 32 addresses this issue and provides methods for clinicians to discuss mistakes with patients and families and to cope with their own emotions. Domestic violence (Chapter 33), a public as well as personal health issue, is often first detected by the primary care provider. This chapter describes its clinical presentation and offers practical interventions. Section V concludes with chapters on chronic illness and death and dying, which offer behavioral and relational perspectives on these challenging areas of patient care.

ACKNOWLEDGMENTS

This book would not have been possible without the support and mentorship of a number of people. We are indebted to Stephen McPhee, MD, for recognizing the need for a book such as this and for continually providing encouragement and advice. We thank Shelley Reinhardt, our senior editor at McGraw-Hill, for providing the vision and support for this second edition. We are very grateful to our contributing authors who, despite busy schedules as clinicians and teachers, have been generous and conscientious in going the distance with us.

Jane Kramer and Julie Burns Christensen and our children, Jake and Hank Christensen and Nina and Jonathan Kramer-Feldman, have continued to be a renewing and cherished presence in our lives. This book would not have been possible without their love and support.

Mitchell D. Feldman, MD, MPhil

John F. Christensen, PhD

San Francisco, California and Portland, Oregon
March 2003

Section I
The Doctor & Patient

The Medical Interview

Mack Lipkin, Jr., MD

INTRODUCTION

The medical interview is the medium—the vehicle—of patient care and is therefore of central importance to practitioners from both a professional and personal perspective. The interview is a principal determinant of the accuracy and completeness of data elicited from the patient. It is the most important factor in determining patient adherence to the plans agreed on—whether to take a medication, take a test, or change a life-style. The interview is also the keystone of patient satisfaction: More than 80% of diagnosis derives from the interview. Interview-related factors have been shown to impact major outcomes of care such as physiological responses, symptom resolution, pain control, functional status, and emotional health.

Quality factors influenced or determined by the medical interview include malpractice suits and their resolution, completeness and accuracy of the information obtained, efficiency, elimination of "door knob" questions, and patient satisfaction. The interview is therefore a major determinant of professional success, yet fewer than 10% of medical practitioners have spent any time since medical school working on their interviewing ability, and when asked, most physicians indicate that they have no plan or approach to monitoring, maintaining, or improving this critical skill.

The interview, which is also centrally important to practitioners' sense of well-being in their work, is the factor that most influences practitioner satisfaction with each individual encounter. Physicians with high career dissatisfaction place unsatisfactory relationships with patients very high on their lists. Physicians with high job satisfaction have a significant interest in the psychosocial aspects of care, relate effectively with patients, and are capable of managing difficult patient situations.

The Ubiquitous Interview

The central importance of the interview derives from its epidemiology. For most physicians (exceptions are non-interventionalist radiologists and pathologists, and some surgeons), it is more prevalent than any other activity in their work or their lives. The average lengths of time per patient visit for internists, average family practitioners, and pediatricians are 15, 12, and 8 minutes, respectively. The average overall for physicians is 6 minutes per visit, a rate curiously constant in the United States, the United Kingdom, The Netherlands, and elsewhere. Some physicians are obviously moving very quickly.

Making conservative assumptions about how many hours a practitioner will work over a 40-year professional lifetime, a generalist will have around 250,000 patient encounters. Each interview can be the source of satisfaction or distress, of learning or apathy, of efficiency or wasted effort (Table 1–1), of personal growth and inspiration or dispiriting discouragement. Few physicians, however, plan, or even think about, how to improve the balance of the desirable goals of satisfaction, learning, and efficiency for themselves.

Each discipline or special interest, such as psychiatry, occupational health, women's health, or domestic violence, has a special set of questions that must be asked of every patient for the interview to be complete and to elicit that patient's particular problems. (If an interviewer were to ask all the questions recommended by each of the dis-

Table 1–1. Gains from improved interviewing techniques.

Increased efficiency in use of time
Increased accuracy and completeness of data
Improved diagnosis
Fewer tests and procedures
Increased compliance
Increased physician satisfaction
Increased patient satisfaction
Decreased dissatisfaction
Increased mutual learning from each encounter

---

parate interests, the interview would go on for hours.) In most cases, these question sets have neither been validated nor shown to be sensitive or specific. Notable exceptions include the CAGE questionnaire (Table 1–2), which is highly specific, sensitive, and efficient as a screening test for alcoholism (see Chapter 20); the two-question depression screen (see Chapter 21), and the one-question domestic violence screen (see Chapter 33).

Rather than using a series of overgeneralized questions, the most efficient approach is to be patient centered, first by eliciting the patient's complete set of concerns and questions, followed by open-to-closed cones of questions to encourage elaboration on the information and complete the needed data about each concern. Open-ended questions elicit information more efficiently than do lists of closed-ended questions. A patient-centered approach also ensures that the patient's concerns are understood and agreed on—a predictor of increased compliance.

This approach is most efficient for several reasons. First, patients usually have a sense of what is relevant and will include some key information and data the interviewer might not think of. If the physician is thinking of the next question rather than listening to what is being said, the ability to attend and hear at multiple levels is compromised. If the interviewer is talking, the patient is not and so is not providing data. The physician can always refer to specific items later and ask other questions to round out the data once the patient's story is told. If the same basic format is used for each interview, variations in responses can be attributed to the patient and themselves provide significant information.

The evidence favoring a patient-centered approach goes beyond its practical advantages in the interview; out-

Table 1–2. The CAGE questionnaire.

C: Have you ever tried to **C**ut down on your drinking?
A: Do you feel **A**nnoyed when asked about your drinking?
G: Do you feel **G**uilty about your drinking?
E: Do you ever take an **E**ye opener in the morning?

---

comes of care are also favorably affected. More complete and higher quality information—with the attendant reduction in procedures and tests—reduces cost, needless side effects, and complications. Increased patient adherence to diagnostic and therapeutic plans leads to greater clinical efficiency and effectiveness. Patients take a more active role in their own care.

Active Listening & Efficiency

A number of factors enhance the interview's efficiency. Efficiency is currently of special concern as the "corporatization" of health care leads both doctors and patients to experience care as more rushed. Actual visit lengths seem to have remained constant—but as each year passes, the tasks to accomplish in a given visit grow—more diseases and risks to evaluate, more treatments to choose among and explain, and more bureaucratic hassles to negotiate. These trends will undoubtedly prove short-sighted: When the visit is effectively cut in length or jammed with too much to do, psychosocial discussion is the first thing omitted, which can lead to unnecessary testing, patient dissatisfaction, and hazardous and needless procedures and treatments. This is exacerbated when behavioral medicine is removed from the benefits provided by the clinician and is provided instead by an external company. Then both sides compete not to care for the patient, and—as might be expected—the relationship and quality of care deteriorate.

Because cost effectiveness and time efficiency are paramount, certain techniques can be helpful. Open-ended questions, as noted earlier, allow patients to elaborate on their responses and thus provide additional information. Active listening refers to listening to all that is being said, at multiple levels, how it is being said, what is included and what is left out, and how what is said reflects the person's culture, personality, mental status, conscious and unconscious motivation, cognitive style, and so on. A skilled active listener acquires such information and other data quickly and continuously. The experienced listener gives these observations their appropriate weight—as clear data, hypotheses, or biases. This enables the efficient creation of a complex and textured portrait of the patient that can be used in generating hypotheses, crafting replies, giving information, relating behaviors, and further questioning to test hypotheses.

THE STRUCTURE OF THE INTERVIEW

The recent literature on the interview runs to roughly 8000 articles, chapters, and books. Although only a modest portion of these derive from empirical bases, sufficient work has been done to describe the interview's conceptual framework as having **structure** and **functions.** Behavioral observations and analyses of interviews have related specific behaviors and skills to both structural elements and functions; performance of these behaviors and skills improves clinical outcomes. The following description of essential structural elements and their associated behaviors, or techniques, although comprehensive, is not so exhaustive as to be impractical. Key behaviors are summarized in Table 1–3. One comprehensive application of this approach developed by the Macy Initiative in Health Communication is shown in Figure 1–1.

Preparing the Physical Environment

Just as some architects and designers believe that form follows function, so the way in which practitioners organize their physical environment reveals characteristics of their practice: how they view the importance of the patient's comfort and ease, how they want to be regarded, and how they as practitioners control their own environment. This last is a key point, as providers often exhort patients to control theirs. Does the patient have a choice of seating? Are both patient and provider seated at a comparable eye level? Is the room easily accessible, quiet, and private?

Preparing Oneself

Humans can process about seven bits of information simultaneously. How many of these bits are consumed because of distractions or trivia in a clinical encounter? The hypnotic concept of *focus* or the recently accepted psychological concepts of centering or flow apply to the clinical encounter (see Chapter 6). If thoughts about the last or next patient, yesterday's mistake, last night's argument, passion, or movie intrude, concentration lapses—and information and opportunity are lost. In contrast, if the practitioner is focused, without external or internal distractions, and expects the interview to be a challenging, fascinating, and unique experience, chances are it will be.

How to achieve such a state of mind is a personal process and is related to each situation. Nevertheless, a few things are common to successful centering: eliminating outside intrusion by having someone else answer the beeper and take phone calls; tuning out other sounds; eliminating internal distractions and intrusive thoughts by resolving not to work on other matters and letting disturbing thoughts simply pass out of consciousness for the moment; and controlling distracting reactions to what is occurring in the interview by noting them, thinking about their origins, and putting them aside if they are not helpful.

Observing the Patient

A great deal can be learned by thoughtfully observing the patient's behavior and body language both before and during the encounter. Although such initial behavioral observations are purely heuristic—used to generate testable hypotheses about the patient—nonverbal behavior can sometimes reveal as much about the patient's state of mind as the patient's verbal responses do. Clinicians who are unaware of being influenced by initial reactions and observations in the patient interview may note that when they themselves get on a bus or an airplane, they—like other people—instantly recognize whom they would prefer—or prefer not—to sit next to. Such responses result from integrating a considerable number of nonverbal cues. Similar input about patients can relate to their overall state of health, vital signs, cardiac and pulmonary compensation, liver function, and more. Observations about grooming, state of rest, alertness, and style of presentation can reveal much about the patient's self-confidence, the presence of psychosis, depression, or anxiety, and the patient's personality style. The physician may also detect signs of possible alcohol or drug use. Escorting patients from the waiting area, letting them walk slightly ahead into the office, allows the practitioner to observe how patients have used their waiting time, note their gait, check on who accompanies them, and look for clues to the relationship with these escorts.

Developing the ability to make and use such clinical observations starts with the intention to do so. A decision to systematically retain and integrate initial observations will provide the physician with important data that have been easily available, but typically overlooked. Asking pertinent questions about behavioral cues, keeping in mind the kinds of observations that are possible, and refining these skills through practice will increase the physician's speed and comprehensiveness of observing. By practicing in crowds, at rounds or in lectures, on the airplane or at parties, it is possible to train oneself to become a more astute observer.

Greeting the Patient

The greeting serves to identify each party to the interaction, to set the social tone, to telegraph intentions concerning equality or dominance, and to prevent mistaken identity. It also allows the practitioner to establish an immediate connection with patients, showing them that they are entrusting themselves to a confident, compassionate professional. It enables the physician to learn how patients assert their own identity—and how to pronounce their names. Using a standard greeting—saying virtually the same thing each time—provides a basis for evaluating a variety of patient responses.

Beginning the Interview

The introductory phase of a medical encounter provides an opportunity for both parties to express their understanding of the purposes and conditions of the encounter,

Table 1–3. Structural elements of the medical interview.

Element	Technique or Behavior
Prepare the environment	Create a private area. Eliminate noise and distractions. Provide comfortable seating at equal eye level. Provide easy physical access.

Prepare oneself	Eliminate distractions and interruptions.
	Focus:
	   Self-hypnosis
	   Meditation
	   Constructive imaging
	Let intrusive thoughts pass.

Observe the patient	Create a personal list of categories of observation. Practice in a variety of settings. Notice physical signs. Notice patient's presentation and affect. Notice what is said and not said.
Greet the patient	Create a flexible personal opening. Introduce oneself. Check the patient's name and how it is pronounced. Create a positive social setting.
Begin the interview	Explain one's role and purpose. Check patient's expectations. Negotiate about differences in perspective. Be sure expectations are congruent with patient's.

Detect and overcome barriers to communication	Be aware of and look for potential barriers:
	   Language.
	   Physical impediments such as deafness, delirium.
	   Cultural differences.
	   Psychological obstacles such as shame, fear, and paranoia.

Survey problems	Develop personal methods to elicit an accounting of problems. Ask "what else" until problems are described.
Negotiate priorities	Ask patient for his or her priorities. State own priorities. Establish mutual interests. Reach agreement on the order of addressing issues.

Develop a narrative thread	Develop personal ways of asking patients to tell their story:
	   When did patient last feel healthy?
	   Describe entire course of illness.
	   Describe recent episode or typical episode.

Establish the life context of the patient	Use first opportunity to inquire about personal and social details. Flesh out developmental history. Learn about patient's support system. Learn about home, work, neighborhood, and safety issues.
Establish a safety net	Memorize complete review of systems. Review issues as appropriate to specific problem.
Present findings and options	Be succinct. Ascertain patient's level of understanding and cognitive style. Ask patient to review and state understanding. Summarize and check. Tape interview and give copy of tape to patient. Ask patient's perspectives.
Negotiate plans	Involve patient actively. Agree on what is feasible. Respect patient's choices whenever possible.
Close the interview	Ask patient to review plans and arrangements. Clarify what patient should do in the interim. Schedule next encounter. Say good-bye.

Begin interview

Prepare
a. Review the patient's chart
b. Assess and prepare the physical environment
   i. Optimize comfort and privacy
   ii. Minimize interruptions and distractions
c. Assess one's own personal issues, values, biases, and assumptions going into the encounter

Open
a. Greet and Welcome the patient and family member present
b. Introduce yourself
c. Explain role and orient patient to the flow of the visit
d. Indicate time available and other constraints
e. Identify and minimize barriers to communication
f. Calibrate your language and vocabulary to that of the patient
g. Accommodate patient comfort and privacy

Gather information
I. Survey patient's reasons for the visit
   a. Start with open-ended, non focused questions
   b. Invite patient to tell the story chronologically ("narrative thread")
   c. Allow the patient to talk without interrupting
   d. Actively listen
   e. Encourage completion of the statement of all of patient's concerns through verbal and non-verbal encouragement ("tell me more", the exhaustive "what else")
   f. Summarize what you heard. Check for understanding. Invite more ("anything more?")
II. Determine the patient's chief concern
   a. Ask closed-ended questions that are non-leading and one at a time
   b. Define the symptom completely
III. Complete the patient's medical database
   a. Obtain past medical and family history
   b. Elicit pertinent psychosocial data
   c. Summarize what you heard and how you understand it, check for accuracy

Elicit and understand patient's perspective
a. Ask patient about ideas about illness or problem
b. Ask patient about expectations
c. Explore beliefs, concerns and expectations
d. Ask about family, community, and religious or spiritual context
e. Acknowledge and respond to patient's concerns, feelings and non verbal cues
f. Acknowledge frustrations/challenges/progress (waiting time, uncertainty)

Communicate during the physical exam or procedure
a. Prepare patient
b. Consider commenting on aspects and findings of the physical exam or procedure as it is performed
c. Listen for previously unexpressed data about the patient's illness or concerns

Fundamental skills to maintain during the entire interview

I. Use relationship building skills
   a. Allow patient to express self
   b. Be attentive and empathic non-verbally
   c. Use appropriate language
   d. Communicate non-judgmental, respectful, and supportive attitude
   e. Accurately recognize emotion and feelings
   f. Use PEARLS Statements (Partnership, Empathy, Apology, Respect, Legitimization, Support) to respond to emotion instead of redirecting or pursuing clinical detail
II. Manage flow
   a. Be organized and logical
   b. Manage time effectively in the interview

Patient education
a. Use Ask-Tell-Ask approach to giving information meaningfully
   -Ask about knowledge, feelings, emotions, reactions, beliefs and expectations
   -Tell the information clearly and concisely, in small chunks, avoid "doctor babble"
   -Ask repeatedly for patient's understanding
b. Use language patient can understand
c. Use qualitative data accurately to enhance understanding
d. Use aids to enhance understanding (diagrams, models, printed material, community resources)
e. Encourage questions

End interview

Close
a. Signal closure
b. Inquire about any other issues or concerns
c. Allow opportunity for final disclosures
d. Summarize and verify assessment and plan
e. Clarify future expectations
f. Assure plan for unexpected outcomes and follow up
g. Thank patient - appropriate parting statement

Negotiate and agree on plan
a. Encourage shared decision making to the extent the patient desires
b. Survey problems and delineate options
c. Elicit patient's understanding, concerns, and preferences
d. Arrive at mutually acceptable solution
e. Check patient's willingness and ability to follow the plan.
f. Identify and enlist resources and supports

*This model is an expansion of the work of the Kalamazoo Consensus Conference held May 1999 supported by Bayer-Fetzer; in addition other models were consulted directly. These included the Brown Interview Checklist, the Three Function Model, the work of the AAPP Courses Committee-Blue Card, Segue, Calgary-Cambridge Observation Guide, Bayer model, and an extensive review of the literature on communications in medicine completed for the Macy Initiative. This model has been prepared by the Macy Initiative in Health Communication. Please address questions to Regina Janicik (212) 263-2304.

Figure 1–1. The medical interview. Developed by the Macy Initiative in Health Communication.

to check each other's expectations, and to negotiate any differences. For example: The patient expects to be seen by the head of the clinic, but the physician is only a year out of residency. The patient wants relief of his back pain and the practitioner is worried about his high blood pressure. The practitioner expects the consultation to lead to cardiac catheterization, whereas the patient thinks the cardiologist's opinions will be sent to his primary care physician for a decision. Or perhaps the physician can spare only 15 minutes, but the patient feels a full hour is needed.

Because one of the best predictors of the outcome of a dyadic relationship is the expectations of each person, clarifying and reconciling these is extremely valuable before beginning the main part of the interview.

Detecting & Overcoming Barriers to Communication

Many factors can interfere with communication between people—and still more place barriers between doctor and patient. There are tangible barriers in patient care: delirium, dementia, deafness, aphasia, intoxication on the part of patient or physician, and ambient noise. Psychological barriers can include depression, anxiety, psychosis, paranoia, and distrust; and social barriers often involve language, cultural differences, fears about immigration status, stigma, or legal problems. It is essential to detect such barriers early in an encounter; failure to do so not only wastes time but can seriously and sometimes dangerously mislead the physician. In addition, detecting a barrier is the first step toward its correction, whether by waiting until delirium or intoxication has cleared; finding a professional interpreter or signer; moving to a quiet, private place; or waiting to deal with the difficult issues until trust is established.

Surveying Problems

Because patients come to medical encounters with multiple problems and may not lead with the most pressing issue, and because physicians typically interrupt very quickly (23 seconds on average), it is vitally important for physicians not to jump in at the first important-sounding problem but instead to survey all problems first. For example, the clinician might ask, "What problems are you having?" or "What issues would you like to work on first?" After getting the initial answer or series of answers, the clinician can then ask what else is bothering the patient until the list of problems ends.

Negotiating Priorities

Once the physician and the patient clearly understand the full list of problems, the patient should then be asked, "Which of these would you like to work on first?" If the physician believes that something else is more important, there should be negotiation about this difference: "Our time is short today, and I think your shortness of breath is potentially more dangerous than your back pain. Suppose we deal with that first and, if we have time, go on to your back pain. If not, we'll take that up on your next visit."

Failure to ascertain and acknowledge patients' priorities will cause them to feel, appropriately, that the physician is not sensitive to their concerns. This can lead to failure to comply with treatment—or failure to return to the office.

Developing a Narrative Thread

Once the physician and the patient have decided which problem has priority, exploration of that problem begins. The most efficient method to use in exploring a problem is to ask the patient to tell the story of the problem. Although many persons will begin at an appropriate point and move toward the present, some patients may need or wish to be guided as to where to start. The physician may have to ask when the patient last felt healthy, when the current episode began, or when the patient thinks the problem started. The patient may not have a feel for the necessary level of detail and may be either too inclusive or too superficial. It may therefore be necessary for the physician to interrupt and indicate a desire to hear more—or less—about the problem. Clarifying questions will show the patient what is needed, and most persons will thereafter provide the appropriate level of detail.

Establishing the Life Context of the Patient

Once the narrative thread is in place, the physician can take the opportunity, when it arises, to inquire about specific points. Such inquiries help the physician learn about and understand the context of the patient's life—spouse, family, neighborhood, job, culture—in more detail. When enough information has been supplied, simply saying, "You were saying . . . ; what happened next?" can return the patient to the narrative.

Creating a Safety Net

Although the problems the patient wishes to discuss have been explored, areas or questions may remain that have not been covered. For these, the physician may choose to ask a series of specific questions or to use a review of systems not already covered. These questions may take the form of the seven dimensions of symptoms described as the location, duration, severity, quality, associations, radiation, and exacerbants and ameliorants or a subset of these dimensions. The final closed-ended questions tie up the loose ends and provide the safety of completeness.

Talking during the Physical Examination & Procedures

During the physical examination, there is a tension between the quiet focusing of the senses and mutually necessary talk.

Practitioners need to use their senses of smell, sight, touch, and hearing to examine the patient. They need to heighten sensory awareness and to think about what they are encountering. Patients need an explanation of what is being done and what to expect (this may hurt), instruction about what to do (please sit here, bring up you knees, hold your breath), and checking on how the patient is doing (does this hurt?). The examination often stimulates patient memory of relevant experiences and problems they had forgotten to mention.

Some physicians like to explain in detail what is happening (I am looking in the back of your eye because it is the one place in the body where blood vessels can be seen). Others do the review of systems during the physical.

In general, it is probably wise to minimize distractions during the physical or a procedure by confining talk to what is necessary for the task and is needed by the patient. Then, at the end, the process of explaining what has been found can benefit from the ability of the physician to observe and respond to the patient's reactions and questions.

Presenting Findings & Options

After the history-taking and physical examination have been completed, it is time for the physician and patient to discuss what the problems appear to be, related findings, the physician's hypotheses or conclusions, and possible approaches to further diagnostic evaluation and treatment. This should be done in language free of jargon and at a level of abstraction that the patient can understand. It is very valuable to foreshadow any bad or potentially upsetting news (see Chapter 3). This preparation helps the patient hear and retain the information better. When bad news is a certainty, it is useful to tape record the explanation and any discussion and give the tape to the patient. This way the patient can review it later, when out of shock. It has been documented that listening to the recording allows the patient to better understand the situation and improves outcomes of care. It is essential not to underestimate the potential impact of both positive and negative findings on the patient; after presenting each item the physician should explore the patient's understanding and reactions. The presentation itself should be problem oriented and systematic—and as simple and succinct as possible. Although the dictum is to be brief, content and empathy should not be sacrificed to brevity.

Negotiating a Plan

Once the patient has been factually informed of the diagnosis and prognosis, it is crucial to involve the patient actively in making choices and in developing diagnostic and therapeutic plans. Such "activation" of the patient has been shown to increase adherence to the plans and improve both the medical outcome and the patient's quality of life.

Where the physician and patient disagree in emphasis or choice, negotiation is necessary. The principles of negotiation can be summarized as finding the areas of mutual interest, emphasizing them, and avoiding the adoption of inflexible positions that can lead only to conflict and defeat. If the physician takes the time to understand the patient's position and respect his or her concerns, the issues can usually be worked out, for example, by agreeing to do a procedure after a grandchild's graduation or agreeing to do noninvasive tests first in the hope they will suffice.

Closing the Interview

The closing should include reviewing the principal findings, plans, and agreements; making arrangements for the next visit and giving the patient instructions for the intervening time; making sure outstanding issues have been covered; and saying good-bye.

THE FUNCTIONS OF THE INTERVIEW

The three functions of the interview (initially described by Bird and Cohen-Cole and subsequently refined and rationalized by Lazare, Putnam, and Lipkin) describe the major purposes of the interview and associated skills and behaviors that improve the interview process and outcomes. The functions—gathering information and monitoring progress; developing, maintaining, and concluding the therapeutic relationship; and educating the patient and implementing treatment plans—are interdependent. For example, patients cannot be expected to reveal personal or humiliating information unless they have developed considerable trust in their physicians. The physician cannot educate a patient effectively without knowing what level of language and which concepts to use, how to frame things for clarity, and which formulations will interpose needless barriers to acceptance—all data derived during information gathering. Therefore, the three functions cannot be pursued sequentially but must be integrated.

Gathering Information & Monitoring Progress

Many physicians consider these medical activities to be the dominant function of the interview. The tasks associated with this first function are to acquire a knowledge base of diseases and disorders and of psychosocial issues and illness behavior; to elicit the data relevant to each problem; to perceive the relevant data; and to generate and test hypotheses relevant to the elicited data. Skills useful in these tasks include starting with open questions such as "Tell me about it" and gradually narrowing the queries down to more specific questions; use of minimal encouragers (eg, "Uh huh," "Hmmm") to facilitate flow; gentle use of direction to steer without dominating; and summarizing and checking ("I think you have said point *a,* point *b,* point *c;* is that right?").

Developing, Maintaining, & Concluding the Therapeutic Relationship

The second function of the interview includes defining the nature of the relationship (short or long term, consultation, primary care, disease-episode oriented); demonstrating professional expertise; communicating interest, respect, empathy, and support; recognizing and resolving relational barriers to communication; and eliciting the patient's perspective. A relationship that engenders trust and safety is pivotal, as it is necessary to gather intimate information and to enable a patient to actively make life style changes or difficult medical decisions.

The belief that relationships cannot be improved, worked on, or manipulated has been disproved by the empirical psychotherapy literature. It is clear that use of appropriate relationship-building skills significantly improves interview outcomes in terms of satisfaction, compliance, data disclosure, quality of life, biological outcomes, and personal growth.

These issues are particularly germane in cases involving mental disorders, in which skill in managing the patient in a manner compatible with the disorder is essential.

In general, naming feelings, communicating unconditional positive regard, expressing empathy and understanding, and being emotionally congruent (what you say is actually what you mean and feel) produce the best outcomes. Other skills include reflection, legitimization, partnership, the nonverbal skills of touch and eye contact, and the avoidance of shame or humiliation (see Chapter 2).

Educating the Patient

Patient education and implementation of treatment plans require being aware of the patient's current level of knowledge, understanding, and motivation and the patient's cognitive style and level, having a receptive patient who is neither in shock nor in disagreement, and using plain language that avoids jargon or undue complexity. The tasks associated with this third function include communicating the diagnostic significance of the problem(s); negotiating and recommending appropriate diagnostic and treatment options and appropriate prevention and lifestyle changes; and enhancing the patient's ability to cope by understanding and communicating the psychological and social impacts of the illness. Involving the patient in making choices, clarifying uncertainties, and expressing fears and concerns markedly improve outcomes. Having the patient actively review what has been discussed and decided is critical to check for understanding, to reinforce memory, and to be sure the patient can and will do what has been agreed (see Chapter 16).

SPECIAL CIRCUMSTANCES & INTERVIEW MODIFICATIONS

Although the preceding principles are applicable to most situations, many circumstances require a modified approach to maximize the usefulness and durability of the interview and relationship. Early detection of special situations is crucial so that the appropriate changes in technique can be made as soon as possible. In most special situations, meticulous attention to the particular relationship needs of the patient is paramount, as, for example, with the paranoid or psychotic patient.

Aids to Diagnosing Mental Disorders

Physicians currently have a variety of aids to use in diagnosing and monitoring mental disorders. The simplest aids have relatively high sensitivity (they detect most of the real cases) but lower specificity (they register as positive cases that do not meet the diagnostic criteria). Among the screening devices for depression are the Beck, Zung, and Hamilton scales. Recently, a two-question screen and a nine-question quantitative scoring method, the Patient Health Questionnaire, have also been shown to be useful in primary care settings (see Chapter 21). Some physicians administer these as part of a packet of materials to be filled out prior to the initial visit. As with other questionnaires, however, these create the additional problem of having to deal with a large number of false positives, which can be extremely time consuming.

One recently developed instrument (with pharmaceutical company support) can screen for the most common mental disorders at the same time. The Primary Care Screen for Mental Disorders (PRIME-MD) is reasonably sensitive and specific and is available for telephone use and for computerized administration. However, empathic physicians have two problems with its use: the program asks about feelings but cannot respond to their expression and scoring it takes several minutes. The role of such devices is still evolving.

SUGGESTED READINGS

Albanese MA, Mitchell S: Problem based learning: a review of literature on its outcomes and implementation issues. Acad Med 1993;68:52.

Balint M: *The Doctor, His Patient, and the Illness.* Pitman, 1957.

Beckman HB, Frankel RM: The effect of physician behavior on the collection of data. Ann Intern Med 1984;101:693.

Fallowfield L, Lipkin M, Hall A: Teaching senior oncologists communication skills: results from phase I of a comprehensive longitudinal program in the United Kingdom. J Clin Oncol 1998;16(5):1961.

Fallowfield L et al: Efficacy of a Cancer Research UK communication skills training model for oncologists: a randomised controlled trial. Lancet 2002;359(9307):650.

Frances V, Korsch BM, Morris MJ: Gaps in doctor-patient communication: patient response to medical advice. N Engl J Med 1969;280:535.

Goffman E: *Stigma: Notes on the Management of Spoiled Identity.* Prentice-Hall, 1963.

Gordon G, Rost K: Evaluating a faculty development course on medical interviewing. In: Lipkin M Jr, Putnam S, Lazare A (editors): *The Medical Interview: Clinical Care, Education and Research.* Springer-Verlag, 1995.

Groves JE: Taking care of the hateful patient. N Engl J Med 1978;298:883.

Hampton JR et al: Relative contributions of history-taking, physical examination, and laboratory investigation to diagnosis and management of medical outpatients. BMJ 1975;2:486.

Kleinman A, Eisenberg J, Good B: Culture, illness and care. Ann Intern Med 1978;88:251.

Kurtz S, Silverman J, Draper J: *Teaching and Learning Communication Skills in Medicine.* Radcliffe Medical Press, 1998.

Lazare A: Shame, humiliation, and stigma in the medical encounter. In: Lipkin M, Putnam SM, Lazare A (editors): *The Medical Interview.* Springer-Verlag, 1995.

Lazare A, Putnam SM: The three functions of the medical interview. In: Lipkin M, Putnam SM, Lazare A (editors): *The Medical Interview.* Springer-Verlag, 1995.

Lazare A, Eisenthal S, Frank A: Clinician-patient relations. II: Conflict and negotiation. In: Lazare A (editor): *Outpatient Psychiatry: Diagnosis and Treatment,* 2nd ed. Williams & Wilkins, 1989, pp 137–152.

Levinson W, Roter D: The effects of two continuing medical education programs on communication skills of practicing primary care physicians. J Gen Intern Med 1993;8(6):318.

Lichstein P: Terminating the doctor/patient relationship. In: Lipkin M, Lazare A (editors): *The Medical Interview.* Springer-Verlag, 1995.

Lipkin M Jr, Quill T, Napodano RJ: The medical interview: a core curriculum for residencies in internal medicine. Ann Intern Med 1984;100:277.

Lipkin M Jr, Putnam S, Lazare A (editors): *The Medical Interview: Clinical Care, Education, and Research.* Springer-Verlag, 1995.

Lipkin M Jr et al: Performing the interview. In: Lipkin M Jr, Putnam S, Lazare A (editors): *The Medical Interview: Clinical Care, Education and Research.* Springer-Verlag, 1995.

Novack DH et al: Medical interviewing and interpersonal skills teaching in U.S. medical schools: progress, problems, and promise. JAMA 1999;269:2101.

Pololi LH: Standardised patients: as we evaluate, so shall we reap. Lancet 1995;345(8955):966.

Putnam SM et al: Personality styles. In: Lipkin M, Putnam SM, Lazare A (editors): *The Medical Interview: Clinical Care, Education and Research.* Springer-Verlag, 1995.

Quill TE: Partnerships in patient care: a contractual approach. Ann Intern Med 1983;98:228.

Quill TE: Barriers to effective communication. In: Lipkin M, Putnam SM, Lazare A (editors): *The Medical Interview: Clinical Care, Education and Research.* Springer-Verlag, 1995.

Reznick RK et al: Large-scale high-stakes testing with an OSCE: report from the Medical Council of Canada. Acad Med 1996;71:19.

Rogers C: Characteristics of a helping relationship. In: Rogers C (editor): *On Becoming a Person.* Houghton Mifflin, 1961.

Roter D: Which facets of communication have strong effects on outcome: a meta-analysis. In: Stewart M, Roter D (editors): *Communicating with Medical Patients.* Sage Publications, 1989.

Roter DL et al: Improving physicians' interviewing skills and reducing patients' emotional distress. A randomized clinical trial. Arch Intern Med 1995;155(17):1877.

Shapiro D: *Neurotic Styles.* Basic Books, 1965.

Smith RC et al: Evidence-based guidelines for teaching patient-centered interviewing. Patient Educ Couns 2000;39:27.

Starfield B et al: Patient-doctor agreement about problems: influence on outcome of care. JAMA 1979;242:344.

Stewart MA: Effective physician-patient communication and health outcomes: a review. Can Med Assoc J 1995;15:480.

Vernon DTA, Blake RL: Does problem-based learning work? A meta-analysis of evaluative research. Acad Med 1993;68:550.

ORGANIZATIONS AND WEB SITES

American Academy on Physician and Patient
AAPP
6728 Old McLean Village Drive
McLean, VA 22101
(703) 556-9222
Fax (703) 556-8729
Email: AAPPatient@degnon.org
http://www.physicianpatient.org

Bayer Institute for Health Care Communication
400 Morgan Lane
West Haven, CT 06516
(800) 800-5907
Fax (416) 240-5391
Email: bayer.institute@bayer.com
www.bayerinstitute.org

Northwest Center for Physician-Patient Communication
The Foundation for Medical Excellence
One SW Columbia Street, Suite 800
Portland, OR 97258-2095
(503) 636-2234
Fax (503) 796-0699
Email: info@tfme.org
www.tfme.org

Empathy

Barry Egener, MD

INTRODUCTION

The concept of empathy dates from the early years of this century, when discussions of the topic were restricted to psychotherapists' analyses of their interactions with patients. More recently, the concept has received renewed attention from a wide spectrum of health practitioners and educators. They believe that empathy can positively affect communication with patients and thus lead to improved therapeutic outcomes. Many of the lay public regard empathy as an avenue to the restoration of compassion and humanism to the doctor–patient relationship, which has been threatened by and has become increasingly impersonal due to technology and financial pressures.

The power of empathy lies in its ability to help us cross, if only for a moment, the divide between clinicians and patients created by their very different circumstances. To briefly bridge that divide and to become simply two humans sharing an experience can help in accomplishing professional diagnostic and therapeutic tasks. We have all experienced the gratitude of patients, isolated by depression or family loss, for our expressed understanding of their sadness.

Succeeding at the greater challenge of putting aside our disagreement with a patient requesting chronic narcotics or perhaps our negative judgment of a patient unable to quit smoking can have proportionally greater rewards. Being willing to imagine what it must be like for these more challenging patients can provide us with insight into what motivates them or what might help them. That's diagnostic information. Communicating that insight may encourage patients to change their behavior. That's therapeutic. Our disclosure also allows us to check the accuracy of what we think we know about the patient's state. We relinquish nothing of ourselves or our role in that moment, we simply expand our perspective.

Empathy can be defined as an intellectual identification with, or vicarious experiencing of, the feelings, thoughts, or attitudes of another. Some have described empathy as a momentary identification with another person in which our human capacity to feel what another feels erodes the boundaries of self. If we in fact temporarily lose awareness of self, the process might better be termed "sympathy for" or "feeling with" someone else. Remaining aware that we are experiencing empathy prevents total dissolution of ego boundaries and permits a more salutary stance. ***Empathy skills*** are behaviors that demonstrate empathy. They may be the clinician's most powerful therapeutic tool.

Research suggests that empathy skills can be taught. This chapter will describe how to develop and improve these skills. Research has recently shed light on the frequency of empathic opportunities in clinical practice, on how physicians respond to or neglect these opportunities, and the implications of such choices. Empathic opportunities occur in more than half of surgical and primary care visits, although there are more opportunities per visit in primary care (2.6) than in surgical care (1.9). Patients initiate most of the opportunities. Contrary to common belief, surgeons respond empathically at least as frequently as primary care physicians, but both miss opportunities to respond more frequently. Empathic behaviors enhance the effectiveness of care as well as patient satisfaction, and their absence may predispose patients to initiate malpractice suits.

There are numerous barriers to discussing emotions with patients, from the impersonal office setting to the disinclination of both physician and patient to address particularly sensitive topics. Nonetheless, appropriate skilled communication can break through these barriers.

OVERCOMING BARRIERS TO EMPATHY

Understanding the feelings, attitudes, and experiences of the patient is the first step toward a more potent therapeutic alliance. Many patients, however, may not be skilled in revealing their feelings to their providers. They need to be made aware that their doctor is interested in their feelings and values them, and that feelings are a legitimate topic for discussion in a medical interview.

Emotions can be difficult for both doctors and patients (Table 2–1), and doctors particularly may prefer the certainty of science. From the patient's point of view, if difficult emotional issues are manifested as a somatic complaint, denial might be the first reaction to a psychological interpretation of the symptoms. The physician must appreciate and mirror the terms in which a patient will speak about illness. In many cultures, emotions are simply not discussed. In the United States, where the biomedical model of disease still predominates over the bio-

Table 2–1. Barriers to discussing emotions.

Doctor
1 Takes too much time
2 Too draining
3 Will lose control of interview
4 Can't fix patient's distress
5 Not my job
6 Managed care is not conducive

Patient
1 Cultural taboo about discussing emotions
2 Preference for interpreting distress in a biomedical model
3 Somatization disorder
4 Desire to meet doctor's expectations
5 Worry about being emotionally overwhelmed
6 Lack of language for emotions

psychosocial model, patients may feel that it is more acceptable to have physical rather than emotional complaints. Because this expectation is often reinforced by their physicians, it behooves physicians to establish a climate conducive to the expression of emotional material and a language useful to that end. Physicians often mention the following barriers to discussing emotions with patients.

1. It takes too much time. In a busy practice, concerns about time are legitimate. Given an organized framework, however, it takes only a few minutes to deal effectively with emotion, and the strategies discussed later in this chapter can prove time efficient for the physician. Recent studies suggest that interviews in which physicians respond to emotions may actually be shorter than those in which they do not. An explanation of this finding is that it may be more time consuming to deal with the indirect effects of unaddressed emotions during the rest of the interview. Moreover, it may be useful to distinguish between "acute efficiency" and "chronic efficiency." "Efficiency" should take into consideration not only the duration of a particular visit, but the total amount of time required to address the patient's concerns. Even if it were to take a few extra minutes to address emotions, that time is more than compensated by fewer phone calls and fewer unscheduled visits.

2. It's too draining. It is unrealistic to expect all providers to be emotionally available at all times to all their patients. A physician who has been awake all night or is emotionally needy may be justified in putting off a discussion of emotions that should otherwise occur. If the physician chooses to defer, it would be wise to return to the topic at another time. Primary care providers sometimes exert a tremendous amount of energy avoiding emotions in the belief that dealing directly with them will be draining. However, it can be far more efficient to make an emotional connection than to expend so much energy in resisting it.

At times, patients may inadvertently raise issues that are emotionally difficult for their providers. Sometimes the clinician can discuss the difficulty with friends, family, or colleagues; at other times it may be most fruitfully addressed in the physician's own therapy. (A longer discussion of this area is beyond the scope of this chapter, but difficult encounters with patients offer physicians an opportunity for personal growth; see Chapter 4.)

3. The interview will get out of control. Although many doctors worry that addressing emotions will cause feelings to escalate, the opposite is often true: Addressing emotions helps diffuse them. Learning a language to handle emotions creates a comfortable distance from the emotions themselves, so that neither the doctor nor the patient becomes overwhelmed.

4. I can't fix it for the patient. Primary care providers are used to "fixing" things. Feelings, however, simply exist, and can't be "fixed." Patients do not expect their feelings to be eliminated; they just want them to be understood.

5. It's not my job. Some doctors believe that their job is to address disease and the psychotherapist's job is to address mental illness. There are several problems with this attitude. Although it is certainly true that collaboration with mental health practitioners may at times be useful, about 65% of mental illnesses are cared for exclusively by primary care physicians. About 26% of primary care patients have mental health diagnoses, and even a higher percentage have important psychiatric comorbidities. Physicians who insist on interpreting the physical symptoms of psychiatric disease such as panic disorder or depression in purely biomedical terms miss the point—and their patients will not get better. Telling a patient who develops chest pain on the anniversary of his father's death (see the section on "The Therapeutic Language of Empathy") that there is nothing wrong with him will help the patient only briefly. Moreover, many physical illnesses have psychosocial sequelae that must also be addressed.

When a patient keeps returning with the same complaint, unimproved by a physician's interventions, the patient is trying to communicate a message. Physicians are often frustrated by these patients; this frustration can be alleviated and the doctor's satisfaction improved by the progress that comes with addressing the underlying problem.

6. I can't be empathic in a managed-care setting. Productivity pressures on physicians present special challenges to the doctor–patient relationship. There is an inherent conflict of interest introduced when the physician has to balance the patient's needs against the financial resources of the plan (or against the physician's income under some arrangements). There is evidence suggesting an erosion of the public's trust in physicians, which has implications for the kind of empathic relationship that this chapter advocates. Nonetheless, at a time when patients and physicians are feeling distanced by the interposition of managed care, empathic skills can help preserve trust. Both doctor and patient may resent having their health care choices constrained by a third party. But physicians who feel obligated to represent the insurer's position to the patient are likely to act defensively if the patient attacks the arrangement. Acknowledging and supporting the patient's feelings offer an alternative that makes the physician a partner again and removes an unwanted burden.

THE ROLE OF EMPATHY IN DIAGNOSIS

Feelings that arise in the provider during an encounter may be useful in forming a diagnostic hypothesis about the patient. For example, a doctor who feels burdened, heavy, or "down" during an interview might consider the possibility that the patient is depressed.

All clinicians have had the experience of trying to help a patient with a behavior change, such as weight loss, only to have each suggestion rejected: "I've already tried that, Doc; it doesn't work." The physician's own feelings of frustration and powerlessness in trying to motivate the patient are often mirrored by the patient's sense of frustration and powerlessness in attempting to accomplish the change in behavior. The physician can confirm the hypothesis that the patient is frustrated, as with any other diagnosis, by testing: "I'm feeling frustrated with this problem, and I'm wondering if you're feeling the same way."

Some patients consistently elicit dislike and rejection from their providers. It may seem that the patient is intentionally trying to manipulate the provider into becoming angry. This may in fact be true. When providers become aware of these feelings, they should consider the possibility that their own impulses to punish the patient may be playing into the patient's self-image as deserving of punishment. This pattern may be consistent with a borderline personality disorder (see Chapter 24).

The physician's experience does not invariably reflect the patient's experience. Rather, physicians should notice their feelings and ask, "Does the way I feel tell me something about the patient or something about myself?" For example, a physician who has recently seen a number of patients seeking drugs begins to feel angry and defensive on noticing that the nurse has recorded "low back pain" as the next patient's chief complaint; these negative feelings indicate more about the physician's recent experiences than they do about the next patient. Feelings are primary data about the person in whom they arise and indirect data about others. The next section clarifies how to test the hypothesis that a patient is feeling a particular emotion and outlines how to respond.

The Therapeutic Language of Empathy

Although empathy is not generally considered a therapeutic tool, discussion of emotional issues can be therapeutic. An empathic relationship is crucial in psychotherapy and enhances the power of all therapeutic relationships. The following sections show how to talk about emotions using specific skills. A premise of this discussion is that biomedical aspects of disease cannot be effectively addressed without considering their emotional consequences. Emotions, whether related to physiological dysfunction or psychosocial issues, color the discussion in the examining room and may be so distracting that the patient cannot fully concentrate on other issues until the emotions are addressed.

A clinical scenario helps to illustrate the usefulness of the emotion-handling skills described here.

 CASE ILLUSTRATION 1

A 35-year-old man presents with a 2-week history of sharp substernal chest pain that occurs at rest, when working in the yard, and while trying to fall asleep at night. He does not smoke but has a positive family history of heart disease. On examination he appears anxious, he has borderline high blood pressure, and he is 5% over ideal body weight. The rest of his examination, laboratory tests, electrocardiogram, and chest x-ray are normal, except for his low-density lipoprotein cholesterol, which is 160 mg/dL.

The doctor reenters the room to review the data.

Patient: Well, Doctor, what did you find?

Doctor: Only some minor abnormalities. I think you need to lose a little weight and perhaps change your diet slightly.

Patient: Is the pain coming from my heart?

Doctor: I don't think so.

Patient: But you're not sure?

Doctor: Nothing in medicine is certain, but your age, the character of your pains, and the fact that antacids help somewhat reassure me that the problem is most likely acid indigestion or muscular pain.

Patient: Don't you think we should do more tests to be sure?

Doctor: With your particular insurance, we need to be very careful about doing unnecessary tests. I think you should resume your normal activities. I'll see you in a month, and we'll see if there's been any change.

Patient: I'm still worried.

Doctor: Don't be. You'll be all right.

Patient: Well, okay, if you say so.

Despite a probably accurate diagnosis of noncardiac chest pain, providing good information, and attempts to reassure the patient, something goes awry in this interaction. The patient still doesn't seem satisfied. Let's look at the effect empathic skills might have.

The techniques discussed in the following sections are adapted from a three-function model of the medical interview developed by Bird and Cole. The goals of the interview are described as gathering medical data, building a relationship with the patient, and educating and motivating the patient (see Chapter 1). The following emotion-handling skills are related to the second function, building relationships with patients (Table 2–2).

REFLECTION

Reflection refers to naming the emotion the doctor sees and reflecting it back to the patient. Reflection communicates the physician's understanding of the patient's experience. It also has the effect of making the feelings behind the patient's behavior or words explicit, so that they can be dealt with directly.

For example, when a patient greets a doctor who is 20 minutes late with, "My time is as valuable as yours," the doctor might say, "I'm sorry I'm late. You seem pretty angry with me." The patient might then ventilate about the doctor's lateness or his treatment at the hands of doctors. He might even deny his anger, since many patients might view an expression of anger at their physicians as unacceptable. In any case, the doctor has a chance to deal with the emotion directly and then proceed with the interview, rather than trying to work with a patient who is angry and has not had a chance to express this anger.

Table 2–2. The empathic skills.

Skill	Example
Reflection	"You seem upset."
Validation	"I can understand your anger with the callous way you were treated."
Support	"You are doing very well handling your grief."
Partnership	"Perhaps we can work together to make you feel better."
Respect	"You have tremendous compassion for your siblings."

After reflecting an emotion, the doctor should stop talking and see how the patient responds. Although the patient will usually elaborate, if the physician keeps talking, the exploration may be prematurely ended.

Sometimes it is clear that a patient is feeling a strong emotion, but it is not clear what that emotion is. It is perfectly acceptable (and perhaps preferable) to treat the emotion as having a differential diagnosis and test a hypothesis as one would for any other medical entity: "I'm wondering if you're upset," or, more tentatively, "It seems that you're feeling something strongly, but I'm not sure what it is. Can you help me out?"

VALIDATION

Validation informs the patient that you understand the reason for the emotion. This has the effect of normalizing the emotion and making the patient feel less isolated. For example, to a somatizing patient who has been to several doctors who have been unable to find a cause for her abdominal pain, you might say, "I can understand how frustrating it's been to be no better after seeking so much help." Some physicians are reluctant to validate emotions in difficult patients for fear of adding fuel to the fire. If reflection is the empathy skill that opens Pandora's Box, validation is the skill that closes it—it is difficult to remain upset with a person who understands how you feel. You don't have to agree with patients to express understanding of their feelings. For example, to a patient with chronic low back pain who has responded angrily when informed that you will not prescribe narcotics, you might say, "Even though I see it differently, I can understand why you would be angry with me." Although disagreeing with the patient such a statement allows you to offer support and enhances your chances of continuing a therapeutic relationship. Validation of feelings emphasizes that the patient and doctor are equals in the human condition, although they have different roles in the therapeutic relationship.

SUPPORT

An expression of support tells patients that the physician cares about them and is willing to be present to their emotion. The expression can be verbal or nonverbal. Examples of nonverbal expression are handing the tearful patient a tissue or touching the patient. In judging whether touching a patient will be perceived as supportive, invasive, or inappropriate, the physician should consider such factors as culture, age, gender, sexual orientation, previous experience of abuse, and the presence or absence of psychiatric symptoms, such as paranoia. In general, putting a hand on the patient's hand or arm will not be misinterpreted. Many physicians prefer to take the lead from the patient by matching the patient's nonverbal behavior.

Some verbal expressions of support are "It's pretty normal to get angry with children when they act out" and "A spouse's death is one of the most difficult life transitions."

Again, these responses are not an attempt to suppress, eliminate, or fix the emotion, but rather an offer to help patients, to reassure them that they are not alone with an uncomfortable emotion. These three skills—reflection, validation, and support—are the most important of the emotion-handling skills and will be involved in most of the work physicians do in this area.

PARTNERSHIP

Partnership implies a team approach, in which the patient and doctor work together toward the same goal. Doctors support and are partners with patients in many ways, but in the context of this chapter, the word *partnership* makes it explicit that you would like to help the patient with the troubling emotion. An advantage of partnership is that it may help motivate patients to take an active role in their improvement and may lay the foundation for a contract for behavior change. This is consistent with the notion, especially important when illness results from patient behaviors, that physicians facilitate the patient's healing rather than curing disease in the passive patient. The physician's use of the pronouns *we* and *us* expresses partnership, as in "Perhaps we can make a plan to help you feel better" or "Let's figure out a way to help you deal with this difficult diagnosis."

RESPECT

This skill honors the emotional resources within a patient. The doctor might say "You've been through a lot" or "I'm impressed with how well you're holding up under the circumstances."

Physicians may not always know what it would be like to be the patient, but they can acknowledge the patient's experience nonetheless: "I'm not a parent, so I can only imagine what it would be like to lose a child. I can see you're feeling the loss quite deeply." On a happier occasion, she might say "What a joy it must be for you to see your grandchild's birth!"

Although it often makes sense to use reflection or validation first when addressing emotion, these skills can be used in any order, and it may be best to go through the sequence several times at different points in an interview.

CASE ILLUSTRATION 1 (CONT.)

Let us return now to the scenario of the 35-year-old man with chest pain to see how that interaction might be improved with a physician who uses empathic skills. The empathic skills used are listed in parentheses.

Patient: Well, what did you find?

Doctor: Only some minor abnormalities that I don't think are significant.

Patient: Then why do I have this pain?

Doctor: You seem pretty anxious. (*reflection*)

Patient: Wouldn't you be anxious if you thought you were working up to a heart attack?

Doctor: I certainly would be. So you're worried you're going to have a heart attack. (*reflection*)

Patient: That's what happened to my father. He was raking leaves and just keeled over. I'm the one who found him.

Doctor: That must have been horrible. (*support*)

Patient: You can't imagine how awful it was. Every time I think of it I get upset. Sometimes it even brings on this chest pain. I've been thinking about him more and more lately, especially when I go to sleep at night. It makes me afraid to fall asleep. I'm afraid I'm not going to wake up.

Doctor: Is there a reason why you've been thinking about him more lately?

Patient: Yeah. I thought I got over his death. But this is the time of year he died. Just raking leaves, which I do every weekend, makes me think of him. Then I get this chest pain and worry about myself. Heart disease runs in families, I don't have to tell you.

Doctor: I'm sorry about your father. It sounds as though there's a pretty strong connection between thinking about your father and the chest pain. (*support*)

Patient: Yeah. I thought maybe being upset stressed my heart. Do you think maybe this is all in my head?

Doctor: I'm sure you really feel the pain, and I suspect your heart still aches for your father—even if only figuratively. It's pretty hard to lose a father. Now, you know there's a pretty strong connection between the body and the mind, and if you've been worrying about your own health, this could be your way of making sure you take care of yourself. (*respect*)

Patient: I never thought of it that way. What you say makes a lot of sense, and I think you're probably right. But I still have this nagging worry in the back of my mind.

Doctor: That's understandable. (*validation*) How about this? Let's work together to reduce whatever risk factors you do have for heart disease to make sure you don't have a problem down the line. (*partnership*) Let me see you again in a month so we can check you over physically to make sure everything's still okay. Right now you're having some pretty strong feelings about your father, and I think that may be the source of your chest pain. See what happens in the next few weeks; if you're still having problems next month, we can talk some more about it.

Patient: That seems reasonable to me. I appreciate your listening to me.

Doctor: Okay, then, I'll see you next month. And if you have severe chest pains, call me immediately; don't wait till the next day.

Patient: Thanks, Doc. See you next month.

Patient satisfaction, as indicated by the patient's responses toward the end of the interview, seems much greater than in the first scenario. Although this scenario is longer than the first, using empathic skills added only approximately 1 minute to the interview, and if that additional minute prevents unnecessary visits by allaying the patient's concerns, the time is well spent. Early in the interview, the doctor does very little talking, and what he does say primarily addresses the patient's charged emotional state. He initially resists the patient's invitation to confirm conclusively that this is all in his head and instead allows the patient to continue to explore his feeling state. There is uncertainty at the end of the medical interview, but it seems to be an uncertainty that both the doctor and patient can accept comfortably, with a sense of partnership.

IMPLICATIONS FOR PROFESSIONAL DEVELOPMENT

Suppose the content of what the patient reveals is upsetting, distasteful, or even abhorrent to the physician. In the previous example of the patient with chest pain suppose that the doctor's mother has just died and his father is scheduled for triple-bypass surgery; the mere contemplation of losing his father is so threatening that the physician withdraws into himself. Psychological defense mechanisms may cause the physician to become distracted from the patient's visit and think about his own concerns.

Suppose, on the other hand, that the patient describes a situation that is emotionally charged, but is so alien to the physician's experience that he cannot empathize. If, for example, a homosexual patient reveals that his partner has become HIV positive, the heterosexual physician may pity (feel sorry *for*) the patient but may be unable to relate to the patient's grief and fears. On the other hand, the physician may be so repelled by the concept of homosexuality that his body language betrays his negative feelings. The patient, feeling judged and embarrassed, is likely to withhold relevant information. Or suppose the physician must present certain treatments to a patient that he considers disgusting or repulsive. His own obvious feeling may prevent the patient from making a truly informed decision.

Finding just the right therapeutic stance is essential; it may be partly intuitive and partly learned, and it may vary from patient to patient—or even with the same patient over time—depending on the patient's needs. Opportunities may be lost when the physician is unable to empathize with the patient, or when the loss of ego boundaries makes a therapeutic stance impossible. The most effective physicians are those whose repertoire permits a rapid interplay of objectivity and emotion.

Calibrating responses to patients requires noticing and understanding when clinicians' own emotional issues prevent them from being maximally effective with patients. The first clue may be that a specific patient or type of patient particularly irks a physician. These "irksome patients" are our teachers. They teach us about ourselves. Personal barriers to effectiveness with patients usually originate in the physician's own family of origin. Numerous tools are available to help physicians overcome these barriers: speaking with a trusted colleague, Balint or other support groups, courses that focus specifically on personal awareness, and personal psychotherapy (see Novack in Suggested Readings).

Empathy in Medical Training

Viewing empathy in this way may have special applications to medical training. It is remarkable how the fresh enthusiasm and caring of medical students can quickly devolve into the wry cynicism of residents. What accounts for this withdrawal? The usual explanation is that insulating oneself in this way is an act of self-preservation in the face of overwhelming demands. It can be torturous to feel another's pain, and if the self is already stressed because of long hours and the other exigencies of training, it may be more difficult to sustain an open posture.

The ways in which doctors withdraw depend on both their personalities and their environment. If the culture around the resident tolerates derogatory labels for patients, it can be easy to see patients as *other,* as not sharing some element of humanity with *us.* Even if such labels are not tolerated and caring for patients is a highly preserved value, dark humor may surface as a means of insulation. To take care of others, one must first take care of oneself. Finding the right balance is a major developmental task of the health-care professions. Perhaps by attending to the well-being of trainees, we will make them better doctors (see Chapter 7). Training programs can demonstrate that caring for others is valuable. Experienced physicians can attend to trainees' growth, help them develop effective and healthy working styles, model those styles, and draw attention to the importance of being aware of one's own development. There is a huge contrast between the concept of residency training as nurturing or mentoring and the concept of residency as "trial by fire." And fire, we know, steels metal, making it harder.

Empathy in the Practice of Medicine

What happens after training? For some practitioners, the pressure becomes less, healthy coping styles develop, and the caring physician reemerges. Far too many, however, are casualties of the training process—or their families are. Gabbard and Menninger have observed that physicians' compulsive personality styles are susceptible to a pattern of delayed gratification. Constantly nurturing others, physicians may have no time left for themselves. Family relationships may atrophy. The most effective physicians may be those who attend to their own needs as well as those of their patients, who understand their own unique struggles, so that these struggles—by making physicians aware of their own humanity—can enhance, rather than detract from, their relationships with patients.

Because the culture of an institution strongly influences the practice of medicine within its purview, physicians who practice together have a unique opportunity to enhance each other's empathic skills. Patient-care conferences can incorporate psychosocial issues into the discussions of difficult cases. Videotaped interviews with difficult patients are a powerful tool that allows physicians to examine their own contributions to the difficulty of such interactions.

Regular videotaped conferences, in which physicians take turns presenting cases, allow them to feel at ease in front of the camera, demonstrate collaboration and mutual support, and reinforce the importance and value of empathy to the group. Balint groups or other types of support groups, which may include nonphysician office staff, can help health practitioners cope with collegial interactions or family relationships that have become stressed by practice. Such groups also show that a psychosocial perspective can benefit both physicians and their patients.

Understanding the interaction between illness and emotion helps us become more effective physicians. Familiarity and practice with the skills in this chapter can make us more comfortable discussing this interaction with our patients. Becoming aware of our own personal response to patients promotes personal growth as well. The emotional demands of the medical profession can be enriching or impoverishing. Using skills of empathy we may become more satisfied and effective clinicians; our patients may become more satisfied and healthier.

SUGGESTED READINGS

Branch WT, Malik TK: Using "windows of opportunity" in brief interviews to understand patients' concerns. JAMA 1993;269: 1667.

Brothers L: Biological perspective on empathy. Am J Psychiatry 1989; 146:10.

Cohen-Cole S, Bird J: Building rapport and responding to the patient's emotions (relationship skills). In: Cohen-Cole S (editor): *The Medical Interview: The Three Function Approach.* Mosby Year Book, 1991.

Gabbard G, Menninger R: The psychology of postponement in the medical marriage. JAMA 1989;261:2378.

Jordan JV: Empathy and self boundaries. In: *A Developmental Perspective.* Wellesley College, No. 16, 1984.

Levinson W et al: A study of patient clues and physician responses in primary care and surgical settings. JAMA 2000;284:1021.

Mengel M, Mauksch L: Disarming the family ghost: A family of origin experience. Fam Med 1989;21:45.

Novack DH et al: Calibrating the physician: personal awareness and effective patient care. JAMA 1997;278:502.

Spiro H: What is empathy and can it be taught? Ann Intern Med 1992;116:843.

Roter D et al: Improving physicians' interviewing skills and reducing patients' emotional distress: a randomized clinical trial. Arch Intern Med 1995;155:1877.

Suchman AL et al: A model of empathic communication in the medical interview. JAMA 1997;277:678.

Wilmer HA: The doctor-patient relationship and the issues of pity, sympathy, and empathy. Br J Med Psychol 1968;41:243.

Zinn W: The empathic physician. Arch Intern Med 1993;153:306.

WEB SITES

American Academy on Physician and Patient
www.physicianpatient.org
Bayer Institute for Healthcare Communication
www.bayerinstitute.org
Foundation for Medical Excellence
www.tfmc.org

Giving Bad News

3

Geoffrey H. Gordon, MD

INTRODUCTION

A debilitating or terminal illness, a catastrophic injury, an unexpected death—these are situations both patients and physicians face, and they are all situations in which the physician must break the news to patients, partners, and family members.

Most physicians in the United States now inform patients with cancer and other serious illnesses at the time of initial diagnosis (a dramatic shift from several decades ago). This reflects greater public awareness of advances in diagnosis and treatment, greater patient autonomy and self-determination, and greater physician collaboration with patients to decrease their isolation and fear and to mobilize their resources and coping skills. Self-report surveys of patients with cancer since 1950 suggest that physicians have always underestimated patients' desire for information.

It seems as if the content of the bad news should be overwhelmingly more important than the process with which it is delivered. This does not appear to be the case. Patients usually have vivid recall of the physician's manner and style but need repeated explanations of the facts. For example, the way that parents are told that their child has a developmental disability affects the emotional state and attitudes of both child and parents. These parents can distinguish the message from the messenger, and one-third to one-half are dissatisfied with how they were given the news.

TECHNIQUES FOR GIVING BAD NEWS

A systematic approach to giving bad news (Table 3–1) can make the process more predictable and less emotionally draining for the physician. The process of giving bad news can be divided into six categories: preparing for the discussion, maximizing the setting, delivering the news, offering emotional support, providing information, and closing the interview.

Cancer as an Example

PREPARING FOR THE DISCUSSION

When cancer or other serious illness is a strong diagnostic possibility, consider discussing it with the patient early in the work-up:

Doctor: That shadow on your x-ray worries me. It could be an old scar, a patch of pneumonia, or even a cancer. I think we should do some more tests to find out exactly what it is. That way, we'll be able to plan the best treatment.

Discuss with the patient how he or she would like to receive the news:

Doctor: Whatever the biopsy shows, I'll want to explain it carefully—is there someone you'd like to have with you when I go over this?

Knowledge of the patient's prior reactions to bad news can be useful—but is not necessarily predictive of the patient's response. Ideally, primary and specialist physicians should decide in advance who will give bad news and arrange follow-up.

MAXIMIZING THE SETTING

All patients in gowns should have the opportunity to dress before receiving bad news. Whenever possible, establish privacy, sit comfortably at eye level with the patient, and minimize physical barriers such as desks and tables. Avoid watching the clock, the chart, or the computer screen. Give the patient your full attention and concern.

If family members are present, introduce yourself and indicate your role and then ask for a few moments alone with the patient. Use this time to establish permission to talk with family members. You can also ask who best understands their views, and who else is important but absent. When you invite family members to return, acknowledge each person individually and learn their relationship to the patient. In large families it may be useful to identify one individual who will coordinate communication between the health care team and the family.

DELIVERING THE NEWS

The next step is to test the patient's readiness to hear the news. Review the work-up to date:

Doctor: You know we saw that shadow on your chest x-ray. When we did the CT scan of your chest, we saw a mass in your lung, and then we looked down your windpipe and took a small sample of your lung. We have the results of that biopsy now.

Some patients immediately ask if the diagnosis is cancer and want to be told promptly and directly. Others will tell the physician, verbally or nonverbally, to go more slowly.

Table 3–1. Techniques for giving bad news.

Category	Technique
Preparation	Forecast possibility of bad news Clarify who should attend the bad news visit Clarify who should give the bad news
Setting	Give bad news in person Give bad news in private Sit down and make eye contact
Delivery	Identify what the patient already knows Give the news clearly and unambiguously Identify important feelings and concerns
Emotional support	Remain with the patient and listen Use empathic statements Invite further dialogue
Information	Use simple, clear words and concepts Summarize and check patient's understanding Use handouts and other resources
Closure	Make a plan for the immediate future Ask about immediate needs Schedule a follow-up appointment

There are at least two ways to slow the message down: To grade the exposure and to present the positive message first.

1. Grade the exposure—Begin with an introductory phrase that prepares the patient for the bad news:

> **Doctor:** I'm afraid I have bad news for you. . . . This is more serious than we thought. . . . There were some cancer cells in the biopsy.

The main challenge with this approach is to finish with a clear, unambiguous statement that the patient has cancer.

2. Present the positive message first—This technique is based on the fact that patients remember little of what they are told after the bad news is given:

> **Doctor:** The main message I want to give you is that the situation is serious, but there's plenty we can do. We'll have to work closely together over the next several months. I wish I had better news, but your tests show that you have a type of lung cancer.

Once the news sinks in, the patient will typically react with a mixture of emotions, concerns, and requests for information and guidance. Devote a few moments to feelings and concerns before giving more information, or patients may be unable to hear and assimilate it.

OFFERING EMOTIONAL SUPPORT

Getting bad news is primarily an emotional rather than a cognitive event. Common, immediate emotional reactions are fear, anger, grief, and shock or emotional numbness. An important challenge for many providers is to stay with patients having strong emotional reactions and to tolerate their distress. There are no magic words or correct responses. Sit near the patient and use empathic statements:

> **Doctor:** I can see this is a terrible blow for you. I can't imagine what it must be like. I want you to know that I'll continue to be your doctor and work with you on this.

Some patients find a touch on the hand or shoulder to be supportive and reassuring. It is also helpful to ask unaccompanied patients if there is anyone who should be called after they receive the news.

Some patients direct anger at the physician:

> **Patient:** You'd better check again—you doctors are always making mistakes!

or

> **Patient:** I've always come in for check-ups; why didn't you find this sooner?

Rather than becoming defensive, the physician should acknowledge that many people in this situation feel cheated and angry. It is important to emphasize that the disease, not the doctor, is the problem and that doctor and patient must work together to deal with it.

Patients who are very reserved or too stunned to communicate their feelings are hard to evaluate because the degree of distress is not always obvious. They may express their grief alone or want to talk with others, such as a friend or spiritual counselor, before sharing their feelings with a doctor. The physician can acknowledge the difficult nature of the news and legitimize future expression of feelings:

> **Doctor:** I know this is hard to believe. You may have some feelings later that you'd like to talk with me about—I'm always ready to listen.

PROVIDING INFORMATION

Remember that most patients consult an informal health advisor (a family member, friend, book, or Web site) at some point during the illness and will already have some ideas about what is wrong, what it means, and what can be done. Eliciting these ideas shows respect for the patient's coping efforts and helps the clinician put new information into a familiar context.

> **Doctor:** What have you already learned about this? Do you know anyone who's had something like this? What concerns you most about it?

Physicians tend to block full disclosure of concerns (except symptoms) with questions, explanations, or premature reassurance. This may help reduce physician anxiety but is rarely helpful for patients who are hearing bad news for the first time. Even with careful explanations, many patients are unable to assimilate much information at the time the bad news is given. Effective educational strategies include using simple, clear words; providing information in small, digestible chunks; and checking the patient's understanding of what has been said ("What message will you take to others at home?"). About a third of the time, physicians and patients have a different understanding of the extent of the disease and the intent of treatment; progress notes in the form of stage-specific treatment plans may help.

Patients often want to know if they really have cancer, if it has spread, if it is treatable or curable, and what treatments are available. Some patients also want to know whether they are going to die and, if so, how much time they have left. Difficult questions should be addressed directly and honestly:

> **Doctor:** First, you're not in any immediate danger, and we have time to plan your treatment together. There are statistics on how long people with this condition are likely to live, and I can share them with you, but they are just statistics. No one can say for sure how long you will live.

CLOSING THE INTERVIEW

The most effective way to reach closure is to provide a plan for the immediate future. This includes asking patients who else needs to know the news and if they want help sharing it. Patients should be reassured of continuity of care even though they will need to see consultants for further testing and treatment. A follow-up appointment should be scheduled within the next several weeks, and patients should be asked to write down questions and concerns that they or their families have between visits.

Some patients have transient anxiety, sadness, or trouble sleeping. A short course of medication for sleeplessness or anxiety may be helpful, but patients should also be told that it is normal to feel upset or to have trouble sleeping after receiving bad news.

A special and problematic type of giving bad news arises when the disease progresses despite all available and appropriate treatment. Over 20% of oncologists report difficulty with these conversations. These physicians are more likely to experience patient death as a personal failure, to regard palliative care as "giving up" or "taking away hope," and to give patients overly optimistic prognoses. Patients and families who reject this news, and health systems that selectively reward technical interventions, are accomplices. In this special case of bad news, physicians must have a clear understanding of comfort care as the active treatment of suffering (physical, psychological, social,

and spiritual) with the goal of improving or maintaining quality of life. They must also appreciate that as care takes on more palliative goals and methods, their roles and relationships with patients become more flexible, the resources on which they can draw expand, and their work often becomes more personally meaningful and rewarding (see Chapter 35).

Death Notification

Some additional considerations apply when notifying family members of the death of a loved one (see Chapter 35). Unexpected or traumatic deaths are most difficult because survivors are unprepared and rarely have a prior relationship with the notifying physician. Physicians should begin by introducing themselves and explaining their role in the deceased person's care. Survivors who must be reached by telephone should be told to come to the hospital prior to the actual death notification, unless they specifically ask if the patient has died.

Once given the news, survivors may want to view the body. This is an important part of the grieving process and should not be discouraged. Survivors are often concerned about whether their loved one suffered or was alone at the time of death and whether they could have done anything to prevent it. They can often be told truthfully that the patient was unconscious prior to death, there was no evidence of suffering, and that maximal efforts were made to help. People also may need to be reassured that none of their actions hastened the patient's death.

Depending on the cause of death and comorbid conditions, the deceased may be a candidate for organ donation. Although some families object, many others find comfort in making an anatomic gift. Many states inquire about and record anatomic donor permission on drivers' licenses, and families may discover that the deceased did, in fact, give such consent. Permission for autopsy can also be requested at this time. Once the notifying physician has brought up these topics, many hospitals have specially trained staff to work further with families. Some hospitals and physicians routinely send sympathy cards or make follow-up calls to recently bereaved survivors.

PROBLEM AREAS

Acceptance

DON'T TELL ME IF IT'S CANCER

Some patients specifically request not to be told their diagnosis. Patients may choose to exercise their autonomy by delegating it to someone else, and they should not have unwanted information forced on them. However, if they are willing to talk further, the physician should ask what bad news would mean to them, and what they are afraid might happen if they were to receive it. These questions can help patients disclose concerns that inhibit their participating in care. Patients can also be told the potential benefits of knowing the diagnosis:

> **Doctor:** One of the ways you can help is to create the best environment for our medicines and treatments to work. This includes planning the best treatment for you, finding which parts of you are healthy and strong, and which areas need some work. Your attitude and interest are important parts of your treatment; they may help you feel better, and in some cases, the treatment may work better. We want you to ask questions about what is happening—remember that there are no stupid questions. If it would help you to talk with someone who has been through this, please let me know.

DON'T TELL HIM OR HER IT'S CANCER

Family members may ask that patients not be told the diagnosis if it is cancer. Families should be thanked for their concern and reassured that information will not be forced on the patient. They should also be told that patients' questions about their conditions will be answered truthfully, that patients usually know or suspect more than they let on, and that keeping secrets in health care settings is difficult. Explain the rationale for the patient knowing the diagnosis, and ask what they are concerned might happen if the patient knows. Some families may benefit from referral to a social worker if they need help finding ways to provide emotional support for the patient and for each other.

I DON'T BELIEVE IT'S CANCER

Some patients are unable to accept the diagnosis, offering such statements as "I just know it isn't cancer. If I can get some rest I'll be fine." This is most frustrating when it delays the early implementation of potentially curative treatment. Physicians often use logical arguments and dire predictions to persuade patients to agree to evaluation and treatment. Paradoxically, this approach makes many patients more resistant. Instead, the physician should try to depict denial as a sometimes useful, but currently maladaptive, way of coping. This can be done by explaining that patients are often of two minds:

> **Doctor:** Many patients find this kind of diagnosis hard to believe. I can see that part of you wants to look on the bright side and stay hopeful, but I wonder if you don't also have times when you realize that problems might arise. Let's think about how to proceed if the diagnosis is more serious.

The physician should offer to answer any future questions the patient might have and expect day-to-day variation in the patient's ability to acknowledge the accuracy of the diagnosis. Conversations should be documented in the patient's chart to notify others of the patient's reaction. Sometimes anticipating future needs helps patients accept the reality of the diagnosis:

> **Doctor:** Let's take a few minutes to think about your plans if your condition worsens. You may want to make decisions and plans now, in case you're unable to handle them in the future.

Different Cultural Values

Attitudes and beliefs about bad news, death, and the expression of grief are determined in part by cultural norms (see Chapter 12). For example, in some cultural groups, bad news about health-related matters is routinely withheld from patients. In other groups, the delivery of bad news to patients is a process that involves the whole family. There are also cultural differences in responding to death; rituals such as opening windows and burning candles may be difficult to accommodate in an acute care setting.

> **Doctor:** Are there any family or cultural traditions I should know about for your medical care?

Cultural differences between physicians and patients or families become problematic when they are not recognized as such and are attributed to uncooperativeness or psychopathology. Physicians from cultural groups with behavioral norms different from their patients or practice environments may find such differences hard to reconcile and therefore may experience role conflicts in caring for patients and families from their own culture. In this case, consultation with a colleague whose background is outside the medical subculture may lend some objectivity.

HOPE & REASSURANCE

Patients and families are fearful of losing hope. Unfortunately, many physicians have never learned how to offer hope and reassurance along with bad news. To physicians, hope and reassurance bring to mind cure, or, at the very least, prolonged survival. To patients and families, hope may initially mean cure but later can mean reconciliation with others, finishing projects, attending a special task or event, staying out of the hospital, or being free of pain.

There are several ways physicians can provide hope and reassurance at the time of bad news:

- Use positive words. Recognize the difference between the uncertain perception of "Your scan is negative" and the clarity of "Your scan showed that your liver is normal and healthy."
- Avoid "medical hexing." Physicians are trained to anticipate, detect, and treat complications of disease and treatment. They should also be prepared to recognize the unexpected good response, and be able to acknowledge and celebrate it.
- Ask patients what they are hoping for now, how close they can get to reaching it, and what they will need.

Then join them to make it happen. For example, a woman with spinal epidural spread of lymphoma began palliative radiation therapy to avoid leg weakness so she could travel to see her granddaughter graduate from high school. Instead, she became too weak to travel. Her oncologist asked her what she hoped to achieve by making the trip; she said she hoped to deliver a special message to her granddaughter. Together they decided that she could make a videotape of her message and have it delivered in time for her granddaughter's graduation.

- Encourage the patient to think of illness as a challenge. Most patients will have faced one or more severe challenges in their lives. Invoke their past successes in coping or mention those of other patients, saying, for example, "I'm always surprised at how well patients do. . . ."
- Work to improve patients' function and participation in their health care. Help them understand that their thoughts, attitudes, and activities affect how they feel, and stress the importance of learning to relax, identifying new sources of pleasure and self-esteem, and learning coping skills from other patients.
- Help patients learn how to face and deal with their illness realistically. Patients who focus exclusively on positive approaches may delay and inhibit their own grieving or feel guilty if they can't laugh or love their cancer away. These patients, and their families, may need permission to accept and grieve their losses. Other patients cope best by consistently fighting the disease and maintaining a positive focus, in the face of all odds, to the very end. Many patients describe alternating days of "giving in" to the disease versus "putting it in its place" and living as normally as possible under the circumstances.

THE HEALTH-CARE TEAM

Although it is the physician's role to deliver the bad news, other team members play important roles.

Nurses are trained to evaluate patients' emotional and physical responses to treatment, their levels of comfort and activity, and their progress toward expected goals. They can be present when bad news is given, help interpret it if necessary, assist patients in verbalizing feelings and questions, and provide emotional support. Some nurses are also skilled at ensuring that treatment decisions are congruent with the overall direction and goals of care.

Social workers are skilled at identifying resources, enhancing coping skills, and working with patients' families. Chaplains can help in identifying and meeting patients' spiritual needs and reconnecting them with a faith, tradition, or community.

Nutritionists, physical therapists, and clinical pharmacists specializing in palliative care can also make important contributions to the management of seriously ill patients.

Occasionally patients and families will need referral for counseling or other mental health services. Indications for referral include prolonged or atypical grief, particularly when it interferes with daily activities or medical care; concern about a patient's suicide potential if given bad news; difficulty communicating within the family or with health-care providers; and assistance in maximizing coping skills. Mental health referrals are most successful when the referring physician explains the goals of the referral to the patient and tells the patient what to expect:

> **Doctor:** I'll do everything I can to work on the disease and symptoms, but Dr. Jones is an expert on helping people manage the impact of this disease on their lives. She will talk to you and then call me to make a care plan.

It is important to ensure follow-up care:

> **Doctor:** I'd like you to make an appointment to see me after you've seen Dr. Jones so we can make some plans together.

Self-Awareness as a Skill

For a physician, checking in with one's own feelings is an invaluable skill. Dissociating from painful feelings protects physicians' psychological equilibrium and allows them to conduct the tasks of medical care objectively. Experiencing and expressing feelings that arise in the course of professional activities, however, are important components of physician well-being. Patients nearly always sense what their physicians are feeling. They often value demonstrations of personal caring and express their appreciation: "I knew the doctor really cared about Jimmy when I saw tears in his eyes when he was talking to us."

Some physicians use tasks such as completing the death certificate as rituals to help them review their relationship with the patient, reflect on what they learned, and reach closure. To deal with cumulative patient deaths, and to better understand their values and attitudes around death, suffering, and the role of medicine, some physicians look to self-awareness groups or spiritual traditions. Most physicians benefit from talking about their own grief with a trusted colleague before—and after—giving bad news (see Chapter 7).

SUGGESTED READINGS

Abrahms EZ, Goodman JF: Diagnosing developmental problems in children: parents and professionals negotiate bad news. J Pediatr Psychol 1998;23(2):87. PMID: 9585635.

Ambuel B, Mazzone MF: Breaking bad news and discussing death. Prim Care 2001;28(2):249. PMID: 11406434.

Baile WF et al: Discussing disease progression and end-of-life decisions. Oncology 1999;13(7):1021. PMID: 10442349.

Baile WF et al: SPIKES—a six-step protocol for delivering bad news: application to the patient with cancer. Oncologist 2000;5(4):302. PMID: 10964998.

Bedell SE, Cadenhead K, Graboys T: The doctor's letter of condolence. N Engl J Med 2001;344(15):1162. PMID: 11302139.

Blackhall LJ et al: Ethnicity and attitudes toward patient autonomy. JAMA 1995;274(10):820. PMID: 7650806.

Coulehan JL: Tenderness and steadiness: emotions in medical practice. Lit Med 1995;14(2):222. PMID: 8558910.

Jurkovich GJ et al: Giving bad news: the family perspective. J Trauma 2000;48(5):865; discussion 870. PMID: 10823529.

Maguire P: Improving communication with cancer patients. Eur J Cancer 1999;35(10):1415. PMID: 10673972.

Module 2: Communicating Bad News. In: Emanuel LL, von Gunten CF, Ferris FD. *The Education for Physicians on End-of-life Care Project (EPEC) Curriculum.* The Robert Wood Johnson Foundation, 1999. At http://www.epec.net/content/participantshandbook.html

Quill TE, Arnold RM, Platt F: "I wish things were different": expressing wishes in response to loss, futility, and unrealistic hopes. Ann Intern Med 2001;135(7):551. PMID: 11578166.

Smith TJ: The art of oncology: when the tumor is not the target. Tell it like it is. J Clin Oncol 2000;18:3441. PMID: 11013287.

von Gunten CF, Ferris FD, Emanuel LL: Ensuring competency in end-of-life care: Communication and relational skills. JAMA 2000;284(23):3051. PMID: 11122596.

Weissman D: Fast Fact #21: Hope and truth telling. End-of-Life Physician Education Resource Center (EPERC), September 2000. http://www.eperc.mcw.edu

WEB SITES

CurrMIT (the AAMC Curriculum Management & Information Tool) is a password-protected, online database, available only to faculty and administrators of LCME-accredited AAMC-member medical schools in the United States and Canada, through their respective offices of medical education and by special arrangement, for osteopathic medical schools that are members of the American Association of Colleges of Osteopathic Medicine (AACOM). Faculty with access to CurrMIT who wish to look for other sources or other faculty delivering this content may wish to review one of the "Existing Reports" in CurrMIT, titled, "ALL_Session_Topic: Breaking bad news." For information on CurrMIT, see http://www.aamc.org/meded/curric/. From this site, AAMC-member faculty who wish to receive access can follow a link to their main CurrMIT contact in the office of medical education.

The End of Life Physician Education Resource Center (EPERC) is a peer-reviewed clearinghouse for educational materials for physicians on all aspects of end of life care, including giving bad news. www.eperc.mcw.edu

Difficult Patients

Howard B. Beckman, MD, FACP

INTRODUCTION

Whenever and wherever health professionals congregate, it doesn't take long before the topic of difficult patients is discussed. Patients and families we experience as difficult increase the personal frustration of delivering care, decrease our satisfaction with work, and make it almost impossible to deliver the person-centered care that is at the heart of high-quality, satisfying, effective health care. Why, we ask, would someone choose to come to the office or hospital and harass, abuse, ignore, or lie to us?

Fortunately, most difficult interactions are both diagnosable and repairable. Aside from the unusual individual who is determined to be difficult, many problematic situations are created by unsatisfactory communication between provider and patient or by personal issues the provider or patient unknowingly brings into these important interactions. Such issues can include similar problems within the provider's own world or negative reactions to the patient's physical condition, sexual orientation, or personality.

Increasingly medical educators are finding that practitioners consider patients difficult based on the patient's similarity to others with whom the practitioner has had interpersonal problems. For example, a physician whose uncle used anger for control may now have problems with older men who similarly express anger. Another common situation is the practitioner who is surprisingly intolerant of patients who won't stop smoking. Perhaps this physician had a close relative who could not be convinced to stop smoking and who, as a result, developed lung cancer. Developing the self-awareness to separate one's own past experience from a patient's current behavior can significantly moderate one's aversive response.

The key to dealing with such situations is to examine them with a critical eye and a more flexible style of communication that includes considerable room for negotiation. Greater self-awareness about one's own feelings, experiences, and beliefs can help practitioners offer more nonjudgmental care to their patients. The case illustrations that follow focus on some of the challenging patients and situations practitioners most frequently find difficult and offer specific approaches to dealing with these. Table 4–1 summarizes some general guidelines for working with difficult patients. Table 4–2 recommends techniques for approaching specific situations.

THE ANGRY PATIENT

 CASE ILLUSTRATION 1

Dr. Swanson enters the room to see her fourth of the dozen patients scheduled for her Thursday morning session. Her patient, Ms. B., a 35-year-old social worker, is sitting with arms crossed, refusing to make eye contact. Dr. Swanson greets the patient by asking, "Ms. B., how are you?" She responds, "I've been waiting 35 minutes! This is no way to run an office." The doctor, who is emotionally drained after spending the last 50 minutes working with a patient newly diagnosed with breast cancer, wonders why she chose medicine as a career.

Diagnosis

Even without this straightforward verbal response, an angry patient is not difficult to recognize. Harsh nonverbal communication such as rigid posturing, a piercing stare, a refusal to shake hands, gritting the teeth, and confrontational or occasionally abusive language provides unmistakable evidence. More subtle behaviors by the patient include refusing to answer questions, failing to make eye contact, or constructing nonverbal barriers to communication such as crossed arms, turning away from the provider, or increasing the physical distance between them.

DIFFERENTIAL DIAGNOSIS

All too often, practitioners assume that the patient is angry with *them,* and, as a result, feel they are being blamed for something they must have done or forgot to do. Although that certainly is one possibility, other important reasons must be considered as the cause for anger. These include but are not limited to the causes listed in Table 4–3.

Table 4–1. General guidelines for working with difficult patients.

Seek broader possibilities for the patient's emotion or problems.
Respond directly to the patient's emotions.
Solicit the patient's perspective on why there is a problem.
Avoid being defensive.
Seek to discover a common goal for the visit.

PSYCHOLOGICAL MECHANISMS

For many patients, the special relationship they develop with their medical practitioner is among the safest and most stable they experience. It is therefore quite common for patients to share emotions they would never consider revealing—let alone discussing—in other relationships. Patients expect to have their concerns investigated with compassion and interest. Any suggestion that the patients' concerns are not taken seriously or are viewed as mundane may transform that feeling of safety into anger.

Patients have lofty expectations of medical practitioners. They expect timely service, relevant and up-to-date information about evaluations and treatments offered, and advice on how to cope with their illness. From their point of view, interactions that fall short can result in feelings of shame and rejection. The resulting humiliation can easily turn to anger.

From the provider's point of view, the patient's expression of anger may trigger feelings as diverse as disappointment at having failed the patient to being insulted by the patient's disrespectful behavior. As a result, practitioners often become defensive, exhibiting reciprocal anger, withdrawal from the relationship, or denial of the behavior the practitioner *assumes* prompted the anger. The difficulties are magnified if the expression of anger is problematic in the practitioner's own family. After recognizing the contributions of one's own experiences, openly encouraging and exploring a patient's anger help create an honest and open relationship, define the problem explicitly, and permit an accurate and timely response.

Management

In most situations involving anger, evaluation and understanding should begin the therapeutic process. Respond-

Table 4–2. Tips for approaching difficult situations or patient behaviors.

Situation	Recommended Techniques
Angry patients	Elicit the patient's reason for being angry: *You seem angry; tell me more about it.* Empathize with the patient's experience: *I can understand why you would be angry.* Solicit the patient's perspective: *What can we do to improve the situation?* If appropriate, apologize: *I'm sorry you had to wait so long.*
Silent patients	Point out the problem: *You're being very quiet.* Elicit the patient's reason for silence: *Why are you being so quiet?* Explain the need for collaboration: *For me to help you, I really need you to talk to me more about your problem.* Respond to cues of hearing impairment or language barriers: *Are you having trouble hearing or understanding me?*
Demanding patients	Take a step back from the demand: *You seem adamant about the MRI. Why do you think it's so important?* Solicit the goal of the demand: *Is there a particular problem you think the MRI will help us diagnose?* Acknowledge emotions unexpressed at the time of the demand: *It must be very frustrating that your back still hurts.* Solicit the patient's perspective: *What do you think is causing your problem?* *In what way had you hoped I could help you?*

Table 4–3. Possible causes of patient anger.

Difficulty in getting to the office
Problems with the office staff
Anger toward the illness from which the person suffers
Anger at the cost of health care
Problems with consultants to whom the practitioner referred the patient
Unanticipated problems from a procedure or medication recommended by the practitioner
Previous unsupportive or condescending treatment by a physician
Anger directed at family members' responses—whether inadequate or overemotional—to the patient's illness
Other significant news or problems unrelated to medical service, such as work- or family-related conflicts

ing calmly, without judgment or projection, with "You seem angry" tests whether the doctor has correctly identified the emotion. Failing to confront anger ensures the collection of superficial information, informs the patient that the provider is impervious to or unsettled by emotion, and discourages any meaningful sharing of feelings. On the other hand, confronting anger is both efficient and medically appropriate.

Although many patients in this situation respond with "You bet I'm angry," some patients deny their anger. Nonetheless, their body language or tone of voice betrays the emotion. In this case, the physician can address the denial: "Maybe 'angry' is too strong a word. It seems to me that you're upset by something; if you'd like to tell me about it, I might be able to help." The practitioner's invitation to explain offers the patient the chance to express explicitly his or her feelings. As a result, the practitioner develops a more complete understanding of the patient's experience. Armed with the patient's point of view the practitioner and the patient can reach agreement on the nature of the problem. This point in the encounter is usually marked by a reduction in the patient's anger, relief on the part of the provider, and the re-creation of patient–doctor collaboration with the mutual goal of solving the identified problem. The subsequent management of the problem depends on the particular cause of the anger.

CASE ILLUSTRATION 1 (CONT.)

In response to the question, "Why are you angry?" Ms. B. responds, "The surgeon you sent me to said she hadn't received your letter. She didn't know why I was there. I had to take half a day off from work—which I could not afford—I drove 2 hours to get

there, and all I did was waste my time. And now you keep me waiting when I'm due in court in an hour."

In response, the doctor apologizes, saying that the letter had been dictated but apparently was not mailed in time. To prevent problems in the future, the practice now faxes a short note to all consultants within 48 hours. She also tells the patient that this morning's delay was unavoidable because of another patient's needs. Ms. B. feels better understood, accepts the apology, and ends by saying, "I hope this doesn't happen again; I have enough stress at work as it is." The doctor says, "I should have asked the receptionist to tell you that I was running late—I'm sorry about that. We're really trying hard to make sure that we communicate more effectively with our patients and our consultants." The total exchange takes 50 seconds—a small cost in time for large gains in the quality of the relationship.

Patient Education

Sometimes patients need to learn that it is not only permissible but important for them and their families to express their feelings. By encouraging the expression of anger, the practitioner helps identify unresolved conflicts that can interfere with the process of delivering appropriate care. Encouraging patients and their families to express concerns or disappointments actually offers the practitioner the opportunity to become more efficient by removing significant barriers to effective, honest collaboration. Encouraging the nursing and office staff to use this approach increases the opportunities to hear patients' thoughts, concerns, and ideas.

Summary

Too often practitioners assume that angry patients are angry with them. Sometimes this is so, but often there are much more complex reasons for a patient's or family's anger, which must be sought directly. Practitioners should not mistakenly project their own assumptions onto the patient. By working hard to avoid becoming defensive, practitioners can acknowledge and then constructively resolve the cause of the anger. Confronted with such a responsive approach, most angry patients become quite satisfied and resume an effective collaborative relationship with their practitioner.

THE SILENT PATIENT

CASE ILLUSTRATION 2

Dr. Cren begins his afternoon office hours; he is scheduled to see Mr. K., a 47-year-old man who has recently relocated to the area. On entering the room, the doctor notices that Mr. K. fails to make eye contact and fiddles with a piece of paper folded over many times. In response to "Good afternoon; I'm Dr. Cren," Mr. K. quietly says, "Good afternoon." When asked what problems he is having, Mr. K. answers, "I've been really tired." After waiting a few seconds, Dr. Cren encourages the patient to speak by asking him to tell him more. The patient responds, "I don't know what to say."

Diagnosis

By definition, silent patients offer little in the way of verbal interaction. In addition to the lack of communication, however, there are a number of important nonverbal cues that deserve attention. The patient may seem withdrawn,

as indicated by sitting a greater distance from the physician than usual, failing to make eye contact, avoiding the physician's gaze, seeming distracted, or not acknowledging the physician's attempts at interaction. Alternatively, the patient may seem anxious, evidenced by nervous or repetitive habits such as nail-biting, pacing, or folding and refolding papers. Finally, the patient may exhibit signs of sadness such as deep sighs, red eyes, or tears.

DIFFERENTIAL DIAGNOSIS

Based on observing the patient's responses to questions and nonverbal behavior, the etiologies listed in Table 4–4 might be considered for the silence.

PSYCHOLOGICAL MECHANISMS

In many families, individuals in positions of authority may demand "silence unless spoken to," which may be transferred to a practitioner–patient relationship. This

Table 4–4. Possible causes of silence in patients.

Cause	Discussion
Adverse reaction to prescription medication (eg, sedation)	*Check for overdose or drug interactions.*
Alcohol or other drug intoxication	*Screen with CAGE questionnaire and elicit history of substance abuse.*
Alzheimer's or other dementia	*Age-dependent; although some dementias strike as early as the mid-40s, most occur in the 65+ age group. Silence is usually a sign of advanced disease associated with withdrawal from the environment.*
Anger	*The patient is feeling wronged or slighted and is trying to elicit an emotional reaction. . . . (see Table 4–3).*
Cultural or language barrier	*Ask whether the patient can understand; use an interpreter or bilingual staff member, if available.*
Depression, dysthymia, or adjustment disorder with depressed mood	*Name the feelings; request elaboration.*
Distraction secondary to depression	*Associated with drawn features, sad affect, lack of eye contact.*
Fear of being told that serious disease is causing the presenting problem	*State clearly that, regardless of the outcome, the practitioner will be there to help.*
Fear of physician authority	*Family background, other experience with domineering authority figures may have demanded submissiveness; a gentle demeanor, reassurance, and an explicit request for collaboration can help win the patient's confidence.*
Hearing impairment	*Use the whisper test.*
Passive or shy personality	*Change to a more direct, closed-ended pattern of questions; encourage descriptions and elaboration.*
Preoccupation with auditory or visual hallucinations	*Request additional information from family or attendant.*
Quiet person	*Usually responds to encouragement, offers to elaborate.*
Stroke, TIA (transient ischemic attack), mass lesion	*Conduct thorough neurologic examination for focal findings.*

deference may also extend to interactions in which differences in gender or social class exist. A history of humiliation or percieved mistreatment in previous medical relationships may also result in withdrawn silent behavior.

When a patient has a serious or potentially life-threatening reason for a concern, silence may represent denial and serve a protective function. For example, a woman can avoid confronting her fears about having breast cancer if she does not mention that she felt a lump in her breast while in the shower.

Silence may also be a sign of a passive personality. These individuals want the partner in the interview to take control and direct the flow of the visit (see Chapter 24). Probably most important, silence may be a profound indicator of a depressed mood or an adverse effect from a psychoactive medication. Those struggling with depression or dysthymia may find it difficult to express their concerns or even find the energy to initiate conversation.

Management

When confronted with a silent patient, exploring the behavior is usually best begun by reflecting "You seem very quiet today." This offers the patient the opportunity to acknowledge the behavior and share the reason for it. Providing time, as much as 3–5 seconds, may encourage a tentative, frightened, or passive patient to begin speaking. When a patient seems passive, it is appropriate to explain the need for the patient to collaborate in the visit: "For me to help you, I really need you to tell me about this problem in more detail."

If the person seems actively distracted, it is fair to ask, "Are you hearing voices or seeing things you think might not be real?" As mentioned earlier, if the patient shows evidence of anger, reflecting the emotion would be appropriate. Especially with older patients, a patient who responds with "What?" most likely has a hearing impairment and the practitioner need only face the patient and speak more loudly. One of the most common complaints by older patients is that their practitioners don't speak clearly or loudly enough.

CASE ILLUSTRATION 2 (CONT.)

In response to "You seem quiet," Mr. K. responds, "Today is 3 months since my favorite aunt died." When Dr. Cren says, "I'm sorry to hear that; would you like to reschedule the visit?" the patient thanks him for the offer, adding that he's concerned about the fatigue and would like to talk about it. With that, the patient becomes more animated and engages in a discussion about his fatigue, which is subsequently diagnosed as being related to depression.

Patient Education

By explaining that silence creates additional barriers to delivering effective care, physicians can invite patients to be increasingly more involved in their treatment decisions. The importance of the patient's or family member's role in evaluating and treating problems and the value of taking an active role in decision making should be emphasized. This discourages the patient from making the practitioner solely—and inappropriately—responsible for evaluation or treatment plans.

Summary

There are many reasons why individuals might be silent in the office. Openly acknowledging the problems silence creates, and then asking for an explanation, offers patients the chance to express a feeling state, an extenuating circumstance, fear of an outcome, or fear of the projected role of the practitioner. Further questioning can also result in a diagnosis of an anatomic cause, such as an acoustic neuroma or a psychiatric condition that causes hallucinations or delusions. Premature testing of an hypothesis runs the risk of insulting patients or driving them further from the relationship.

Silent patients are often distressing, particularly for individuals who value the social and interpersonal aspects of medical practice. Learning to encourage a more mutual collaboration is usually both beneficial and rewarding. Sometimes we struggle with particular types of patients because they remind us of others from previous experiences. These reminders can evoke strong negative responses. For example, someone easily frustrated by silent patients may be reminded of a father who died because he didn't let anyone know he was having exertional chest pain. Recognizing the sources of our intense personal responses can help us remain focused on a patient's problem or response and avoid unproductive replays of unsettling past experiences. Acknowledging the power of these prior experiences allows the practitioner to decide how to confront or address these important personal issues.

THE DEMANDING PATIENT

CASE ILLUSTRATION 3

Dr. Hartwick is seeing Mr. G., a 48-year-old bricklayer, her fifth patient of the afternoon. Mr. G. is being seen for back pain that began after a day of particularly heavy work on the job. In the initial visit, after taking a history and excluding points suggestive of an underlying cancer or spinal cord injury, Dr. Hartwick had prescribed limited activity, exercise as tolerated, analgesics, and the application of heat. Two weeks later, Mr. G. returns, and when asked how things have gone in the last 2 weeks, responds, "I'm no better. I've checked into a web-based back pain chat room and everyone agreed I should have an MRI [magnetic resonance imaging]." Dr. Hartwick leans back in her chair, anticipating an extremely frustrating encounter.

Diagnosis

When a demand is made, the practitioner may quickly identify the signs of anger. Alternatively, the patient's actions—nail-biting, repetitive movements, or poor attention—might suggest frustration or anxiety. A grimacing facial expression, an inability to move, or obvious pain with movement suggests an unacceptable level of pain. A focus on a seemingly unrelated article—a medical device such as a cane or brace, internet search results, or an advertisement—can represent a clue that an important issue has yet to be resolved.

DIFFERENTIAL DIAGNOSIS

Although a patient's demand is usually tied to dissatisfaction with the current plan for evaluation or treatment, there are many possible causes of the dissatisfaction. As a rule, if there is disagreement about treatment, the problem results from a concern about the accuracy of the diagnosis. If the problem involves a diagnostic test, the problem often arises either from the prior evaluation or a failure to solicit important aspects of the history. On the other hand, a recommended test or treatment may trigger a memory of a family member or friend's similar and unpleasant experience. The consequence is that the patient projects an undesirable outcome on the current plan.

Sometimes the reason for an unexpected demand involves secondary gain, such as a workers' compensation, a disability claim, or a lawsuit. Another possibility is that the patient has read something in the press, listened to a friend, or found something on the internet that suggests a simplistic or "right" way to solve the problem while attacking other approaches. Finally, the patient may be frustrated with the lack of relief because additional treatment is actually indicated. By listening carefully to a patient's dissatisfaction, the practitioner may rethink the diagnosis and seek alternatives to the current treatment plan. An example would be the patient, presumed to have a sprained wrist, who returns with unremitting pain. The increased severity of symptom reporting prompts a search for a fracture—which is subsequently diagnosed by x-ray.

PSYCHOLOGICAL MECHANISMS

The demand for additional intervention can be triggered by any of the feelings listed in Table 4–5.

Individuals are often isolated from family and friends during times of illness. Such a person may begin to doubt that the practitioner is sufficiently interested in the problem to ensure the best possible outcome. As distrust of the physician grows, the patient feels increasingly responsible for the outcome of his or her care and begins to seek alternative sources of care. The result can become a more fearful and demanding patient. On the other hand, if secondary gains are connected with the illness, the patient may demand testing to demonstrate levels of disability or prove that the problem is as severe as claimed. This is especially true in pain syndromes in which testing is generally unrevealing. The employer, lawyer, or insurance company begins to feel that the problem is "all in the patient's head." As a result, the patient seeks evidence of a severe condition capable of causing his or her incapacitating symptoms.

Practitioners often experience feelings of rejection, distrust, blame, or humiliation in response to demanding patients. As a result, the practitioner often becomes defensive. By prematurely assuming this defensive posture, the practitioner loses the opportunity to explore the pa-

Table 4–5. Possible reasons for demanding additional interventions.

Feeling	Discussion
Anger	*The patient is feeling wronged or is reexperiencing a previous bad outcome (see Table 4–3).*
Fear	*The patient may be afraid that the illness is terminal, serious, horrible, disfiguring, etc., if not attacked quickly.*
Frustration	*The patient may feel that no—or insufficient—progress has been made.*
Personal responsibility for health outcome	*Previous experience may have convinced the patient that physicians are not trustworthy, competent, or interested.*
Doubt	*The patient may wonder if economic reasons are driving decision making or if the practitioner is skilled enough or up to date with current evaluation and treatment technologies.*

tient's subtle clues to the reasons for a demand. For example, casual asides, postural shifts in response to a topic, and expressions of fear, agitation, and grief are often ignored.

Management

Rather than respond to a presumed cause for the demand, the first step in evaluating or reevaluating the demand is to identify and explore the patient's affect appropriately. Let us consider case illustration 3. Because Mr. G. seems frustrated, Dr. Hartwick reflects the feeling: "You seem frustrated." The patient responds, "I am frustrated. My father had a similar condition, and 2 years later they found he had a herniated disk which was successfully treated surgically. I don't want to wait that long to find out what I have."

In response to an acknowledgment of affect, the patient usually confirms or denies the practitioner's hypothesis. If the patient responds affirmatively (eg, "I am angry, frustrated, sad, nervous"), the practitioner would ask, "Why are you. . . ." This permits the patient to explain and share the experience that surrounds the emotion. Often this prompts a story or a piece of information that is instrumental in allowing the physician to ask and the patient to answer pertinent questions. In Mr. G.'s case, hearing what the patient fears better prepares Dr. Hartwick to understand what prompted the request for an MRI and determine to what extent education, a redescription of the results of evaluation or treatment, another examination, or discussion about possible secondary gain might be most appropriate. As all aspects of a demand are explored, an appropriate response can be constructed.

When this approach is less successful, a number of probing questions are useful. One is to ask patients what they think is causing their problem; often patients do not offer their opinions without being asked. Given the opportunity, patients frequently say that after an evaluation they were told the test results were all negative, but the cause of the problem they perceived was not addressed. This point cannot be stressed enough: *To provide meaningful reassurance, the patient's attribution for the symptom must be elicited and confronted.*

Another useful question is: "How had you hoped I could help you?" This gives the patient the opportunity to express dissatisfaction with the extent of evaluation, treatment, or commitment by the practitioner; it often lightens the practitioner's burden, as the patient's request may be significantly less difficult than anticipated by the practitioner. A typical example might be the arthritic patient who complains bitterly about the pain in his hip. When the physician asks, "How had you hoped I could help you?" the patients responds, "I'd like a prescription for a cane." The physician had anticipated a request for additional imaging and narcotics.

CASE ILLUSTRATION 3 (CONT.)

In response to Dr. Hartwick's question, Mr. G. says, "I want to know how I can find out exactly what I have and make sure I don't have any problems with my disk." The doctor then describes recently updated back pain guidelines that support the use of MRI testing only for determining operability in patients with prolonged pain or defined neurologic syndromes, such as radiculopathy or cauda equina syndrome.

By offering alternatives to the demand that would accomplish the same goal—while taking into account the patient's reason for the demand—the practitioner has begun the process of collaborative negotiating. Respecting the patient's point of view generally provides the basis for construction of a mutually satisfactory plan.

Dr. Hartwick further explains to Mr. G.: "I've examined you again and I find no evidence of nerve root involvement. From what you've said about your father's symptoms, his back problem was quite different from what you're experiencing. Let's put off doing any tests for now. What I would like to do is continue our present course of treatment, since in 90% of cases the symptoms you describe resolve within 12 weeks. If at the end of that time you're still having these symptoms, I'll refer you to a neurologist for another opinion on what we might do. I appreciate your telling me about your dad, because it's obviously causing you some distress and making you wonder whether I was doing the right thing. Looking at things from your perspective helps me do a better job." The time cost of this explanation is 38 seconds; the reexamination adds only 2 minutes.

A practitioner who believes that the demand is related to secondary gain (for example, a desire to remain away from work for an extended period), can confront the patient and offer a plan that provides ample time for recovery.

Patient Education

Patients respond to instruction when they believe it will be helpful in solving their problem. Until there is agreement on the need for education by practitioner and patient, the patient might perceive education as the practitioner's way of controlling the visit. The patient's usual response in such an encounter is either to tune out the information or to construct mental barriers to implementing the practitioner's recommendations. On the other hand, once the patient's concerns have been successfully addressed and a partnership has been formed, the patient often asks for and benefits from the information supporting the practitioner's point of view. In Case Illustration 3, recent web-based guidelines that support the doctor's plan served to educate and reassure the patient that his physician's plan was consistent with best medical practice.

Summary

A patient presenting what appears to be unreasonable demands is a clue that previous interactions have been unsuccessful. Exploring the reason for the demand in a nonjudgmental fashion allows most demands to be understood and addressed. Knowing the cause of the demand allows the practitioner to negotiate a plan that is mutually agreeable. When it becomes clear that such a negotiation is not possible, the patient should be informed of realistic limits to what the practitioner can offer. The patient can then decide whether he or she is willing to accept the practitioner's boundaries or needs to seek the services of another practitioner.

THE "YES, BUT . . ." PATIENT

 CASE ILLUSTRATION 4

Mrs. M. is a 58-year-old woman who is being followed for obesity and poorly controlled high blood pressure. Her doctor is frustrated because his continued attempts to get Mrs. M. to lose weight have been unsuccessful. As a result, he is pessimistic about their ability to work together to treat her hypertension, which he feels is a clear risk to her health. When the doctor notes that Mrs. M.'s blood pressure is still elevated, he asks whether she is still taking her medication.

She responds, "Oh, I'm sorry doctor, I ran out of my medicine 3 days ago and didn't want to bother you for a refill." Later in the visit the doctor asks, "Did you join that exercise program you said you would last time?" Mrs. M. replies, "I've been so busy. I'll do it next week." The doctor pulls back in his chair, thinking to himself, "This will never go anywhere."

Diagnosis

When problems are being discussed, the nonverbal behavior of patients in this group is usually engaged and active: leaning forward, bright affect, and dynamic gestures. As recommendations for evaluation and treatment are made, however, the patient typically becomes withdrawn,

eye contact diminishes, and language becomes significantly less animated. Verbally, during the discussion of evaluation and treatment, the patient becomes quiet, volunteers little, and characteristically offers no solutions to problems. In fact, as the practitioner makes recommendations, the patient often responds with the classic, "I'd like to do that but. . . ."

DIFFERENTIAL DIAGNOSIS

Frequently, this behavior indicates a passive-aggressive personality. The practitioner initially feels encouraged to offer suggestions to the patient, who then invariably rejects the offer or agrees to the plan but does not carry it out.

There are other possibilities, however, that are often not explored. Probably most important is that the practitioner's plan has not taken the patient's perspective into account and is therefore unrealistic or economically or logistically impossible. Another consideration is that the patient comes from a highly controlling family and is attempting to follow the recommendations but for psychosocial reasons is unable. Lastly, the patient's previous experiences with practitioners may have been so hierarchical and paternalistic that the thought of disagreeing or negotiating a position with a practitioner does not come to mind, even when the suggested approach is not acceptable.

PSYCHOLOGICAL MECHANISMS

Passive-aggressive behavior is used by persons who do not feel capable of asserting themselves directly. They become skilled in positioning themselves so that others feel they want to—or must—save them. The practitioner's attempt to solve the problem is invariably followed by the patient's frustrating failure to collaborate. The patient successfully transfers responsibly for his or her problem to the practitioner and then rejects each solution offered. Continued failure results in repeated visits, offering the patient continuing attention and increasing the practitioner's frustration.

Other patients who are unable to offer an opinion may have been emotionally, verbally, or physically abused earlier in life or may have had family or other personal experiences that taught unquestioning submission to authority.

Most people who enter the healing professions have a desire, even a need, to be helpful. Passive-aggressive patients' solicitations for practitioners to save them can be extremely seductive, luring practitioners into believing that these patients will singularly benefit from their expertise. The extent to which practitioners use a patient's recovery to validate their competence or professional value may determine how frustrated and angry they will become when treatment is unsuccessful. Rather than focusing initially on outcomes, the physician is better served by answering the following questions: "Am I encouraging patients to take a more active role in their care?" and "Am I giving patients the chance to say why they're not using the treatments on which I thought we agreed?"

Management

In working with individuals who are interested in having their practitioner take responsibility for solving their health problems, it is important to communicate clearly that only the patient can solve his or her problems. To help differentiate patients who are dependent and unable to carry out plans from those with a definable personality disorder, the physician can confront the patient and offer, "I'm frustrated with how things are going. Let's start again and see if what I see as a problem is really a problem for you."

Treatment is dependent on agreeing on the diagnosis or the problem. If there is disagreement, questions such as "What do you think the problem is?" or "What do you think should be done?" should be asked explicitly. If agreement is not reached, practitioner and patient must work to resolve the conflict.

If the patient agrees with the problem statement, the next step is to ask what he or she thinks would be helpful in solving the problem. Again, to distinguish patients who are unable to collaborate successfully from those who have a personality disorder, one can ask, "Do you think you can really do this?" If the question is asked in a supportive fashion, many patients who initially agreed to an unrealistic plan (perhaps to please the practitioner) respond more honestly, acknowledging that they are unable to fully adhere to the plan. If asked respectfully, they generally share their reasons. Once patients have honestly shared their opinion regarding evaluation and/or treatment, the practitioner can encourage collaboration by saying, "Let's explore what we *can* do to solve this problem together. It will certainly help if you tell me what's possible for you and what's not." The approach to patients with personality disorders, which is beyond the scope of this chapter, is covered in Chapter 24.

If the patient displays passive-aggressive behavior, the practitioner can seek agreement on the nature of the problem and then make very specific contracts for what the patient will do. They can be as simple as "So, until our next visit, you will remain abstinent from alcohol," or "Between now and our next visit, you'll keep a diary and record when, and under what conditions, your headaches occur." The physician's support and enthusiasm can be directly tied to the degree to which both parties carry out the requirements of the contract. In this way, the physician can promote the patient's autonomy and offer support, without taking full responsibility for the patient's behavior. Over time, patients learn to respond to the support offered and begin to take a more active role in their care. Of course, there is always the risk that a passive-aggressive individual attempting to control the relationship will choose to seek another practitioner who can be more easily manipulated.

Patient Education

Patients who are unfamiliar with a collaborative model can be given specific information about the practitioner's understanding and particular style of collaborating. Explicit requests for patients' opinions about doctor–patient collaboration can be extremely useful. Over time, given the opportunity to state opinions and formulate plans, most individuals find such an approach satisfying, engaging, and motivating. Indeed, there is convincing evidence that patients taught to be more assertive improve their health outcomes, such as lowering blood pressure and controlling diabetes.

Educating patients who exhibit passive-aggressive behavior about such behavior can begin a process of introspection and self-awareness. Encouraging individuals to explore the origins of these behaviors and consider a therapeutic relationship that facilitates the process can be rewarding for both patient and practitioner. Descriptions of behavior that hit home can provoke emotional responses in patients, but penetrating long-held psychological defenses can spur growth. The physician might say, for example, "You say your mother was overbearing and controlling and withheld praise. Isn't that what your children are telling you?" In most instances, the benefits outweigh the risks.

CASE ILLUSTRATION 4 (CONT.)

The doctor leans forward and says, "Mrs. M., your actions tell me I'm pushing you to do something you don't want to do. I'm concerned about your weight—what are your thoughts on this?" Mrs. M.'s eyes moisten and she responds, "I want to lose weight, but I can't do it. I've tried for years, and it's so frustrating." The doctor nods and says, "Let's hold off on the weight control for now. How about taking one thing at a time and focusing on your blood pressure?"

Mrs. M. agrees to take her medication and to return for a blood pressure check in 2 weeks. The doctor gives her a card so that she can record her own blood pressure when she checks it at the drug store or the mall.

Summary

Setting limits and providing explicit feedback can teach patients to collaborate more effectively in their own care. Being aware of "yes-but" patterns can help the practitioner initiate a strategy to develop shared responsibility, preventing the ultimately unhelpful rescuing behaviors that leave all parties frustrated and dissatisfied and interfere with successful treatment.

INDICATIONS FOR REFERRAL

Indications for referral of individuals with whom interactions are difficult include the practitioner's inability to make a diagnosis, negative personal feelings that create a barrier to a therapeutic relationship, an objective assessment that the patient is not benefiting from evaluation or treatment, or the practitioner's feeling of being threatened or in danger.

With particular reference to a practitioner's negative feelings, when an inability to work together significantly impairs the provision of effective care, outside assistance and advice are required. Interestingly, because negative feelings often relate to a practitioner's previous family and life experiences, a patient who is difficult for one physician is often not difficult for another.

Once the decision to refer is made, framing the referral in a positive way is particularly valuable. One strategy is to acknowledge the need for assistance in managing difficult situations or problems. The dialogue might take the following form:

Doctor: Mrs. S., for the last 2 months I've been trying to figure out how to make your headaches better. I think it would help us if you could be evaluated by a psychologist; we might be able to get a better handle on what else we could do to deal with the problems.

Mrs. S.: Are you saying that I'm imagining this? Do you think it's all in my head?

Doctor: No, not at all. But nothing we've tried has stopped your headaches. It often helps me to have another person listen to the story and maybe find a new direction to take. Dr. F. has helped me with a number of people in the past, and I'm hopeful she can help us here as well.

Mrs. S.: What do I have to do? I really do want these headaches to end.

Doctor: Great. In addition to the referral, I'll schedule you for two visits with me over the next 12 weeks to see how things are going and help answer any questions you or Dr. F. may have.

Proposing a positive outcome from the referral can be remarkably useful. In addition, scheduling a visit for the person to return after the referral reassures the patient that the referring physician is truly seeking assistance rather than simply "dumping" the problem on someone else.

Learning to understand the person's perspective, negotiating for realistic plans of evaluation and treatment, and being aware of and responsive to verbal and nonverbal evidence that a recommendation was misunderstood or rejected create a collaboration that can be remarkably satisfying for both participants.

Underused skills such as soliciting the patient's attribution for a problem, offering praise and support, listening carefully to the patient's description of a problem, and explicitly confronting problematic or confusing behavior inform the patient that a serious attempt is underway to understand and work with the patient's concerns.

By exploring their own expectations and feelings, practitioners become more self-aware and recognize who else is in the room. Clearly, to the extent practitioners improve their self-awareness and learn to confront their feelings, their effectiveness as physicians will improve.

SUGGESTED READINGS

Beckman HB et al: The doctor-patient relationship and malpractice: lessons from plaintiff depositions. Arch Intern Med 1994;154:1365.

Lazare A: Shame and humiliation in the medical encounter. Arch Intern Med 1987;147:1653.

Levinson W, Gorawara-Bhat R, Lamb J: A study of patient clues and physician responses in primary care and surgical settings. JAMA 2000;284:1021.

Quill TE: Partnerships in patient care: a contractual approach. Ann Intern Med 1983;98:228.

Suchman AL et al: A model of empathic communication in the medical interview. JAMA 1997;277:678.

WEB SITE

Bayer Institute for Healthcare Communication:
www.bayerinstitute.org

Sexual Issues and Professional Development: A Challenge for Medical Education

5

Richard M. Frankel, PhD, Sarah Williams, MD, & Elizabeth A. Edwardsen, MD

INTRODUCTION

Sexuality and sexual feelings are omnipresent parts of life that do not disappear when individuals become doctors, nurses, or therapists, or when professionals interact with patients or colleagues. Despite the importance and complexity of this aspect of medicine, most health care professionals enter practice quite unprepared to deal with these sexual issues.

Professional education and clinical practice address many aspects of human existence such as health, illness, dying, and death. At the same time, each professional is independently and collectively striving to achieve personal goals, often with deep-seated desires and dreams. Searching for the meaning of life, professionally and personally, and clarifying core values and priorities often intensify the medical experience. Not unexpectedly, intense emotions and issues of sexuality and intimacy arise and continue to be present over the course of one's career. Medical education, including continuing education, needs to address these issues directly so that meaningful guidance can be offered.

HISTORICAL PERSPECTIVE

Ethical codes of conduct for physicians have existed for thousands of years. In the modern era, the doctor–patient relationship has been viewed as a type of contract, with both legal and ethical standards against which behavior may be judged. Ethical standards of behavior based on contract are an important and much-discussed aspect of providing medical care. Less well described is the relational basis of appropriate behavior and the personal consequences that ensue when relational boundaries between physicians and patients are crossed. Such a description is particularly important for physicians who must balance legal and ethical concerns with caring and compassion.

A DEFINITIONAL FRAMEWORK

Sexuality

Defined narrowly, sexuality means engaging in sexual activity with another person. Sexuality of this sort has been widely discussed and is generally considered to be inappropriate in the medical workplace. As such, this aspect of sexuality will not be further explored in this chapter. There has been far less discussion, however, of a more comprehensive understanding of sexuality. This broader definition includes thoughts and feelings about sex that are part of a physician's daily work life; sexuality as a part of an individual's identity, the desire and capacity for intimacy; and sexuality as an integral part of an individual's physical and emotional vitality.

Relationship Boundaries

The concepts of personal and relationship boundaries are pivotal to discussions of sexuality and intimacy. One useful definition of relationship boundaries has been offered by Peterson: "the limits that allow for safe connection based on the client's needs. When these limits are altered, what is allowed in the relationship becomes ambiguous. Such ambiguity is often experienced as an intrusion into the sphere of safety." The narratives reported here describe a range of ambiguities, from boundary confusion to boundary crossing and violation, and their impact on patient care and relationships.

Boundary confusion occurs when one (or more) element of the doctor–patient relationship becomes ambiguous. The physician or patient becomes aware of ambiguous feelings about sexual issues in the relationship. The majority of our case examples are of this nature, involving situations in which the physician becomes aware that something about a patient or an encounter is different or unusual in terms of sexuality.

Boundary crossings occur when physicians or patients begin acting upon their ambiguous feelings. The physician–patient relationship appears to have become increasingly sexualized, but nothing explicit has been said or done. As each person's perceptions become clouded by his or her own desires and fears, it becomes increasingly difficult to "read" the other's behavior or understand its meaning.

Boundary violations occur as the sexual dimension of a doctor–patient relationship becomes more explicit, understood, and acted upon. Gutheil and Gabbard suggest that sexual misconduct, the most serious form of boundary violation, usually begins with relatively minor boundary crossings that "often show a crescendo pattern of increasing intrusion into the patient's space that culminates in sexual contact. A direct shift from talking to intercourse is quite rare." Peterson suggests that "In every story of a (boundary) violation . . . four motifs surface: 1) a reversal of roles (the patient takes care of the doctor), 2) a secret (shared intimate feelings), 3) a double bind (it is impossible to stay in or get out of the relationship), and 4) an indulgence in professional privilege (the doctor prevails upon the patient to meet a personal need)."

The actions defined above describe a stepwise sequence of increasingly risk-laden behaviors that can seriously impair both the relational and legal nature of the doctor–patient covenant. Conceivably, recognition of boundary confusion and subsequent intervention could help prevent progression to boundary crossing and violation. This may require that power structures and limitations of the medical system be addressed. Of note, sexual harassment is reported to be fairly common in medical settings, particularly in training.

METHODS & MATERIALS

For 3 years (1991, 1993, 1994), a small group workshop, "Sexual Issues in the Workplace," was conducted by two of the authors (R. Frankel and S. Williams) in which sexuality and professionalism issues were explored with practicing physicians, faculty, and trainees. To date, the workshops' participants have numbered 100, mostly internists and family physicians at various levels of training, and a small number of other health professionals.

The workshop design permitted narrative data to be collected for research purposes. At the very beginning of the workshops, participants were invited "to write a five-minute narrative about sexual issues in the workplace." At the conclusion of the workshop, the "uncontaminated" written narratives were requested on a strictly voluntary basis to become part of an ongoing research database. Of the 100 participants who attended the workshops, 73 (73%) volunteered their stories for inclusion in the research database that forms the basis for this analysis. No information is available about those participants who chose not to include their narratives in the database.

Once the written narratives were completed, participants were divided into small groups, and those who were willing shared and discussed their stories. At the conclusion of the workshop, the groups came together for a discussion of the workshop experience and to plan "next steps" in teaching and learning about sexual issues in the workplace.

The stories that were collected from each workshop session were transcribed and coded by date and participants' level of training. The narratives were then added to the database. Between 1991 and 1995, data were collected from three Society of General Internal Medicine (SGIM) National Meetings (1991, 1993, and 1994), three groups of Family Medicine and Internal Medicine Fellows at the University of Rochester, and four groups of residents and medical students at New York University and the University of Rochester.

Once collated, the entire set of narratives was reviewed independently by members of the research team to identify common themes. An iterative approach was used in which the independent judgments about common themes were compared, differences were noted, and attempts to reach consensus followed. Using this process, agreement was eventually reached on the classification of all the narratives. Although this method does not ensure statistical validity, it does follow a well-recognized set of procedures for ensuring the trustworthiness of qualitative narrative data.

ANALYSIS OF NARRATIVE THEMES

Ambiguity

The most frequently mentioned theme in the narratives was ambiguity involving sexuality and the heightened tension and confusion that ambiguity caused in personal and professional roles. In the following example, the sexual nature of a patient's presentation produced mixed (ambiguous) feelings of discomfort and enjoyment. Despite recognizing the ambiguity, the provider reports that he was either unwilling or unable to redirect or clarify the nature of the relationship:

 CASE ILLUSTRATION 1

One of my patients, a young attractive buxom blonde woman has been incredibly suggestive toward me. . . . I have actually only seen her in the office a few times, but each time she comes in with low-cut outfits that cling to her body. She speaks in a soft, seductive voice and makes completely inappropriate suggestions like: "Can't we go some place and be alone?" or "I've always wanted to be a doctor; can you show me how to do it? You can't

blame a girl for trying." I always tell her no, but I haven't really clamped down and confronted her with how inappropriate this is and how uncomfortable this makes me. The problem is that I kind of enjoy it.

Another physician describes her awareness of sexual ambiguity in her relationship with a male patient, the role confusion it caused, and her lack of a clarifying response, presumably for fear of insulting or angering the patient and losing companionship:

CASE ILLUSTRATION 2

I had a 65-year-old male patient who was wonderful to take care of. He was funny, charming, and had led an interesting life. He was also alone—I couldn't imagine why. I enjoyed spending a few minutes after dealing with the complaint talking with him. Usually, he left with a warm handshake. One Christmas he hugged me, and that was fine. Come the New Year, he kept hugging me when he left the office— no more handshakes. I was confused. I was attracted to him but not intensely. I also loved his company. I just wasn't convinced these hugs were appropriate, but I did nothing, afraid of confronting him.

Connectedness

For some, sexuality and "connectedness" or energy at work were related. The presence or, more characteristically, the absence of sexual feelings at work was found to be related to work satisfaction and broader questions of identity. One participant writes:

CASE ILLUSTRATION 3

This year I lost the joy of living for a time. I know myself by this quality—it is the core of me to wake up excited about a new day or know that it could be [exciting]. It had to do with feeling paralyzed to change. The work is incredibly important to me as are the people with whom I've connected in the process, and so even the thought of leaving stopped me cold and stopped me inside—including sexually. I didn't desire or hope. Ultimately, I felt that no work,

no matter how "meaningful," is more important than the capacity to hope, to feel joy, and to feel sexual and alive, and [so] I have left the job that I was in.

Identity

Another participant describes the experience of losing her identity as a sexual woman, which she identified as necessary to feel energy and enthusiasm for work:

CASE ILLUSTRATION 4

For the first time in my life since I was a teenager, I am without a sexual partner. . . . Now, with my husband gone, I find I am very visible as a person, but invisible as a woman. Somewhere I crossed the line from desirable to undesirable. Maybe not that, maybe just "not considered." All my colleagues are much younger. I'm currently cut off from what I'd always thought would be mine—my femaleness!

Intensity and Physical Intimacy

Sexuality in medical training often goes unaddressed. Learning to be a doctor involves intense contacts and physical intimacy that can heighten sexual feelings and tensions. The setting becomes so routine for practicing professionals and teachers that its impact on trainees may be overlooked. One participant, a clinical teacher, describes an experience that brought this issue vividly to consciousness:

CASE ILLUSTRATION 5

I was precepting two male medical students. They were sitting in with me while I saw a young female patient. . . . I wanted to examine her spleen, which had been enlarged. One of the students couldn't "appreciate" the spleen so I took his hand and placed it over the splenic area and we spent a few seconds in this position. Then we stepped out in the hallway to "discuss the case." Within a second the med student was swaying and then dropped to the floor, hitting his head . . . he had fainted! I was so frightened and impressed by the enormity of what happened and with how intimate the physical examination is . . . and how little we acknowledge the sexual issue. . . .

The residency training years also present a variety of situations that can intensify issues of sexuality. Working long hours, associating with peers in all aspects of daily living (work, meals, sleep), and sharing call rooms inevitably create compromising situations. One participant writes about his internship year:

CASE ILLUSTRATION 6

I was sitting with my resident in a call room at 2:00 A.M. Another resident entered for a second to say that she was going to the emergency room to do a pelvic exam. She jokingly said she was going to "tickle the vagina" of this patient, then she left (leaving me, a single male, with my female resident). My resident then looked over at me and said, "Gosh, I wish someone would tickle my vagina . . . that hasn't happened in so long." I chuckled, wondering if this was a solicitation/proposal or what? Since we were all alone in a room with a bed, I excused myself to go get some coffee.

The intern maintained the relationship within professional boundaries by finding a way to diplomatically terminate a sexually charged encounter.

In the following story, a female physician describes how a relationship, fueled by the emotional needs of both members, slowly progressed beyond the boundaries of resident comraderie:

CASE ILLUSTRATION 7

It was March of my junior residency year. I was running the ward team—height of power in my program. The team was "tight" . . . we spent from 7:30 A.M. to 11:00 P.M. on the wards, in our back room, eating takeout food at night, running codes together, and laughing.

She then goes on to describe the close relationship that developed between herself and the intern who eventually disclosed that she was gay and had never had a romantic relationship:

CASE ILLUSTRATION 7 (CONT.)

We immediately developed an intense bond with an intense edge and secrecy not unlike that of a new romantic relationship. She came over to my apartment, as I was still playing the role of a confidant/resident/ therapist. We talked into the early morning and at one point I held her and she cried. She declared her love for me.

The unexpectedly rapid and intense escalation from boundary confusion to boundary crossing described in this story was very surprising and frightening to the storyteller, and caused her to abruptly sever the relationship by avoidance of her intern. The cut-off in this relationship parallels the relationship break that may occur in patient care, as will be seen in the subsequent doctor–patient case illustrations. This disruption in a relationship is a common outcome of boundary confusion.

Developmental Experiences

Developmental experiences of physicians can have an impact on workplace sexual issues. How individuals handle the sexual tensions of collegial and provider–patient relations is often influenced by their personal history, including developmental issues, past sexual experiences, and sexual attitudes and beliefs. In the following narrative, one participant describes her struggle to define the role of sexuality in her work life:

CASE ILLUSTRATION 8

When I was younger, I was a very seductive person and I had a lot of sexually charged interactions with colleagues and teachers. In some ways I valued these because I felt—especially during medical school and training—that they humanized what was otherwise an incredibly repressed and interpersonally barren environment. At the same time, I think my abilities to be seductive were bad for me because they reflected and reinforced my sense that they were the only valuable part of me. As I began to change and feel more self-confident about other parts of me, I began to see my sexuality as a bad thing and to feel ashamed about it. As a result I began to keep this aspect of myself totally out of my workplace self. After a while, I realized that this sort of "repression" was making me feel bad about my sexuality in general, and also it took away an important part of my pleasure and energy at work. So, more recently my struggle has been to let these feelings back into my sense of myself, including my professional self. I have also realized that I really like feeling sexy and feeling sexual attractions, but at the same time, the nice part now is that I don't feel any pressure to act on those feelings.

The cold, often unfeeling, reality of the work environment was a form of repression that negatively impacted on the performance and feelings of this physician.

Another participant, a medical educator, describes how an adolescent experience of being sexually molested by a teacher "sensitized" him to the importance of these issues for his residents and motivated him to discuss sexuality and professionalism in the workplace.

 CASE ILLUSTRATION 9

When I was in the ninth grade, I was invited by a popular science teacher on an overnight camping trip. It was just the two of us and when I woke up in the morning, I found his hand on my penis trying to arouse me. I told him to take his hands off me and to drive me home, which he did, but I never said anything to my parents, friends, or the school authorities. I was too embarrassed and ashamed. Five years later at a reunion of some high school friends the subject of this science teacher came up and it turned out that all of us had the same experience and that none of us had done or said anything to bring the situation to light. It has now been 32 years since my victimization and I have a wonderful 5-year-old son. It troubles me that in my own silence, I may inadvertently be making him more vulnerable to being victimized as I was. As a result of this experience I take an active interest and role in working with medical students and residents around issues of sexuality, professionalism, and the workplace.

A female resident describes the effects of early "boundary violations" on her professional life and her approach to the work environment:

 CASE ILLUSTRATION 10

I feared being physically violated by my stepfather, and was so fiercely determined to keep this from happening that it affected the way I present myself to the world. Only once did he come close: I was wrapped in a towel after bathing and he was "showing" me how to rub alcohol on my chest above my towel. At that time I thought, "I just dare you to do something, I'll finally have real evidence against you and get you thrown out of here." He did not pursue to active violation, although I was scared, angry, and determined. As a result I . . . go to what might be extremes (ie, rarely wear skirts) to avoid appearing vulnerable. I've taken karate to . . . marshall my sense of confidence to "potential" violators. . . . I attribute the fact that I have no memorable encounters of inappropriateness with patients to the fact that I give no room for these things to happen.

Awareness

When boundary confusion occurs, the provider often masks his or her awareness of its effect. A male resident describes the effect taking a sexual history had on him:

 CASE ILLUSTRATION 11

I was working at the adolescent clinic where I had been told that it was my obligation to talk about sex with my patients. There was this young, attractive black teenager who came to see me and the discussion got very detailed and explicit about sexual positions and arousal and things. And I couldn't help it. I was trying to be very professional about my questions but the more she talked, the more aroused I felt myself become. It was embarrassing sitting there with an erection, but I just couldn't help it.

Note that despite having an erection and feeling embarrassed (confused) the physician inappropriately continued to elicit additional sexual history from the patient. Had he had more skill training in dealing with these issues, he might have been able to redirect the interview more effectively.

Some boundary crossings are brief, episodic, and unilateral as the following case illustrates:

CASE ILLUSTRATION 12

I recall an elderly gentleman who was homeless and indigent that I saw in the emergency room as a medical student. After he received his care, he asked if he could have a kiss and pulled me down to kiss me (not sexual, but more intimate than I wanted to be with this patient).

In some cases, boundary confusion around sexual issues may create enough tension to have a negative impact on patient care. Uncomfortable situations may inhibit or prevent a physician from providing appropriate care as the following case illustrates:

CASE ILLUSTRATION 13

I was working in the emergency room and here comes an attractive 20- to 21-year-old lady with a complaint of severe abdominal pain. She has a history of pancreatitis in the past, and I know that I have to do a pelvic/rectal on her in order to be complete and not to miss any other etiologies for her abdominal pain. But I opted not to, hoping that her amylase and lipase would come back positive so I wouldn't have to do them.

Progression to Termination of Relationship

Generally, the boundary crossings described in our case illustrations developed over time and followed a certain developmental trajectory in which both the physician and patient (and sometimes the staff) are aware that something more than the normal doctor–patient relationship is emerging. Characteristic in these illustrations is an abrupt "cut-off" of the relationship at the point at which a suggestion (such as having sex) would move the relationship from a boundary crossing to a violation of the physician's ethical code. One participant described it this way:

CASE ILLUSTRATION 14

A young, attractive woman presented to the emergency room for evaluation of asthma. After initial treatment by me, she was given an appointment for follow-up in my General Medicine Clinic. Over the course of the next several months, she presented to clinic unexpectedly several times with complaints of breast problems and genitourinary symptoms, requesting breast and pelvic exams. During the course of these she regularly made seductive comments. These episodes progressed to the point of frequent calls to me during office and nonoffice hours. I obviously enjoyed the encounters—yet when, finally, I was explicitly solicited, I declined sexual participation, after which the patient was never heard from.

In the next case illustration, a physician describes his growing awareness of his own attraction to a female patient, his position of power, his inability to change his course of action, and his perception or assumption of reciprocation on her part. At the point at which the physician brings explicit attention to the sexual dimension of their relationship, the patient responds with anger and terminates the relationship. Was it the resident's fantasies and interpretation of the patient's behavior that characterized their relationship or mutual sexual attractions?

CASE ILLUSTRATION 15

There was a patient that I saw recently. She's 19 and came in with complaints of irregular periods, wanting a pregnancy test and pelvic exam. I went ahead and did a pelvic exam. . . . I did a thorough exam, but maybe I was a little too thorough. Sometimes I don't do a breast exam when I do a pelvic exam, but in this case I did and it was extra thorough. And I thought to myself, am I toying with this patient because she was kind of . . . very flirtatious and I knew I had this position of power and I was kind of struggling with that in the long run, but I didn't resolve it. I didn't step outside and try to collect my thoughts and stuff. It made me feel really clouded, you know.

I gave her my card and told her to call me at my regular clinic . . . and she's been here twice and she made several phone calls. And initially I was kind of friendly, you know, maybe a little too friendly. You know there was probably some mutual flirtation going on here. . . . She came to me another time for a rash. When I asked her to show me the rash, she took off her sweatshirt and jeans and underneath it all she was wearing this sexy "teddy." Well, the next time she came back, about a week later, she had a different "teddy" on and I said in a flippant sort of way, "That's an interesting way of dressing to come to see the doctor." Well, she got really angry and basically walked out of my clinic and hasn't been back since. I know I wasn't completely blameless in this situation, but still I was surprised that she got so angry and never came back.

These kinds of situations, which were common in residents' stories, show how interpersonal confusion and lack of self-awareness prevent physicians from effectively reading and dealing with patients' behavior. The therapeutic relationship was often the casualty, and abrupt termination of the relationship was a frequent outcome.

Relationships with Colleagues

Sexual tensions/relationships between colleagues, rather than patients, become more prominent as medical careers advance. In workshop sessions with residents and students, stories of boundary issues tended to focus on patients and the sexual tensions surrounding the care delivery process. In sessions with more senior physicians, stories were increasingly likely to address sexual attractions and relationships between colleagues. Several of these stories focused on sexual needs outside of work affecting relationships in the workplace. The following narrative is illustrative:

CASE ILLUSTRATION 16

While in a prior relationship, I had sexual feelings for a couple of women with whom I worked, which I proceeded to act upon. In neither case did I feel guilty. In both cases, everyone involved was under a lot of stress and seeking outside comfort. In both cases, the relationships ended amicably and at mutually agreeable times. Subsequently, my primary relationship dissolved and it was clear that the relationship had been lacking sufficient sensuality and sexuality, among other problems, which led to my acting upon these prior feelings.

Another story conveys the intensity of sexual feeling that can arise between colleagues. Note that the physicians

involved were away from their normal work routine, a situation that often creates boundary confusion.

CASE ILLUSTRATION 17

I was taking a trip—with my new boss. We were there to attend some meetings but mostly to write a grant that was due shortly after we got back. I know I was attracted to him and hadn't thought about the feelings being reciprocated until we were on our way to a show and I realized he had his arm around me the way boys used to do when I'd go out on a date as a teenager. When we walked up to join a group of people he knew, he quickly jerked his arm away. I was surprised and amazed. Later when we each went back to our respective hotel rooms which happened to be next door, fantasies kept crowding into my concentrated efforts to write a portion of the grant. I did a lot of yoga just to cool down, but recognized that if he had made a move, I would have said yes willingly and lived with the negative consequences for my marriage later. He never asked.

Although the preceding incident occurred between a faculty member and her boss, the power differential between them does not seem to have played much of a role. Often, however, when boundary crossings occur between people of unequal power, the consequences are intensified and potentially more dangerous.

Power Differences

Power differences can be explicit, as in the formal hierarchies of medical teaching institutions, or implicit, based on differences in age, gender, social status, access to knowledge, resources, and the like. The doctor–patient relationship and the teacher–learner relationship are often good examples of an implicit power differential. Adult learner–teacher relationships can involve formal or informal power relationships, depending on the situation. (For a more extended discussion of this point, see Gordon, Labby, and Levinson, 1992.) The following story, written by a female attending physician, describes the complex interaction of sexuality in a semiformal teacher–learner relationship:

CASE ILLUSTRATION 18

Several years ago at a seminar, I had a facilitator with whom I had very charged interactions. . . . I saw us as being very similar in style and personality; we were both somewhat dramatic, a bit flamboyant and flirtatious, and expressive about our reactions and feelings. Initially, the experience was positive and added energy to the process; but as the week wore on, we began to clash and irritate one another. . . . Ultimately, he, in front of the group in which we both participated, accused me of being seductive and "sucking him up." I felt shamed, humiliated, and angry. Some time later, we discussed the incident and he apologized. Our relationship remains amicable but still strained when we've interacted since in various professional ways and subsequent courses.

Note the similarity of this type of collegial relationship based on an asymmetry of power to boundary confusions in the doctor–patient relationship in which the provider denies any role in encouraging, or at least not discouraging, increasing sexual tension in the relationship.

Narratives of sexual harassment were rarely reported in our sessions. The only sexual harassment story reported in our data illustrates how power in an academic medical hierarchy allowed a department chairman to devastate a junior faculty member personally and professionally:

CASE ILLUSTRATION 19

First job out of residency, at a teaching hospital. My direct supervisor was also the chairperson of the department. He began keeping me late after hours to discuss new directions in the department, which he wanted me to be involved in. Then, it was multiple phone calls to my office almost every day for after-hours dinners, which I refused for 3 months. Day after day, he still would call. I explained that I would meet him over lunch to discuss pertinent issues, but he refused these counteroffers. He began to "question my loyalty to the department." He spontaneously began to relate stories of his past career— talking without bridges to inappropriate issues, eg, how he could sky-write with his penis. He next wanted me to join him in coffee houses to meet Friday to Sunday every week to do intensive "group" work. When I refused all these advances he began to write memos of my "uncooperativeness." I felt forced out of the workplace by his threats to fire me.

Shame and Humiliation

The following narrative illustrates the extent to which lack of sexual awareness and sensitivity on the provider's part can cause shame and humiliation in the patient.

CASE ILLUSTRATION 20

The only really uncomfortable experience I had was a rectal exam I did on a young man about 17 or 18. . . I was just going through my list, it was very mechanical. And I told him what I was going to do and he went, "Oh, wow!" And it just didn't click, you know. I just should have backed off and instead I just said, "Okay, well just go ahead, bend over and we'll get this done." And afterward, just the look on his face of horror and embarrassment and humiliation and tears almost in his eyes just made me feel awful. And he just said, "I don't believe you did that." He left and I thought that probably was not the best thing I could have done. I felt really bad after that.

Similarly, as one participant's narrative illustrates, feelings of shame or public humiliation can occur when professional boundaries are breached:

CASE ILLUSTRATION 21

I was a third year medical student on a surgery rotation scrubbed in the operating room. My resident came up behind me and reached around my waist and untied my scrub pants. Because I could not leave the sterile field I stood holding my pants with my elbows until a nurse took pity on me and helped me out—I was very humiliated.

Finally, shame and embarrassment may accompany encounters in which cultural differences in values and orientations exist. The narratives that touch on this theme include one from a Pakistani physician who describes the embarrassment of being kissed and hugged by a nurse. Although the behavior described would seem innocuous in an American or western context, it caused significant embarrassment for the resident in whose cultural context such behavior is considered highly inappropriate:

CASE ILLUSTRATION 22

While working as a pharmacy intern in a hospital pharmacy, a nurse called from the intensive care unit (ICU) for some medication for a patient. I collected the medication and ran to the ICU and she became maybe so excited or happy about my prompt action that she gave me a big hug and kiss on the cheek. I turned very red and nervous. It was kind of a culture shock to me, and I felt very embarrassed with that particular nurse for at least 1 week.

Integrating Principles of Awareness, Acceptance, Separation of Feelings and Actions

The following story eloquently embodies the basic principles of dealing with sexual tensions (and many other emotionally laden issues) in the doctor–patient relationship: being aware of one's feelings and accepting them, distinguishing one's own feelings or needs from the patient's, and separating feelings from actions to permit completion of a therapeutic history and physical and treatment plan.

CASE ILLUSTRATION 23

Some years ago, as a Fellow, I had a patient referred to me by another patient. She was my age, stunningly dressed, with all the physical characteristics I have found to be beautiful. I was unmarried and, at the time, searching for a mate. When I met her in my office, there was an unforgettable moment of heightened tension. She was the paradigm of physical beauty to me. I was the doctor who her closest friend had spoken so highly of. I wondered if I could get through the session while maintaining my professionalism—and—without compromising my ability to care for this person.

My questions were the same ones I ask every new patient. They included inquiries about education, work, professional aspirations, significant relationships, principal stressors, past use of or desire for professional counseling . . . and what one does for fun. As my questions were asked, her attraction for me seemed to meet my initial attraction for her. Fortunately, in yet another fateful moment, I realized that this was a terribly sad, lonely, needy, albeit beautiful, woman. She needed counseling more than a boyfriend. The last thing she needed was an intimate

relationship with her new doctor. My composure regained, I sighed a sigh of relief and mustered enough courage to proceed with the physical exam.

DISCUSSION

Clearly, the sample of narratives reported here is not representative of all physicians or other caregivers, nor are the numbers sufficient for any statistical analysis. Rather, these stories are a rich source of qualitative data that can be used to begin to examine the intriguing, relatively unexplored territory of sexuality and professionalism and suggest guidelines for increasing awareness and education.

Clinical care is often intensely intimate as patients share their innermost feelings, fears, and secrets. It is generally assumed and taught that most of the needs and vulnerabilities expressed in clinical interactions are the patient's. This inequality of power and vulnerability is an important issue when sexual relationships develop between patient and doctor. It is apparent from the stories we analyzed that physician vulnerabilities and needs frequently come into play when sexual issues arise. Such needs reflect the physician's own personal and developmental history and are shaped, as well, by educational and institutional policies, commitments, and values.

Caregivers' own developmental experiences (conscious and unconscious) with issues such as dependency, aggression, sexuality, self-esteem, and autonomy can have an impact on professional conduct and attitudes. For example, deLahunta and Tulsky found that 12% of responding faculty and medical students at one university reported a personal history of sexual abuse (6% as children, 7% as adults). Of note, several of the study participants acknowledged that they had never been in an intimate relationship in their lifetime. In a recent study of residents, 73% of the responding women and 22% of the men reported being sexually harassed at least once during their training. Another study revealed that 39% of female and 25% of male residents reported sexual harassment directed at them, with 75% of the residents reporting that the harassment was initiated by a faculty member. In yet another study of first year postgraduates, 36% of residents reported experiencing sexual harassment or discrimination. Finally, a survey of 1480 residents in 1991 revealed that 65% of female and 9.6% of male respondents reported having been subject to sexual harassment.

The effect of these types of experiences on professional development and conduct is currently unknown and deserves further study. Given the evidence that early developmental experiences shape adult behavior patterns, we would expect that a similar pattern would be obtained in professional development. Whatever the case may be, understanding and mastering the distinction between feelings and actions and sparing patients from assault and abandonment are important factors in maintaining healthy professional relationships and reducing negative influences of personal history. Working toward continuous self-awareness is also important.

Many training programs outside of medicine have incorporated material on sexuality into their curricula and initiated efforts to overcome the separation of sex-related content from other course content. However, when nurses' practices related to sexuality were examined using the Survey on Sexuality in Nursing Practice (SSNP), only 12% addressed sexuality with a majority of their clients even though the nurse/subjects consistently identified sexuality as a necessary part of nursing practice. In *Nursing Clinics of North America,* Schuster describes how Life Enrichment Opportunities, Inc. was created to fill a need and correct a deficiency of individuals and organizations prepared to serve as sex educators, consultants, counselors, or therapists. Within medicine, the results are much the same. A questionnaire distributed to 1128 residents entering the field of obstetrics and gynecology throughout the United States showed that a large majority desired greater understanding of sexuality.

Each doctor–patient relationship must develop its own appropriate boundaries, which may be difficult. When, for example, is a caring hand on a patient's shoulder a welcome gesture of comfort, and when is it an unappreciated boundary crossing? Based on the complexities and variety of the interpersonal skills of the physician, the needs of the patient and the realities of the clinical environment, each clinical encounter may have a different approach. Hopefully, medical education can address proper assessment and negotiation of the doctor–patient relationship to be therapeutic.

From the stories we analyzed, it is apparent that sexual feelings and conflicts inform many aspects of providers' interactions with patients and colleagues. When these issues are recognized and accepted (and worked through as needed), they need not be harmful and may in fact enhance work satisfaction and effectiveness. On the other hand, when providers are uncomfortable with their sexual feelings or conflicts and try to avoid or ignore them, negative consequences for patient care, and perhaps for the providers themselves, are much more likely. Some specific negative consequences include the following:

- *Avoidance of the patient generally or not performing important services* such as asking about sexual risk behaviors and/or not providing appropriate counseling to minimize sexual risk. This is an especially egregious omission in an age of widespread human immunodeficiency virus (HIV) infection.
- *Not performing indicated examinations,* particularly genital, breast, and rectal examinations, due to embarrassment or avoidance.

- *Inability to effectively manage patients' sexual advances or sexual attraction between doctor and patient.* As many of the case illustrations reveal, this leads to tensions and confusion in the encounter, preventing the development of an appropriate, therapeutic doctor–patient relationship, and may cause the patient to terminate care prematurely.
- *Increased risk of boundary confusion or violation.* Intense emotions (sexual or otherwise) are much more likely to distort our perceptions or behaviors when they are unacknowledged or ambiguous. Providers who are unaware of or feel clouded about their sexual feelings are less able to separate feelings from actions and more likely to engage in inappropriate behaviors that allow professional boundaries to become blurred. Medical education that addresses peer exploitation, harassment, humiliation, and cultural insensitivity can help to avert delayed consequences.
- *An erosion of professional satisfaction and well-being because of unresolved sexual issues.* Sexuality in its broadest sense is an integral part of personal and professional identity, energy, and engagement in work and relationships. Hence, we cannot ignore issues of sexuality without cutting off parts of our selves and our vitality.

Shame and humiliation seem to accompany a significant number of the interactions reported in participants' narratives. The fact that much of the potential for shame and humiliation appears to go unrecognized is of particular relevance. (Lazare notes that there is a high, and generally unrecognized, potential for shame and humiliation in medical encounters.) Some of these feelings may be potentiated by the nature of medical care, particularly the physical examination, and the inability of many physicians to deal with sexual issues, a tendency reinforced by years of ignoring or denying sexual feelings in medical education. Cross-cultural aspects of care are another problematical area in which increased attention and heightened awareness would be beneficial in medical education. Support groups and targeted clinical exercises can be useful in bringing to light the potential for shame and humiliation in medical encounters, as well as helping clinicians develop the requisite skills to deal with this issue appropriately.

Sexuality and sexual feelings are present in many types of workplace interactions in medicine including training, patient care, and peer relationships. The majority of narratives in this sample focused on a type of sexual issue that we have defined as "boundary confusion." The most salient feature of these cases is the awareness or perception of another's behavior (patient, supervisor, or peer) toward the doctor as being potentially sexual in nature, creating an ambiguous or "clouded" interactional field. In our data, there were many fewer examples of boundary crossings in which more explicit behavior was initiated by one or the other party, and no examples of true boundary violations in which the provider deliberately exploited a patient's vulnerability and indulged in inappropriate professional privilege.

Although this is not a representative sample, it is conceivable that the vast majority of sexual boundary issues in the medical workplace involve confusion around personal and professional identity and role, particularly for residents. Learning about appropriate personal and professional boundaries is one of the most important and challenging developmental tasks for inexperienced physicians, one that relates to all aspects of emotional involvement with patients.

Residents struggle with difficult questions such as: How close should I get to patients I like or with whom I identify? How much can I be personally affected when my patients do not do well or die? Providing information in the context of guidelines and structured instruction may assist with role development, boundary definitions, and the merging of professional and personal identities. Graduate medical education programs must also allow for personal time for physicians in training to maintain their physical and emotional health and to create a personal life separate from their professional life.

Boundary confusions and crossings in patient care that dominated resident sessions seemed less common with increasing experience. Perhaps, as physicians become more confident and comfortable with their professional identity and have opportunities for fulfilling personal lives, they project a clearer sense of boundaries. They also may have learned to relate to patients within the boundaries of a caring but professional relationship, without needing, for example, "to be the patient's friend," a typical conflict experienced by medical students.

Senior physicians' narratives focused more on relationships between colleagues. Several revealed clear parallels between physicians' personal issues regarding intimacy, loneliness, etc, and behavior at work. It is not entirely clear why collegial stories dominate among more senior physicians. Conceivably, as physicians mature, marry, and begin their own families, they focus more on peer relationships and experiences. For academic physicians, there may be less intense exposure to patients and more emphasis on interactions with colleagues. Whatever the reasons, workplace issues involving sexuality seem to correspond with different levels of training and expertise. Continuing medical education programs should reflect these differences.

The narratives reflect an apparent lack of insight by physicians as to the reasons patients may attempt to test or cross sexual boundaries in a medical encounter. It may be useful to explore with physicians (and especially with residents) a range of possible reasons that a patient "comes onto" a physician. These may include a physician's own needs and communication patterns, a patient's need to

control, and feelings of anxiety and psychiatric impairment. Again, facilitated opportunities for self-reflection and discussion are useful in improving awareness of the complex nature of these interactions.

Some physicians do acknowledge enjoying their sexually charged interactions with patients, at least initially. Others express discomfort or anxiety with patients' boundary crossings, but don't know how to set limits in an appropriately caring way. This may reflect the confusion noted earlier about caring and personal involvement. Unfortunately, there seems to be little opportunity in undergraduate medical education or residency to discuss these important issues. Little guidance is available to help physicians-in-training acquire appropriate limit-setting skills. As a consequence, students and residents often are left to their own devices in developing healthy approaches to boundary setting. In addition to preventing some physicians from eliciting pertinent clinical information and providing necessary care (as previously discussed), the lack of opportunity to discuss sexually confusing situations may have other negative effects, such as encouraging boundary crossings and violations.

Providing regular opportunities for students and residents to discuss personal feelings and role play difficult or challenging situations can help in the development of healthy approaches to sexuality in the medical workplace. In other professional training environments such as clinical psychology and psychiatry, specfic attention is paid to the issue of sexual feelings in psychotherapy that are addressed in publications sponsored by professional societies. Workshops, clinical demonstrations, case discussions, and observed interviews with "difficult" patients over time are useful in teaching limit setting. Open acknowledgment of issues of sexuality and their impact on interpersonal encounters of all kinds may lead to greater understanding, improved educational modalities, and more therapeutic doctor–patient relationships.

Encouraging healthy mentoring relationships is another opportunity to address issues of sexuality in the workplace. The classic definition of a mentoring relationship is a close, intense, mutually beneficial personal relationship between a person who is usually older, wiser, more experienced, and powerful with someone who is usually younger, less experienced, and less powerful. The mentoring relationship is characterized by intense feelings. There are many parallels with other intense human relationships and, in fact, with love relationships. Healthy mentoring relationships can provide an important context for discussion and exploration of professional relationships, including sexuality. Further, they represent a pinnacle along a continuum of developmental relationships that carry increasing amounts of intimacy and influence for the mentee and an involvement that is clearly mutually beneficial.

The ideal mentor is able to nurture, love, care, teach, listen, protect, show kindness and empathy, and share wisdom. In turn, these qualities become part of the mentee's armamentarium of skills in working with others. Although the potential for boundary violations is increased by the intensity and intimacy of mentoring relationships, expecially with mixed gender mentoring, it is generally acknowledged that the benefits of such relationships outweigh the risks. Recent work in this area suggests, and we agree, that it is important not only to create individually satisfying mentoring relationships but a culture of mentoring that is community-wide, safe and supportive, and allows trainees to acquire skills and healthy professional identities.

CONCLUSIONS & RECOMMENDATIONS

- It is important for physicians-in-training as well as practicing physicians to recognize, acknowledge, and talk about the importance of sexual feelings in all aspects of medical work.

- Acceptance of one's own sexual feelings (founded in past and present experiences) is a subset of acceptance of feelings in general. This requires awareness of the physician's own feelings and needs, as well as those of the patient.

- Most apparent sexual issues in patient care involve confusion about appropriate ways to demonstrate caring, or confusion between physician and patient needs.

- True boundary violations are more likely to relate to power and vulnerability than to the physical act of sex.

- It is important to be able to separate sexual feelings from sexual actions and to work through issues of guilt, shame, and personal needs.

- For medical providers, rigid boundaries based on legal and ethical codes alone are insufficient guides to behavior. A relational and developmental approach is more helpful in understanding appropriate boundaries in any particular relationship.

- The use of facilitated discussion groups, workshops, mentoring relationships, support and personal awareness groups, as well as individual and group therapy approaches to encourage open discussions of sexual issues in the workplace is recommended. These approaches can increase self-awareness, prevent unconscious acting out of sexual needs, help distinguish feelings from actions, and help trainees and practitioners develop appropriate personal and professional boundaries.

SUGGESTED READINGS

Andrew L: Mentoring relationships: an evolving model, Part 1. ACEP News June 1996;8.

Baldwin DC Jr, Daugherty SR, Rowley BD: Residents' and medical students' reports of sexual harassment and discrimination. Acad Med 1996;Suppl 10:525.

Bauer, S: *The Intimate Hour: Love and Sex in Psychotherapy.* Houghton Mifflin, 1997.

Council on Ethical and Judicial Affairs, American Medical Association: Sexual misconduct in the practice of medicine. JAMA 1991;266:19:2741.

Daugherty S, Baldwin DC Jr: *Report to the AMA-ERF: Survey of Resident Educational and Working Conditions.* American Medical Association, 1991.

deLahunta EA, Tulsky AA: Personal exposure of faculty and medical students to family violence. JAMA 1996;275:1903.

Farley MM, Kozarsky P: Sexual harassment in medical training. N Engl J Med 1993;329:661.

Gabbard GO, Nadelson C: Professional boundaries in the physician-patient relationship. JAMA 1995;273(18):1445.

Gordon G, Labby D, Levinson W: Sex and the teacher-learner relationship in medicine. J Gen Intern Med 1992;7:443.

Grady-Weliky T et al: The mentor-mentee relationship in medical education: a new analysis. In: Wear D, Bickel J (editors): *Educating for Professionalism: Creating a Culture of Humanism in Medical Education.* University of Iowa Press, 2000.

Gutheil TG, Gabbard GO: The concept of boundaries in clinical practice: theoretical and risk-management dimensions. Am J Psychiatry 1993;150(2):188.

Johnson JD, Shore DA: Teaching human sexuality and social work values. Health Social Work 1982;7(1):41.

Kilborn PT: In a rare move, agency acts swiftly in a sexual harassment case. New York Times January 1995;A-16.

Komaromy M et al: Sexual harassment in medical training. N Engl J Med 1993;328:322.

Lazare A: Shame and humiliation in the medical encounter. Arch Intern Med 1987;147:1653.

Levinson DJ: *The Seasons of a Man's Life.* Alfred A. Knopf, 1978.

Lincoln YS, Guba E: *Naturalistic Inquiry,* Chapter 11, *Establishing Trustworthiness.* Sage, 1995.

Margolis AJ, Greenwood S, Heilbron D: Survey of men and women residents entering United States obstetrics and gynecology programs in 1981. Am J Obstet Gynecol 1983;146(5):541.

Matocha LK, Waterhouse JK: Current nursing practice related to sexuality. Res Nurs Health 1993;16(5):371.

Novack DH et al: Calibrating the physician: personal awareness and effective patient care. JAMA 1997;278:502.

Osler W: *Aequanimitas: With Other Addresses to Medical Students, Nurses, and Practitioners of Medicine.* The Blakiston Company, 1943.

Peterson MR: *At Personal Risk: Boundary Violations in Professional-Client Relationships.* W.W. Norton, 1992.

Pope KS et al: *Sexual Feelings in Psychotherapy: Explorations for Therapists and Therapists-In-Training.* American Psychological Association, 1995.

Schuster EA, Unsain IC, Goodwin MH: Nursing practice in human sexuality. Nurs Clin N Am 1982;17(3):345.

Sheehan KH et al: A pilot study of medical student abuse: student perceptions of mistreatment and misconduct in medical school. JAMA 1990;263(4):533.

Sherman C: Behind closed doors: therapist-client sex. Psychol Today May/June 1993;64.

Silver HK, Glicken AD: Medical student abuse: incidence, severity, and significance. JAMA 1990;263(4):527.

Suggestion & Hypnosis

John F. Christensen, PhD

INTRODUCTION

The history of hypnosis as a healing art has varied from acceptance as a treatment modality to dismissal as a parlor trick. Discredited in 1784 by a French royal commission appointed to investigate the healing techniques of Mesmer (although commission chairman Benjamin Franklin did note that belief might influence bodily effects), hypnosis has since regained respectability. Hypnosis appears to be a special manifestation of the mind–body system's ability to process information by transducing it from a semantic to a somatic modality. Its therapeutic effectiveness is supported by both research and clinical experience. Today, hypnosis is widely used to treat a variety of conditions—pain, airway restriction, skin lesions, burns, and anxiety—as well as for preparation for surgical procedures and habit change (such as smoking cessation or dieting).

Trance and suggestion occur naturally throughout human experience and are a function of how the mind works. Becoming absorbed in a novel and being unaware of surrounding sounds or daydreaming while driving and not remembering the last few miles are common experiences that illustrate the ubiquitous nature of trance. Responding to subliminal messages in advertising by thinking about purchasing a product—or actually doing so—represents ordinary reactions to suggestions made in a carefully crafted trance. These common experiences of trance and suggestion also occur with patients in health care. The power of certain somatic sensations (eg, abdominal pain) to evoke a trance (a restriction of the field of the patient's awareness to the abdominal region), coupled with autosuggestion as to the meaning of the symptom (eg, "I wonder if that could be cancer"), increases attention to the sensation and may prompt a visit to the doctor.

The medical encounter can be considered to be similar to a trance phenomenon; patients are naturally absorbed in their somatic symptoms, and the clinical environment concentrates their focus of awareness. Because patients in this naturally occurring trance may be in a hypersuggestible state, it is important to avoid making negative suggestions and to be alert to opportunities for making positive, health-promoting suggestions. Because clinicians, too, can be induced into a trance in which they focus on pathology, they must be alert to finding ways of shifting their awareness to the larger context of the clinician–patient relationship.

DEFINITIONS

Derived from a Greek word meaning "sleep," hypnosis is in fact a therapeutic procedure that requires active cooperation on the part of the patient. The following definitions, used in this chapter, describe the states and processes involved:

Trance: A state of focused attention, in which a person becomes uncritically absorbed in some phenomenon and defocused on other aspects of reality. Trance states can be positive or negative.

Suggestion: A communication that occurs in trance, with special power to elicit a particular attentional, emotional, cognitive, or behavioral sequence of events.

Hypnosis: A communicative interaction that elicits a trance in which other-than-conscious processes effect therapeutic changes in the subject's mind–body system. Hypnosis can be other- or self-induced.

Induction: The process by which a trance is initiated. This can occur naturally or as the first phase of hypnosis.

Utilization: The therapeutic use of trance to achieve desired outcomes and the phase of hypnosis following induction in which this occurs.

TRANCE & SUGGESTION IN THE MEDICAL ENCOUNTER

Both patient and clinician undergo a mutual trance induction that, depending on the self-awareness of the participants, can leave either more susceptible to suggestion. This state is neither pathological nor unwarranted, but part of the natural pattern of human awareness in this environment. Generally, because of the power imbalance inherent in help-seeking situations, the patient is more vulnerable to suggestion. Being cognizant of trance and suggestion can give clinicians greater flexibility and influence in leading their patients to more positive outcomes.

Many patients waiting in an examining room are in a trance that has developed through a series of events that started with the onset of the symptom. The patient's awareness of this stimulus then leads to an internal search for meaning. Prior beliefs, personal experience, or the prompting of family or friends may lead the patient to attribute a particular meaning to the symptom. This attribution constitutes the initial suggestion, which in turn increases awareness of the sensation and further restricts the patient's attentional field. Increased absorption in the symptom and decreased awareness of other sensations are the essence of the trance.

The decision to see the doctor further deepens the trance, and this process continues as the patient, waiting first in the doctor's office and then in the examining room, rehearses how to describe the symptom and discuss it with the doctor. As noted earlier, this process of trance induction around a symptom is not pathological, but is part of the natural unfolding of awareness surrounding a medical visit.

By the time the physician enters the examining room, the patient is in a trance and consequently susceptible to suggestion. Whatever the clinician says or does not say in the course of the interview can, because of the power generated by the patient's suggestibility, further develop the patient's trance, shift its focus, augment or diminish the patient's somatic awareness, and influence ongoing patient emotions, cognitions, and behaviors surrounding the symptom.

The clinician is also susceptible to trance. Patients can sometimes unwittingly induce a trance in the clinician through a combination of verbal and nonverbal techniques such as the initial verbalization of the problem, hand gestures, grimacing, and changes in voice tone and tempo. These all contribute to focusing the attention of the clinician on the problem or on what hurts. This narrowing of the physician's focus (even while a differential diagnosis is being developed) may preclude other internal images, such as the future good health of the patient or a positive doctor–patient relationship, that could otherwise give rise to helpful discussions. A too-rapid response by the physician results in premature closure on the nature of the patient's problem and solidifies the clinician's initial trance. However, attending to and eliciting the whole story from the patient (see Chapters 1 and 2) keeps that focus fluid. Sometimes patients induce a recurrent negative trance in the provider, leading to antagonism or aversion for the patient or to feelings of powerlessness in the face of the patient's problem (Chapter 4).

 CASE ILLUSTRATION

A 55-year-old single woman was being followed by her primary care physician for chronic chest pain after a thoracotomy. The pain affected the patient's life by causing her to withdraw from social activities. The complaints, which continued for several months, *appeared inconsistent with the progress of healing around the surgical wound, however. Various pain-management strategies that the physician proposed, including physical therapy, acetaminophen, and a tricyclic antidepressant, had little effect on the complaints. Both patient and doctor became frustrated, with the patient feeling that nothing new was being done for her pain and the physician feeling powerless to alleviate the patient's suffering.*

Eventually, seeing this patient's name on the appointment schedule would produce a sinking feeling and tightness in the physician's stomach, and his breathing would become more shallow. As he walked into the examining room and observed the patient's slumped posture and grim facial expression, he could predict how the discussion would go:

Doctor: How have you been doing since our last visit?

Patient: (*pointing to her chest, and responding with slow speech and long latencies*) This pain really has hold of me, and I can't escape it.

Doctor: (*anticipating a negative answer*) Did you try any of the exercises the physical therapist recommended?

Patient: (*grimacing, shifting position, looking down and then back at doctor*) I've tried that before, and it only makes the pain worse. (*eyes filling with tears*) Can't you do something for me?

This case illustrates several components of trance in both patient and doctor. The patient's recurring chest pain induces a trance in which her attention becomes narrowly focused on her suffering and disability. Anticipation of a visit to her doctor further restricts her focus, and her rehearsal of how she can convince the doctor of how bad it really is further heightens the trance. She has learned to associate the image of her doctor's face and the sound of his voice with frustrating discussions about the intractable nature of her pain. Her continued presence at these appointments corresponds with a belief that the power to alleviate her suffering lies outside of herself—this doctor, if only he knew everything there was to know about her pain, would be able to help. This expectation keeps her in a hypersuggestible state.

The doctor, too, has shifted into a negative trance by the time he enters the examining room. The induction begins as he anticipates seeing the patient and continues as his accompanying somatic responses shift his focus from his habitual openness to the field of possibilities to his own powerlessness to effect change. His trance is deepened by the patient's nonverbal and verbal communications about her continuing pain. The doctor becomes more vulnerable to suggestion, and the patient's plea to do something for her creates the expectation in him that he must. This expectation, in the face of the patient's persistent pain, deepens his sense of powerlessness.

Therapeutic Uses of Trance & Suggestion in the Medical Encounter

The clinician can use the patient's trance to make specific suggestions that enhance therapeutic outcomes. The language used in medical encounters can lead to unintended patient beliefs and behaviors that influence both illness and healing. For example, the prediction of continued problems for a patient with a weak knee—"You'll probably always be bothered by some pain in that joint"—in the first postsurgical visit has enhanced power to influence the patient's future awareness of and belief in the knee's integrity. The warning becomes a self-fulfilling prophecy as the patient unwittingly guards the knee and develops a compensatory gait. A positive suggestion—"Whatever residual discomfort you feel, in time you will notice more freedom of motion and activity"—can create expectations that are more likely to enhance healing and the resumption of activity.

A more subtle consideration is the use of positive images and avoidance of negative modifiers. Consider the following statement to a patient after surgery:

Doctor: Your ankle ought to hurt less in a few weeks.

The unconscious mind tends to delete negative modifiers, in this case "less." The embedded suggestion becomes: "Ankle . . . hurt . . . in a few weeks." A positive suggestion would be:

Doctor: You will notice much more freedom from pain within a few weeks.

Because the primary words of the sentence are positive, the suggestion might be incorporated as:

Doctor: You will notice . . . freedom . . . within a few weeks.

In the context of discussing sleep hygiene with an insomniac patient, the well-intended suggestion, "When you go to bed, try not to worry about staying awake," might contain several unintended messages leading to disturbed sleep. The word "try" connotes effort; it becomes associated with "bed"; the negative modifier "not" is deleted by the unconscious mind, leaving the additional message to "worry about staying awake." The suggestion could be positively restated:

Doctor: After you get into bed, I want you to enjoy a few minutes of deep relaxation before falling soundly asleep.

Clinicians can also use temporal clauses to embed suggestions that lead to positive patient expectations. For example, linking pain with expectations for healing can be accomplished by the following statement:

Doctor: When you first experience postoperative pain, it is important to realize that the healing has already begun.

Predicting positive change that precedes the patient's awareness of it can build positive expectations—even if the discomfort continues. For example, the physician might predict the course of recovery as a patient responds to antidepressant medication:

Doctor: Your spouse and others close to you will notice the changes in you long before you begin to feel better.

The implied suggestion is that you will begin to feel better, and when you do, positive changes will already have occurred.

The provider can also reframe uncomfortable side effects of some medications as an indicator of their potency, thus enhancing the placebo effect. In prescribing an antidepressant, the physician could disclose the anticipated side effects:

Doctor: If you notice this kind of discomfort as you begin to adjust to the medication, keep in mind that this is a potent drug that has the capability of achieving the results we want.

The message contains two positive associations with the side effects: adjustment to the medication and movement toward the desired outcome.

The clinician who appreciates the trance-like nature of the medical encounter can use the patient's openness to suggestion not only to present positive suggestions and avoid those that are negative, but also to promote healing. This is true for both the clinician's own trance and that of the patient.

Shifting from a Negative to a Positive Trance

Clinicians have several options to shift a dysfunctional trance that runs counter to the goals of healing in a more open direction.

CHANGING BODY POSITION

This works directly with the somatic configuration that maintains a trance state. A depressed patient may have a frozen, slumped posture, downcast eyes, and shallow breathing. This frozen posture amplifies negative images and self-statements and inhibits any focus on possibilities for change. The physician can comment on this posture and suggest modifications, such as raising the eyes to observe cloud formations, birds, or airplanes, and shifting breathing to the abdomen. The physician might also suggest that the patient occasionally put on some music and dance—even alone—at home. Clinicians, too, can use a shift of physical position to break an unwanted trance in themselves. A physician who feels ineffectual in the face of an inordinately blaming or demanding patient and reacts physically with chest tightness and throat constriction can stand up, say "Excuse me while I adjust the light," walk to the window, adjust the blinds or shade, move the chair to a slightly different location, and then sit down. During this activity, the physician can shift breathing to the abdomen and prepare to open a new line of discourse with the patient:

> **Doctor:** It's quite obvious how frustrated you are with the way things are going. Let's refocus for a moment on our goals and how things will look for you then.

CONFUSION

Confusion can be helpful in breaking a pattern that locks patient and clinician into repeatedly acting out a script whose negative outcome both can predict:

> **Patient:** Fix me.
>
> **Doctor:** Try this.
>
> **Patient:** That won't work.
>
> **Doctor:** What do you think will work?
>
> **Patient:** I don't know. You're the doctor.

When the clinician becomes aware of such a pattern, it is helpful to ask "What is the patient anticipating I will say or do next?" If at this point the clinician can do something unpredictable, the result will be temporary confusion, which can be used to shift the patient's trance in a more resourceful direction. The unpredictable action might be the "Columbo technique" (named for the television detective). In this technique, the physician suddenly and dramatically remembers some minor personal problem (eg, forgetting a spouse's birthday gift), asks the patient's forgiveness for the distraction, and requests the patient's aid. The momentary confusion that ensues (whether or not the patient is able to offer any help) breaks the previous trance and allows the formation of a new one. This temporary role reversal is only one example of the use of unpredictable behavior to induce confusion, interrupting the pattern, and allowing greater rapport and more effective communication.

MINING FOR GOLD

This phrase refers to a technique that shifts the focus of discussion away from distress and toward an exploration of the patient's resources. Useful at any time, this is especially helpful when the tone of meetings with the patient is persistently hopeless, when the patient appears to legitimize the visit by focusing exclusively on somatic complaints, or when the patient's continuing complaints make the clinician feel ineffective or frustrated. In mining for gold, the physician may inquire about things the patient is proud of—past successes, hobbies, travels, relationships, and obstacles overcome. The clinician observes when the patient becomes animated or otherwise shifts out of the negative trance and notes the topic in the chart, returning to this topic briefly in subsequent sessions. Sometimes the change in the patient's state leads to a change in behavior, emotions, or outlook that had been precluded by the "what's wrong with me" trance. Similarly, the clinician's

feeling about the patient may change; renewed interest and curiosity about the patient's personal resources may transform a previously difficult relationship.

ELICITING TARGET STATES

Here the clinician engages the patient in thinking and talking about a future well state, asking the patient to describe what things will be like when the medical problem is resolved or no longer interferes with the patient's life. It is important that the patient be able not only to name the target state ("I want to feel good again" or "I want to be free of pain"), but also to generate visual, auditory, and kinesthetic images of activities associated with that state. This discussion helps physician and patient establish criteria for knowing when the problem is resolved; it also engages the patient in imagining a well state unrelated to and incompatible with present suffering. This trance shift may be accompanied by positive physiological changes and increased animation and hope.

 ## CASE ILLUSTRATION (CONT.)

In the case of the woman with postthoracotomy pain, the physician tried using the technique of eliciting a target state to alter the patient's trance.

Patient: (*grimacing*) I feel trapped. I never imagined it would hurt this bad.

Doctor: How do you imagine it will be when you've completely recovered from your surgery?

Patient: Well, I hope I'll feel better.

Doctor: Well, let's think about what that would be like for you. Once you're feeling better, what do you see yourself doing differently?

Patient: Fly fishing.

Doctor: (*smiles; eyebrows raised, voice more animated*) You like to fish? (*the doctor is a fly fisherman and has shifted automatically into a state of high interest*)

Patient: (*looks at doctor, smiles*) I used to enjoy being out on the river in my waders, fishing for steelhead and Chinook salmon.

The doctor and patient proceeded to discuss various rivers they had fished. The patient had momentarily shifted her mental imagery and her kinesthetic state away from the pain trance toward future health. This created a context in which she could construct a full sensory image of that future well state that was incompatible with the pain behaviors she had displayed. In addition, her image of the doctor, previously associated exclusively with her pain awareness, became, in subsequent visits, associated with images of recovery and hope. The doctor's impression of the patient also changed, so that he looked forward to their meetings instead of dreading them.

MEDICAL APPLICATIONS OF HYPNOSIS

Hypnosis can be an effective therapeutic option for a variety of problems. The neurophysiological processes by which hypnosis can effect change in such a wide range of complaints are still open to debate. One current theory uses information processing as a heuristic model, with the body, brain, cells, and organs regarded as an information-processing system. In the brain, semantic information (encoded in language) is transduced into molecular information, which uses neurochemical and neurohormonal channels to cause changes in diverse organ systems.

In deciding whether to use hypnotic procedures with patients (or to refer them to a hypnotherapist), it is important to consider patients' beliefs about hypnosis, their openness to other therapeutic modalities, and their locus of control. Some religious groups (eg, Jehovah's Witnesses) forbid use of hypnosis, and some patients may fear that they will surrender control to a powerful "other," who can then control their minds. Brief education by the physician about the nature of hypnosis and its usefulness as a tool to help patients increase control over their symptoms may correct these beliefs. If the patients are not convinced, they are probably not good candidates for hypnosis.

Furthermore, some patients may resist hypnosis because they infer that the physician thinks the problem "is all in their head." For such patients, anything other than a biomedical intervention may be viewed with suspicion. Assuring them that hypnosis is simply part of a comprehensive medical management of their problem may increase their openness.

Locus of control—internal or external—is also a significant factor. Patients with an internal locus of control believe that they can influence many of life's rewards or punishments, and they may be better candidates for hypnosis than those with an external locus of control. This latter group may respond better to biofeedback, which relies on equipment that is external to the patient.

In the following brief descriptions of clinical situations, hypnosis can be considered as an adjunctive or, in some cases, primary treatment.

Relaxation & Stress Management

One of the physiological effects of therapeutic hypnosis is stimulation of the parasympathetic nervous system. Several stress-related conditions have been attributed to hyperstimulation of the sympathetic nervous system, which is modulated by the parasympathetic nervous system in a dynamic interrelationship. Sympathetic activation can be part of the fight-or-flight response to perceived threats.

Given the plethora of real or perceived threats in today's world, stress-related illnesses may be a common primary care presentation of patients' habitual levels of sympathetic arousal (see Chapter 29). Sympathetic responses include tachycardia, muscle tension, adrenaline release, pupil dilation, inhibited intestinal mobility, shortness of breath, and sweating. This autonomic activation is reversed during hypnosis, and with parasympathetic stimulation the individual becomes relaxed, leading to energy restoration, conservation, and renewal.

Anxiety

Hypnosis can be quite effective as a primary or adjunctive treatment for anxiety. Patients with an internal locus of control will find self-hypnosis an especially satisfying alternative to anxiolytic medication. When introducing this as an alternative treatment, the physician can say:

> **Doctor:** You have a powerful pharmacy in your brain that can produce significant healing effects. Through hypnosis you can learn to mobilize that pharmacy and let it work cooperatively with the other approaches we use.

The clinician can devote 15–20 minutes to inducing a trance, suggesting that the patient imagine being in a relaxing place. If the session is audiotaped, patients can take the tape home for daily practice, learning to self-induce trances and regulate their own levels of autonomic nervous system arousal.

Pain Management

Because cortical elaboration of nociception is a component of pain, hypnosis can be used to shift the focus of attention away from pain sensations. In some surgical or dental procedures, hypnosis can be used as an adjunct to, or instead of, anesthesia. In addition, patients with chronic pain can be taught to relax the muscles they tense around areas of pain as part of their "guarding" or bracing efforts. This hypnotic relaxation reduces the component of the pain that is due to muscle contraction. Patients with migraine headaches can be taught to dilate blood vessels in their hands and feet through hand- and foot-warming imagery—sitting in front of a campfire, for example. In the early prodromal stage of migraine, this procedure can sometimes reverse the progress of the headache. Temporomandibular disorders, pain from repetitive strain injuries, and tension headaches have also been treated effectively with hypnosis.

Hospice & Palliative Care

Hypnosis has been used adjunctively with other therapies to help patients with chronic and terminal illnesses. Relaxation, overcoming insomnia, pain relief, and enhancing relationships with relatives and other support persons are some of the benefits of this modality in the hospice setting.

Cancer

There is strong evidence that hypnosis is effective in alleviating the chronic pain associated with cancer. In addition, hypnosis can control symptoms such as nausea, anticipatory emesis, and learned food aversion; it is also helpful in managing anxiety and other emotions associated with cancer. There are indications that some patients can use hypnotic imagery to retard the progression of cancer tumors and, in some cases, achieve remission; controlled studies, however, have not yet demonstrated this.

Skin Problems

Certain dermatological conditions, such as warts and alopecia, have been treated successfully with hypnosis. While in trance, patients are given the suggestion to experience tingling or flushing in the affected area. Warts may respond to these suggestions by shrinking in size or—in some cases—disappearing. Burns have also responded to hypnotherapeutic suggestion, both in lessening the degree of the burn and in controlling pain.

Immune System Function

Hypnosis has been used successfully to treat genital herpes, both in reducing the number of flare-ups and in decreasing the duration of flare-ups. Hypnosis has been shown to decrease blood levels of herpes simplex virus and to increase T-cell effectiveness, NK-cell activity, secretory immunoglobulin A, and neutrophil adherence. The clinical application of these findings is yet to be determined.

Respiratory Problems

Patients with asthma have been taught to use self-hypnosis to expand airways and minimize stress-induced attacks. Some patients are able to decrease their bronchodilator use with daily self-hypnosis. Weaning patients off a ventilator in the intensive care unit has been facilitated by the use of hypnosis.

Hypertension

Hypnosis for relaxation can be a useful adjunct to other therapies for hypertension. Daily practice, perhaps using an audio tape made in the doctor's office, can help patients reduce their blood pressure.

Gastrointestinal Problems

Problems such as irritable bowel syndrome, ulcerative colitis, and peptic ulcer, which can be stress related, are amenable to adjunctive treatment with hypnosis. In one study on the use of hypnosis with irritable bowel syndrome, 85% of patients showed significant reduction or elimination of symptoms of abdominal pain, abdominal distention, diarrhea, and constipation. The primary approach is to reduce anxiety, induce relaxation, incorporate abdominal breathing, and suggest warmth in the abdomen and proper functioning in the bowels. Preoperative suggestions have been used successfully to promote an early return of gastrointestinal motility following intra-abdominal surgery, leading to shorter hospital stays.

Sleep Problems

Sleep-onset insomnia—associated with anxiety, obsessive worrying, or sympathetic arousal conditioned to the cue of getting into bed—can be treated with hypnotherapy. By making an audiotaped recording of an induction in which the patient is led into a relaxed state and invited to form positive associations with lying in bed before falling asleep, the clinician can give the patient a new nightly ritual that will enhance relaxation. A relaxing trance can also help the patient return to sleep more quickly after waking up.

Pediatrics

Pediatricians and family physicians skilled in hypnosis find it a useful adjunct in the treatment of children. Children are often amenable to the use of imagination and storytelling as trance induction techniques. Some of the conditions that respond well to primary or adjunctive use of hypnosis include nocturnal enuresis, night terrors, functional abdominal pain, surgical and other office procedures, chronic dyspnea, and symptoms related to cystic fibrosis.

Pregnancy

Hypnosis has been used successfully to reduce symptoms of hyperemesis gravidarum. Habitual aborters have been helped to relieve anticipatory anxiety and lessen the psychogenic risks of spontaneous abortion when organic etiologies have been ruled out. Hypnosis has also served as an aid for relaxation during childbirth.

Preparing for Surgical and Other Difficult Procedures

Patient expectations appear to play a role in the degree of pain and distress felt with surgery and procedures such as colonoscopy. Hypnosis has been used to anesthetize patients who are allergic to anesthetic drugs and to decrease the use of postoperative pain medication. Usually hypnotic anesthesia requires a deep level of trance, which calls for advanced skill on the part of the hypnotist along with the patient's ability to be hypnotized. Using the naturally occurring trance of patients anticipating surgery, physicians can make simple suggestions to enhance surgical wound healing and reduce postoperative pain. Referring to pain as "discomfort" or an "unusual sensation," the physician can offer a patient a statement such as:

> **Doctor:** No matter what you've been thinking about the time after surgery, you'll be pleasantly surprised at how little discomfort you have.

Presurgical hypnosis can also decrease disorientation and confusion following surgery.

Habit Change

For patients in the determination or action stage of readiness to stop smoking or to change eating behavior (Chapter 15), hypnosis can be a useful ally. The ritual pattern of patient behavior around smoking can be viewed as a trance phenomenon. There is an automatic, other-than-conscious sequence of kinesthetic (tactile, visceral, emotional, and postural) awarenesses and behavior usually set in motion by contextual cues (eg, finishing a meal, drinking coffee or alcohol, talking on the telephone). Hypnosis can be described to patients in the determination stage as a useful tool "to help you come out of the smoker's trance and into a more satisfying, health-promoting trance." The clinician can call patients' attention to the automatic behavioral sequence while taking a smoking history (Table 6–1). Asking patients to describe in detail which hand they use to pick up the cigarette pack, take the cigarette out of the pack, hold the lighter or strike the match, and so on will call their attention to the automatic, trance-like nature of their behavior. After inducing a hypnotic trance, the clinician can suggest that patients visualize in slow motion the entire sequence prior to lighting each cigarette. When the previously automatic behavior is raised to the level of awareness, patients are able to break the previous pattern and approach each episode of smoking with increased deliberation. Once patients are in the action stage of cessation, the parasympathetic effects of self-hypnosis can be used as an alternative stress-reducing activity.

SELF-HYPNOSIS

With proper training, patients who respond well to hypnotic trances can learn to self-induce hypnosis to achieve both relaxation and specific therapeutic effects. A useful transition to confidence in self-hypnosis is the patient's regular use of a taped hypnotic induction made by the clinician (primary care provider or referral specialist) in the office, thereby extending the clinician's presence into the patient's milieu. As the patient gains experience going into therapeutic trance by listening to the tape, the clinician can teach the patient one of several self-induction protocols, such as the one shown in Table 6–2 (this can

Table 6–1. Hypnotic smoking-cessation interview.

The following questions are designed not only to gather information about the patient's smoking behavior and its parameters, but also to raise the patient's awareness about behaviors that are usually automatic and unconscious. The interview presupposes that the patient has already expressed a desire to stop smoking.

- Have you ever quit smoking before? How long were you successful at curtailing your smoking? What allowed you to succeed at not smoking for that long?
- What other habits have you overcome? How have you done that?
- What brand of tobacco have you been using?
- What motivates you to continue smoking?
- Where do you have your first cigarette of the day?
- Where do you have your second cigarette?
- What is the sequence of activities that precede the first cigarette of the day?
- Describe the different situations in which you are likely to smoke.
- Describe the mood or emotional state that usually precedes smoking.
- Describe the urge to smoke in detail.
- Describe how you light a cigarette (if the response is vague, offer the following prompts):
  - Which hand do you use to reach for the pack?
  - Which hand do you use to pull the cigarette out of the pack?
  - Which hand do you use to put it in your mouth?
  - Which hand do you use to light it?
  - Which hand do you use to continue smoking?
- Will you describe in detail all of the reasons that you can think of for not taking a first puff after you have stopped smoking?
- How long will you have to stop before you realize that you are permanently free of smoking?
- How will you tell people that you have stopped smoking?

also serve as a handout). Some patients are able to develop their skill at self-hypnosis and retain it as a life-long health resource.

REFERRAL FOR TREATMENT WITH HYPNOSIS

The various medical applications of hypnosis described above require one or more sessions with a trained hypnotherapist. Skilled hypnotherapists spend time with patients prior to hypnosis discussing their understanding and expectations of the hypnotic experience and addressing their anxieties and misconceptions. The aim here is to establish rapport and raise positive expectations in the patient's mind. When this preliminary discussion is completed, the clinician proceeds to the induction of a trance,

Table 6–2. Eyeroll technique for self-hypnosis.

1. Find a relaxed, quiet place to sit or lie down.
2. Open yourself to a few minutes of inner renewal and refreshment.
3. Use a one-two-three count:
   One: Roll your eyes up to the top of your head.
   Two: Slowly close your eyelids over raised eyes. Inhale deeply.
   Three: Slowly exhale while you relax your eyes.
4. Continue breathing in a relaxed way from your abdomen.
5. Imagine yourself in some pleasant scene or experience for a few minutes.
6. Imagine the sights, sounds, feelings, and smells.
7. While imagining this scene, focus on the desired outcome of this trance (relaxation, pain reduction, etc).
8. To alert yourself, use a three-two-one-zero count:
   Three: Tell yourself, "I'm ready to be alert."
   Two: Roll your eyes up under your closed eyelids.
   One: Slowly open your eyes and make a fist.
   Zero: Relax your eyes and your hand. Enjoy reorienting yourself to your surroundings.

using one of several approaches. (The specifics of these inductions are too numerous and complex to be discussed properly here, and special training is required to use them appropriately and with flexibility to the patient's responses.) Once the patient exhibits signs of a trance, the clinician proceeds to the utilization of that trance for the specific benefit desired. This involves offering suggestions for the patient to imagine changes in somatic sensations, emotions, or future behaviors. The clinician then concludes by alerting and reorienting the patient to the external surroundings. After the procedure, the hypnotherapist can discuss the patient's subjective experiences and answer questions.

As noted earlier, some primary care providers become trained in hypnosis (see the section titled "Training in Hypnosis") so they can integrate this treatment seamlessly into their medical practices. Others may choose to refer patients to a specialist (psychiatrist, psychologist, clinical social worker, or psychiatric nurse practitioner) trained in hypnosis and familiar with its medical applications. To maximize the therapeutic outcome, it is essential that the referring practitioner communicate with the specialist—before the visit—about the nature of the medical problem, the desired clinical outcome, and the patient's expectations about treatment. It is also important to prepare the patient by explaining the nature of therapeutic hypnosis and by explaining that its intent is to increase the patient's control over both symptoms and their impact.

TRAINING IN HYPNOSIS

Clinicians who are interested in developing their own skills in hypnosis are encouraged to receive formal training from an accredited training program or receive supervision from a licensed health professional with formal training in hypnosis.

- The American Society of Clinical Hypnosis (ASCH)
  http://www.asch.net
  Publication: *American Journal of Clinical Hypnosis*
- American Psychological Association
  http://www.apa.org/divisions/div30/
  Publication: *Psychological Hypnosis: A Bulletin of Division 30*
- The Milton H. Erickson Foundation
  e-mail: office@erickson-foundation.org
  http://www.erickson-foundation.org
- Society for Clinical and Experimental Hypnosis
  e-mail: sceh@pullman.com
  http://sunsite.utk.edu/IJCEH/scehframe.htm
  Publication: *International Journal of Clinical and Experimental Hypnosis*
- International Society of Hypnosis
  e-mail: ish-central.office@medicine.unimelb.edu.au
  http://www.ish.unimelb.edu.au/

SUGGESTED READINGS

Anbar RD: Self-hypnosis for management of chronic dyspnea in pediatric patients. Pediatrics 2001;107:1.

Christensen JF, Levinson W, Grinder M: Applications of neurolinguistic programming to medicine. J Gen Intern Med 1990; 5:522.

Douglas DB: Hypnosis: useful, neglected, available. Am J Hospice Palliative Care 1999;16:665.

Galovski TE, Blanchard EB: The treatment of irritable bowel syndrome with hypnotherapy. Appl Psychophysiol Biofeedback 1998;23:219.

Gonsalkorale WM: The use of hypnosis in medicine: the possible pathways involved. Eur J Gastroenterol Hepatol 1996;8:520.

Levinson W: Reflections: mining for gold. J Gen Intern Med 1993; 8:172.

Miller GE, Cohen S: Psychological interventions and the immune system: a meta-analytic review and critique. Health Psychol 2001;20:47.

Mind-Body Interventions for Gastrointestinal Conditions. Summary, Evidence Report/Technology Assessment: Number 40. AHRQ Publication No. 01-E027, March 2001. Agency for Healthcare Research and Quality, Rockville, MD.(http://hstat.nlm.nih.gov/ftrs/directBrowse.pl?collect=epc&dbName=mindsum)

Moore LE, Wiesner SL: Hypnotically induced vasodilation in the treatment of repetitive strain injuries. Am J Clin Hypn 1996;39:97.

NIH Technology Assessment Panel on Integration of Behavioral and Relaxation Approaches into the Treatment of Chronic Pain and Insomnia. JAMA 1996;276:313.

Patterson DR, Goldberg ML, Ehde DM: Hypnosis in the treatment of patients with severe burns. Am J Clin Hypn 1996;38:200.

Rossi EL: *The Collected Papers of Milton H. Erickson on Hypnosis, Vols I–IV.* Irvington, 1980.

Rossi EL: *The Psychobiology of Gene Expression: Neuroscience and Neurogenesis in Hypnosis and the Healing Arts.* Norton, 2002.

Rossi EL: In search of a deep psychobiology of hypnosis: visionary hypotheses for a new millennium. Am J Clin Hypn 2000;42:178. (Available on-line: http://home.earthlink.net/~rossi/InSearch OfDeepPsychobiolg.htm)

Schafer DW: Hypnosis and the treatment of ulcerative colitis and Crohn's disease. Am J Clin Hypn 1997;40:111.

Simon RP, Schwartz J: Medical hypnosis for hyperemesis gravidarum. BIRTH 1999;26:248-254.

Syrjala KL, Cummings C, Donaldson GW: Hypnosis or cognitive behavioral training for the reduction of pain and nausea during cancer treatment: a controlled clinical trial. Pain 1992; 48:137.

Zilbergeld B, Edelstein MG, Araoz DL: *Hypnosis: Questions and Answers.* Norton, 1986.

Physician Well-being

7

Anthony L. Suchman, MD, MA, & Gita Ramamurthy, MD

INTRODUCTION

 CASE ILLUSTRATION

Don, a 38-year-old primary care physician, sighs as he sees Mrs. D.'s name as a last-minute addition to his patient list. It is midafternoon on Friday, and he had blacked out the last hour of the day to attend his son's final softball game. "Of all the days for one of her 'crying headaches,'" Don mutters to himself, "why today?"

Don's skill in handling patients with somatoform problems is respected throughout the health center. Since he assumed responsibility for Mrs. D.'s care, her emergency-department visits have fallen by 90%, and she has even taken a part-time job. Don has almost always been able to help her through these spells by sitting with her, holding her hands, and letting her talk.

When he was growing up, Don was always a leader; he was the pride of his home town, the young man people always thought would "make it out of this place." Now he is back home, as a founding partner in a successful regional health center—and with a waiting list of residents from the university hoping to rotate through his thriving primary care practice.

"Hey, Don!" The greeting comes from Grace, one of Don's partners. Briefcase in hand, she is moving toward the door. "What a great afternoon! My last patient just canceled—I'm going to go home, pour myself a glass of white wine, sit out on the deck, and catch up on some journals. Hope you have a great weekend."

The door opens, the door closes, and frustration, sadness, loneliness, and anger come together as Don watches Grace leave.

Primary care practice can be both an enriching source of personal growth and meaning and an unmerciful and depleting taskmaster. It provides us with access to a broad range of human experience—an intimate view of the characters and stories of a thousand novels—and an opportunity to have our very presence matter to others. At the same time, it makes constant demands and surrounds us with perpetual uncertainty; it relentlessly confronts us with our limitations of time, energy, knowledge, and compassion. It is a job that is never done; at best, problems are stabilized until something else goes wrong.

The balance each of us strikes between our own enrichment and depletion is critical to our own physical, emotional, and spiritual health and to our ability to care for others. All too often, however, we lose sight of this balance. We become so outwardly focused, attending to clinical problem solving, that we do not tend to our own renewal. This lack of balance is not surprising; our education has taught us much more about how to care for others than how to care for ourselves. The socialization processes of medical school and residency have cultivated a variety of unrealistic self-expectations and attitudes, especially concerning control and self-sufficiency.

Over time, this imbalance produces a vague but increasing sense of demoralization. The joy of work is lost; patients seem increasingly annoying and adversarial. Work becomes the means to some other end—skiing trips or a vacation house—rather than meaningful in its own right. When the root causes of this dissatisfaction are invisible to us, we blame external sources such as the government, insurance companies, or lawyers. Although there are many legitimate complaints about restrictions and bureaucracy, the most fundamental determinants of satisfaction and well-being are not external but rather are found within.

This chapter discusses important values, attitudes, skills, and healthy work environments, but it must be remembered that simply reading a chapter is not enough to meet the personal challenges that practitioners face. It can, however, help foster practitioners' awareness of important underlying issues that affect their satisfaction and well-being.

BASIC NEEDS OF PRACTITIONERS

The foundation of our well-being is the acknowledgment that we are human, that we have needs and limits, and that to keep on giving we must know and have reliable access to those things that sustain and revitalize us. Unfortunately, the notion that clinicians have needs has been virtually off-limits. An excessively narrow interpretation of the scientific model that guides our work has called on us to be detached and objective observers, leaving no

4

room for our own subjective experience. Moreover, we are exposed early and repeatedly to the ideal of the clinician who is selfless, invulnerable, and omnipotent (the "iron man" model). This ideal is at best unrealistic and at worst dangerous to both ourselves and our patients. Each of us has a variety of needs, both universal and neurotic, that will ultimately assert themselves. The more we are aware of these needs and attend to them, consciously and purposefully, the healthier our lives will be.

Among our most fundamental needs are those for human connection, meaning, and self-transcendence—experiencing ourselves as part of something larger than we are. Clinical work is particularly rich with opportunity for human contact and appreciation. Many studies have shown the patient–clinician relationship to be the single most important factor contributing to physician satisfaction (mirroring its central importance to patients). When we are working under excessive pressure or in situations for which we are not adequately prepared, however, clinical work can interfere with the satisfaction of these needs, resulting in depersonalization and alienation from and hostility toward our patients.

Clinical work can also threaten the fulfillment of transpersonal needs through family and community life. Family and career often compete intensely for time and attention, too often to the detriment of the former. Moreover, we sometimes have difficulty shedding the white coat—leaving our professional caretaking role and expressing the spontaneity and vulnerability necessary for intimacy. As tensions build at home, putting more time into work can provide a short-term escape. In the long term, however, avoidance of difficult relationship problems leads to alienation and potentially to the breakdown of crucial personal support systems.

In addition to our universal needs for connection and meaning, we also have very individual neurotic needs—born of pain and conflict—that are intimately related to our medical work. These needs influence both our motivation to go into medicine in the first place and the way we practice. Out of a need to feel loved or appreciated, we often find ourselves in the role of overfunctioning caretakers, and our difficulty saying no quickly leads to overcommitment. Feelings of impotence engendered by childhood experiences of illness—our own or that of a close friend or relative—may be relieved through our work with patients, but the wishful fantasy of controlling disease is constantly challenged by reality. Voyeuristic desires, fear of death, and the fulfillment of parental expectations are other factors, conscious or unconscious, that can motivate our careers.

These darker, neurotic needs are no less legitimate than those less hidden; they, too, are a normal part of life. When these needs operate outside our awareness, however, they can drive us to work excessively, assume unrealistic degrees of responsibility, and otherwise distort our work lives, thereby causing us to suffer. If we invest ourselves in unrealistic solutions that must inevitably fail, we risk chronic anxiety, substance abuse, and even suicide. Through various processes of self-exploration (such as psychotherapy, peer support groups, or self-awareness workshops), we can become more aware of these needs that underlie our work and find healthier ways to satisfy them. We ignore them at our own peril.

PERSONAL PHILOSOPHY

Another important but underrecognized determinant of our well-being is our personal philosophy—the deeply held beliefs and values that address the most fundamental questions of our lives: the meaning and purpose of life, death, joy, and suffering; why things happen the way they do; the nature of our relationship to other people and to the world; and the nature of our goals and responsibilities as human beings. Our personal philosophies define our expectations of ourselves and other people. They guide the way we perceive and respond to our world and help us identify our place in it. They define the framework by which we imbue things in our lives with meaning, joy, or pain and by which we determine what seems right and what seems wrong.

Developing a personal philosophy tends to be a subliminal process—a gradual internalization of attitudes and values from family, culture, education, and life experience. This process makes it possible for us to be entirely unaware of our core beliefs as an ideology; we may take them so completely for granted that they just seem to be part of the way things are. If we do not understand how these beliefs filter our perceptions and shape our behaviors, then we are unable to subject them to critical reflection and to decide which parts work well for us and which parts need to be changed.

The Control Model

An aspect of personal philosophy with special importance to clinical practice is our attitude toward control. Through the influence of Western culture in general and medical culture in particular, we often perceive being in control (of disease, of patients, of the health-care team) to be the ideal state (Table 7–1). We use specific intellectual tools for gathering and applying knowledge: *reductionism:* "Sickle cell anemia is attributable to the substitution of a single nucleotide"; *linear causality:* "*A* causes *B*"; and *moving away from the particular toward the general:* "This is a case of asthma." All have a distinctly controlling, outcome-oriented focus, that is, to manipulate *A* so as to control *B*. Although this approach has led to important technological advances, it also has important adverse consequences.

EXPECTATIONS

The control model creates unrealistic expectations that limit our opportunities to feel successful. Consider, for in-

Table 7–1. A comparison of control- and relationship-based personal philosophies.

Attribute	Control	Relational (I–Thou)[1]
Phenomenon of interest	Thing-in-itself	Thing-in-context
Epistemologic strategy	Reductionist; linear causality	Emergent; systems model
Clinician's stance	Detached observer	Participant observer
Information deemed relevant	Objective data only	Subjective and objective data
Model for patient–clinician relationship	Hierarchy	Partnership
Focus of attention	Outcome-oriented	Process-oriented

[1] Terms are from Martin Buber: *I and Thou*. Scribner, 1970.

stance, how our expectations of good control in caring for a diabetic patient allow us to feel successful only when the blood sugar is tightly regulated. The patient's blood sugar, however, is influenced by many factors over which we have no control, the patient's own behavior being foremost among them. We become angry at the patient whose noncompliance stands in the way of our success. If success for us is defined only in terms of controlling disease, we are precluded from feeling successful in many, if not most, situations. Accepting responsibility for outcomes over which we have little or no control is highly stressful and leads us to feel helpless, anxious, and angry.

DISTANCE AND DETACHMENT

Our quest for control also creates distance and detachment in the patient–clinician relationship, which, as we have already seen, is an important factor in professional satisfaction. A strong orientation toward control leads to hierarchic relationships. This, coupled with the reductionism and labeling of medical thinking, turns patients into objects, and we find ourselves working more with *things*—organs, diseases, medications, tests—than with people. We, too, become depersonalized in this process, leaving no room for our subjective experience.

The Relational Model

An alternative philosophy that avoids many of these problems emphasizes relatedness rather than control. This model does not reject the insights of reductionism, but rather builds on them by adding an appreciation of context and relationship. Therefore, although *A* may seem to cause *B*, there are also other mediating factors and bi-directional interactions (*A* and *B* influence each other). For example, the tubercle bacillus causes tuberculosis, but not everyone who is exposed to this bacterium becomes ill; environmental and socioeconomic factors also contribute to the process. The illness, in turn, affects those contextual factors; no portion of the system exists in isolation.

In the relational model, we seek to be with and to understand the patient in a number of dimensions simultaneously—biological, experiential, functional, and spiritual. As we come to understand patients' experiences, we may or may not identify opportunities to recommend

strategies or undertake treatments to ameliorate their suffering. We are mindful that patients are ultimately responsible for their own lives; they may or may not accept our suggestions. In some cases, we may have no suggestions or treatment to offer, but we can still find success in offering empathic witnessing, honoring the patient's need for connection—a healing intervention in its own right.

This relational model helps us avoid unrealistic expectations of ourselves. It offers us the opportunity to feel successful in situations, such as untreatable illness or a patient's refusal to accept our good advice, that would seem like failures under the control model. The relational model also leads us to more effective action. In contrast to the control model, which attends exclusively to outcomes, this model calls for explicit attention to process, to the quality of communication, and to the values embedded in the way we work together. Paradoxically, it is by letting go of outcomes and focusing more on making the process as good as possible that we achieve the best outcomes. The relational model also gives us more room to look outside ourselves for guidance and solutions—and to admit our own limitations or powerlessness.

Whereas the control model creates barriers between clinicians and patients, the relational model keeps us closer to the experience of both our patients and ourselves, thereby increasing the opportunities for our work to be meaningful and decreasing the potential for frustration, alienation, and burnout.

SKILLS

There are a number of skills that can make the difference between depletion and thriving in practice.

Time-Management Skills

These skills are essential both within the office visit and in arranging work schedules (see the Suggested Readings at the end of the chapter). Negotiating an agenda at the start of each visit focuses attention on the issues that are most important to the patient and the clinician, minimizes time spent on unnecessary tasks, and vastly reduces the emergence of last-minute topics ("Oh, by the way, Doc, I've got this chest pain. . . .") that lay waste to office schedules. Informing patients at the outset how long their visits will last and reminding them a few minutes before ending allow them to share responsibility for using time effectively. On a more global level, time-management skills can help preserve the balance among work, family, community, and recreation that is so important to life satisfaction. Keeping time logs for several days can help us discover whether we are apportioning our time in accordance with our personal goals and priorities. Time logs can also point out time wasters (eg, unnecessary interruptions) in daily work habits and help us devise more efficient office procedures.

Communication

Given the important contribution of the patient–clinician relationship as a source of meaning, communication and relationship skills become critical tools for well-being. Learning to *be with* the patient requires broadening the goal of the interview from making a diagnosis to understanding the story of the patient's illness as a lived experience. We need to understand the meaning of the illness to the patient—why this disease in this particular patient at this particular time, what its functional effect is, and what role it might be playing in the patient's life. Thus, we need skills for eliciting deeper levels of patients' stories and responding to their emotions. As we become more able to do this, it becomes apparent that there are no longer routine or uninteresting cases—each patient is unique.

Coaching & Negotiation

Sharing responsibility more effectively and more realistically with patients requires both coaching and negotiation skills. Specifically, we must know how to facilitate patients in articulating their own values, goals, and opinions, including their feedback about their medical care. We must be willing to relinquish our traditional—and burdensome—role of unquestioned authority and adopt instead a more flexible stance, trying to combine synergistically our own knowledge of medicine with patients' knowledge of themselves and the patterns, problems, and balances of their daily lives. We must learn to see patients' increasing capacity for gathering information and making their own decisions not as a threat but as a sign of our success. Knowing how and when to set firm boundaries without being judgmental and how to discuss communication and relationship problems openly can help to resolve impasses with many seemingly difficult patients, making their care less frustrating and more rewarding.

Self-Reflection & Self-Care

We need to be able to reflect on our own feelings and actions, to acknowledge our vulnerabilities and needs, to seek and courageously follow our sense of calling, and to act in support of our own health. Rather than shutting out as "unprofessional" and "unobjective" feelings such as anger, attraction, or insecurity that must inevitably arise in

us, we can learn to use them to gain insights about ourselves and our patients. Through solitary reflection and honest conversation with trusted colleagues (informally or in more organized formats such as Balint groups, workshops, executive coaching, or psychotherapy) we can listen more closely to what our hearts are telling us about the state of our lives. These opportunities to shed the mask of the iron man and disclose our vulnerabilities to each other are also key resources for working amidst uncertainty and coping with mistakes. And finally, we can make choices to limit our work hours, simplifying our material needs to gain more time for whatever it is that truly gives us joy and meaning.

HEALTHY WORK ENVIRONMENTS

Our workplaces have an important effect on our well-being. The local culture of the institutions in which we work—be they hospitals, individual practices, or medical communities—subtly reinforces values through both formal educational processes and everyday policies and practices. The local culture can determine whether we feel able to disclose uncertainty and vulnerability to one another or feel constrained always to maintain the iron man facade; whether we can discuss mistakes and ask for help or be forced to work in perpetual isolation; whether we receive encouragement and respect for setting reasonable limits on our workload so we can be present in our families or feel shamed for being lazy.

The Person-Centered Environment

Creating environments that support relationship-centered care is a large topic; a few general principles must suffice for this discussion.

- As clinicians, we tend to treat patients in the same way that we ourselves are treated within our institutions. Core values such as respect, partnership, honesty, and accountability must be explicitly articulated and embodied in institutional policies and procedures. Clinicians and administrators alike may need to learn new communication and relationship skills, and redesign processes for making decisions and maintaining accountability.
- Respecting values and attending to the quality of process must be embraced as the most effective means to high-quality outcomes at the organizational level, just as at the clinical level. This requires a departure from traditional, hierarchic approaches of top-down decision making and control of the work process.
- We can replace the current culture of rugged individualism with a culture of teamwork, accountability, and mutual support. Support groups for all staff, including physicians, may encourage self-awareness, increase sensitivity to patients' concerns, and diminish the isolation and depersonalization that both

characterize and accelerate burnout. We can be vigilant to ways in which the local culture reinforces work addiction and inhibits collaboration and work to improve it.

In this time of concern about health care costs and patient safety, clinicians, administrators, patients, and families need to work together in partnership to redesign our medical institutions, making them more respectful and humane, more collaborative in terms of care, and more responsive to the needs of the people they serve and the people who work within them. Clinical outcomes, financial performance, patient satisfaction, and staff satisfaction have all been associated with factors that create healthy work environments for health care providers; institutions thus have a direct stake in maintaining the well-being of their clinicians and staff.

Whether the rigors of clinical work become sources of meaning or exhaustion depends on a number of factors. We must be able to know and address deliberately the personal needs that affect our work. The need for connection and meaning is particularly important and when met is sustaining. A more mature perspective of balance, acceptance, and relation must replace the current preoccupation with control. The latter leads only to unrealistic (hence unachievable) expectations and the ongoing specter of inadequacy or failure. Skills must be acquired for working with uncertainty, sharing responsibility, and promoting relationship. We must become more attentive to the values expressed subliminally but powerfully in our work environments and begin to make necessary changes so that our environments call forth the best and healthiest of what we have to offer, both as professionals and as human beings. These approaches can help us to appreciate fully the privilege of caring for patients and to realize our best potential for personal fulfillment and growth.

SUGGESTED READINGS

Committee on Quality of Health Care in America: *Crossing the Quality Chasm: A New Health System of the 21st Century.* Institute of Medicine, 2001.

Elovainio M, Kivimaki M, Vahtera J: Organizational justice: evidence of a new psychosocial predictor of health. Am J Public Health 2002;92:105. PMID: 11772771.

Epstein RM: Mindful practice. JAMA 1999;282:833. PMID: 10478689.

Gabbard GO, Menninger RW: The psychology of postponement in the medical marriage. JAMA 1989;261:2378.

Hobbs CR: *Time Power.* Harper, 1987.

Novack DH et al: Calibrating the physician: personal awareness and effective patient care. JAMA 1997;278:502. PMID: 9256226.

Palmer P. *Let Your Life Speak: Listening for the Voice of Vocation.* Jossey-Bass, 2000.

Quill TE: Partnerships in patient care: a contractual approach. Ann Intern Med 1983;98:228.

Quill TE, Williamson PR: Healthy approaches to physician stress. Arch Intern Med 1990;150:1857.

Remen RN: *My Grandfather's Blessings.* Riverhead Books, 2000.

Suchman AL: Control and relation: two foundational values and their consequences. In: Suchman AL, Botelho RJ, Hinton-Walker P (editors): *Partnerships in Healthcare: Transforming Relational Process.* University of Rochester Press, 1998.

Suchman AL: The influence of healthcare organizations on well-being. West J Med 2001:174:43. PMID: 11154668.

Vaillant G: Some psychologic vulnerabilities of physicians. N Engl J Med 1972;287:372.

Wetterneck TB et al: Worklife and satisfaction of general internists. Arch Intern Med 2002;162:649. PMID: 11911718.

Williamson PR: Support groups: an important aspect of physician education (editorial). J Gen Intern Med 1991;6:179.

ORGANIZATIONS & WEB SITES

Center for Physician Renewal
Bellevue, WA
(253) 351-8577
Email: MDRENEW@aol.com

The Center for Professional Health
Vanderbilt University Medical Center
1107 Oxford House
Nashville, TN 37232-4300
(615) 936-0678
Website: www.mc.vanderbilt.edu/cph/cph.html
Email: cph@mcmail.vanderbilt.edu

Center for Professional and Personal Renewal
Palo Alto, CA
(800) 377-1096
www.cppr.com
Email: pmoskowitz@batnet.com

Meaning in Medicine Outreach Program for Physicians
Institute for the Study of Health and Illness
http://www.commonweal.org/outreach.html

Medical Spouse Association
http://www.medicalspouse.org/

Medical Student Well-Being
http://www.amsa.org/well/ttp.cfm

Menninger Clinic's Professionals in Crisis program
Topeka, KS
(800) 351-9058
www.menninger.edu

Northwest Center for Physician Well-Being
The Foundation for Medical Excellence
One SW Columbia Street, Suite 800
Portland, OR 97258-2095
Tel (503) 636-2234
Fax (503) 796-0699
Email: info@tfme.org
Web: www.tfme.org

Positive Psychology
http://www.apa.org/releases/positivepsy.html

Relationship Centered Administration
http://www.groups.yahoo.com/group/lead-org-health

Society of General Internal Medicine
Personal-Professional Balance Interest Group
http://www.sgim.org/balance.cfm

Section II
Working with Specific Populations

| Families | 8 |

Steven R. Hahn, MD

INTRODUCTION

Our experience of health, illness, and health care, as patients and as doctors, occurs in a social context. The "family" is the heart of that context. Making the patient's family and social context an explicit part of medical care affects every step of the clinical process, from basic assumptions about who the patient is, to the conceptual framework for the database, theories of causality, and the implementation of treatment. Consider the following vignettes:

1. Despite wondering whether he could have done something more for Joe, his now deceased patient who had gastric cancer, the doctor is gratified and reassured by the family's overwhelming thanks for the "wonderful care" he provided for the past 10 years and in particular during the time preceding the patient's death. The family is grateful for his help in family discussions about end-of-life care and for helping them make the initially counterintuitive decision to appoint the eldest son rather than the patient's spouse as health care agent.

2. Gina is a 40-year-old woman with diabetes who has extraordinary difficulty following a reasonable diet. Her husband has been unwilling to change his expectations about their meal plans and she has been unable to persist in negotiating a change with him.

3. Mary, 50 years old and previously without complaints, presents with headaches that have been ongoing for 2 months. She's afraid she has a tumor or "something bad." A brief discussion about her family reveals that her 60-year-old husband has been depressed and forgetful for at least 6 months. Two months ago he got lost on his way home from the hardware store. After her doctor listens to her story, she agrees that she too is depressed and very concerned about her husband. She's upset that he has refused to see a doctor. She accepts her doctor's offer to help her get him evaluated, but she is still worried that her headache is something bad.

4. Edith is a 60-year-old woman with two daughters and six young grandchildren. She has polyarthralgia that is much worse than can be explained by organic disease. The mystery of her excess impairment is resolved by assessing the family situation. The doctor concludes that Edith has intuitively evolved the only possible strategy that can fend off her daughters' requests that she provide childcare for the grandchildren and still be acceptable to her own internal sense of duty and obligation—that she is too ill. The doctor does not share his causal hypothesis with her, but does point out that her emotional distress about her daughters' expectations are an important problem "in addition to" the joint pains. He tells her that "even if she were the picture of health, she would still be entitled to be a grandmother and not a nanny." The patient happily accepts a prescription for acetaminophen after the doctor promises that "although it will help, it probably won't make the pain go away completely."

5. Eva, who is 27 years old, has multiple changing physical complaints and panic disorder. She was raised by her grandmother after her mother died, and when her grandmother died 4 years later, by an aunt 20 years

her elder. She and her aunt became very close, "almost like sisters, we did everything together." After completing college she returned to live with her aunt, who had recently begun the first serious relationship of her life. Eva doesn't understand why her aunt needs a boyfriend, and reports that her many symptoms and panic attacks often interrupt her aunt's plans to spend time alone with her fiancé.

In every case, the family context is critical to understanding the situation. In the case of Joe, the doctor has attended to both patient and family and the family is a partner in care and grief. Family function has become a significant barrier to critical self-care for Gina. Mary is having a psychophysiological reaction to family stress. Edith needs to be in the "sick role" to cope with family pressures that she can't respond to more directly. Eva is a vulnerable young woman with two mental disorders that are not only a response to her aunt's perceived abandonment but also a high-cost and inadequate "solution."

All physicians have a latent and intuitive understanding about "the family" and how families work and develop. However, lack of clinically useful tools for making the family an explicit part of care may prevent successful application of this knowledge. Caring for the patient in the context of the family goes beyond involving the families of some patients in the management of care. Two case illustrations are presented throughout the chapter that will illustrate the conceptual foundation and basic skills of family assessment and intervention in primary care.

THE FAMILY AS THE CONTEXT OF ILLNESS

The family is the primary social context of experience, including that of health and illness. The individual's awareness and perception of symptoms are shaped by the family, as are decisions about whether, how, and from whom to seek help. Use of health care services and acceptance of and adherence to medical treatments are all influenced by the family.

Reciprocal Relationships

There is a reciprocal relationship between healthy family systems and the physical and mental health of its members. There is also a reciprocal relationship between the health of the family and the health of its individual members. Ample research has demonstrated that physical symptoms and illness significantly influence the family's emotional state and behavior, often causing dysfunction in family relationships. At the same time, dysfunction in the family system can generate stress and lead to physical illness. Dysfunctional family systems can incorporate a physical illness and symptoms into the family's behavioral

patterns, thereby reinforcing the sick role for one or more members and sustaining or exacerbating illness and symptoms. In these "somatizing" families, the presence and persistence of the symptom or illness cannot be understood without examining its meaning in the context of the family.

What Is a Family?

Our intuitive sense of family is based on our intimate personal experience with our own family and familiarity with the families of others. Despite this considerable personal knowledge, it is difficult to define the family because of the diversity of family structures. The variety of groups that are experienced as family is enormous: two-parent nuclear families, single-parent families, foster parents with children from different biological families, families of divorcees blended through remarriage, families with gay or lesbian couples as parents, and married or cohabiting couples without any children. Isolated elderly individuals may think of their home health attendants as family, and for other solitary individuals the only family they may know is their pets.

All of these groups can be experienced as families. They share similarities in the structure of the relationships between their members and the role that the family group plays for the individuals and for the society in which the group exists. So, rather than define the family in terms of its members, we describe it as a *system having certain functional roles.*

The Role of the Family

Family relationships are described more by their roles than by the labels traditionally applied to individuals. For example, in one family an elderly woman may obtain companionship and emotional support from a home health attendant, a friend at the local senior citizen's center, and a daughter, whereas a woman in another family may find these needs met by her marital partner. In one society, the primary education and socialization of children may be accomplished in the household of the child's parent(s) and in community schools. In another society, a boarding school or unrelated individuals may accomplish these educational tasks, and play a more prominent, family-like role in childrens' lives. Hence, for physicians, the patient's family context must be understood as the individuals in the social system who are involved in the roles and tasks that are of central importance to the patient (Table 8–1).

The Family as a System

An understanding of the system properties of families is the theoretical foundation for most schools of family therapy and "family systems medicine." Families as systems are characterized by

Table 8–1. The role of the family: A partial list.

Reproduction
Supervision of children
Food, shelter, and clothing
Emotional support
Education: technical, social, and moral
Religious training
Health care—nursing
Financial support
Entertainment and recreation

1. external and internal boundaries
2. an internal hierarchy
3. self-regulation through feedback
4. change with time, specifically family life cycle changes

The qualities of these four system characteristics in a particular family help shape the family's internal milieu and functioning.

BOUNDARIES

The family is partially separated from the outside world by a set of behaviors and norms that creates a "boundary." Family boundaries are created by norms that determine who interacts with whom, in what way, and around what activities. Different parts of the family system (ie, subsystems), such as "the parents" and "the children," or each "individual," are also separated from one another by boundaries. Teaching children "not to talk to strangers" creates a boundary around the family. Internal boundaries work in the same way: children who speak back to a parent may be told that they "don't know their place"; they have crossed a boundary that defines their role. Healthy boundaries balance the individual identity of family subsystems with the openness required for interaction and communication across boundaries. Boundaries may be excessively rigid, prohibiting communication between individuals and the world outside the family.

INTERNAL HIERARCHY

Subsystems of the family, including the individual, relate to one another hierarchically: parents have authority over the children, the older children over the younger children, and so on. A healthy hierarchy is clear and flexible enough to evolve with the needs of the family, and localizes power and control in those who are the most competent. Hierarchies may become dysfunctional when they are unable to adapt to change, when the allocation of power or authority is not consistent with the location of expertise or competence in the family, or when the lines of authority are blurred and effective decisions cannot be made.

SELF-REGULATION THROUGH FEEDBACK

Relationships within the boundaries of the family system and its subsystems are regulated by "feedback." Each individual act sets a series of actions in motion that in turn influences the original actor. All behaviors in the family have some effect on other members as feedback.

Feedback maintains the integrity of the family system as a unit, establishes and maintains hierarchies, and regulates the function of boundaries in accordance with the individual family's norms and style. This tendency toward maintaining "homeostasis" is critical to the integrity of the family. The need for stability, however, must be balanced with the inevitable need for change as families evolve.

CHANGE AND THE FAMILY LIFE CYCLE

The family must continually adapt as its members evolve through the biological and social stages of individual development (Table 8–2). For example, the family with young children must keep them safely within the boundaries of the family's protective circle (or that of specific delegates, such as the schools). When the children become adolescents, they need to achieve a degree of independence and the ability to function without immediate adult supervision. To facilitate this, the family must develop new norms of behavior and relax the boundary between the child and the world and redraw the boundaries between parent and child (eg, provide more areas of autonomy and privacy). Each stage of the family life cycle presents new challenges, and healthy families are able to change their hierarchic relationships and boundaries as they arise. Families whose boundaries, hierarchies, and self-regulatory feedback are dysfunctional have difficulties at each transition.

HEALTH AND ILLNESS IN FAMILIES: THE "SICK ROLE"

Behavior in social settings can be understood in terms of "roles" that are shaped by shared expectations, rules, and beliefs. All roles have prerequisites, obligations, and benefits or dispensations. One such role is the "sick role," which is temporarily and conditionally granted to individuals when they have a medical condition perceived to be beyond their control, seek professional help and adhere to treatment, and accept the social stigma associated with being sick. Individuals in the sick role are exempt from many of the obligations of their usual roles and entitled to special attention and resources. The sick role therefore has a profound effect on relationships within the family.

The exemption from obligations that is part of the sick role is critical to recovery from illness and adaptation to disability. The obligations and stigmatization of the sick role are important to protect others from abuse. Physicians play a critical role in establishing the legitimacy of the sick role by certifying the prerequisite illness or disability, and attesting to adequate adherence to

Table 8–2. The family life cycle.

Life Cycle Stage	Dominant Theme	Transitional Task
The single young adult	Separating from family of origin	Differentiation from family of origin. Developing intimate relationships with peers. Establishing career and financial independence.
Forming a committed relationship	Commitment to a new family	Formation of a committed relationship. Forming and changing relationships with both families of origin.
The family with young children	Adjusting to new family members	Adjusting the relationship to make time and space for children. Negotiating parenting responsibilities. Adjusting relationships with extended families to incorporate parenting and grandparenting.
The family with adolescents	Increasing flexibility of boundaries to allow for children's independence	Adjusting boundaries to allow children to move in and out of the family more freely. Attending to midlife relationship and career issues. Adjusting to aging parent's needs and role.
Launching children	Accepting exits and entries into the system	Adjusting committed relationship to absence of children in the household. Adjusting relationships with children to their independence and adult status. Including new in-laws and becoming grandparents. Adjusting to aging or dying parents' needs and role.
The family later in life	Adjusting to age and new roles	Maintaining functional status, developing new social and familial roles. Supporting central role of middle generation. Integrating the elderly into family life. Dealing with loss of parents, spouse, peers; life review and integration.

Source: Adapted, with permission, from Carter and McGoldrick (1980), Doherty and Baird (1983), and McDaniel, Campbell, and Seaburn (1990).

treatment. Because the sick role has such a profound effect on the family of the sick individual, physicians' obligate role in establishing the sick role makes the physician a powerful actor in the patient's family system, and makes the family system an intrinsic part of the doctor–patient relationship, whether the physician is aware of these ramifications or not.

The Doctor–Patient–Family Relationship & the Compensatory Alliance

The doctor–patient relationship is part of the patient's larger social system, and is influenced by the other members of the family. The apparently dyadic doctor–patient relationship is actually part of the doctor–patient–family relationship, called a "therapeutic triangle" by Doherty and Baird. A positive relationship with an active and concerned family can be one of the physician's most powerful tools and enjoyable clinical experiences. In these circumstances working with the family seems quite natural and the complexities of the doctor–patient–family relationship are not apparent. On the other hand, when significant family problems exist, the doctor–patient relationship can become entangled in the family system's dysfunction.

When the family system has induced one or more members to assume the sick role in response to family problems, the task of providing appropriate care for the patient's medical problems may be subverted and subsumed by family dysfunction. Some families can achieve internal stability and meet the needs of their members only when one or more individuals is perceived as being sick. Edith, for example, can regulate the balance between being a grandparent and a nanny only by invoking the sick role. Eva can keep her aunt at home when she has physical symptoms or a panic attack. Ultimately Edith and Eva's sick role will be effective only if it is validated by a physician.

The physician's role in determining that the patient is entitled to the special prerogatives and dispensations of the "sick role" makes the physician a central and powerful member of these family systems. The authority to prescribe changes in role function for the patient further involves the physician in the life of the entire family. In effect, the physician and patient develop an alliance that compensates for the dysfunction and deficit at home. Hahn, Feiner, and Bellin have termed this a *compensatory alliance.*

When the physician is unaware of underlying family dysfunction, the compensatory alliance can become dysfunctional and contribute to somatization and noncompliance, and support the ultimately inadequate coping mechanism afforded by the sick role.

PATIENT CARE IN THE CONTEXT OF THE FAMILY: FAMILY ASSESMENT & INTERVENTION FOR PRIMARY CARE

General Considerations

Treating the patient in the context of the family requires a practical method that can be learned and used by primary care providers in real world practice and training. The large number of tasks that occupy the primary care provider places limits on the complexity of and time available for family assessment and intervention. A primary care family assessment and intervention method must be focused, time efficient, and consistent with the general scope of care.

All patients in primary care should receive a "basic" family assessment that allows the doctor to understand how the patient's family milieu will influence the basic tasks of care, and that identifies family problems requiring intervention (Table 8–3). Basic family assessment consists of two processes: (1) conducting a genogram-based interview and identifying the relevant family life cycle stages and (2) screening for family problems that are associated with family life cycle stage tasks, or the patient's medical problems. A subset of patients with problems rooted in serious family dysfunction will then require the four-step primary care family intervention described below.

Treating the patient in the context of the family does not necessarily mean bringing the family into the examining room with the patient and physician, and in adult medicine usually does not. In theory, primary care family assessment and intervention can be accomplished by meeting exclusively with the patient. Meeting with other family members is very often desirable, sometimes necessary, and almost always enhances the physician's ability to provide care. Using a family systems orientation without meeting directly with other family members requires the

Table 8–3. Goals of basic family assessment and intervention in primary care.

Understand the pattern of family involvement with the patient's medical problems.

Communicate with other family members about the management of patient's medical problems.

Recognize the presence of problem behaviors (eg, alcohol or drug abuse, somatization, domestic violence, physician experience of the patient as "difficult") and family dysfunction affecting the patient's medical problems or functional status, which require further assessment and intervention.

Assess the family's behavioral and emotional response to the patient's problems, and provide emotional support to the patient and family.

Provide counseling to enhance the family's emotional and functional adaptation to the patient's medical problems.

Perform a preliminary assessment of the doctor–patient–family relationship and recognize a "dysfunctional compensatory alliance" when present or developing.

Refer the patient or family for further assessment and intervention, or obtain a family systems consultation.

Understand the triangular relationships and repetitive patterns of interaction between members of the family system, including the development of a "dysfunctional compensatory alliance" in the doctor-patient-family triangle.

ability to explore the life of the family and bring the family into the room through the patient's narrative.

The genogram-based interview, described below, is a powerful technique for accomplishing this goal. However, the task of understanding the patient's family system in this way can be complicated by the fact that patients often give a distorted and incomplete presentation of family life. Such distortion may be conscious, unknowing, or some of both. Therefore clinicians need to learn to infer what is going on at home—to "see the family over the patient's shoulder"—by imagining how members of the patient's family might be reacting or behaving in ways that the patient doesn't understand or won't report.

BASIC FAMILY ASSESSMENT: CONDUCTING A GENOGRAM-BASED INTERVIEW, IDENTIFYING FAMILY LIFE CYCLE STAGE ISSUES, & SCREENING FOR PROBLEMS

 CASE ILLUSTRATION 1

The patient, Ariana, is a 40-year-old Italian-American woman with multiple somatic complaints. She has complained of chronic diarrhea but had normal stool collections and colonoscopy; dyspepsia, but with normal endoscopy; severe polyarthralgia without physical or serological evidence of inflammation; and asthma, but without documented wheezing or abnormal spirometry. She has made multiple visits to her primary provider and to an urgent care clinic, and has been seen in several subspecialty clinics. She has made an average of 15 visits per year for the past several years and 40 visits in the past year.

Constructing a Genogram

The first step to treating the patient in the context of the family is to literally create a picture of the family by conducting a "genogram-based interview." A genogram is a graphic representation of the members of a family. It uses the iconography of the genetic pedigree (Figures 8–1 and 8–2) and can be used to record data ranging from family medical history to life events and employment, as well as family issues. The overall objective of the genogram interview is to help the patient tell the family's story.

CONDUCTING A GENOGRAM INTERVIEW

Begin with a blank page, or a designated section of the patient's chart. Place the genogram where the patient can see it. Draw a family tree with the patient looking on and

helping. Note important dates such as marriages, divorces, and deaths, and the general location of individuals in other households. Family systems data can be recorded using lines to enclose household boundaries, double lines between individuals to indicate strong relationships or coalitions, jagged lines to indicate conflict, and triple lines to indicate dysfunctional overinvolvement. At subsequent visits take a brief look at the genogram to recall the patient's family context, and expand or alter the genogram as the family changes or new issues arise.

FOCUSING THE GENOGRAM

The type of information explored, the number of generations, and the level of detail included in the genogram depend on an initial sense of the importance of family issues. A detailed, comprehensive genogram interview going back more than one generation can be a powerful clinical tool but is impractical in everyday practice. The genogram must be "focused" on the most clinically useful information while providing the foundation for treating the patient in the context of the family. As with most clinical databases, it is harder to know what can safely be excluded than it is to include the entire range of family-oriented data. However, skillful parsimony is acquired with experience, and efficiency is produced by following three principles:

1. Engage patients' active participation—they will take you to the heart of the story.

2. Focus the interview on family life cycle tasks and issues—they are almost always the focal point of stress and dysfunction.

3. Draw and examine the genogram—a picture is worth 1,000 words (eg, picture a single mother, six children, parents and siblings in another country, three different fathers in various places, and a new boyfriend).

Focus the genogram by beginning with the core members of the family, ie, household members, parents, children, and past and present spouses. Identify the family life cycle/stage of the patient's family from the ages, relationships, and household composition of the nucleus of the patient's family. As described below, the family life cycle stage will almost always predict the locus of stress, challenge, or conflict in the patient's family system.

Inquire about the family's responses to any known or presenting problems, and to issues identified using the family life cycle screening questions described below. If no significant major problems or dysfunction are identified, stop the focused genogram interview when you understand the family well enough to take the family into consideration in addressing the patient's medical and other problems. If significant family problems are discovered, continue with the four-step family intervention described below.

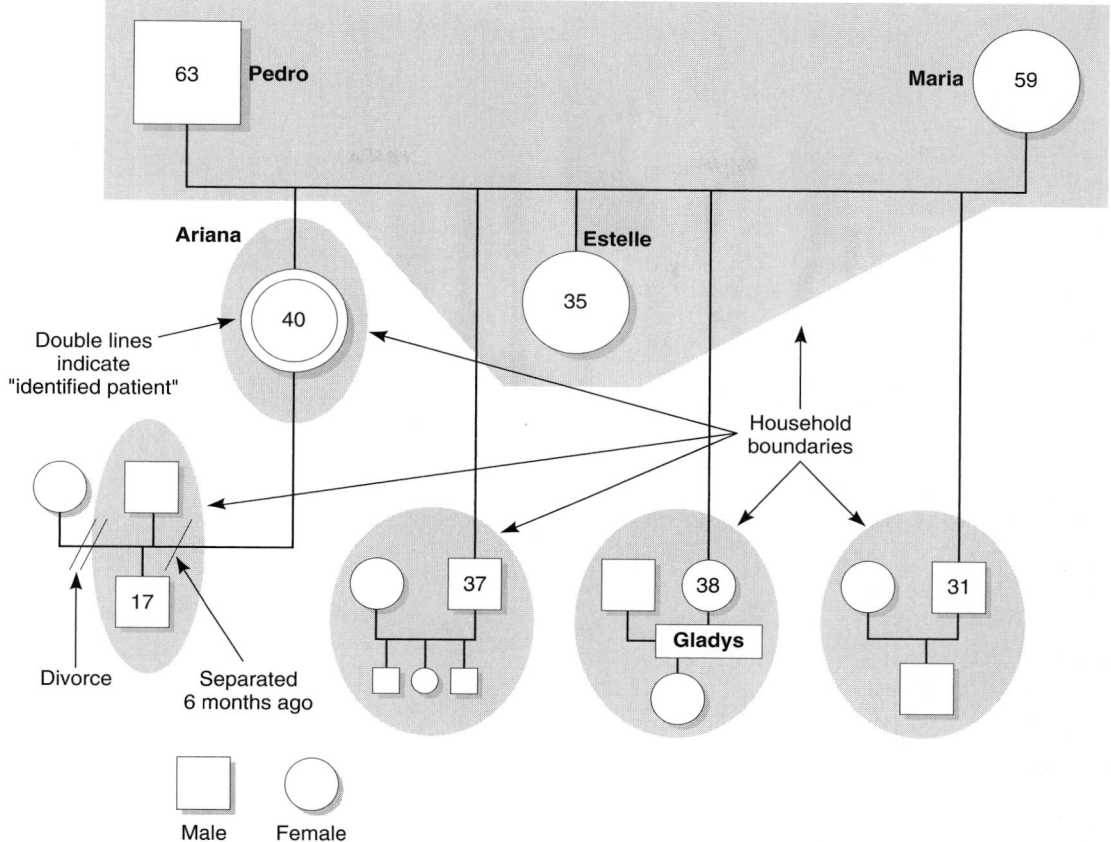

Figure 8–1. Genogram showing household composition and key family members in Ariana's family (Case Illustration 1).

Figure 8–1 shows the skeleton of the genogram for Case Illustration 1. The amount of information you gather about each individual and the family should be guided by the evolution of your hypotheses about family function as you go along. When major family issues emerge from the shape of the genogram or the patient's narrative, exploration of family relationships and history can be very focused. If the nature of family issues is initially obscure, but you suspect something important is going on, expand the genogram to include more peripheral family members and examine individual relationships more completely.

In general, it is useful to obtain brief descriptions of family members and important relationships, the history of major life events, immigrations, and comings and goings from the household(s). Record important information on the genogram as the interview progresses to create a picture of the family as the patient watches. Remember, the greatest efficiency in the genogram interview comes from the patient's active participation. As soon as patients realize what you are after, they will very often take you straight to the heart of the story.

Identifying the Family Life Cycle Stage & Predicting Stress & Conflict

FAMILY LIFE CYCLE STAGE ASSESSMENT

Determining the life cycle stage of the family is the first task of a genogram assessment. The stages of the life cycle are a road map for exploring the important issues in the life of a patient and family.

The family life cycle consists of six stages (Table 8–2). Each stage is grounded in biologically driven and socially shaped patterns of individual development. The cycle "begins" with the separation of the individual from the family of origin (stage 1), followed by the formation of a new family of procreation (stage 2), the raising and "launching" of children into the world (stages 3, 4, and 5),

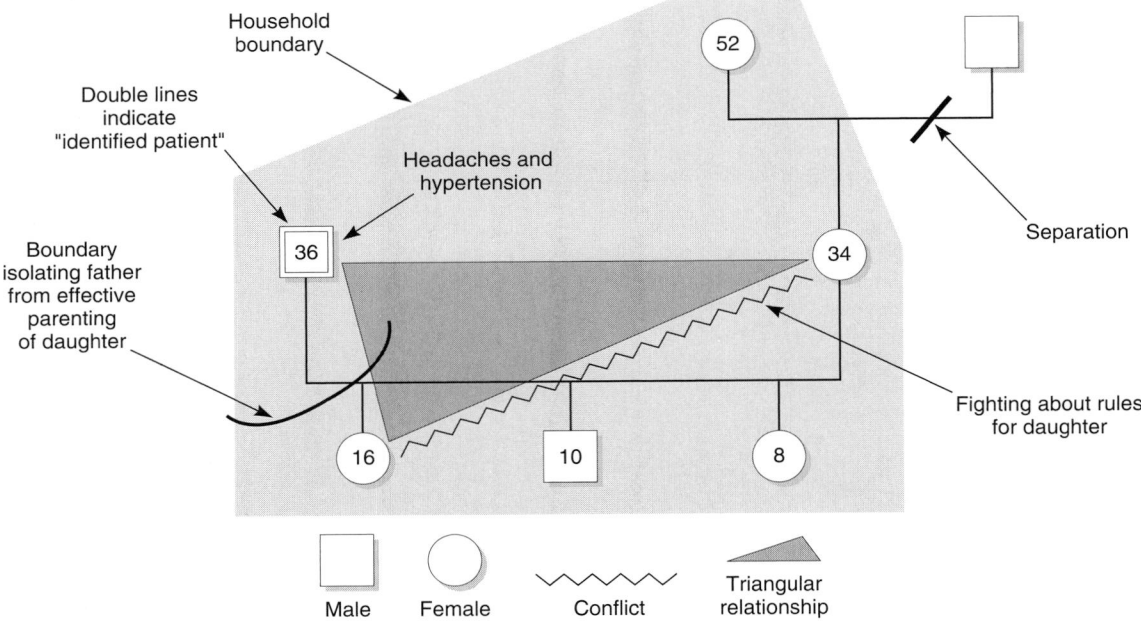

Figure 8–2. Genogram of the family of Case Illustration 2.

and the family later in life (stage 6). Each of these stages is dominated by a theme and principal task. Each task requires two to four major changes in family structure and function. More often than not, family problems revolve around difficulty with one or more of the developmental tasks of the family's life cycle stage.

THE FAMILY LIFE CYCLE: ROLES AND GENERATIONS

With each stage of the family life cycle individuals acquire new roles: from single adult to husband or wife *and simultaneously* to son or daughter-in-law. As you and the patient scan the genogram, look up, down, and sideways and note these roles. Each has the potential for being a wonderful source of gratification, the bane of one's existence, or both. A directed open-ended question to screen for problems in each role is an efficient way of exploring the patient's relationships: "What's it like being a grandmother of six? Joe's wife? The daughter of a 95 year old?" If the patient is suitably activated, the whole story may come out after the first inquiry: "Being a grandmother is great, it's being a mother-in-law that I can't stand!"

THE LIFE CYCLE AND PATTERNS OF PARENTING

In probing for life cycle problems be sensitive to the influence of culture, ethnicity, and social class on norms and expected patterns. Pay particular attention to the structure of the parental subsystem: the adaptational strategies of families with one parent, one "working" and one "child-care" parent, two working parents, families with extended-

family parenting, and blended families have differences that can be anticipated.

CASE ILLUSTRATION 1: DISCUSSION

Ariana (see Figure 8–1) is in the first stage of the family life cycle, an unattached young adult, in her case between families. Her divorce from her husband suggests difficulty forming a new family and moving on to the second stage of the family life cycle. It is noteworthy that the patient's sister Estelle is still at home and having difficulty with the first phase of the life cycle.

Screening for Family Function

After drawing the genogram and determining the life cycle stage of the family, the next step is to screen for family problems (Table 8–4). An activated patient will do the work of screening for you and immediately describe the "real problems." If the patient is reticent or the problem more obscure the following strategies should aid the exploration.

GLOBAL FAMILY FUNCTION

Begin screening for family problems with open-ended questions about global family function (Table 8–5). The tone and content of the questions should be nonjudgmental, and even normalize the presence of family problems, for example, "All families have their ups and downs, how's yours doing these days with all that is going on in

Table 8–4. Presentations and problems associated with family dysfunction that should trigger screening for family dysfunction.

Noncompliance with self-care regimens
Alcohol or substance abuse
Mental disorders, especially psychotic, mood, and anxiety disorders
Unexplained medical symptoms and somatization
Physician experienced difficulty in the doctor–patient relationship, ie, the "difficult patient"
Health-related habitual behaviors—smoking, eating disorders
Newly diagnosed, rapidly deteriorating, or frightening illnesses, eg, HIV infection, cancer, end-stage renal disease, myocardial infarction
Disruptions and change in the family system—divorce, separation, death, immigration or emigration
Natural and social disaster or trauma—fires, floods, earthquakes, crimes
Sexually transmitted illness
Anniversary dates and important holidays
Domestic violence
Reproductive health: pregnancy, termination of pregnancy, family planning

your life?" An effective initial inquiry directs the patient's attention to family issues in general leaving the patient free rein to respond.

SCREENING FOR FAMILY LIFE CYCLE PROBLEMS

If a question about global function doesn't provide the necessary information, ask a few screening questions about the life cycle tasks that confront the patient's family. For

example, the genogram in Figure 8–2 indicates that this family will be dealing with the tasks of "the family with young children" and "the family with adolescents" (see Table 8–2). Six questions, one for each of the three tasks in these two different life cycle stages, can screen for life cycle problems in this family (Table 8–6). However, it is likely that not all of these six questions will have to be asked to identify sources of difficulty, especially if the unique features of any particular family are used to select the initial questions.

SCREENING FOR FAMILY DIFFICULTY WITH THE PATIENT'S MEDICAL PROBLEMS AND SYMPTOMS

The presence of somatization is one of the most important indications for exploring the patient's family because it is usually driven by the patient's and/or family's need to have the patient occupy the sick role. An effective strategy for exploring the role of symptoms and medical problems in families is to follow the sequence: *symptom—function—family response. Symptom*—"Tell me about your symptom." *Function*—"How does your symptom affect your functioning, your normal activities and ability to do what is expected?" *Family response*—"If you can't do these things, who does? What does your family do and say?"

SCREENING WITH RED-FLAG PROBLEMS

Whenever a problem often associated with family dysfunction is present, the physician should screen for the family's reaction and response (see Tables 8–4 and 8–5). Many of these problems are emotionally charged and stigmatizing. Nonjudgmental, normalizing, and directive rather than closed-ended questions are therefore critical. Many of these issues have immediate clinical and legal implications and raise issues of confidentiality that need to be discussed.

Table 8–5. Family assessment screening questions.

Category	Example
Open-ended assessment of family problems	"How are things going with your family? How is everyone getting along?" "Are you having any problems with (name the key individuals in the genogram)?"
Family problems with the patient's medical problems	"How is your family dealing with your medical problems?" "How is (name the key individuals in the genogram) dealing with it, what is their reaction?"
Problems associated with family dysfunction (see Table 8–4)	"I know you have been feeling quite depressed lately, how has your family reacted to that?" "What has (name the key individuals) said or done about your depression?"
Family life cycle problems	"I see you have a houseful of adolescents. I know that can be quite difficult. How have you been bearing up?"
Problems in the doctor–patient–family relationship: the compensatory alliance	"What does your family think and feel about the suggestions I have made?" "What were you hoping I might say to or do about your family?"

Table 8–6. Family life cycle screening questions for families with young children and adolescents.

Stage 3—The family with young children.
How are you doing with making time and space in your lives for three children?
How are you and your wife managing with child care responsibilities?
How are you getting along with the children's grandparents, *particularly your mother-in-law,*[1] and your other in-laws?

Stage 4—The family with adolescents.
How are you doing with a teenager, *your daughter,* in the house, and setting rules and expectations?
How are you and your wife doing with your work or careers?
Your youngest is going to go to school all day now. Will that change you or your wife's responsibilities or activities?
What concerns do you have about the health or functioning of your parents or in-laws, *particularly your mother-in-law?*

[1] Generic questions for this stage of the family life cycle are shown in regular type, questions or elements in italic are modifications *specific for the family of the father* (see Figure 8–2).

SCREENING FOR PROBLEMS IN THE DOCTOR–PATIENT–FAMILY RELATIONSHIP

Throughout the family assessment consider what role you may be playing in the family system and be alert to the formation of a dysfunctional compensatory alliance. Ask the patient or other family members what reactions the family has had to your or other health care providers' suggestions or interventions. It is also useful to determine what the patient wants you to say to other family members. Often these hopes and expectations are implied by patients' words or behavior rather than stated, because patients are not fully aware of what they want, are too embarrassed to ask for it, or do not feel they have permission to make the request explicit.

 CASE ILLUSTRATION 1 (CONT.)

In response to an open-ended question about how things are going at home, Ariana immediately identifies as the major problem the stress that Estelle's illness places on her mother and the pressure her mother puts on her (Ariana) to help out. Regarding her family's reaction to her own medical problems, Ariana says her mom has difficulty un-derstanding why she's always so sick. Ariana's sister Gladys has come right out and said that she doesn't think Ariana's problems should be taken seriously. Ariana admits to difficulty with the life cycle task of forming a new family, and although she feels lonely, the pressure of her mother's demands makes it difficult to think about getting involved with any-one. She blames her divorce on her ex-stepson's wildness and her ex-husband's inability to control him. Ariana thinks her mother is depressed about Estelle's illness, and suspects that she resents Estelle's continued dependence but can't admit it to herself or anyone else. Asked what she would like her physician to do in terms of her problems at home, Ariana says that she would like the physician to make her family understand that she really is sick. (Figure 8–3 shows the genogram at this stage of the family assessment.)

Treating the Patient in the Context of the Family: Communicating about & Caring for the Patient's Medical Problems

After completing the basic genogram, assessing the family life cycle stage, and screening for problems in family function, the physician should be able to provide basic primary care for the patient in the context of the family (Table 8–7). With the majority of families, the interventions described in this step accomplish the basic goals of family assessment and no further intervention is needed (see Table 8–3). A basic family assessment will, by itself, facilitate the following.

ENHANCING THE THERAPEUTIC ALLIANCE

Perhaps the most important consequence of conducting a family systems assessment is to enhance the therapeutic alliance between the patient, physician, and other family members. Patients' perception that their physician cares for them is probably the single most important variable in the formation of a successful doctor–patient relationship. Few things accomplish this better than talking to patients about the most important people in their lives.

COMMUNICATING WITH THE FAMILY

Family assessment promotes better communication with the family about the patient's medical problems. Communications with the family may involve educating them about the patient's condition, discussing self-care regimens and monitoring family involvement with the medical regimen, facilitating the family's role in decision making and advance directives, and helping the family adjust to changes in the patient's functional capacity.

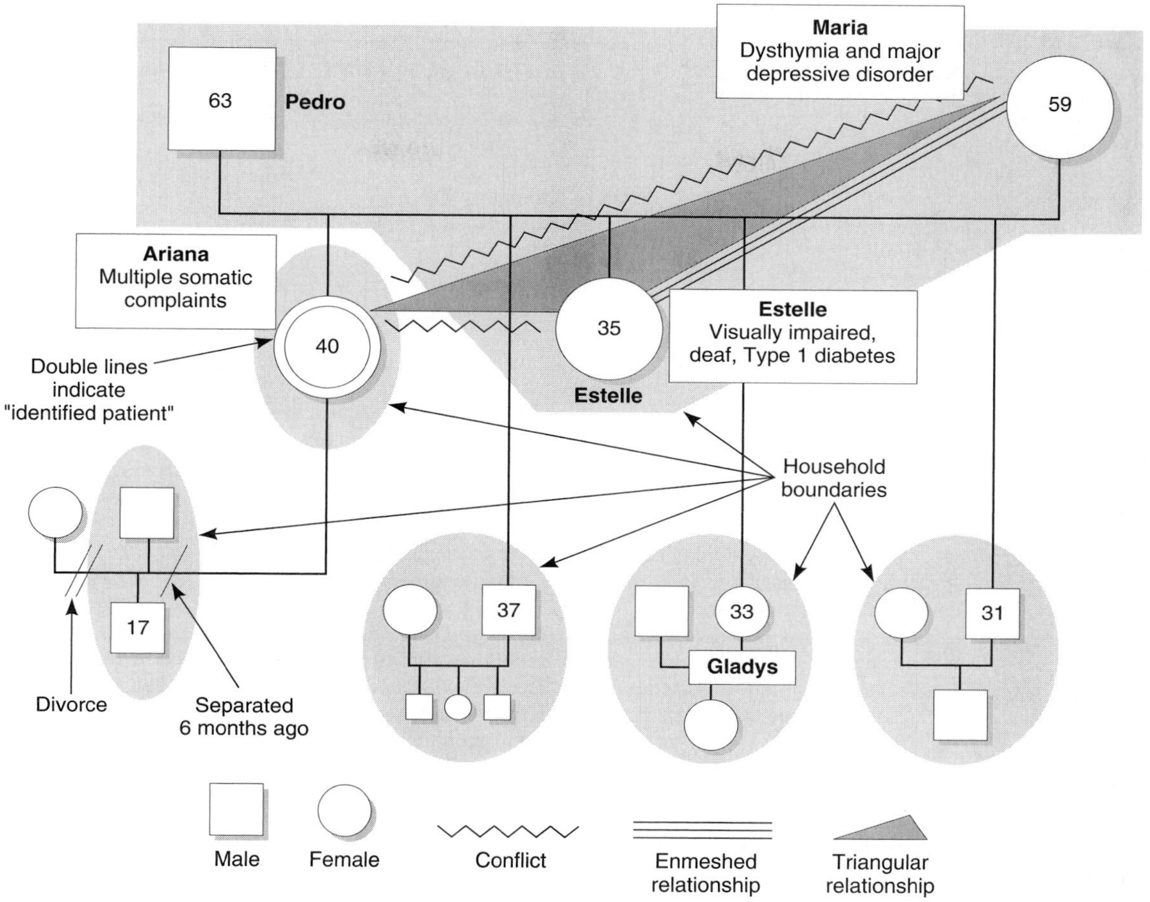

Figure 8–3. Annotated genogram for Ariana in Case Illustration 1.

ASSESSMENT AND SUPPORT

Assessing the family's emotional response to the patient's problems and providing needed support are challenging and rewarding family-oriented tasks. It is often difficult for the physician to witness the emotional distress experienced by patient and family in the face of serious medical problems. The temptation to "stick to the facts" and restrict attention to biomedical issues is both strong and understandable. Perhaps one of the greatest barriers to providing emotional support to the family is the physician's perception that he or she "can do nothing" about the emotional pain. It is important to understand that empathically listening to the family and the patient is a powerful therapeutic intervention in itself—even if it appears to "fix" nothing (see Chapter 2).

It is often possible to make simple family systems interventions by suggesting that families try new behaviors.

CASE ILLUSTRATION 2

A 36-year-old man with hypertension presents to a walk-in clinic with tension headaches that have been going on for 2 weeks. The genogram interview (see Figure 8–2 and Table 8–6) reveals that he is distressed by ongoing conflict between his wife and teenage daughter about rules governing her behavior with peers outside the home. At home the father remains silent until the fights between mother and daughter become intolerable. Their fights stop only when he complains about the headaches the fights have given him. He has never discussed his own ideas about rules for his daughter's behavior—or of family arguments—or negotiated a common position with his wife.

Table 8–7. Basic family interventions in primary care.

Enhancing the therapeutic alliance by demonstrating interest and concern about the patient's family and life situation
Communicating with the family about the patient's medical condition
Providing information about the patient's problems: Discussing prognosis and answering family members' questions about medical problems
Discussing self-care and enlisting family assistance with medical management
Facilitating the family's participation in decision making about therapeutic options
Discussing and mediating the effect of the patient's loss of function on the roles of other family members
Providing emotional support to the patient and family
Counseling the family about simple family system problems
Identifying problems requiring attention from the family
Preparing for further family assessment, intervention, and referral for further family interventions
Working in collaboration with family therapists or other mental health specialists

The suggestion that the patient and his wife discuss the situation before the fights begin and try to develop a plan on which they both agree would be an appropriate intervention. If the family has the flexibility to respond to this suggestion, it may help them with the developmental life cycle challenge. If this intervention fails to help sufficiently, it may be a sign that further family assessment and intervention are required. It is important that suggestions be based on at least as thorough an evaluation as that produced by the preceding steps of this method; premature suggestions based on incomplete assessment are likely to fail.

CAREGIVER COLLABORATION

If the patient or family is receiving treatment from mental health specialists, the physician should actively collaborate. It is important to maintain boundaries between the roles of the mental health specialist and the primary care provider. Patients may attempt to play one health care provider against the other; for example, they may present somatic symptoms to the mental health specialist and attempt to engage the primary care provider in issues being examined in therapy. Patients or family members may complain about the therapist, especially when the family or patient is being challenged to change. The primary care physician and mental health specialist need to keep lines of communication open to prevent this kind of splitting, and use one another as resources when issues come up that are relevant to the other's expertise.

FOCUSING ON THE DYSFUNCTION

Many problems have an obvious and potentially devastating effect on the family. Focusing the family's attention on the problems associated with family dysfunction is a crucial clinical task. For example, if a patient or a member of the patient's family has a problem with alcohol abuse or dependence, it is important to assess the family's response, help the family accept the reality of the problem, and support their need to address it. Many families

are waiting for just the kind of professional, extrafamiliar attention that the physician can provide. Validating their feelings, and providing information about resources such as Alcoholics Anonymous (AA), may be all that it takes to precipitate action.

On the other hand, the patient's and family's resistance to change may be so strong that basic family assessment is not enough to help them take action. In these cases it is sometimes possible to refer the patient to a mental health specialist without further primary care family intervention. However, it is often necessary to proceed to the next level of primary care family intervention to make a successful referral.

 CASE ILLUSTRATION 1 (CONT.)

Ariana greatly appreciated the opportunity to describe the situation at home, especially when the physician expressed sympathy for the burden that Estelle's illness placed on everyone and for the disappointment resulting from Ariana's failed marriage. The physician now had a general feel for Ariana's family. It was clear that Ariana needed to be labeled as "sick" and that every diagnostic test, referral to a specialist, and symptomatic treatment helped create a compensatory alliance establishing the sick role. Ariana, clearly feeling that the physician was on her side after the genogram interview, readily agreed to a family meeting.

FOUR-STEP PRIMARY CARE FAMILY ASSESSMENT & INTERVENTION

If serious family dysfunction is interfering with medical management, the doctor–patient relationship, or the patient's functional status and quality of life, a more intensive, four-step evaluation and intervention is required (Table 8–8). The goals of family assessment and intervention in primary care, as described here, differ from the structural systems changes that are employed in family therapy. Even if primary care physicians had the time and training, they could not treat families with commonly employed techniques that require forming alliances with different family members during treatment, because this process can threaten the trust required to deal effectively with the patient's medical problems.

There is one goal of family therapy that is uniquely appropriate for the primary care provider: to refocus the patient's attention on family problems so that they can be addressed. Therapists ultimately wish to facilitate change in family systems, but the patient must engage in treatment first. Therefore the primary care physician's role in "reframing" the patient's attention is the critical first step in helping patients and families change. The overall strategy of primary care family intervention with dysfunctional families is to make the nature of the dysfunction—as well as the pain and the impairment it causes—so palpable and real to the patient and family that they have little choice but to shift their attention to the family problems. If this can be coupled with hope that things can change, the primary care intervention will accomplish its objective and become an effective bridge to the interventions of mental health specialists.

Step 1: Assessing the Family: "Bringing the Pain into the Room"

The previously described basic family assessment is the core and foundation of the first of the four steps of primary care family intervention with dysfunctional families (Table 8–8). The difference lies in the need to achieve three goals that go beyond a basic understanding of family functioning. The physician must (1) have a relatively complete understanding of the major conflicts or issues in the family; (2) understand how the sick role, if present (and it usually is), is functioning as a coping strategy for the patient and the family; and (3) conduct the interview so that patients can bring the full intensity of their feelings about the family problems out, ie, "bring the pain into the room."

The first step of family assessment and intervention is complete when you can say, with confidence that the pa-

Table 8–8. Family intervention in primary care.

Step	Objectives	Statement
Analyze, and "bring the pain into the room"	1. Understand the major conflicts in the family system. 2. Understand how the sick role functions in the family system. 3. "Bring the pain into the room," ie, help the patient (and family if present) experience the pain of their problems during the interview.	"Your [family problems] are serious and painful, and you have not been able to resolve them on your own."
Reframe	1. Direct the patient's (and family's) attention to the underlying family problems and away from the sick role establishing somatization, excessive functional impairment, or dysfunctional self-care behavior. 2. Endorse the patient's objectives while separating them from the use of the sick role to obtain them.	"*In addition to* your [symptom/problem] these family problems are equally worthy of attention." "*Even if you were in perfect health* I could understand why you would want your [family problem] resolved in a way that meets your needs."
Empathically witness	1. Provide emotional support and empowerment to the patient. 2. Enhance the therapeutic alliance.	"I am so impressed with how well you are doing despite all your problems."
Refer	1. Provide access to and educate patients about psychotherapeutic intervention. 2. Address resistance to psychotherapeutic treatments.	"You have important questions about how to improve your family situation; therapy is a way of answering those questions."

tient will agree, "It seems to me that the family problems we are discussing are extremely painful, and that you have been unable to resolve them until now." Bringing the pain of the patient's life "into the room" during the interview is an important part of the process because the shared knowledge of the pain will provide the rationale and impetus for the second step of the process, ie, reframing attention to the underlying family problems. The following techniques will help accomplish the task of analyzing the system and "bringing the pain into the room."

Two features of the way in which family systems work, triangles and circles, can help guide exploration of family relationships. First, all dyadic interactions ultimately triangulate. We fully understand the way individuals interact only when we understand the series of triangular relationships they belong to. Second, families that are having difficulty, that are "stuck," engage in a repetitive or "circular" sequence of behaviors that represents the best they can do to cope with their problems. For example, in their study of adolescents with brittle diabetes or poorly controlled asthma, Minuchin and colleagues often observed the following pattern: unresolved marital conflict erupts into an argument between the adolescent's parents; the adolescent, in response to the stress of the fight, becomes acutely ill; the parents stop fighting and focus on caring for their child; the exacerbation of the child's illness resolves; the unresolved marital conflict erupts into another fight, and the process is repeated. From this point of view, it is clear that the outcome of the seemingly dyadic parental conflict cannot be understood without knowing that the child and the illness are "triangulated." It is impossible to understand the behavior of any member of this triangle without examining the interaction with both of the other two.

The triangular relationships among family members are caught up in circular patterns of interactions. The sequence of events that takes place in the adolescent's family may be described in a linear fashion, that is, parents argue, the child is upset and gets sick, the parents stop arguing to help the child, the child gets better. The interruption of the fight, however, also prevents the parents from "finishing" their fight and resolving their problems, thus, the pattern inevitably repeats. Dysfunctional families are almost always stuck in such a repetitive, self-sustaining pattern. If they could modify the pattern, they would not be stuck, and they would not be dysfunctional.

It is important to understand how the "sick role," created by the patient's symptoms, is embedded in the family system, and how the whole family participates in it. There are no pure victims or villains in such a system: The adolescent is not merely the "victim" of marital discord; the child's sick role and the acute exacerbations of illness have a powerful controlling influence on the inability of the spouses to resolve their conflicts. Looked at from a more positive vantage point, the child's illness is per-

forming the important function of modulating a marital conflict that might otherwise threaten the integrity of the family system more completely. The symptom is the product of and serves the needs of the entire family system. Though the price is high for all involved, and this "solution" is likely to fail in the long run, the circular, dysfunctional, family dance is the best that the family can do at the moment to cope with the totality of their problems.

Patient-centered emotion-supporting interviewing techniques can be instrumental in "bringing the pain into the room" during the interview. A "one-two punch" that couples a statement giving permission to express feelings, combined with an open-ended question about an emotionally charged issue, is often effective. For example, you might say to a new grandmother whose single-parent daughter is hoping for childcare for her new baby, "setting limits with your children so that you can be a grandparent rather than a nanny can be difficult and even cause a lot of guilt. How's it been for you?"

Conducting a family meeting is a powerful technique for analyzing family systems and "bringing the pain into the room." With patients who have established a compensatory alliance, and "play their cards close to their chest" when alone with the physician because they don't want the doctor to know the other side of the story it may be necessary to have a family meeting. The objective of the family meeting is to have the family enact their interactions, and have other members directly report their responses to the patient's sick role symptoms and behavior. If they enact "the pain in the room" so much the better. The physician merely stops the action when it reaches its peak, concludes Step 1 with the statement, "It seems to me that the family problems we are discussing are extremely painful, and that you have been unable to resolve them until now," and moves on to Step 2, "reframing."

 CASE ILLUSTRATION 1 (CONT.)

During the family interview, the tremendous burden placed on the family by Estelle's visual impairment, deafness, and diabetes became painfully clear as the physician struggled to communicate with her, a process that required writing notes in letters six inches high, or having Ariana or her mother slowly and carefully speak so that Estelle could read their lips (Estelle was unable to read anyone else's lips, and the family had tried but failed to learn sign language). It became clear how much the family depended on Ariana and how she stepped ambivalently into the fray whenever Estelle needed attention.

When the subject turned to Ariana's failed marriage and social life, the mother (Maria) expressed some hope, immediately labeled as ridiculous by Ariana, that she (Ariana) would get back together with her ex-husband. Ariana said, "with all this," meaning the problems with Estelle, "how can I find time to get involved with anyone?"

Further discussion revealed that Maria was a worrier and was constantly preoccupied with whichever of her children was having difficulties, especially medical problems. Next to Estelle, Ariana was labeled as being the most in need of attention by everyone except Gladys. Gladys had been the most successful of the children in separating from her parents' household (she did not come to the family meeting despite being invited). In fact, Ariana made it clear that her own illnesses had no effect on Gladys' or anyone else's willingness to help out with Estelle. The family seemed to concur that Gladys' child and Ariana's brothers' jobs were legit imate reasons for them not being able to help out with Estelle. On the other hand, Ariana's medical problems did elicit emotional support and sympathy from her mother, who suggested that since Ariana was no longer married, she should move back into the family house.

Ariana immediately rejected the offer and said that her medical problems were the primary reason she could not move back into the house; she didn't want her mother to see her when she was sick because her mother would worry too much. Ariana added that when she was feeling sick, she needed to stay home by herself, and at these times she didn't even answer the phone or know what was going on in her parents' house.

The physician concluded that Ariana's somatization was embedded in the repetitive pattern of events dominated by her triangular relationship with Estelle and their mother. Ariana's physical symptoms allowed her to remain connected to and receive attention and emotional support from her mother, and simultaneously allowed her to control the family's expectations that she would always be there to help with Estelle. It seemed to be critical that Ariana's reason for remaining away from her mother and Estelle was an illness, that is, something beyond her control. Ariana needed a reason as compelling and acceptable to the family and herself as Gladys' childcare responsibilities or her brothers' jobs. The desire to devote more of her life to herself, even though it was closer to the truth, would not be acceptable to either Ariana or the family.

Step 2: Reframing Attention to the Underlying Family Problems

The goal of Step 2 of family intervention, "reframing," is two-fold (Table 8–8): (1) Focus the patient's and family's attention on the underlying family problems, and away from physical symptoms and sick role-justifying problems. (2) Separate the patient's (or family's) objective in using the sick role from the use of the sick role as a tactic

to achieve the goal. This is done by recognizing the objective that the patient is pursuing and endorsing it as something that the patient is "entitled to even if [they] are in perfect health."

REFRAMING, "IN ADDITION TO YOUR PAIN . . ."

The transition from Step 1 to Step 2 occurs when the interview has "brought the pain into the room," and patients are in touch with their distress, ie, when they cannot fail to agree with the first critical reframing statement, "It seems to me that the family situation you have just described is extremely painful, and that *in addition to* your [problematic symptom or behavior], this family problem is also worthy of attention."

A critical component of the first reframing statement is *"in addition to"* in contrast to either "instead of" or "because of." Even if your understanding, based upon a psychosomatic hypothesis, is that family stress is "causing" the somatoform presentation, you must resist saying so. This is because the legitimacy of the sick role and coping strategies that the patient and family currently need to function depends upon there being a "disease beyond one's control" to justify the sick role. If the family intervention begins to have effect, and healthier coping strategies are adopted, then the family will be able to relinquish sick role-based coping. Until that time they must be allowed to retain the sick role strategy. Therefore, the goal of reframing is to establish a *parallel* concern directed at the underlying family problems. Occasionally a patient or family member will be able to make the connection themselves: "Doctor, do you think that maybe my headache is being caused by all these problems?" In such cases the psychosomatic hypothesis can be endorsed. The mistake is to make the connection before the patient and family are ready. This will result in the all too familiar, "Doctor, you think it's all in my head. It's not in my head, my pain is real!"

REFRAMING, "EVEN IF YOU WERE THE PICTURE OF PERFECT HEALTH YOU WOULD BE ENTITLED TO . . ."

Unless your patient's objectives in occupying the sick role are antisocial you should be able to identify an essential core of their objective that you can endorse—a new grandmother who doesn't want to be mistaken for a nanny, a father who wants peace in his home and rules for his teenage daughter, a young woman who does not want to become her sister's home health aide, etc.

The second objective of reframing is to separate the objective from the tactic of occupying the sick role, and to empower the patient and family to adopt other, healthier strategies. This can be done by telling the patient, *"if you were the picture of perfect health, you would be entitled to—* be a grandmother not a nanny, have your daughter follow some agreed upon rules, set limits on your role in taking care of your sister, etc." This part of the reframing addresses the fundamental function of the sick role, which is to establish entitlement, and uses the authority of the physician to legitimate the desired entitlement on other, healthier grounds.

CASE ILLUSTRATION 1: DISCUSSION (CONT.)

It was relatively easy to reframe the burden of caring for Estelle as a problem worthy of attention after the painful demonstration of just how difficult it was to just have a conversation with her. It was also easy to reframe Ariana's desire to have some time for herself—a need she was unwilling to claim on her own—as something that would be important for "a woman her age" *even if she was not ill.* Ariana was willing to accept the suggestion that her failure to develop the kind of intimate relationship she desired was also a problem worthy of consideration.

Step 3: Empathic Witnessing: "I Am So Impressed with How Well You Are Doing Despite . . ."

The most immediate way to ensure that family intervention has a positive and therapeutic effect is to "empathically witness" the patient's and family's problems and their efforts to cope (Table 8–8). If the interview has succeeded in exposing the family's distress and their best attempts to deal with their problems, the patient and family will recognize that the physician knows the family in a very intimate way. If the physician acknowledges the special nature of this awareness, and responds empathically to the patient and family, the effect can be very therapeutic. The general format for empathic witnessing is to say to the patient (or family) that having heard their story, and seen what they have to cope with, *"I am very impressed with how well you are doing despite all your problems and difficulties."* It is helpful to remember that even if you cannot praise the patient's behavior or accomplishments, you can usually empathically witness their efforts: "I am impressed that you *want to be* a good mother to your children."

CASE ILLUSTRATION 1 (CONT.)

The family admitted that the current situation was indeed painful and that they had not been able to solve the problem despite their best efforts. The physician was able to tell Ariana and her mother: "I am so impressed with how well you are both doing despite the tremendous problems you have had to deal with." The physician also remarked on the magnitude of the sacrifice Ariana had made, neglecting her own social life to be available to the family, and commented that developing the social aspect of her life was just as important to Ariana at her stage of life as caring for children was for Gladys. The physician also commented that it was easy to understand how this area of Ariana's life might be difficult for her to deal with because of her past problems.

Step 4: Referral for Family & Psychotherapy

Referral for therapy is not always indicated. Very often a primary care family intervention can empower patients and their families to address their difficulties with new energy, insight, and courage to change. However, when mental health intervention is indicated and proposed, patients and families may not readily accept it (Table 8–8).

OVERCOMING RESISTANCE

Resistance to referral for psychotherapeutic intervention is common and is often one of the reasons family assessment and intervention are required. Success in analyzing, reframing, and empathically witnessing is the foundation of patients' acceptance of referrals to mental health providers. Referral for therapy may make sense to the provider long before it does to the patient. Resistance to referral shows that the patient does not share that understanding. Successfully reframing attention to the underlying family problems addresses this discrepancy and is critical to addressing other causes of resistance to engaging in therapy. Framing family problems as "in addition to" will help patients feel comfortable that therapy does not threaten their use of the sick role before they are ready to give it up. Resistance to therapy may be due to fear of dealing directly with painful and powerful emotions. Empathic witnessing and reframing can make this challenge seem more surmountable. Finally, patients may accept the reality of family problems yet not accept the fact that therapy will help: "What's talking going to accomplish?" The process of therapy may indeed seem obscure to patients and a little education can be helpful. It may be useful to restate problems as questions and describe therapy as the process of looking for answers. For example, "you have a serious question to answer. You have to determine how much childcare you actually want to provide, and then figure out how to talk to your daughter about it. Therapy can help you find answers to these questions."

Despite the physician's best efforts, resistance to therapy can be persistant. It may take years before the reframing and empathic witnessing bear fruit. It is not unusual for patients and families to finally go to a therapist only after they feel they have had no choice because there has been some further crisis or deterioration in family functioning. Sometimes it is forced on them, for example, by the courts in criminal or custodial cases, or employer-mandated treatment for substance abuse. The first family intervention you do will help create a stronger therapeutic alliance, and the second round of intervention will be more effective when the next crisis does arrive, as it inevitably will.

Sometimes, patients and their families never get to therapy. Even in that case, the reframing and empathic witnessing of the patient's family story have a positive effect. Aside from the intrinsic therapeutic benefit mentioned earlier, repeated empathic witnessing offers a therapeutic response to the patient who continues to present with somatoform symptoms, neglect of self-care, or destructive health-related behaviors. *After* performing a family assessment and intervention, the physician may say the following to the patient who has not followed through with referral for therapy and who returns with persistent or recurrent symptoms (as did the father in Case Illustration 2):

CASE ILLUSTRATION 2 (CONCLUSION)

"I am sorry that your headache is still bothering you. Your wife and daughter are still fighting, aren't they? It's too bad that you haven't gotten to the therapist yet. I truly wish that there was more that I could do for you. Now, why don't we check your blood pressure."

The patient—aware that the physician has witnessed the family conflict—knows that the clinician understands the importance of the conflict at home and that this understanding is empathic. Hence, the physician does not have to repeat the assessment and intervention interview, merely recall it for the patient. The physician is in a position to respect the meaning of the patient's symptoms without allowing them to divert the process of care into unnecessary testing, medication, or referrals for more evaluation. The physician is therefore able to maintain an emotionally supportive alliance with the patient, while avoiding a dysfunctional compensatory alliance. This is accomplished by responding to the patient's symptoms in three ways: (1) making a therapeutic suggestion, (2) clarifying the limits of the provider's capacity to help, and (3) pointing out the patient's responsibility and opportunity to act on his own behalf.

CASE ILLUSTRATION 1 (CONCLUSION)

The physician (1) referred the family for family therapy to explore better approaches to coping with the burden of Estelle's medical problems; (2) suggested that Ariana would benefit from individual counseling to explore her difficulties in forming a satisfying

intimate relationship; (3) asked Maria's physician to consider the diagnoses of dysthymia and major depression; and (4) recommended that the family try to obtain a home health aide for Estelle to give Maria a break. The family agreed to all four of these suggestions. When Ariana returned for her next visit, she still had somatoform symptoms but spoke of them only briefly, allowing the physician to turn the discussion to what was going on at home. Ariana reported that the family had taken no steps toward family therapy and that she was still considering whether to go to individual therapy. She did report feeling more comfortable setting limits on her mother's expectations of assistance in dealing with Estelle, and reported success in obtaining a home health aide for Estelle. Maria had been placed on an antidepressant, made a few visits to a community mental health center, and was much less symptomatic.

Eight months later, Ariana entered individual therapy for about a year. Her somatization decreased dramatically and her limit-setting improved. Eventually she started dating and entered a steady relationship but has not married. The family subsequently weathered some major upheavals, including further deterioration in Estelle's physical and mental status and the death of a brother and sister-in-law from AIDS, leaving Ariana with custody of their son. The family never entered family therapy.

SUGGESTED READINGS

Carter CA, McGoldrick M (editors): *The Family Life cycle: A Framework for Family Therapy.* Gardner Press, 1980.

Doherty WJ, Baird MA: *Family Therapy and Family Medicine.* Guilford Press, 1983.

Doherty WJ, Baird MA: *Family-Centered Medical Care: A Clinical Case Book.* Guilford Press, 1987.

Doherty WJ, Campbell TL: *Families and Health.* Sage Publications, 1988.

Hahn SR, Feiner JS, Bellin EH: The doctor–patient–family relationship: a compensatory alliance. Ann Intern Med 1988;109:884.

Haley J: *Problem Solving Therapy.* Jossey-Bass, 1976.

McDaniel S, Campbell TL, Seaburn DB: *Family-Oriented Primary Care.* Springer-Verlag, 1990.

McGoldrick M, Gerson R: *Genograms in Family Assessment.* Norton, 1985.

Minuchin S: *Families and Family Therapy.* Harvard University Press, 1974.

Minuchin S, Bosman BL, Baker L: *Psychosomatic Families.* Harvard University Press, 1987.

Children

Howard L. Taras, MD

INTRODUCTION

This chapter reviews common childhood behavioral problems and suggests some management guidelines. Pediatric behavioral medicine cannot be easily disassociated from child development because many problematic childhood behaviors have developmental roots.

UNDESIRABLE BEHAVIOR AS A NORMAL PART OF DEVELOPMENT

A child's ability to understand and interact with the environment is constantly evolving. To learn more about the world, a child experiments with ways of interacting with it. Most often, children test the reactions of the people to whom they are closest, their parents. Colloquial phrases such as *"the terrible twos," "She's going through a stage,"* and *"Boys will be boys"* indicate that undesirable childhood behaviors are commonly accepted as "normal." But when an undesirable behavior is manifesting in your child, the normalcy can be difficult to accept. And even when the cause is well understood, many parents still need the knowledge and skills to respond to the problem behavior.

EXTRAORDINARY STRESS

Behavioral problems associated with normal childhood development must be distinguished from problems with more complex causes. Aberrant childhood behaviors are often secondary to extraordinary life stresses. This applies to children who witness violence, are exposed to continuous marital discord, have a chronic illness or a chronically ill sibling, or who don't feel wanted. Children living under any condition that seriously threatens healthy and successful transition through a developmental stage are likely to pose serious behavioral problems.

Children, like adults, may appear to be the dysfunctional member of an otherwise healthy family unit even though the problem actually stems from family issues. This is particularly the case with childhood behaviors, because children are dependent on adults in almost every way. Take, for instance, the child who refuses to attend school. Classically, this behavior occurs when one or both parents send subliminal messages to the child to remain home. Although the primary problem is parental anxiety about separation, it is the child who exhibits the apparent symptoms.

INHERENT DISORDERS

In addition to childhood behavioral problems stemming from normal development and extraordinary life stresses, a third general category involves problems caused by disorders inherent to the child. Attention deficit disorders are the most common and well known, but conduct disorders, depression, pervasive developmental disorders, and other psychiatric diagnoses may manifest during childhood. A complete history, observation, and response to treatment help the primary care clinician distinguish these from other causes of behavioral problems.

SCREENING FAMILIES FOR DIFFICULTIES WITH CHILDHOOD BEHAVIORS

Pediatric primary care providers must screen families for difficulties with undesirable childhood behaviors, sort out probable causes for the behaviors, recognize when a mental health referral is appropriate, and manage those problems that are likely to respond to simple environmental changes or to elementary behavioral management techniques.

Practitioner Concern versus Time Constraints

Many parents do not know where to seek help for behavioral problems such as their baby's night awakenings, their toddler's tantrums, or their fourth grader's class-clown behavior. They do not realize that their child's clinician can assist them. To overcome these barriers, health care providers should take every opportunity to talk about behavioral issues, although time constraints may limit the practitioner's ability to listen to extensive histories. Therefore clinicians need to screen for behavioral information in ways that are expedient and that leave time to reflect on issues that can be discussed more fully at another time.

Trigger Questions & Questionnaires

One way to elicit information from parents is to ask a preset list of key questions, specific to each age group. An excellent source for such "trigger" questions is Green's *Bright Futures: Guidelines for Health Supervision of Infants, Children, and Adolescents* (see Suggested Readings).

Another option is to routinely use formal, standardized questionnaires that are designed so that parents can respond to them by mail in advance of an appointment or in the clinician's waiting room. They enable parents to take the time to respond thoughtfully to physician inquiries and they include the input of both parents—often exposing differences in parents' opinions. These questionnaires also minimize parents' discomfort with verbalizing certain family problems. They often yield information from a wide range of potential problem areas and do so effectively. Many of these tools are accompanied by a separate set of questions for teachers, which are useful when a problem has been identified.

Table 9–1 lists four behavioral screens that are popular and appropriate for use by primary care clinicians. Other available questionnaires were reviewed by Stancin and Palermo (see Suggested Readings). This review is a useful guide for clinicians who wish to identify which tool is most suitable to their needs.

To effectively screen for childhood behavioral problems, practitioners also need to develop their skills of observation and to learn to apply their natural intuitions. Parent–child interaction in the office can be an excellent indicator of problems occurring at home. Incidents in the office that induce parents to discipline their child are opportunities for clinicians to better understand the parent–child relationship and to bring behavioral management issues into discussion. Experienced clinicians have learned to become aware of subtle signs in the office that are indicative of a family's dynamics, such as how a mother holds her baby. A mother who seems uncomfortable feeding her baby, a pattern of noncompliance, or suspicion about the levels of interest mother or father show are all indicative of issues that should register concern with the clinician. Involvement of grandparents and other extended family, references parents make about their own upbringing, and other family characteristics are also worth noting.

Although signs for concern do not always indicate problems, this information is often useful in evaluating a child behavioral issue, although sometimes not until months or years later. Positive impressions that clinicians form about families also provide clinically useful information.

INTERVIEWING YOUNG CHILDREN

Primary care providers can find themselves in a quandary when they try to elicit information directly from the child. Most children by age 2½–3 years are capable of communicating certain thoughts and feelings to an inquiring health provider. But children do not typically divulge such information to clinicians when questioned directly. Children freely offer their honest opinions on just about any topic, sensitive or banal, but they often do so when it is unsolicited. Parents themselves are often surprised when their children first reveal their feelings about a delicate personal issue to an adult with whom they are not ostensibly very close (a preschool teacher, a friend's mother in their car pool, etc).

Primary care providers should therefore use tools that help children more freely and predictably disclose what's on their minds. One way is to ask children old enough to understand and comply to draw a picture, for example, to draw "anything they want," "something scary," "their

Table 9–1. Behavioral screening tools.

Name	Author/Reference	Characteristics
Achenbach Child Behavior Checklist	Achenbach TM: *Manual for the Child Behavior Checklist/4–18 and 1991 Profile.* University of Vermont Department of Psychiatry, 1991.	112 items ages 2–18
Conners Parent Rating Scale	Conners CK et al: The revised Conners' Parent Rating Scale (CPRS-R): factor structure, reliability, and criterion validity. J Abnorm Child Psychol 1998;26(4):257.	Brief, but only valuable when ADHD is suspected, less valuable as a general screen
Eyberg Child Behavior Inventory	Eyberg S: The Eyberg Child Behavioral Inventory. J Clin Child Psychol 1980;9:22.	36 items/ages 2–16
Pediatric Symptom Checklist	Jellinek et al: Pediatric symptom checklist: screening school-age children for psychosocial dysfunction. J Pediatr 1988;112:201.	5 minutes/35 items for grades 1–12

family," or "the worst day at school." The position of the characters in the drawings, facial expressions, and choice of colors can yield important information about what they are thinking and may be indicative of how they are feeling and can be used as a starting point for discussion. Children often find it easier to speak about themselves when the conversation is in the third person, such as "Why would that little girl in the picture want to hit her mommy?"

To avoid alienating parents, you may go through a few such questions when both parent and child are in the room. But many children, and most of those older than age 4 years, respond differently when their parents are in the room. Explain to parents that you would like to interview the child in the same way without them. The general nature of children's responses can be discussed later with parents. Parents should be notified that this will occur. But the interviewer need not feel compelled to reveal children's specific responses to each interview item, particularly if information may be hurtful and not of therapeutic value at that time. Parents and children should know that too.

Other oblique ways of eliciting information from children are to ask open-ended questions using questions that children like to respond to: "Pretend a magical genie in a bottle wanted to grant you three wishes, what would they be?" And "If you could magically turn into any animal you wanted, what would it be?" To their response to the last question, then ask, "Well that's wonderful! And why would you be happy as that animal?"

Sentence completion games are also useful. The clinician begins the first few words of a sentence and asks the child to complete the sentence by making something up. Examples of some are given in Table 9–2, and these (and others like them) can be typed onto colorful cards so that children can choose one at a time and perceive it as a game, not a real interview. Allow the child to be imaginative with responses, and indicate that their responses can be the truth but don't have to be.

Toddlers and school age children are often aware of the clinicians' actual intent when these interviewing techniques are used. Despite this, children seem to enjoy going along with this format of questioning and appreciate having an easy way to express themselves. Children respond best when they are comfortable with the clinician. Arranging a number of office visits can help to establish that relationship.

When using drawings, questions in the third person, or questions evoking the child's imagination, it is important not to read too deeply into children's responses. Children have active imaginations: they play around with frightening ideas and with wishful thinking. Sometimes they are merely obsessed with speaking about what they've recently seen on television. To be taken seriously, responses of young children should fit into a general pattern of what the clinician suspects from parent interview and symptoms. One or two worrisome responses should not stand on their own as proof for the etiology to a problem.

BEYOND THE PHYSICIAN–CHILD–PARENT TRIAD

Many toddlers are placed in the care of a day-care provider, baby-sitter, or relative. Virtually all children older than age 5 spend a large portion of their waking hours in school. Yet despite this, clinicians traditionally rely almost exclusively on parents (and the children themselves) to gather a behavioral history. Some clinicians send questionnaires to school staff to elicit information, or they ask parents about their children's progress at school or day care. It is rare, however, for clinicians to routinely engage in direct telephone contact with child care providers and teachers. Yet these people occupy many, and occasionally most, of children's waking hours. The value of attaining parental permission to speak directly with educational professionals in a child's life cannot be overstated. Teachers and child care providers can provide valuable insight. Many have numerous years of experience with all types of children, and their observations rarely include the emotional biases that sometimes confound a parent's interpretation and recollection of details. Once a behavior plan has been recommended, a relationship with daytime caretakers may extend the plan's implementation to that setting and render it more effective.

NORMAL CHILD DEVELOPMENT

To attribute an undesirable behavior to a developmental stage of childhood, health care providers need to be knowledgeable about stages of normal childhood development (Table 9–3).

Maturational Theory

This theory teaches that behavioral sequences occur by a process of unfolding in all children, that these sequences are regulated by genes, and that detrimental environmental factors could impede this sequence.

Table 9–2. Samples of "sentence completion" items for interviewing young children.

I really like it when . . .
I am ashamed . . .
I worry a lot about . . .
My mother . . .
I hate . . .
It makes me sad to . . .
It makes me happy to . . .
People think that I . . .
I really hope one day that I . . .

Table 9–3. Highlights of child characteristics during stages of development.

Theory	Ages 0–2	Ages 2–6	Ages 6–12
Kohlberg (Development of moral judgment)	*Premoral Stage* Egocentric, no moral concepts Satisfaction of own needs	*Moral Stage* Desires to please others	*Moral Stage* Obligation to duty Respect for authority
Piaget (Cognitive development)	*Sensorimotor/Preverbal* Emergence of purposeful activities Learns that objects and people exist even when out of sight	*Preoperational/Prelogical* Can deal with one aspect of a problem at a time Learns to use symbols for language, etc	*Concrete Operational/Logical* Can deal with multiple aspects of a problem, if not abstract Ability to classify things
Erickson (Psychosocial development)	*Oral Stage (early on)* Initially gaining trust Once gained, seeks independence Uses words like "no" and "me" *Anal Stage (2nd year)* Initially learns self control Then, can develop self-esteem and good will Learns autonomy but struggles with shame and doubt	*Phallic Stage* Takes initiative, is curious Becomes more aggressive and competitive Starts to plan ahead Struggles with guilt	*Latency Stage* An industrious stage Focused on performance and producing results Struggles with inferiority/ inadequacy when meeting some meritable failures

Freudian Psychoanalytic Theories

Freud's theories emphasize unconscious and conscious mental processes that children go through. For example, in the anal stage at 1½–3 years of age children are personally focused on elimination and interpersonally focused on "rebellion versus compliance" with parental demands. At this stage, they may fear loss of parental love.

Erikson's Stages of Child Development

Erickson's stages are an expanded version of psychoanalytic theory, and his teachings help clinicians understand children's psychosocial development.

Piagetian Theory

Piaget's staging of children's cognitive development describes, for example, that a child cannot be expected to see a situation from a perspective other than his or her own until school age.

Kohlberg's Theory

Kohlberg's theory of children's moral development describes, for example, how young toddlers understand their actions to be good or bad based on the presence or absence of a resulting punishment or reward.

Each of these theories presents a different view of a single multidimensional entity we call "child development." Each describes child development from another perspective. If one theory illuminates a given child's behavior more than another, then try using it to explain an undesirable behavior and to help guide parents toward a proper response.

MANAGEMENT & REFERRAL

Primary care providers must often evaluate and manage common child behavior problems in their own offices. In addition, mental health referrals are usually unnecessary since so many undesirable child behaviors are maladaptations or manifestations of normal child development. There are occasions when the need for psychiatric assessment, psychotherapy, or play therapy is apparent from the start. But for most problems that present to primary care practitioners, children respond well to brief, solution-focused strategies. Although no single behavioral management technique works well for all children with similar problems and similar etiologies to their problems, clinicians can quickly learn to tailor their management plans to suit the individual needs of each family. These plans should be based on families' cultural characteristics, size, work schedules, and other factors. A management failure should always first be considered a problem with the behavioral management technique prescribed, not with the child or family.

PREVENTING SUBSTANCE ABUSE, VIOLENCE, & OTHER MALADAPTIVE BEHAVIORS

Primary care clinicians who treat children have the opportunity and responsibility to intervene during these early years to prevent maladaptive behavior. This prevention can take two forms. First, clinicians can work with individual families and patients as they visit the practice for preventive screens and episodic care. Second, clinicians have the power to help modify the environment in which children spend time in their communities, such as schools, playgrounds, and child care centers. This second role of the primary care clinician is an example of "Community-Oriented Primary Care," which is a model that addresses the emerging roles of current and future health care providers as they evolve to meet changing societal needs. Clinicians can select from several existing preventive theories as they work with children, their families, and communities to thwart the adoption of violence, substance abuse, and self-destructive life-styles in the children's futures. Two are described here.

Emotional Intelligence

Emotional intelligence is defined as the ability to identify one's own feelings, to identify the feelings of others, and to solve problems that involve emotional issues. The extent to which this "intelligence" is innate versus learned is unknown. Although this field is in its infancy, some components of this theory warrant clinicians' attention. For example, parents who provide their child with "tools" to handle emotional challenges may increase the emotional intelligence of their child. By teaching a vocabulary of words that describes emotions, such as "frustrated," "anxious," and "envious," children may become more likely to use them in lieu of acting these behaviors out. Parents are also encouraged to foster an environment in which children will want to describe their feelings. Naturally, this is more easily accepted in theory by parents in your office than at home. Clinicians can ask about specific and recent situations at home that demonstrate the child's personality and point of emotional maturation. By understanding these details, a clinician can offer step-by-step suggestions that are most pertinent to that family's issues and that child's age.

Many classroom programs that are designed to encourage conflict resolution and prevent violence are based on similar theories. Children are taught that anger is an emotion that can be recognized before it is acted upon irrationally. Children discuss and even act out situations that evoke their own anger and those of others. They also learn how to temper these emotions and how to de-escalate a situation. Clinicians have some responsibility to encourage schools and other agencies to make these programs available to children in their neighborhoods.

Developmental Asset Theory

Another preventive theoretical construct is to provide children with a large number of assets in their lives; this will make them less likely to adopt maladaptive behaviors now and in the future. Lists of 40 assets have been developed for various age groups, including preschool and elementary age children. Cumulatively, these assets are purported to foster healthy development (Search Institute, Minneapolis, MN; www.search-institute.org). Examples of assets for school-age children are doing service for others in the community or having a supportive relationship with an adult in addition to their parents. For a preschooler, a parent must also have support from people outside the home.

Despite the early stages of research for this theory, promoting these assets is likely harmless and potentially very beneficial. Clinicians have some opportunity to promote such assets with families in their practices. Moreover, they can help assess the range of opportunities in their communities for children to acquire such assets.

EXAMPLES OF COMMON BEHAVIORAL ISSUES

Infancy: Night Waking

 CASE ILLUSTRATION 1

Parents of a 12-week-old girl complain that their daughter rarely sleeps more than a total of 4–5 hours between 8 P.M. and 6 A.M. She may fall asleep at 8 P.M., only to awaken an hour later. She seems to fall asleep during or after short feeds and then remains awake for hours later on. Each night is a struggle of long awakened periods between short spells of sleep. Her parents note that she cries when left alone. She seems content at night when parents walk around with her.

Child development in early infancy is characterized by large fluctuations in temperament and schedules. In the first few weeks of life, infants often sleep as much during the day as at night. In the first 2 months of life, two night awakenings are common, but by 3 months of life most infants are sleeping for 5–6 hours uninterrupted. In this case, the child did not naturally "learn" the difference between night and day, and parents did not train her to do so. But if clinicians ask parents to let their young infants cry themselves to sleep, they set parents up for feelings of inadequacy or guilt. This, in turn, strains the relationship of attachment that parents are forming with their children.

CASE ILLUSTRATION 1 (CONT.)

On further questioning in this case, the parents reported that their baby falls asleep immediately after daytime feeds and sleeps for 3–5 consecutive hours thereafter. This baby did not adapt to an acceptable or optimal day/night schedule. In this case their doctor recommended waking the baby up after no more than 2–3 hours of daytime sleep. Parents were to try to occupy their infant's daytime hours by walking around, talking, playing music, and offering other playful activities. It was recommended that nighttime feeds be made minimally stimulating: soften the lights, produce minimal noise, and avoid "fun" interactions at night. Although sleeping and feeding "on demand" need not always be discouraged, in this case the infant's pattern needlessly disrupted parents' well-being and this justified modification. After 5–6 days of compliance with this schedule, it became easier for parents to keep their daughter awake during the day and the parents settled for a nighttime feed at 11 P.M. before they retired and another feed at 4 A.M.

It is important to note that likely causes for night awakenings change with developmental stages. This same sleep history told by parents of a 9-month-old child would be more likely related to the child's cognitive ability to recognize that parents still "exist" after they leave the room. At that age, if there were no other likely cause, other recommendations would be in order. A nightlight or a transitional object (favorite blanket or teddy bear) could prove to be helpful. The clinician, in this case, should devise a careful behavioral intervention schedule that includes parental reassurance for the child but may also include an allowance for the child to "cry it out" for a couple of nights.

Toddlers: Aggression

CASE ILLUSTRATION 2

The parent of a 3-year-old boy reports that her son throws himself on the floor, throws objects, and screams . . . usually when he doesn't get his own way. This seems to happen daily. At his child care center,
he has begun to bite other children when he is angry, and other parents have begun to complain about him.

Assessment of this behavior begins with elucidating, through history gathering, the extent of the child's aggression and its likely etiology. Angry outbursts are common at 3 years of age, when children often begin to direct their anger at others. Parental response to a given level of aggression differs widely from family to family. Parental expectations of children's behavior, not solely the magnitude of the child's behavior, help define whether a behavior is a problem. Large discrepancies between childhood behaviors and parental thresholds may predict that a child will continue to be problematic in the future. A child who explores the environment very actively may be described as "curious" in one family but as "always climbing the walls" in another. A "difficult and stubborn" child in one family is "persistent—just like his successful grandpa" in another. Perhaps the more positive perspective creates a better self-image for a child and leads to fewer problems later on.

Certain questions may help clinicians assess the etiology of aggressive behavior: Is the child a cruel or unhappy child? Is the child exposed to frequent violent (physical or verbal) outbursts from others at home? Are the incidents that induce these behaviors unpredictable? Is the child cognitively not acting consistently with his or her age? Positive responses to these questions make a normal developmental etiology less likely.

When development is still the most likely cause, there are a number of possibilities to consider. First, children with well-developed cognitive abilities, but with comparatively delayed language abilities, often become frustrated with limited ways of expressing themselves. Second, children at this stage often strive for adult attention and have found aggressive behaviors to be a certain way of getting it. Third, children at this stage need to express their independence, yet some adults have not found enough acceptable ways to allow the child to do this. To ascertain the likely cause(s), clinicians should explore events surrounding these incidents of aggression. Detailed examples of what instigated the last one or two aggressive behaviors are more revealing than letting the parent say, "Oh it happens for just about anything." Always ask parents how they feel when their child acts out. Feeling like "I just don't have time for this" may be a good indication that the child is trying to get attention. If their first reaction is to feel that this is a power struggle, then the child's strivings for independence may be his or her primary incentive. Also ask what parents have done in response to a misbehavior and whether this reaction worked.

CASE ILLUSTRATION 2 (CONT.)

In this case, the child's degree of aggression was within reason for a child at his developmental stage. His tantrums began as a result of typical frustrations experienced by children his age. Over a period of months as his parent became busier with other family needs, however, he discovered that expressing anger was an excellent way to get adult attention, and the frequency of these behaviors increased. As part of the management plan, his parent was instructed to ignore his anger and put him in his room for a few minutes when he became physically violent with others. Concomitantly, she was to increase time spent doing happier things with him, like playing games, going on walks, and having him help around the house. At day care, he was given increased individual attention during times he was behaving well. Child care providers were asked to ignore him when he attacked other children and to shower a "noticeable" amount of attention on the attacked child. Within a couple of weeks he stopped biting and seemed happier. Although he still had a terrible temper, these strategies gave his mother the feeling that she had some control over the situation.

Toddlers: Oppositional Behavior

CASE ILLUSTRATION 3

A 3-year-old boy refuses to go to bed on time. He prolongs bedtime rituals by making numerous requests (eg, for water, use of bathroom, adjusting the door, etc). He repeatedly leaves his bed. On many nights he finally falls asleep in the living room or his parents' bedroom while spending time with his parents.

CASE ILLUSTRATION 4

A mother solicits your opinion on vitamin supplements to counterbalance her 28-month-old daughter's picky eating habits. She drinks apple juice and eats hot dogs and Honey-Nut Cheerios, and little else. When these foods are not offered, she protests violently and eats nothing.

The behaviors described in these cases are typical for this age group. Toddlers commonly oppose parents for many sorts of issues, including the eating and bedtime cases illustrated here (eg, getting dressed, putting toys away, wearing seat belt, etc). A tendency to challenge parents' instructions subsides naturally as children grow older. But they need to be dealt with properly for those months or years they are present. When parents mistake a child's behavior as a personal offense, they react to the behavior in a way that creates additional conflict and heightens oppositional behavior. Therefore it is important for clinicians to emphasize the developmental component. Children in both illustrative cases have learned to exploit their parents' uncertainty with what exactly is in their child's best interest. In both cases, the clinician should rule out deeper problems by interviewing the parent and, to whatever extent possible, the child. Look for unusual fears, nightmares, and other symptoms that may indicate an unusual etiology to the oppositional behavior. None was found in these two cases.

CASE ILLUSTRATION 3 (CONT.)

In the first case, the pediatrician recommended to the parents that they explain to the child that from now on after his bedtime ritual he must remain in his bedroom whether he is able to sleep or not. They were to routinely ask their child before leaving his bedroom if he needed anything else. Thereafter, if the child cried, screamed, or tried to carry on a conversation with his parents, they were to ignore him. When he left his bed, they were to physically put him back without talking to him and with expressionless faces. They were to do this even in the middle of the night. They were warned that their child's behavior would likely worsen for one or two nights before improving. In less than a week, this boy resigned himself to making only one unenthusiastic, "face-saving" attempt to stay up before he fell asleep.

Parental persistence must be designed to outlast the child's. It is almost always effective within 2 weeks, and often within 2 nights. If this child shared a room with a sibling, it would have been suggested that the sibling sleep in the parents' room until the index child's behavior became less disruptive.

CASE ILLUSTRATION 4 (CONT.)

In the second case, the same principles were applied to other behaviors. The child was offered three whole-

some meals and one snack at preset times of the day. After telling their daughter once, parents were not to engage in any discussion with their child about the volume eaten. No other foods in the house were made available to her during this behavioral management period. Between meals this girl was allowed an unlimited quantity of water, but nothing else. After a difficult period of $1^{1}/_{2}$ days (thrown silverware, persistent crying, etc), she began to nibble at new foods and to enjoy the positive attention for doing so. Although the patient still enjoyed only a limited range of foods, parents were able to expand her repertoire to include broccoli, milk, and pasta.

Parents often worry about harming their child by restricting access to food after a missed meal, so they need to be reassured that this is not harmful and will ultimately improve nutrition. It is all too common for a well-meaning grandparent who resides in the home to "save" the child by sneaking her a cookie between meals (case 4) or lying down with the child after a designated bedtime (case 3). Such kindly motivated behaviors unwittingly prolong the child's maladaptive behavior, extending the period of inadequate nutrition and sleep. It is imperative that clinicians invite all adult household members to their offices when prescribing a management plan to ensure that all involved endorse both the intent and methods. It is useful to write behavioral management "rules" down on a prescription pad to be taped to the refrigerator door. This helps prevent conflict among adult household members that may arise later. Clinicians should also routinely recommend follow-up visits to their offices once the management plan has been implemented to monitor progress.

Toddlers: Toilet Training

Children must be developmentally ready before toilet training is initiated by parents. First, physiological sphincter control is necessary. This usually develops between ages 1 and 2 years, and parents often know when their child is beginning to sense a bowel movement because of a characteristic grimace or stance. The ability to follow sequential instructions, the motivation to imitate parents, and the patience to sit on a potty should also be present. It is reasonable to try toilet training at age 2 years if these milestones have been achieved. But disinterest or undue difficulty should alert parents to terminate their attempt and wait 2–3 months before trying again. Some children may not be ready until age 3. Others are ready at 18 months.

Although a number of effective toilet training methods exist, only one method is described here. Place the potty in the bathroom the child typically uses and explain what it is for by drawing parallels with the toilet parents

use. The child should be encouraged with praise to sit on the potty for a couple of minutes a day, initially with diaper and pants on and after a few days, without them. The child should accompany the parent to empty soiled diapers into the potty. Parents should avoid commenting on the foul odor of the stool, as some children identify what they've produced as extensions of themselves. Gradually, the child should be asked to sit on the potty more frequently during the day, particularly if there is a time when bowel movements are likely to occur. Encourage the child to let the potty "catch" the stool. Parents should never scold a child for an inability to do this or for any "accidents." Night training, standing at urination, and using a larger toilet are secondary skills that should be introduced only after the child has mastered the basics or if the child expresses interest.

School Age: Primary Nocturnal Enuresis

One workable definition for enuresis is at least one bed-wetting incident weekly for a boy older than age 6 or a girl older than age 5. It is considered secondary enuresis if a child had been dry previously for a period greater than 6 months. By this definition, 15% of children have this condition, making it one of the most commonly asked questions of pediatric health care providers. Absence of other urinary tract problems (infection, neurogenic bladder, etc) can be ruled out with a basic medical examination and history. It is important to recognize that the only problems with primary nocturnal enuresis are the reactions of the child and the parent. Otherwise, it is a self-limiting condition that resolves spontaneously. If a child and his or her parents are not bothered by it, then no treatment is necessary. This is worthwhile to point out to families whenever the option for intervention is offered.

To treat this condition, it is necessary that children themselves, not only their parents, are motivated. Verify that a child is truly motivated and determine the source of motivation by interviewing the child separately. When a child is not genuinely motivated to try something new in order to be dry, clinical efforts should be directed toward other family members. Gauge parental actions and anxieties and if necessary influence them so that their actions and anxieties are not causes of unnecessary stress for their child. Children should never be punished for their enuretic disorder. Even if parents insist that their child help to change wet bed sheets, this task should be carried out with the same attitude as other household responsibilities the child has been expected to take on.

Commercially available alarm devices assist clinicians and parents in instituting "conditioning therapy." This method is of clinically proven use. With this device, an alarm awakens the child with the first few drops of urine. Eventually this teaches the child to awaken with the sensation of a full bladder. The child is still responsible to get to the bathroom. The alarm is usually effective when used nightly for a couple of months. Setbacks occur after removing the alarm, but these are often corrected more permanently by one further trial period with the device.

Desmopressin (DDAVP), an analogue of antidiuretic hormone, is a pharmacologic therapy of choice. If children respond to this nasally administered medication they usually do so within 2 weeks. Relapses after withdrawal are not uncommon, however, and this therapy is best offered when the alarm device has failed. Imipramine has also been shown to be useful in certain circumstances. Sphincter control exercises, fluid restrictions in the evening hours, and urine retention training may be tried, but these methods have shown only limited success.

School Age: Attention Deficit Disorders

Unlike the behavioral problems described earlier, attention deficit/hyperactivity disorder (ADHD) is not a manifestation of normal child development but a disorder described in the *Diagnostic and Statistical Manual of Mental Disorders,* 4th edition (*DSM-IV*) of the American Psychiatric Association. It is characterized by inattention or hyperactivity/impulsivity for a period of at least 6 months. Symptoms begin prior to age 7 years. There must be clear evidence of clinically significant impairment in social or academic functioning with some impairment evident in more than one setting. Its diagnosis and management (and misdiagnosis and mismanagement) have become so popularized in the public press that clinicians are sometimes confronted with an unexpectedly emotionally charged situation when the diagnosis is being considered. Many school teachers and parents have strong opinions on both sides of the spectrum, that is, that medications for this disorder are either grossly underprescribed or overprescribed. The American Academy of Pediatrics has prepared two statements on ADHD for the primary care clinician: one that focuses primarily on diagnosis and the other on treatment (see Suggested Readings). The first role of a clinician is to bring a level of pragmatism to the diagnostic process and to the management of the disorder. Clinicians need to carefully explain the rationale behind their investigative and management plans. Some useful strategies are described here.

Often it is classroom problems, not problems at home, that instigate a referral to a health care provider for suspected ADHD. Yet paradoxically little emphasis is placed on establishing direct communication between clinicians and appropriate school staff. Parents should be encouraged to provide consent to exchange such information and be reassured that they will participate at each stage of the process. Most elementary schools have multidisciplinary teams consisting of resource teachers, school psychologists, counselors, and so forth, whose function is to review students with learning or behavior problems. Clinicians are well advised to contact their patient's school to inquire about such teams and then suggest that their patient's case

be presented there. This team's report can save the patient, the parent, and the clinician large amounts of time by avoiding unnecessary investigations. Multidisciplinary school teams provide excellent insight into children's behavior and help to assess the likelihood of an associated or an alternate diagnosis, such as a learning disorder. This strategy is of particular importance economically because diagnoses and effective management occur after fewer office visits, and because third-party payers and managed health care plans frequently do not cover psychological tests to investigate learning disorders.

As with learning disorders, emotional and environmental problems can be mistaken for ADHD, or they may coexist with ADHD but exacerbate the symptoms. Primary care providers can usually fulfill their roles as diagnosticians by conducting thorough patient and family interviews (Table 9–4). Existing published questionnaires

Table 9–4. A differential diagnosis of attention deficits.

Primary

Neurobiologically based
Inherited or secondary to factors affecting early brain development
Dysfunction of varying combinations of neural systems with varying clinical presentations (subtypes)

Secondary

Symptoms secondary to, associated with, or mimicked by
  Cognitive/processing disorder
    Language disorder
    Learning disorder
    Cognitive impairment/mental retardation
  Medical disorder

Neurologic	Metabolic
Seizures	Endocrine
Infections	Toxins
Choreiform disorder	Iron deficiency
Neurodegenerative conditions	Sensory impairment

  Emotional/psychiatric disorders
    Anxiety
    Depression
    Autism
    Personality/behavioral factors
  Environmental factors
    Disruptive/chaotic home situations
    Inappropriate school placement
    Mismatch of neurobehavioral styles and environmental expectations

---

Source: Reprinted, with permission, from Kelly D: Attention deficits in school-aged children and adolescents. Pediatr Clin North Am 1992;39(3):487.

and rating scales simplify the elicitation of histories from educators and parents.

As management is being contemplated, a number of factors need to be considered to enhance parent, child, and school acceptance for the management plan—including medication. It must be explained that ADHD is a chronic condition and that specific outcomes will drive your management. Although stimulant medication has been well researched, it is wise to start the medication on a trial basis only. Some clinicians do this by alternating one week on medication with one week without for a period of a month. Keep the teacher blinded to this regimen, but ask the teacher for weekly feedback. It is reassuring to patients, families, and prescribing physicians when the worth of a medication is demonstrated in this way. Emphasize to patients that medication serves only to help them perform as well as they want. It is important that improvements are attributed to the child's efforts, not only to the medication. Medications should be prescribed only as one part of a larger management plan. Classroom strategies that assist students with attention deficits should be concomitantly implemented. Examples of these are listed in Table 9–5. These are best implemented through strong home–school–clinic communication lines. These techniques are most readily accepted in schools with programs that encourage teachers experienced with students with ADHD to assist teachers who are new to these children. Always follow the child in the context of the expected outcomes. Reconsider both the management choice and the diagnosis if expected outcomes are not achieved. Other diagnoses and/or unaddressed coexisting conditions may be the cause.

CONCLUSION

With the elicitation of a good history and an understanding of child development, primary care clinicians can develop reasonable hypotheses about childhood behavioral problems. Clinicians who manage childhood behavioral problems become very comfortable with a set of behavioral management protocols that can be applied to many common misbehaviors. Most problems of a serious nature that require psychiatric or psychological intervention become apparent early in the process. It is not only cost-effective to avoid unnecessary referrals; assisting families with behavioral issues that arise with their children in the primary care office improves the relationship that families develop with their primary care clinicians.

Table 9–5. Examples of classroom strategies for students with ADHD.[1]

Seat the child close to teacher, or ask the teacher to circulate around classroom near to student.

Teacher should frequently signal student to get on task.

Use signals classmates may not notice (eg, hand on shoulder).

Find enclosed spaces for student to work (cubicles, if possible).

Make frequent topic changes during the day for student (or class as a whole).

Reward progress and effort, not only achievement.

Avoid long written assignments (replace with oral examinations) and have tolerance for poor handwriting.

Break all tasks (tests, assignments, and worksheets) into smaller parts.

Regard inconsistency as part of ADHD, not student attitude.

Devise a behavioral modification plan for classroom behaviors (eg, impulsive behaviors like blurting out answers).

Be prepared to revise behavioral modification techniques frequently (eg, change reinforcements).

Specifically target organizational skills as a learning objective.

Minimize clutter on blackboard, desk, handouts, etc.

---

[1] Attention deficit/hyperactivity disorder.

SUGGESTED READINGS

Benson PL: *All Kids Are Our Kids: What Communities Must Do to Raise Caring and Responsible Children and Adolescents.* Jossey-Bass, 1997.

Committee on Quality Improvement, Subcommittee on Attention-Deficit/Hyperactivity Disorder; Clinical Practice Guideline: Diagnosis and Evaluation of the Child with Attention-Deficit/Hyperactivity Disorder, American Academy of Pediatrics. Pediatrics 2000;105(5):1158.

Glascoe F, Dworkin P: The role of parents in the detection of developmental and behavioral problems. Pediatrics 1995;95:829.

Green M (editor): *Bright Futures: Guidelines for Health Supervision of Infants, Children, and Adolescents.* National Center for Education in Maternal and Child Health, 1994.

Longlett SK, Kruse JE, Wesley RM: Community-oriented primary care: critical assessment and implications for resident education. J Am Board Family Pract 2001;14(2):141.

Mayer JD, Salovey P, Caruso, DR: *Models of Emotional Intelligence.* In: Sternberg RJ (editor): *Handbook of Human Intelligence,* 2nd ed. Cambridge University Press, 2000.

Nevin JE, Gohel MM: Community-oriented primary care.

Primary Care; Clin Office Pract 1996;23(1):1.

Roehlkepartain JL, Leffert N: *A Leader's Guide to What Young Children Need to Succeed; Working Together to Build Assets from Birth to Age 11.* Free Spirit Publishing, Inc., 2000.

Stancin T, Palermo TM: A review of behavioral screening practices in pediatric settings: do they pass the test? Dev Behav Pediatr 1997;18(3):183.

WEB SITES

American Academy of Pediatrics: "You and Your Family"
http://www.aap.org/family/

"Kids Health for Parents"
http://kidshealth.org/parents/emotions/

National Library of Medicine: "Child and Teen Health Topics"
http://www.nlm.nih.gov/medlineplus/childandteenhealth.htm/

Adolescents

Lawrence S. Friedman, MD

INTRODUCTION

This chapter offers a practical behavioral framework to assist those who provide health care to teenagers. Stages of adolescent development along with behavioral correlates are discussed, and suggestions for effective patient–doctor communication, interviewing, and provision of health services are presented.

DEFINITION

Adolescence is not a disease. From a physiological perspective, adolescence is the interval between the onset of puberty and the cessation of body growth. Because *physical change* does not adequately describe cognitive, emotional, psychological, or behavioral development, a purely physiological definition is too confining. In psychosocial terms, adolescence is the period during which adult body image and sexual identity emerge; independent moral standards, intimate interpersonal relationships, vocational goals, and health behaviors develop; and the separation from parents takes place. Ultimately, this should lead to a firm sense of individual identity, self-esteem, and community attachment. Although some of these tasks may begin prior to puberty and continue evolving into adulthood, they provide the foundation for understanding adolescent behavior.

Health Status & Trends

Most teenagers are healthy. Compared with other age groups, mortality rates for teenagers are low. Even teenagers with serious chronic illness usually survive into early or middle adulthood. The majority of serious health problems in this population are behavior related. They include unwanted pregnancy; sexually transmitted diseases; weapon carrying; interpersonal violence; suicidal ideation; alcohol, cigarette, and illicit drug use; and dietary patterns. Nationally, accidents are the leading cause of death for most populations of teenagers, although homicide (mostly gang related) leads in some geographic locations. Socioeconomic status and population density, rather than ethnic or racial grouping, define the neighborhoods most at risk for gunshot deaths. Despite these significant problems, however, the most common reasons for acute office

visits for teenagers are routine or sports physicals, upper respiratory infections, and acne. Eliciting a history leading to health risk behaviors requires provider skill and motivation. Traditionally, health care resources have been allocated for established diseases rather than prevention. Because most adolescent mortality and morbidity are preventable and because many behaviors such as sexual practices, diet, exercise, and substance use that result in adult disease begin in adolescence, ignoring this age group means missing a major public health opportunity.

In 1992, the American Medical Association produced the first set of developmentally and behaviorally appropriate comprehensive health-care guidelines for adolescents. These guidelines emphasize anticipatory, preventive, and patient-centered services. They suggest that promotion of adolescent health and prevention of disease involves a partnership encompassing patients, parents, schools, communities, and health-care providers. Although these guidelines have existed for nearly a decade, have been well disseminated, and have been shown to be valuable as care standards and as quality measures, there is little evidence that they are being widely implemented.

Adolescent health outcomes—perhaps more than for any other population—are closely linked to cultural, educational, political, and economic policies. Handguns and tobacco are both relevant examples. For example, the availability of handguns is not a problem that the physician can resolve during an office visit, yet making them less available would substantially benefit the health of many teenagers. Many more teenagers would never begin using tobacco if cigarette prices were significantly higher and advertising were not designed to attract teenagers. There is compelling evidence that teenagers who feel connected to parents, school, and community are less likely to participate in health-compromising behavior than teens who feel isolated or disconnected.

STAGES OF DEVELOPMENT

Medical services for teenagers need to be developmentally appropriate. Each of the three recognized developmental stages in adolescence is distinguished by physical, cognitive, and behavioral hallmarks. Not all adolescents fit perfectly into each phase, and they often progress at different rates from one phase to the next. In addition, rates of physical, cognitive, and behavioral development may not be congruent. For example, a 14-year-old girl who is physically mature may be emotionally unable to decide about sexual intimacy and the consequences of pregnancy—or even its possibility.

Early Adolescence (Ages 11–14)

PHYSICAL

Rapid growth causes physical and body-image changes. Many teenagers question whether their growth is "normal," and commonly there is a good deal of somatic preoccupation and worry. Gynecomastia, for example (a common transient problem for boys), may cause anxiety and concern, and prevent participation in physical education class. Because the topic may be too embarrassing for an already self-conscious teenager to raise, physician-initiated reassurance is essential when the condition is identified during a physical examination. Early or later onset of puberty has widely variable effects. Early puberty may be associated with the increased likelihood of weight concern and excessive dieting and other eating disorders in girls, but it may result in greater self-esteem and athletic prowess in boys. Because self-esteem is linked closely with physical development and peer-group attractiveness, teens who develop later than their peers may have self-esteem problems. Among early adolescents, questions and concerns about menstruation, masturbation, wet dreams, and the size of their breasts (too large or too small) and genitals are common. These questions need to be anticipated and specifically and carefully addressed. Endocrine disorders related to sexual maturation are likely to emerge; early diagnosis and treatment will improve self-esteem.

SOCIAL

Peer-group involvement increases, and family involvement decreases. Friendships are idealized and are mostly same gender. Close peer relationships coupled with curiosity about body development may result in homosexual and other sexual experimentation, anxiety, and fear. Although some heterosexual relationships are initiated, contact with the opposite sex frequently occurs in groups.

COGNITIVE

The transition from concrete to abstract thinking begins. Because experience and emotion play important roles in decision making, improved cognition alone is not enough to prevent many teenagers from making impulsive decisions with little regard for consequences. Increased cognitive ability linked with the search for identity often leads teenagers to test limits both at home and at school. Daydreaming is common.

Middle Adolescence (Ages 15–17)

PHYSICAL

The issues of early adolescence may continue, although most physical development is complete by the end of this phase.

SOCIAL

The struggles involving independence, identity, and autonomy intensify. Peer groups may become more important than family to some teenagers and result in increasing teen–parent conflict. Experimentation with alcohol, drugs, and sex is common. A sense of invincibility coupled with impulsiveness leads to high rates of automobile accidents and interpersonal violence. Unfortunately, suicide, impulsively linked to failed love relationships, or poor self-esteem because of difficulty finding peer group acceptance also occurs during this phase. Despite adhering to peer-group norms regarding music, dress, and appearance (including body piercing, hair color, and makeup), the expression of individuality is common. Many teenagers find identity and support in school, sports, community, or church activities. For teenagers whose support systems or community resources are inadequate, gangs may supplement personal strength and provide a sense of identity. Teenagers from alienated and disenfranchised ethnic groups are at particular risk for gang activity.

COGNITIVE

Improved reasoning and abstraction allow for closer interpersonal relationships and empathy in this group. Evaluation of future academic and vocational plans becomes important. Poor school performance may heighten anxiety and concern about vocational choices and lead to "escape" in drugs and alcohol. Practical guidance that identifies strengths and builds self-esteem can help avoid frustration and failure.

Late Adolescence (Ages 18–24)

PHYSICAL

Body growth is usually no longer a concern. The quest to become comfortable with one's physical appearance, however, usually continues throughout adulthood.

SOCIAL

If the adolescent's development has occurred within the context of a supportive family, community, school, and peer environment, individual identity formation and separation will be complete. In reality, however, at least some developmental issues usually remain unresolved into adulthood. Late adolescents typically spend more time developing monogamous interpersonal relationships and less time seeking peer-group support. Ideally, decision making, based on an individualized value system, is mediated by setting of limits and compromise.

COGNITIVE

Vocational goals are now set in practical terms, and there should be realistic expectations about education and work.

ADOLESCENTS & THE MEDICAL INTERVIEW

Flexibility and a sense of humor may be the most important qualities of the interviewer. A general health assessment should include a review of systems and an evaluation of health-related behavior, such as risk factors for accidents; sexually transmitted diseases (STDs), including human immunodeficiency virus (HIV); pregnancy; interpersonal violence (including past physical or sexual abuse); diet; substance use; exercise; learning; and mental health problems. Guidance about promoting healthful behaviors and preventing disease should be integrated into the discussion. From the patient's perspective, the provider's inquiries and assessment of some behaviors may be viewed as embarrassing, intrusive, or trivial. It is therefore helpful to explain, prior to questioning, that (1) the same questions are asked of all patients and that (2) the encounter goal is patient self-awareness and education. This preamble is especially reassuring to teenagers, who are usually preoccupied with their bodies. During the interview it is important to reinforce healthy decisions, such as sexual abstinence, with praise.

Confidentiality

Certain ground rules are important. Ensure the adolescent that, unless homicide or suicide is threatened or ongoing abuse is reported, all conversations are confidential, and the information will not be shared with parents, teachers, or other authorities without permission. Discussions about sex and drugs should always occur in private unless otherwise requested by the patient. If the patient is accompanied by a parent, solicit parental concerns, then ask the adult to leave the room and conduct the interview in private.

Although teenagers want to receive information and discuss sexual behavior, pregnancy prevention, AIDS prevention, and substance use, these discussions must generally be initiated by the physician. Most teenagers are not accustomed to interacting in such participatory conversations with adults. The willingness of a teenager to share personal or intimate information depends on the perceived receptiveness of the provider. Teenagers need to feel that they have permission to share this type of information. For example, it is usually not difficult for patients and providers to discuss routine chronic medical conditions such as diabetes or asthma. Control of these conditions in some teenagers, however, may be related

more to dietary indiscretions and marijuana or cigarette consumption, respectively, than to insulin or inhaler use. Such health-compromising behaviors must be identified before they can be dealt with; comments, facial expressions, or body language indicating disapproval can undermine the patient's willingness to disclose confidential behavior (Table 10–1).

Legal Issues

Many practitioners worry about the legality of evaluating and treating teenagers without parental consent. Because laws vary by state, it is important to become familiar with the applicable local statutes. Almost all states permit the diagnosis and treatment of teenagers with sex, drug-, and alcohol-related problems without parental notification or consent. Likewise, most states also permit medical care to be provided to teenagers if the condition is potentially life-threatening. In reality, because it is often impossible to determine whether a condition is potentially life-threatening until after taking the history and performing a physical examination, there is usually some legal leeway in this area. For instance, it is easy to justify evaluating a 15-year-old girl with abdominal pain, because, until determined otherwise, the pain may be from an ectopic pregnancy.

The Interview Organization

A comprehensive health-risk assessment should cover issues concerning Home, Education, Activities, Drug use,

Table 10–1. Suggestions for dealing with adolescents.

---

1. Ensure doctor–patient confidentiality. Don't inquire about health-related behaviors in front of parents.
2. Use the HEADSS format to organize the interview.
3. Assess the patient's cognitive and developmental level through interactive dialogue.
4. Initiate discussions about behavior and offer anticipatory guidance that is culturally and developmentally appropriate.
5. Listen actively to patients' opinions and perspective.
6. Be familiar with and refer to local resources for cases of domestic violence, runaways, and substance abuse.
7. Include patients in discussing and making all diagnostic and therapeutic decisions.
8. Review the behavioral stages of development with parents. Emphasize the importance of instilling confidence and building self-esteem in their children.
9. Reinforce good behavior. Congratulate teenagers who do not use drugs and who are not sexually active.
10. Address all teenagers with respect, and be nonjudgmental about their behaviors and traits.

Sexual practices, and Suicidal ideation (HEADSS). Using the HEADSS format helps with organization and standardization. Assessing cognitive ability, using interactive dialogue, needs to be done in the first few minutes of the interview. The following interview goals and questions facilitate communication.

HOME

1. Goal—Determine the family's structure and function, its conflict-resolution skills, the possibility of domestic violence, and the presence of chronic illness in the family (see Chapter 8).

2. Questions—"Who lives where you live?" If only one parent is at home, the interviewer should inquire about the other parent's whereabouts, visitation pattern, and reasons for leaving (especially domestic violence and substance abuse) and whether the teen moves back and forth between parents. Teenagers caught between divorced parents or those who feel neglected may "act out" and get into trouble to gain parental attention, sometimes in the hope that their problems will reunite separated parents. For single-parent families, the patient can be asked, "Does your mom or dad date? How do you get along with the people he or she dates?" Questions about domestic violence should include "What happens when people argue in your house?" and "Does anyone get hurt during arguments? How about you?" and "What if someone has been drinking or using drugs and they argue?" and "Have you ever seen your mother hit by anyone?" Ask about siblings, including their health and whereabouts. Somatization may be learned by observing a family member who receives attention for a chronic medical condition.

EDUCATION

1. Goal—Identify attention deficit hyperactivity disorder (ADHD) and other learning disabilities, and evaluate the patient's declining grades (if applicable), cognitive ability, and vocational potential.

2. Questions—"What grade are you in?" "What type of grades do you get?" "How do they compare with your grades last year?" Falling grades may indicate family, mental health, or substance-abuse problems. "Have you ever been told you had a learning problem?" "Can you see the blackboard?" Most teenagers respond that everything in school is okay. Specific questions about courses and content need to be asked, including the student's favorite and worst subjects and his or her career aspirations. Generally, teenagers who perform well in school are less likely to participate in multiple risk behaviors. The physician should ask about attendance, and truancy or other school troubles. Teenagers with chemical dependency may enjoy going to school because, although they may rarely attend class, school is where they can visit friends and purchase drugs. Students who get all "A's" should be asked about school-

related stress and what would happen if they didn't receive high grades. Some suicides are related to unrealistic grade expectations by teenagers and their parents.

ACTIVITIES

1. Goal—Evaluate the patient's social interactions, interests, and self-esteem.

2. Questions—"What do you do for fun?" "Are you involved in school, community, or religious activities, such as youth groups, clubs, or sports?" Self-esteem is often related to successful participation in these activities. Teenagers actively involved in "productive" activities are less likely to participate in delinquent behavior. The clinician should ask about gang or fraternity or sorority membership, either of which can be a source of inappropriate peer pressure. Gangs may provide the strongest sense of family or community that is available to some teenagers.

Questions should be asked about dietary habits, including the frequency and amount of "junk" food, who cooks, and dieting or self-induced vomiting (see Chapter 19). It is also important to inquire about patients' physical activities and to educate them and make recommendations about regular exercise.

DRUGS

1. Goal—Evaluate the patient's current habits and patterns of use and the genetic or environmental risk factors (Table 10–2). Distinguish those who drink because of social, cultural, and peer pressure from those who are genetically predisposed and from those who drink or use illicit drugs because of comorbid mental health problems.

2. Questions—It is less threatening to begin by asking, "Are you aware of alcohol or drug use at your school?" and "Do any of your friends drink or use drugs?" followed by "Have you ever tried alcohol or drugs?" The physician should inquire specifically about cigarettes, alcohol, marijuana, "pills" (ecstacy, ketamine, etc.), cocaine, LSD, crystal methamphetamine, anabolic steroids, and heroin. The quantity, frequency, circumstances, and family patterns of use are important. To learn about family drinking, ask specific questions about each parent and both maternal and paternal grandparents, including whether anyone in the family attends Alcoholics Anonymous (AA) or other

Table 10–2. Substance-abuse risk factors for adolescents.

1. Family history of use
2. Low self-esteem and body image
3. Depression or thought disorder
4. Antisocial personality traits
5. Peer and cultural pressures

self-help groups. When parents do not recognize or admit to a problem, a child may not identify them as "alcoholics." The teenager should be asked to describe the parent's pattern of alcohol use. "Have you ever seen your mother or father drunk?" If the answer is yes, "When and how frequently?"

Recognition of a parental problem is essential. Even the best treatment program will fail if a teenager is discharged back into the home of an actively using parent. The willingness of parents to change either their own drinking or family behavior patterns is one of the best predictors of adolescent treatment success.

Among many teenagers, the use of drugs and alcohol is often not considered abnormal or dangerous. In fact, only 5–10% of teenage drinkers or drug users develop substance-abuse problems as adults. Because serious physical consequences, other than accidents, usually do not occur until later in life, there is little negative association with alcohol or drug use. Abused, neglected, disabled, or chronically ill teenagers may consider drugs or alcohol one of the few things that, at least temporarily, make them feel good. If legal involvement, school problems, or family conflict are present, it is important to assess the role of alcohol and drugs. Even if use seems minimal, it should be pointed out that problems are best solved sober.

Referral to a substance-abuse expert is indicated when use significantly interferes with school, family, or social functioning. Frequently, all aspects of the teenager's life are negatively affected by significant abuse or dependency. Anticipatory guidance should address age-appropriate concerns. Advising teenagers to stop smoking cigarettes because of the possibility of future lung cancer and heart disease is meaningless to most of them. Talking about wrinkled skin, bad breath, and yellow teeth is much more relevant to body-image concerns and far more likely to prevent or stop cigarette use. Similarly, the association between alcohol and date rape is more important to teenage girls than are other far-off consequences.

Sex

1. Goal—Determine the level of the patient's sexual involvement and sexuality, use of birth control, protection against STDs, and any history of abuse.

2. Questions—An opening question such as "Have you ever been sexually involved with anyone?" is preferable to "Are you sexually active?" The word *active* is notoriously misinterpreted. Questions need to be open-ended and should not assume heterosexual orientation. Assumptions about boyfriends or girlfriends inhibit discussion or questions about homosexual partners or feelings. Because teenagers frequently practice serial monogamy, the sequential number of different partners and their ages should be determined. A 15-year-old teenager with a peer-group partner is at less risk for STDs, especially HIV, than

is one with a substantially older partner. Most HIV infection in teenage girls is through contact with older intravenous drug-using partners. For the sexually involved, discuss birth control techniques and condoms. One of the most common reasons for not using a condom is the belief that birth control pills provide adequate protection against STDs. Many teenage boys report using condoms to prevent partner pregnancy rather than out of concern about STDs. The physician, however, should not expect every teenager to be sexually experienced and should reinforce sexual abstinence with congratulations and support.

Sexual abuse is unfortunately common, and a history of sexual abuse should be sought by asking, "Have you ever been touched sexually when you did not want to be?" Obtaining this history may be pivotal in helping a teenager who has developed abuse-related behavioral problems, such as sexual promiscuity, depression, substance abuse, delinquency, or an eating or a somatization disorder.

Although in decline over the past decade, teenage pregnancy is still at epidemic proportions. Risk factors are complex but include ignorance, lack of access to family-planning services, cultural acceptance, and poor self-esteem. Some girls fantasize that having a child will heighten their self-esteem and ensure their getting attention.

Suicide

1. Goal—Identify serious mental health problems and distinguish them from normal adolescent affect and moodiness. Primary risk factors are listed in Table 10–3.

Distinguishing significant psychiatric disease from normal fluctuations in a teenager's affect is challenging. In spite of the general perception to the contrary, most teenagers are not maladjusted, and the rates of mental health problems are no higher than in adults. Few teenagers announce that they are feeling depressed or are in emotional turmoil. Depression is instead often reflected in sexual promiscuity, in drug and alcohol abuse, or in the commission of violent and delinquent acts. Chronic somatic complaints such as headache, abdominal pain, or chest pain without an identifiable biological explanation may also indicate depression.

Table 10–3. Risk factors for major depression and suicide.

1. Prior episode of serious depression or suicide
2. Family history of suicide or mental health problems
3. History of victimization
4. Substance abuse or dependency
5. Gay or lesbian sexual identity
6. Availability of handguns (increases rate of success)
7. Recent loss of significant friends or family
8. Extreme family, school, or social stress

2. Questions—The physician should identify vegetative signs of depression, such as sleep disturbance, decreased appetite, hopelessness, lethargy, continuous thoughts about suicide, hallucinations, or illogical thoughts. It should also be noted that many of these symptoms may also be caused by substance abuse. Evaluation of lethargy should be done from the patient's perspective. Energy may be low relative to the parents' desires or expectations—but sufficient for the teenager. There may be insufficient energy to clean, help with household chores, or complete homework but plenty of energy available to play sports, go on a date, party with friends, or travel miles and wait for hours to obtain concert tickets.

CASE ILLUSTRATION 1

Two days after being injured in a traffic accident, Jeff, a 16-year-old teenager, comes to the physician's office complaining of left shoulder pain. He is accompanied by his mother, who is concerned because Jeff was recently arrested for driving under the influence of alcohol. There is no history of medical or behavioral problems, although, on questioning, his mother describes a 12-month history of moodiness and falling school grades. Using the HEADDS format assessment, the physician assesses Jeff's health risks:

Home: Jeff lives at home with his biological mother and father. The parents are first-generation immigrants who both work full-time. There are few arguments at home, and Jeff describes both parents as stoic, religious, and unemotional.

Education: Although he was an above-average student until last year, Jeff's education is now being adversely affected by his truancy and lack of interest.

Activity: Although Jeff previously played several sports at school, watching television is now his favorite activity.

Drugs: Jeff admits to using drugs frequently. He drinks alcohol at least twice a week and smokes marijuana on the other five days. Since this use is no more frequent than that of his friends, he does not consider it excessive.

Sex: Jeff has no steady sexual partners, but he has had several short-term relationships.

Suicide: Jeff denies being suicidal or depressed. When asked about significant losses, however, he becomes tearful and talks hesitantly about his older brother, a construction worker, who died accidentally 2 years ago. Since the religious burial, his brother was never talked about at home.

The connection between increased substance use, declining grades, and the brother's death seems obvious. Because the substance use began insidiously, and significant trouble did not occur until more than a year after his brother's death, neither Jeff nor his parents associated the events. Furthermore, this is a family that does not share emotions, and Jeff never learned how to discuss his feelings. In this case, simply learning about his drug use, home situation, school performance, and activities was not enough. The facts all confirmed his substance abuse but did not explain it. With a teenager who previously has been without significant behavioral problems, it is crucial to search for personal or family events, including losses, that underlie and precipitate the change in behavior.

Both Jeff and his parents must be made aware of the connection between the substance use and the brother's death. It is imperative that Jeff acknowledge his drug problem and be referred to a practitioner experienced in treating adolescents with substance-abuse problems (see Chapter 20). Although Jeff should respond to psychotherapy that addresses his grief and loss, psychotherapy may not be effective if mind-altering substances are being used, and their discontinuation must be emphasized.

SPECIFIC AT-RISK POPULATIONS

Homeless & Runaway Teenagers

There is a heterogeneous group of between 500,000 and 2 million homeless teenagers in the United States. Some are homeless because their families are homeless, some live on the streets for brief periods of time, and others find shelter with friends or relatives. Runaways who leave home, do not return, and no longer depend on parents for financial support or shelter constitute a significant proportion and may be more precisely called *throwaways*. Before they leave home, these teenagers have usually had repeated contacts with social service agencies and have histories of severe parental conflict and high rates of physical and sexual abuse. Family abandonment because of sexual orientation is not uncommon. The social network designed to protect them has failed, and their experience of neglect, abuse, and abandonment results in a distrust of adults and institutions.

Leaving home and living on the streets may initially be a liberating experience. Once on the street, multiple substance use is common, often becoming a short-term pleasant escape from an otherwise dismal existence. Survival often depends on trading sex for drugs, food, or shelter. Other survival techniques, such as selling drugs and theft, create risks for interpersonal violence and victimization. Poor self-esteem, depression, and suicidal ideation are common in this group. Usually—within weeks or months— the liberating experience of independence becomes one of desperation and hopelessness.

The initial medical evaluation may seem overwhelming. Most of these patients qualify for emancipated-minor legal status and may be eligible for Medicaid or other entitlements. Distrust of adults, the inability to navigate a complicated health system, and reluctance to disclose personal information may, however, keep them from receiving benefits and proper health care. It is important for the provider to prioritize such a patient's health issues and be familiar with community referral sources. Shelter, food, safety, social support, substance-abuse and mental health counseling, and medical evaluation are all usually necessary. Developing a trusting working relationship is essential and may require several visits. Keeping medical appointments and complying with referrals may be complicated by a reversed sleep–wake cycle. As with other teenagers, questions about sex and drugs are best kept in a medical context; it should be made clear that they are raised solely because of their health implications. Rather than asking whether a teenager has been a "prostitute," asking, "Have you ever had sex in order to obtain drugs, food, or a place to sleep?" is nonjudgmental and will be readily understood. Questions about sexual orientation may be confusing to a teenager with a history of sexual abuse and survival sex and may provoke anxiety and shame. These issues are best raised after a stable living situation and support system have been established. Runaway youth exist in every community, and they seem to be increasing in both number and diversity. Health-care providers must support local and national efforts to reverse this disastrous national trend.

Chronic Disease & Disability

At least 2 million teenagers in the United States have chronic disabilities or diseases. Although this is a diverse group, its members share some similar behavioral issues. Unlike other teenagers whose identity and self-esteem are molded by the acceptance of their peer group, chronically ill or disabled teenagers have a limited ability to conform and often suffer poor self-esteem. Too frequently this leads to depression, family conflict, and social isolation.

Concerns—like those of other teenagers—usually revolve around physical, social, and sexual development. Frank discussions, including realistic assessments of their hopes and expectations, need to be initiated by the physician. It is crucial to identify and encourage the interests and skills that may realistically be expected to strengthen self-esteem and lead to peer recognition and companionship. Predictors of successful coping include friendships with healthy as well as ill or disabled peers, parents who are not overly protective, involvement with family activities, and appropriate household responsibilities.

Chronically ill teenagers are often "noncompliant" with medical regimens. Adolescence is no less a time of experi-

mentation, self-discovery, and testing of limits for the chronically ill teen than for other teens, and chronically ill teenagers—like other teenagers (and many adults)—are often noncompliant. Issues about compliance are often issues about control and of testing of limits. The struggle for independence runs head first into the limitations placed by the disability as well as those placed by parents and health-care providers. Table 10–4 lists some suggestions for ways of improving compliance.

Gay & Lesbian Youth

Gay and lesbian teenagers are at risk for social isolation, depression, STDs (including HIV), substance abuse, and interpersonal violence. The relationships they develop with their health-care providers may help avoid the severe negative stereotyping they will receive from many parts of society. A nonjudgmental and supportive attitude helps lessen the weight of such cultural negativity.

Although some teenagers may volunteer information about their homosexual concerns or ideation, many do not unless they are specifically asked or "given permission to do so." Some teens may have feelings of anxiety, shame, and guilt about same-sex experiences. Such experiences are common, especially among young adolescents who have not yet recognized a sexual identity, and do not necessarily reflect sexual orientation. The risk of HIV infection increases when gay teenage boys have older partners, who themselves may often have had multiple partners and may

Table 10–4. Strategies for improving compliance.

1. Have patients participate in all therapeutic and diagnostic decisions.
2. Discuss developmentally appropriate consequences of noncompliance. For instance, the renal or neurologic complications of poor diabetes control will not seem very important to a 14-year-old teenager. Emphasize the positive instead—such as how proper glucose control will allow continued participation in sports and other peer activities.
3. Parents need guidance on how to balance protectiveness with their teenager's need to make independent decisions. Role-playing in specific scenarios may be helpful.
4. When possible, communicate directly with the patient without using the parent as a conduit. Let patients know that their opinions and questions are important.
5. Refer patients and parents to local peer support groups such as diabetes, asthma, and epilepsy societies. Support groups exist for almost all chronic illnesses and can usually be found through local telephone directories or agencies such as United Way.

Table 10–5. Recommendations for addressing needs of gay or lesbian youth.

---

1. Assess the patient's level of comfort and self-acceptance.
2. Evaluate and discuss external stressors, such as parents, school, and the patient's social and religious environment. Refer the patient (and parents, if necessary) to mental health experts if the stressors are severe and interfere with daily activities.
3. Reassure the patient that from a medical perspective, homosexuality is a normal variant like left-handedness.
4. Refer patients to local gay youth groups for peer support; most cities and colleges provide resources for lesbian and gay youth, and telephone directories usually list local resources. Refer parents to local parent support groups, especially the local chapter of Parents and Friends of Lesbian and Gay Youth (P-FLAG).

---

provide easier access to alcohol and drugs. Table 10–5 lists some suggestions for working with gay and lesbian youth.

SUGGESTED READINGS

Bethell C, Klein J, Peck C: Assessing health system provision of adolescent preventive services: The Young Adult Health Care Survey. Med Care 2001;39(5):478. PMID: 11317096.

Centers for Disease Control and Prevention: Youth Risk Behavior Surveillance—United States. MMRW 2000;49(SS05):1.

Dixon SD, Stein MT: *Encounters with Children: Pediatric Behavior and Development,* 3rd ed. Mosby, 2000.

Elster AB, Kuznets NJ (editors): *AMA Guidelines for Adolescent Preventive Services (GAPS).* Williams & Wilkins, 1994.

Emans SJ, Laufer MR, Goldstein DP: *Pediatric and Adolescent Gynecology,* 4th ed. Little, Brown, 1998.

Friedman SB et al (editors): *Comprehensive Adolescent Health Care,* 2nd ed. WB Saunders, 1998.

Newacheck PW et al: Adolescent health insurance coverage: recent changes and access to care. Pediatrics 1999;104(2):195. PMID: 10428994.

WEB SITES

American Academy of Pediatrics: position papers on adolescent health
www.pediatrics.org

Society for Adolescent Medicine: official position papers on multiple relevant topics
www.adolescenthealth.org

Older Patients

Clifford Milo Singer, MD, Linda Ganzini, MD, & Stephen R. Jones, MD

INTRODUCTION

We are an aging society. By the year 2020, one in five Americans will be over the age of 65, compared to a little over one in eight today. The number of oldest old, those over 85, is increasing rapidly; these frequently frail patients can make up large proportions of primary care practices. Providing optimal care to these patients requires special knowledge of normal aging and common diseases of old age.

Although temperament (ie, energy, intensity, reactivity) remains remarkably stable throughout adult life, personality (learned behavior patterns) undergoes refinement and change over time in most healthy adults. Mental illnesses and neurodegenerative diseases take their toll, but the majority of elderly persons actively continue to seek pleasure, to be curious, and to learn throughout their lives. Predictable changes in intellect occur in most people as they age. Although judgment, knowledge, and verbal skills increase through the lifespan, mental functions relying on memory and processing speed are adversely affected by aging.

Successful adaptation to old age is difficult to define and is variably expressed. Signs of successful aging that clinicians might notice include acceptance of change, affectionate relationships with family and friends, and a positive view of one's life story. Another indicator might be the ability to find new sources of self-esteem independent of raising children, career, physical strength, or beauty. Factors that promote successful adaptation are luck (good genes, avoiding injury), good health behaviors, enough money for basic needs, a culture that values old people, available confidants, strong kinship and extended family bonds, and, for many people, spirituality. Opportunities to be productive and assist younger generations often provide a sense of connection to one's community and a feeling of completeness. Conditions that contribute to demoralization in old age include highly mobile and rapidly changing communities, youth-oriented aesthetics, the deaths of friends and family members, and forced retirement.

Declining hygiene, poor nutrition, falls, alcohol abuse, social withdrawal, chaotic finances, and denial of severe health problems are clues that an older person is failing at home because of diminishing physical, emotional, or intellectual function. Recognizing these problems can be difficult. Health care practitioners may not detect problems if older patients are reclusive, try to look their best in the office, or avoid discussion of problems they face functioning at home. Often it is family members, friends, neighbors, and others who first recognize a person's functional decline. Their impressions can be very helpful to the clinician.

Elderly patients experience obstacles to obtaining medical care. They may also deliberately avoid seeking help, particularly for emotional and cognitive problems. People in the current older generations may not view emotional distress as something to discuss with physicians. They suffer silently or disguise their distress with physical symptoms or irritability and withdrawal from family, friends, or caregivers. Unfortunately, the prejudicial attitudes of physicians and mental health providers about mental and emotional problems in old age play into this silence and contribute to the underrecognition and treatment of these disorders. Clinicians may be reluctant to prescribe treatment for problems viewed as inevitable parts of aging or they may simply consider treatment to be futile.

Providing expert medical care to elderly patients requires an understanding of normal changes in mental and emotional functioning in old age and skill in determining when intervention is needed. Addressing the concerns of family and caregivers, accessing community services, and advising patients about end-of-life and long-term care options all require sensitivity and skill. Diagnosing mental disorders in older people is challenging as multiple clinical syndromes—including both mental and medical—often overlap. Given a basic knowledge of clinical geriatrics, time to adequately assess symptoms, strategic use of all sources of information, and a sense of optimism in treating chronic disease, clinicians can provide substantial help to their older patients and ample gratification for themselves.

Case Examples

CASE ILLUSTRATION 1

Martha is an 87-year-old woman who never married and who lives alone in her own home, as she has for 48 years. Her doctor is a family physician who has been asked to see Martha by her niece Joanne, a current patient. Martha's sister (Joanne's mother) died not long ago and was the only person with whom Martha had significant contact in recent years.

Joanne tells the doctor that she recently went to see her aunt and was appalled by her living conditions. Martha had more than 20 cats, many of whom appeared sick. The house reeked of cat urine and the entire first floor was full of trash and newspapers. Cat food, soda pop, cookies, canned spaghetti, and candy bars were the only food in the house. Although the house had gas, electricity, and running water, there was no phone service. Unpaid bills, bank statements, a social security check, and some cash were stuffed into a coffee can in the kitchen sink.

The following week, Joanne brings her aunt to the doctor's office. Martha is a thin, disheveled, and foul-smelling woman with poor dentition. She shakes the doctor's hand and comments pleasantly on how nicely she has been treated by the office staff. She has not seen a physician in 30 years and has no physical complaints. She cooperates with the physical examination that reveals she is 5 feet 4 inches tall and weighs 82 pounds. Her blood pressure is 180/98. The remainder of the neurological and physical examination is unremarkable. Her blood work is normal except for a hematocrit of 30 and an albumin of 3.0.

The doctor asks Martha how she is managing at home. This seems to irritate her, and as he is about to proceed with a mental status examination, she politely but firmly states that the interview is complete, that she feels fine, and she has no need for his services. She dresses herself and says she will be sitting outside in the waiting room. When she is out of earshot, Joanne says, "See what I mean? Even when she was young she was off and now she's totally unreasonable. Can you help me get her into a nursing home?"

The doctor must now consider what other information is needed to determine whether Martha has a mental disorder and how different diagnoses would affect his approach to the situation. Some important issues need to be addressed: Can Martha safely remain in her home? What else does the doctor need to know about her cognitive function? What is Joanne's role?

CASE ILLUSTRATION 2

Mr. and Mrs. J. have been patients in this internal medicine practice for several years. Mr. J., a retired engineer, is 89 years old. Mrs. J., also 89, is a retired teacher who until recently had volunteered as a church secretary. In their retirement they have been very active, particularly in church-related activities. The couple has two daughters living in the area, but one is in ill health, and the other, a single mother, has a demanding job and children to care for. Neither of the daughters is in a position to care for their father, who has been diagnosed with Alzheimer's disease.

Now, 3 years later, he has almost caused a fire by leaving a glue gun burning in the garage and has had to give up woodworking, his favorite activity. Mrs. J. is also concerned because her husband has wandered away from the house several times, and on one occasion had to be brought home by the police. His personality changes have been particularly difficult. At church several months ago, Mr. J. began swearing loudly during the service and his wife had to take him home. Mrs. J. has been too embarrassed to return. Nights are also difficult in that Mr. J. gets up and wanders. Sometimes at night he doesn't recognize his wife and demands she leave his house.

Today Mrs. J. brings her husband in for an evaluation. During the appointment she begins to cry, saying she cannot go on much longer. She believes God is punishing her for being a bad wife and she feels guilty because she has been losing her temper with her husband. The physician discovers that Mrs. J. has lost 15 pounds and is suffering severe sleep deprivation.

What interventions might help Mr. J. become more manageable? What services could help Mrs. J. gain respite from the burden of care for her husband? Does Mrs. J. need treatment herself?

CASE ILLUSTRATION 3

Mr. L. is a 79-year-old man whose wife of 45 years died unexpectedly 2 months ago. The marriage was not an easy one: Mr. L. drank heavily, had numerous affairs, and was verbally abusive to his wife. Since his retirement at age 65, however, their relationship improved and Mr. L. treated his wife with more respect and affection.

Mr. L.'s daughter, Eleanor, calls her parents' long-time physician to say she thinks her father is becoming "senile." He seems to be at a complete loss since his wife died: He has not paid any bills, and the only food in his refrigerator is what neighbors and Eleanor bring. He hasn't changed his clothes or bathed for at least a week. One of the neighbors called Eleanor last week to say her father was wandering around the yard at night. Even more alarming to Eleanor, she has found him talking to his deceased wife as if she was there.

Eleanor makes an appointment for her father. When they come in for the office visit the doctor is taken aback by Mr. L.'s haggard appearance.

Although he seems distracted on mental status examination, Mr. L. proves to be oriented to year and month but not the date or day of the week. His thinking and speech are very slow. Everything he is asked reminds him of his wife and makes him tearful. Mr. L. complains of insomnia and asks for sleep medication.

What is happening to Mr. L.? Is he developing dementia or mental illness? Is this just normal bereavement? What assessment and interventions should the physician consider?

DIAGNOSTIC TECHNIQUES

The Clinical Interview

THE CLINICAL SETTING

Environmental conditions in the office can impair communication and rapport between elderly patients and health care providers. Clinicians should be sensitive to noise, glare, and physical layout. Rooms must be wheelchair accessible and large enough to accommodate family and caregivers when necessary.

PATIENT INTERVIEW

Extra time should be allowed for elderly persons to move into the examination room and to tell their stories. Current generations of elderly patients grew up in more formal times and many prefer to be called by their last names. Clinicians should inquire early in the interview whether they are being heard and understood. Projecting one's voice and speaking distinctly are helpful for many older persons, but clinicians should not assume this is necessary and shout at all patients just because they are very old. Active listening methods, such as maintaining eye contact, nodding, and paraphrasing the patient's questions and statements should be used (see Chapter 1). Shorter more frequent visits for patients with many symptoms or greater need to talk will reduce the physician's frustration, improve communication, and better meet the patient's emotional needs for contact with the physician.

FAMILY AND CAREGIVER INTERVIEW

Most frail elderly patients should be accompanied by a family member or caregiver so that the clinician can obtain a complete view of the problem. Patients with dementia may not be aware of their memory impairment and can actively deny they have any problem. They may also have limited insight into depressive symptoms or paranoid thinking. Delusional thoughts may seem perfectly logical until the family or caregiver is consulted (sometimes, of course, the patient is correct—abuse and exploitation must be ruled out). The health care practitioner may alienate the patient while interviewing family and caregivers, so family consultation must be pursued with sensitivity to the patient's feelings. One approach is to see everybody together in the first few minutes of the visit in order to establish the nature of the problem. Then the clinician can spend time alone with the patient for physical, neurological, and mental status examinations, asking about special concerns the patient may have been unwilling to mention in the presence of others. Meanwhile, a second staff member, after obtaining the patient's permission, can interview the family and caregiver to obtain a more detailed history or description of symptoms they do not feel free to describe in the presence of the patient. It is during these separate interviews that clinicians can obtain more candid reports of functional impairment, psychiatric symptoms, and memory problems.

Assessment

HISTORY

The health care practitioner should inquire about past episodes of symptoms similar to the chief complaint, recent changes in function, the time course of symptoms, modifying factors, and all prescribed and over-the-counter medications. Vitamins, food supplements, and homeopathic remedies are used by a significant percentage of older patients and need to be surveyed as well. Alcohol use should be evaluated. A useful acronym that we have developed for a geriatric review of systems (MOMS AND DADS) is presented in Table 11–1.

PHYSICAL ASSESSMENT

General appearance, weight and nutritional status, hygiene, vital signs, and physical and neurological examinations help determine whether the patient is medically stable, well cared for, or taking care of themselves adequately. Evidence of abuse, such as suspicious bruises or injuries, or evidence of medical neglect should prompt an adult protective services referral through the local Area Agency on Aging.

MENTAL AND COGNITIVE STATUS EXAMINATIONS

An assessment of orientation, recent memory, problem-solving ability, judgment, insight, initiative, mood and affect, and the presence of suspiciousness, paranoia, or unusual beliefs is essential for ruling out dementia, depression, or delusional disorders. Judgment and insight are the most subtle and subjective of these aspects of mental function to assess, but health care behavior and decision-making ability provide the clinician with clues about these functions, although these things must be interpreted in light of the patient's cultural and religious values. Use of standardized mood rating scales, such as the Geriatric Depression Scale, can dramatically improve detection of depression in primary care settings. Cognition rating scales

Table 11–1. The "MOMS AND DADS" geriatric review of systems.[1]

M	Mobility	Gait and balance, recent falls, use of aides
O	Output	Bowel function, urine output, bladder continence
M	Memory	Emphasis on recent memory function
S	Senses	Changes in hearing and vision
A	Aches	Pain survey
N	Neuro	Neuro sx such as dizziness or weakness
D	Delusions	Psychotic symptoms, paranoia, hallucinations
D	Depression	Dysphoria, anxiety, fearfulness, irritability, hopelessness
A	Appetite	Food and fluid intake
D	Dermis	Changes in skin color, integrity, dental problems
S	Sleep	Problems initiating or maintaining sleep, daytime alertness, abnormal nocturnal activity

[1] This offers a helpful supplement to the standard organ-system-based review of systems.

should be used routinely to screen for cognitive impairment. The Folstein Mini-Mental Status Exam is the most widely used, but many others are available.

FUNCTIONAL ASSESSMENT

The ability to do activities of daily living (ADLs), such as bathing, dressing, grooming, eating, transferring, and toileting can be affected by medical illness and mental disorders. Instrumental activities of daily living (IADLs) such as telephone use, money and medication management, shopping, cooking, driving, and transportation are impacted by even mild dementia. Status of ADL and IADL function needs to be assessed to determine a person's safety at home. Improvements in ADL and IADL status will demonstrate response to medical treatments and allow patients to remain at home and independent for as long as possible.

SOCIAL SYSTEM ASSESSMENT

When frail patients are dependent on caregivers, the caregiver's capacity and coping become the clinician's concern. Caregiving is associated with depression and health problems. The clinician should tactfully probe for indicators of stress, feelings of burden, and breakdown in the caregiver's

ability to provide care. The potential for abuse should also be assessed with an awareness that hostile remarks and impatience are problematic in themselves and may be risk factors for physical aggression and neglect. Many states require physicians to report suspected abuse and all communities are required by federal law to have Area Agencies on Aging that provide adult protective services.

ENVIRONMENTAL ASSESSMENT

Community nursing and senior care agencies can assist health care providers by making home assessments and evaluating patients' safety in their own environment. Fall risk, fire safety, medication management, and hygiene concerns are among the many things that can be evaluated. Home visits by the physician or practitioner can also have great benefits by providing first-hand observations, as well as increasing patient trust and rapport.

DIAGNOSIS

Major Mental Disorders of Old Age

DEPRESSION

Major depression is common in older adults, occurring in 2–4% of community-residing elderly. The prevalence of depressive symptoms is much higher in the chronically ill. Major depression in geriatric patients manifests in all the usual ways seen in younger adults (see Chapter 21), but nonspecific and atypical symptoms are common and may dominate the clinical presentation. Although depressed mood and hopelessness have diagnostic value, less specific symptoms may be prominent and give valuable clues to the underlying diagnosis. Anhedonia, anxiety, fearfulness, irritability, cognitive impairment, apathy, dependency, and numerous somatic complaints should prompt the consideration of depression even when the patient denies feeling depressed. As stated previously, depression-rating instruments such as the Geriatric Depression Scale are helpful for screening in primary care settings. The prognosis for depression in old age is fairly good and patients need to be told this to counter the hopelessness they feel. However, partial remissions and relapses are common, especially in patients with previous episodes of depression. Other negative predictors include persistent health problems that compromise function or comfort and ongoing psychosocial stressors. Antidepressant medication and psychosocial support are known to improve outcomes and reduce the risk of relapse in older adults. Cognitive impairment associated with depression may improve with remission of the mood disorder, but is predictive of an underlying neurodegenerative dementia. Such patients need close follow-up to catch the dementia early.

Many older people look and act depressed but do not feel sad or meet the diagnostic criteria for major depression. These so called "masked depressions" often occur in the context of chronic medical illness, weight loss, and functional decline, creating the clinical syndrome of "failure to thrive." Some of these patients experience a slow recovery from an acute physical illness, with poor oral intake and little motivation to regain strength. Standard treatments for depression can be targeted to improve initiative and motivation, appetite, and pain tolerance in failing patients when there are many or unclear underlying causes of the syndrome. Psychostimulants such as methylphenidate or *d*-amphetamine may be helpful as short-term adjunctive treatments.

It is not unusual to make the diagnosis of bipolar affective disorder in older patients, either as a primary mania or hypomania developing for the first time or previous illness that went undiagnosed. Secondary mania from stroke, epilepsy, neurodegenerative diseases, and medical conditions is also seen. Mood is frequently dysphoric and irritable (prompting a misdiagnosis of "agitated depression" in some patients), although classic euphoria is seen too. Impulsivity, talkativeness, and intense, labile affect are clues to the correct diagnosis. Hyperactivity, reduced sleep, paranoia, and hypersexuality are very suggestive of the diagnosis but are not always present. Rapid cycling with several episodes of depression and mania every year is common in elderly bipolar patients. Treatment must include mood stabilizers such as divalproex and the newer antipsychotic drugs rather than antidepressants.

ANXIETY DISORDERS

Elderly patients have the highest per capita use of antianxiety medications. These figures are probably higher than necessary, considering that many of the anxious elderly are actually suffering from depression. Apart from depression, the differential diagnosis of anxiety in the elderly includes transient apprehension and fear about changes in the environment, adjustments to life changes, phobic avoidant behaviors, obsessive-compulsive disorder, panic, and generalized anxiety disorder. Secondary anxiety disorders are also very common; medications, chronic obstructive pulmonary disease, and endocrinopathies are often implicated.

DELUSIONAL DISORDERS

Delusional thinking arises from a number of disturbances in old age. A primary delusional disorder of unknown etiology, previously known as paranoia, is typically seen in elderly women who live alone. Although these patients describe persecutory delusions of an intense nature, highly suggestive of schizophrenia, they do not have other the other manifestations of this disease, such as hallucinations, loose associations, disorganized behavior, and functional decline. Elderly persons who do exhibit these cardinal symptoms of schizophrenia have usually had the disease for many years, although it can develop in late life on rare occasion. Paranoia and delusions can also be the presenting

symptoms of dementia, depression, mania, and alcohol abuse.

DEMENTIA

The prevalence of dementia increases with age, approaching 20% at age 80 and 50% by age 90. The diagnosis of dementia is made when intellectual impairment is severe enough to affect independent functioning (see Chapter 25). Alzheimer's disease (AD) is the most common cause of dementia in the elderly, and can be diagnosed with fairly good accuracy by using formal diagnostic criteria (Table 11–2). The presence of progressive decline in recent memory, normal motor examination (without weakness, ataxia, or parkinsonism), and deficits in at least one other higher cortical function (language, praxis, visual-spatial, calculations, and executive functions), is highly supportive of the diagnosis. Mild cognitive impairment (MCI) is diagnosed when memory is impaired but other cognitive functions remain intact. MCI gradually progresses to AD in most individuals, but the diagnosis of AD is delayed until dementia is actually present: ie, more than just memory is impaired and independent function is lost. Medical treatment of AD includes long-term maintenance on acetylcholinesterase inhibitors to slow functional decline, high dose α-tocopherol (vitamin E 800–2000 IU/day) to slow disease progression, treatment of neuropsychiatric symptoms when necessary, and attention to comfort (especially pain), continence, and caregiver distress.

Anther common dementia of old age is Lewy body dementia (LBD). This is diagnosed when a patient manifests a progressive dementia, parkinsonism (especially bradykinesia), daily fluctuations in symptoms, and visual hallucinations. Sleep disturbance is common. LBD accounts for 5–10% of cases of old age dementia, and may occur mixed with AD. Treatment of LBD involves trials

Table 11–2. Diagnostic criteria for Alzheimer's disease.[1]

- The patient develops multiple cognitive deficits, including both of the following: memory impairment *and* impairment in at least one other higher cortical function (language, complex motor tasks, visual-spatial functions, executive function)
- The cognitive deficits cause significant impairment and a decline from a previous level of function
- The cognitive impairments are not due to another known neurodegenerative disease, acute illness, medications, intoxication, delirium, or a major mental illness
- The course of the illness is characterized by gradual onset and progressive decline in function

[1] Adapted, with permission, from American Psychiatric Association: *Diagnostic and Statistical Manual of Mental Disorders,* 4th edition. American Psychiatric Association Press, 1994.

of acetylcholinesterase inhibitors and psychotropic medications for targeted neuropsychiatric symptoms. Older antipsychotic medications such as haloperidol must be rigorously avoided. The parkinsonism can respond modestly to L-Dopa and dopamine agonists, but care must be taken to balance the doses against worsening neuropsychiatric symptoms.

Vascular dementia is another common cause of intellectual and functional decline in old age, accounting for about 5% of dementia cases and contributing to worsening dementia in many more patients as a comorbid condition with AD. Large cortical strokes produce a stepwise decline with noticeable points of change associated with strokes (multi-infarct dementia). Small vessel disease producing lacunar infarcts in subcortical structures is associated with hypertension and diabetes. Also known as Binswanger's dementia, this condition produces a more gradually progressive dementia that looks similar to AD, but with more obvious gait impairment, incontinence, parkinsonism, and affect lability. Circulatory problems in the absence of stroke (ie, congestive heart failure, hyperviscosity states, etc) can also produce cognitive impairment.

DELIRIUM

Delirium is characterized by the acute (within hours) or subacute (within days) development of disorientation and confusion. Inability to focus and sustain attention are key to the diagnosis. Hallucinations, fearful or paranoid perceptions, fluctuating awareness, and alterations in the sleep–wake cycle are other frequent symptoms. In patients with mild delirium, the decreased level of alertness may not be obvious. Patients will often have psychomotor slowing, withdrawal, listlessness, and apathy. These patients are frequently misdiagnosed as depressed. Delirium is often the first symptom of medical illness in frail elderly people. The most common causes of delirium in older patients are infections (usually urinary tract and pulmonary), medications, metabolic abnormalities, alcohol or sedative intoxication and withdrawal, stroke, seizures, and heart failure. In patients with dementia, problems such as pain, fecal impaction, and urinary retention can cause rapid changes in mental status and behavior that look like superimposed delirium.

SUBSTANCE ABUSE AND POLYPHARMACY

Often overlooked, substance abuse is very common in the elderly; alcohol abuse is the third most common mental disorder in elderly males. Unexplained falls, ataxia, confusion, malnutrition, burns, head trauma, and depression should prompt questions about surreptitious alcohol abuse. Sedative-hypnotic medications and over-the-counter remedies for constipation, sleeplessness, and pain, and numerous vitamins and supplements are also overused. Seeing multiple physicians and practitioners and patronizing several pharmacies are clues to the clinician that prescription abuse is likely.

Because of their greater number of chronic medical conditions, older patients generally take more prescription medications than younger patients. Although often necessary, polypharmacy increases the risk of adverse drug reactions, a leading cause of confusion, depression, falls, and functional decline. An ongoing effort to evaluate the current need for everything being taken is prudent (see Chapter 20).

SOMATIZATION

Geriatric patients are not immune to somatic perceptions for which there are no known physical causes. The clinician must avoid unnecessary interventions while continuously supporting the needs of the patient to be heard and understood. Although regularly scheduled appointments with brief, focused examinationinations that allow the "laying on of the hands" continue to be the most effective interventions, major depression and anxiety disorders commonly underlie hypochondriasis. Antidepressants and psychotherapy may improve function and sense of well-being in somatically focused patients (see Chapter 23).

TREATMENT
Caring for Elderly Patients
HELPING OLD PEOPLE STAY AT HOME

The focus of treatment planning with the frail elderly patient is always the provision of comfort and the maintenance of independent functioning. Although there are clearly times when safety becomes the paramount issue, as in the case of the elderly driver who is becoming a hazard behind the wheel, independence is usually the shared goal of patient and clinician. To achieve this in the face of aging and progressive disease, treatment planning must include utilization of community care resources, skillful medical management, and rehabilitation therapies.

COMMUNITY CARE OPTIONS FOR THE FRAIL ELDERLY

Clinicians should become familiar with the services available in their community that provide case management, in-home assistance, and emotional support to elderly patients and caregivers. Local and county agencies providing services for seniors, private case management firms, local chapters of the Alzheimer's Association, and home health care agencies will be resources to you and your patients in arranging the services necessary to keep your patients at home longer than would otherwise be safe. In rural areas without these resources, family, neighbors, and lay networks of helpers can sometimes fill in the gaps and keep frail elders cared for at home.

Patients with round-the-clock care needs will eventually exhaust many family caregivers. Some patients with dementia-associated agitation, delusions, and misperceptions can be combative and make caregiving frustrating and occasionally dangerous. Caregivers, family, and paid professionals all face depression and health risks beyond their peers. There comes a time when placement in a long-term care facility becomes necessary for both the patient's as well as the family's well-being. Physicians, nurses, and other practitioners play important roles in assisting patients and families through this transition. Clinicians can help them anticipate the need to leave home for supervised living settings, familiarize them with different long-term care options in the community, and also help families with feelings of guilt experienced when they have to make the decision on the patient's behalf. This role requires clinicians to know what the patient's care needs are and what type of facility can safely meet those needs. People who need assistance only with housekeeping and cooking will do fine in residential care facilities. Some of these facilities can also administer medications and provide assistance with ADLs for additional cost. A few states allow people to provide care for up to five frail elders in a private home. Such "adult foster homes" provide a home-like alternative to residential care facilities. Additional care needs may be met by an assisted living facility. Assisted living facilities may provide some nursing supervision and occasionally may even have a medical director. However, the amount of nursing and medical involvement varies greatly based on state regulations and the management philosophy of the owners. These facilities are very popular with patients and families and are increasingly seen as alternatives to skilled nursing facilities because they are less expensive and much less "hospital like" than nursing homes. Many assisted living facilities allow patients to "age in place" and even allow them to receive hospice-level care at the end of life without having to move to a skilled nursing facility. However, it is important to inform patients and families that these facilities cannot generally provide the same level of nursing assessment and care that skilled nursing facilities provide. Many patients with complex care needs will still need nursing homes, but there are now many other options for less frail patients.

MEDICAL TREATMENT PLANNING

The motto of the British Geriatrics Society, "Adding Life to Years," is useful to keep in mind when treating elderly patients. Comfort and increased activity become the goals of treatment. Providing adequate pain relief, physical therapy, and treatment of depression are all integrated into comprehensive treatment plans.

Immunizations, stress reduction, smoking cessation, exercise, and proper nutrition should continue to be a focus of preventive care in the elderly. It is also important to explore the expectations of both the patient and the caregiver and to discuss end-of-life treatment decisions. If possible, this discussion should take place before an

acute medical condition forces interventions that may be invasive, futile, or unwanted. These "advance directives" should extend beyond cardiopulmonary resuscitation and include the patient's goals of care. If the decision is to forego these interventions, the clinician should provide assurances that the comfort of the patient will be maintained.

Given the high prevalence of mental disorders in old age, it is not surprising that the elderly are prescribed psychotropic medications at a higher rate than younger adults. Whereas many of the older agents were as efficacious as their modern counterparts, they frequently extracted a cost of diminished function through sedation, postural hypotension, anticolinergic effects, and in the case of some antipsychotic agents, parkinsonism and dyskinesia. It is now possible to choose a therapeutic agent from every class to minimize or avoid these side effects in high-risk elderly patients. Special care must still be taken, however, to start most medications at a lower dose in older patients (generally half the usual starting dose in young-old patients, ie, 65–80 years, and a third the usual dose in old-old patients, ie, over age 80). In the case of benzodiazepines, antipsychotics, and mood stabilizers, the effective treatment dose will also usually be one-half to one-third the dose used in younger patients. However, in the case of antidepressants, the eventual effective doses are frequently at the same levels used in young adults.

FUNCTIONAL REHABILITATION

Functional rehabilitation of elderly patients with mental disorders following stroke, fracture, or medical illness ideally involves a multidisciplinary team approach. The goal is to treat the mental disorder and primary disability, while preventing secondary disabilities such as immobility and incontinence, and complications such skin breakdown and infection. The composition of the team varies widely and may include rehabilitation professionals such as physical, occupational, and speech therapists. The rehabilitation plan, like the medical plan, must have realistic goals that are individualized to the patient.

CASE DISCUSSIONS

 CASE ILLUSTRATION 1

Despite her niece's concerns, Martha may only be an eccentric person, and not one with a neurodegenerative condition or mental illness. The so-called "Senior Squalor Syndrome" or Diogenes Syndrome, however, is often due to underlying dementia, depression, paranoid disorder, schizophrenia, or alcoholism. Occasionally, fear of losing autonomy and being forced from the home will lead seniors to cover-up their

physical incapacity to keep up at home. Knowing whether this represents a change in personality and a recent decline in function inconsistent with past habits will allow the clinician to determine whether this is just eccentric life-style preferences in an otherwise healthy person or a pathological condition of old age. A mental status examination and functional assessment would be helpful. Knowing she is paranoid or has memory and self-care deficits will alter the clinician's approach to eliciting her cooperation. Documenting specific ADL and IADL deficits in the patient's abilities and safety hazards in the home (fire, food safety, fall risk, ability to summon emergency services) are key to determining whether intervention is necessary. Martha has apparently been paying electricity and water bills, which indicates some preservation of cognitive function. Perhaps she could remain home safely if she received help with housekeeping, shopping, and nutrition. Phone service would also be helpful, assuming she could afford a phone and be able and willing to use it.

Several things will determine the success of the physician's efforts to intervene. First, because Martha seems to be sensitive and defensive, the doctor needs to approach her thoughtfully, emphasizing the shared goal of her staying healthy and independent. Second, Martha's financial status may limit her options. She needs a social worker or case manager to help sort out her finances and arrange necessary community services. Treating the dementia, depression, or psychosis may have a large impact on function.

The local humane society or animal protection league needs to take some of the cats away. The remaining ones need veterinary care and neutering. Because the cats are important to Martha, if she did have to leave the home, placement in a facility that allows her to have a cat or two would be important for her well-being.

Joanne is Martha's only living relative and if Martha is found to have impaired decision-making capacity, she will need to assume a formal role as power-of-attorney, guardian, or conservator. Her ability to represent Martha's interests will need on-going assessment by the clinician and the court.

CASE ILLUSTRATION 2

Like many caregivers, Mrs. J. is overwhelmed by the problems she faces and needs to use more support services. Options available in most areas include caregiver support groups, respite care, day programs, and housekeeping and home health services. Learning how to manage the behavioral symptoms of her husband's dementia will decrease her feelings of helplessness. Involvement with the local chapter of the Alzheimer's Association should be strongly recommended. If agitation and delusions become severe, the newer antipsychotic medications can be very effective. Antidepressants and anticonvulsants can be effective with agitation as well. Sleep medication for Mr. J. may give both the patient and caregiver some rest.

Mrs. J. may be depressed. She is also at risk for other caregiver stress-related health problems. Treatment for the depression and counseling focused on grief and anger management would be very helpful. Even with treatment of the depression, Mrs. J. may no longer be able to effectively care for her husband in their home and a discussion with the family about Mr. J. moving to a dementia-care facility will help prepare them for what may be necessary in the future.

CASE ILLUSTRATION 3

The major diagnostic considerations in Mr. L.'s case are bereavement, major depression, dementia, and alcoholism—which can all coexist. His symptoms are consistent with bereavement: disorganization, dishevelment, talking to the deceased, and poor sleep. Although medications to aid sleep may be helpful, benzodiazepines are a risky choice for him given his past alcoholism, advanced age, and cognitive impairment. Antidepressant medication might be indicated if the severe symptoms of dysphoria persist. Grief counseling and in-home support services could both be helpful. Although making major life decisions should be avoided during a period of acute grief, a move to a residential care or assisted living facility might provide a balance of privacy, socialization, independence, and support for daily activities.

CONTINUING EDUCATION RESOURCES

The American Geriatric Society (770 Lexington Avenue, Suite 300, New York, NY 10021), The Gerontological Society of America (1275 K Street NW, Suite 350, Washington DC 20005-4006), the American Association of Geriatric Psychiatry (PO Box 376A, Greenbelt, MD 20768), and the American Medical Director's Association (10480 Patuyent Parkway, Suite 760, Columbia, MD 21094) publish outstanding journals, have useful websites, and sponsor educational conferences for physicians and other healthcare providers.

SUGGESTED READINGS

Coffey CE et al (editors): *Textbook of Geriatric Psychiatry,* 2nd ed. American Psychiatric Press, 2000.

Salzman C (editor): *Clinical Geriatric Psychopharmacology,* 3rd ed. Williams & Wilkins, 1998.

WEB SITES

American Association of Geriatric Psychiatry
www.AAGPGPA.org
American Geriatric Society
www.American.Geriatrics.org
American Medical Director's Association
www.AMDA.com
British Society of Gerontology
www.britishgerontology.org
Canadian Association of Gerontology
www.cagacg.com
Gerontology Society of America
www.Geron.org
Journal of Gerontology
http://biomed.gerontology.journals.org

Cross-Cultural Communication   12

Thomas Denberg, MD, PhD, Melissa Welch, MD, MPH, & Mitchell D. Feldman, MD, MPhil

INTRODUCTION

Effective clinician–patient communication involves verbal and nonverbal sharing of information across cultural and linguistic boundaries. In the medical arena, these boundaries are populated on the one side by clinicians, who represent the at times esoteric world of biomedicine, and on the other side by patients and families, who often lack familiarity with biomedical concepts and procedures and may have their own strongly held beliefs about illness— what it means, how it should be diagnosed, and how it should be treated. The goals of effective cross-cultural communication (or "cultural competency," as it is sometimes called) are three-fold: (1) to understand illness from the perspective of the *patient;* (2) to assist patients in understanding diseases and treatments from the perspective of *biomedicine;* and (3) to help patients and their families navigate, express themselves, and feel comfortable within large, complex, and often impersonal health care organizations. These activities require some awareness of the wider context of patients' lives, and of how the worlds of biomedicine and the lay public interact and, oftentimes, conflict and misunderstand each other.

Cross-cultural communication skills are best developed through practice, reflection, and reading about and interacting with diverse patient populations. Knowing a few facts about the beliefs regarding illness of an immigrant group or ethnic minority is not enough. It is also important to develop ways of perceiving and interpreting what *individual* patients say and do in the context of their previous experiences with illness, structural positions within society, and membership within particular ethnic and religious communities. True cultural awareness also involves understanding how biomedicine is itself a cultural system, and how it is likely to be perceived and (mis)understood by patients.

As the dominant form of health care in the United States, biomedicine is practiced by highly specialized professionals and relies on detailed, scientific information about the human body and the use of pharmaceutical and surgical interventions to treat or prevent anatomical and physiological disorders and their associated symptoms. It has a definite body of knowledge, set of practices, strengths, non-evidence-based biases, and inherent limitations. Each of its many specialties and subspecialties has unique conventions, systems of knowledge, and ways of making sense of people and events. To patients of all backgrounds, much about biomedicine is obscure; difficulties agreeing with and accepting medical explanations and recommendations are commonplace. Thus, although cross-cultural communication is especially important and challenging for immigrant and minority patients, it has relevance to *all* patients. Such is the perspective that orients the discussion in this chapter, the purpose of which is to review general concepts and themes related to cross-cultural communication in primary care settings.

CULTURE & SOCIAL LOCATION

Culture

Culture refers to beliefs, values, rituals, customs, institutions, social roles, and relationships that are shared among identifiable groups of people. Typically, our own culture is taken for granted; it feels entirely natural, consisting of those assumptions and routines that make the world what it is "supposed" to be. Unconscious learning and modeling play important roles in the acquisition of cultural assumptions and routines. Within the family, one of the most influential cultural systems, there generally arises a clear-cut division of labor, regular routines such as meal and work times, explanations (or myths) about family origins, and strategies for fulfilling common goals and passing down shared values. It is also within the family that beliefs are first developed about the causes of illness, acceptable ways of expressing symptoms, and strategies for diagnosing illness and restoring health. Individuals are also, of course, shaped by, and participate in, cultures related to work, school, worship, political affiliation, social clubs, and so on, each of which may also have important—and sometimes contradictory or inconsistent—influences on beliefs about and responses to illness.

Cultures are neither pure nor static, but constantly intermix and evolve. Particularly in the United States—a highly mobile, diverse, and media-saturated society— millions of people move in and out of a multiple domains, borrowing and adapting ideas and customs from other groups. Because cultural change over time and across generations is so considerable, it should not be *assumed* that particular patients have certain beliefs or engage in certain behaviors solely on the basis of their last name, physical appearance, or national origin. Inferences—always open to revision—should be based on detailed knowledge of patient attributes that go beyond race and ethnicity alone.

THE RELATIONSHIP OF CULTURE TO RACE, ETHNICITY, AND NATIONAL ORIGIN

In some cultural competency training classes various racial, ethnic, and national groups are said to possess distinctive cultural traits with which the clinician should become familiar in order to render more effective care. Commonly cited examples include beliefs in "fallen fontanelle" and "evil eye" among Latinos and "high blood/low blood" among African-Americans, as well as values such as "individualism" among North Americans and "family centeredness" among Asians. Although these generalizations may illustrate a wide spectrum of cultural influences on illness and healing, this approach is too simplistic. It implies that race, ethnicity, and national origin are the most important determinants of an individual's understanding of and response to illness, and ignores the tremendous heterogeneity among individuals *within* each of these groups.

Take the case of the United States, in which the primary racial/ethnic categories include black, white, Asian, American Indian, Pacific Islander, and Latino. Some people may self-identify using these terms, and the labels are often important politically, but there are significant differences among people within each of these categories in terms of age, place of birth, religion, social class, level of education, and so on. Conceptualizing differences in health beliefs and behaviors on the overarching levels of race and ethnicity promotes stereotyping and does little to advance more effective medical care. In general, assumptions about cultural beliefs and practices should be based on more specific identification of group membership, such as recent immigrants; particular U.S. subpopulations such as the homeless or southern, rural African-Americans; or inhabitants of particular city neighborhoods.

Social Location

As we move beyond ideas of culture determined solely by race and ethnicity, knowledge of patients will be enhanced by awareness of their *social location.* Social location specifies one's position in society relative to others and is based on an amalgam of characteristics that include not only race and ethnicity, but also gender, age, immigration status, language(s) spoken, neighborhood of residence, length of time and number of generations in the United States, educational attainment, income, occupation, religion, and prior experiences with racism. Gender and age are two fundamental variables that influence how patients give meaning to illness and express themselves in relation to it. Men and women, and people over the age of 50 and under 20, although from the same city or region, will generally belong to distinctive subcultures: they may share certain core beliefs, values, and customs, but not others. Another fundamental influence on disease risk, health behaviors, and familiarity with biomedicine is degree of acculturation. One's neighborhood of residence, with its quality of housing and schools, population density, associated level of crime, and access to public transportation, also dramatically shapes one's understanding of the world and strategies for dealing with adversity. Religion, faith, and membership in a community of like-minded believers also have significant bearings on attitudes toward health and illness. Historical experiences of racism can engender feelings of helplessness, anger, and distrust that can, in turn, significantly affect attitudes toward medical providers as well as interpretations of illness. Finally, the elements of social class—education, income, and occupation—have a profound effect on people's beliefs about illness and opportunities and strategies for restoring health.

The attributes of social location are more complete, specific, and clinically relevant than race and ethnicity alone. In this way, a clinician will not simply note that a patient is Latino, or even Mexican-American, and then attempt to remember "typical" cultural traits that apply to members of this group. Instead, they will observe that the U.S.-born patient is 20 years old, unemployed, has completed high school, speaks little Spanish, and lives with her Mexican-born, primarily Spanish-speaking, rural-origin parents in a mixed race, working-class neighborhood. Each of these characteristics, alone and in combination, provides important clues about *this* patient—clues that help in interpreting the patient's statements and symptoms and that facilitate patient education and tailored treatment.

Obviously, the more experience practitioners have with patients from a specific, narrowly defined population or community, the more they will become aware of the health problems and themes important to that group as a whole. The ability to communicate effectively with patients from such groups can be enhanced by spending time in the local community—in senior citizen centers, at cultural and sporting events, churches, and schools—as well as by reading relevant neighborhood newsletters, ethnographies, social histories, census reports, novels, and biographies. Although such activities and materials do not constitute the normal corpus of medical duties or references, they can powerfully sensitize the clinician to the issues that are important to patients—in their own terms and from their own points of view. Detailed knowledge of a specific population can also help the clinician understand not only the literal sense of a patient's words, but other kinds of meanings contained in what the patient says (or chooses not to say), and in what the patient does (or chooses not to do), such as adhere to prescribed treatments.

IMMIGRANTS & ETHNIC MINORITIES

Recent immigrants bring a number of unique issues and challenges to medical cross-cultural communication. Relocating to a new country often results in dramatic alterations in social status, occupation, and daily routines, isolation from previous friendships and networks of social support, and the upending of traditional roles as older individuals rely on those who are younger to support the family, locate housing, and interpret local events. Anomie (a sense of purposelessness) and alienation (lack of feelings of belonging) can contribute to anxiety, depression, and a decreased ability to cope with the new stresses of daily life. Refugee experiences of war and natural catastrophe exacerbate these problems. The astute clinician will be aware that many individuals somatize this distress.

Immigrants are the most likely to hold beliefs and practices that to "western"-trained physicians seem colorful or strange. These beliefs about illness are often cited in discussions of cultural competence but are generally most applicable to elderly and/or recently arrived immigrants. Processes of globalization, including the growth of tourism, the opening of commercial markets, and the spread of popular culture from the United States and Europe, have familiarized large numbers of third-world immigrants with life in industrially advanced, capitalist societies. In addition, a substantial proportion of first- and second-generation residents quickly accommodate themselves to U.S. society, often because of a keen desire to "fit in" or "become American." Even among individuals who speak English poorly, are poorly assimilated, or actively resist assimilation, many will have had a significant amount of experience with biomedicine in their countries of origin. Although they may not have previously encountered the technological and organizational complexity that characterize biomedicine in the United States, they may be reasonably familiar with its reductionistic, scientific foundation, status as a profession, and its conventions for diagnosing and treating illness. It is difficult, if not impossible, to accurately gauge a patient's level of sophistication about biomedicine and "western" disease categories through visual inspection or knowledge of the patient's race and ethnicity alone; the clinician should avoid assumptions and instead learn by observing and asking questions of the patient.

BIOMEDICINE AS A CULTURAL SYSTEM

Focusing on "culture" primarily in relation to immigrant or minority patients may reinforce the notion that biomedicine is itself without culture. In fact, though biomedicine is informed by scientific knowledge, it is also shaped by the politics of government funding, insurance reimbursement, rivalries among specialties, as well as by competing ideologies of profit versus altruism, changing fashions and trends, best guesses, and regional biases. Biomedicine comprises many cultural worlds—primary care, cardiology, surgery; the hospital, the clinic; nursing, physicians, pharmacists; and so on—that for many patients are strange, potentially threatening, and difficult to understand. Awareness of how different kinds of patients are likely to experience and interpret biomedicine is a prerequisite to enhancing cross-cultural communication. It is equally important for clinicians to be aware of their own roles in perpetuating the culture of biomedicine, and to realize the extent to which they are both the products and practitioners of this cultural system. Table 12–1 lists several characteristics that have been associated with biomedicine and its practitioners.

Tensions and misunderstandings between practitioner and patient are often strongly rooted in many of the attributes listed under (A) in Table 12–1. Often most problematic from the perspective of patients is biomedicine's well-described tendency to sharply differentiate body from mind and to emphasize organic pathophysiology over the psychosocial ramifications and origins of illness. Nonetheless, many of biomedicine's major successes have been achieved despite—or often because of—such tendencies. For the most part, these are the characteristics that make biomedicine unique and set it apart from other systems of healing. They are also quite resistant to change. The clinician's goal should be to act as a cultural broker, making these features of biomedicine more accessible and understandable to the patient while at the same time exploring and attending to the psychosocial dimensions of illness from the patient's perspective.

Individual practitioners vary greatly in the degree to which they conform to the attributes of professionalism listed under (B) in Table 12–1. Although common, none is a *predictable* feature of biomedicine in the same way as those listed under (A). A central problem, however, is that many patients have difficulty understanding or sympathizing with the attributes in either category, compounding communication difficulties and leading some to hold many of the negative impressions listed under (C) in Table 12–1. This is especially true when patients desire a more personal and less professional relationship with their physicians, or when social distance compounds the patient's feelings of powerlessness. The culturally competent clinician will understand these common features and negative patient perceptions of biomedicine, recognizing when they contribute to misunderstandings and impair the patient's ability to feel at ease, communicate, and benefit from biomedical approaches to conceptualizing and treating illness.

COMMUNICATION

Communication involves the exchange, processing, and interpretation of messages both verbal and nonverbal. In this complex process, there are myriad opportunities for miscommunication: messages can be incomplete, confusing, and contradictory; language barriers as well as emotional and physical distractions can interfere with the receipt and relaying of information; and unspoken

Table 12–1. Characteristics of biomedicine and its practitioners.

(A) Biomedicine *as a system of healing rests upon and esteems the following:*

• Empiric science	• Reductionism (pathophysiology is molecular and anatomic; symptoms are expressions of underlying disease rather than diseases themselves)
• Written knowledge as opposed to oral tradition	
• Rigorous and lengthy training	
• Technological sophistication and innovation	• High levels of bureaucratic organization and subspecialization
• Action orientation and interventionism ("doing something rather than nothing")	• Efficiency
• Materialism (disease in the individual, physical body rather than in the family, social group, mind, or spirit)	• Cost containment
	• "Defensiveness" or avoiding malpractice
• Differentiating among acute illness, chronic illness, and prevention	• The prolongation of life

(B) *Many* **clinicians** *value these traits:*

• Hard work	• Punctuality
• Self-sacrifice	• The physician as *the* expert
• Self-reliance and autonomy	• Deliberateness
• Strong career orientation	• Articulateness
• Status consciousness	• A clear separation between personal and work lives
• Respect for authority and hierarchy	• Conservatism in dress and expressions of emotion
• Hygiene	• Quality judged by one's colleagues

(C) *Common attributions that* **patients** *have about biomedicine and its practitioners:*

Negative	Positive
• Arrogant	• Highly competent
• Elite	• Honest
• Judgmental	• Careful
• Remote and inaccessible	• Thorough
• Narrow minded	• Methodical
• Difficult to comprehend	• Caring
• Money hungry	• Accurate
• Rushed	• Reliable
• Dogmatic	• Responsible
• Rigid	• Impartial
• Uninterested in the patient as a person	• Putting the patient's welfare first and foremost

assumptions can influence the meaning one person attributes to another's statements or actions. Much of this takes place outside of conscious awareness. With this in mind, this section reviews three fundamental aspects of communication to which the clinician should direct particular attention: (1) attempting to understand the illness from the *patient's* perspective; (2) ensuring that the patient understands, as much as possible and at an appropriate level, *biomedical* explanations of the illness and its treatment; and (3) guiding patients through the *ritualized* clinical encounter and the health care bureaucracy in ways that increase their familiarity and comfort with it.

The Patient

Barriers to health care affecting both immigrants and disadvantaged minority groups, including lack of insurance and other financial resources, physical distance, and low literacy, often make biomedical treatment an option of last resort. Clinical consultations for such patients will frequently be more time consuming and require increased patience by the clinician. Extra effort may sometimes be needed to teach such patients to be assertive, ask questions, and raise concerns. Clinicians who treat large numbers of such patients will benefit the most from reading about and becoming personally familiar with them outside of medical settings.

EXPLANATORY MODELS

Explanatory models refer to theories of disease causation, prognosis, typical symptoms, and appropriate treatment. Although biomedical explanatory models tend to be highly technical, elaborated, and specific, those of patients are typically much vaguer, sometimes contradictory, and may change over time. Nonetheless, eliciting patients' explanatory models of disease offers unparalleled insight into their sense of self and relationships with significant others while yielding clues about how they are likely to interpret, resist, or accept biomedical explanations and treatments. Knowledge of the patient's own perspective also facilitates the ability to ease patient fear and anxiety. Understanding the patient's *explanatory model* of illness is especially important when treating potentially debilitating chronic conditions, where nonadherence is a common concern and where the psychosocial dimensions of illness loom large.

Typically, the most important component of a patient's explanatory model is the idea of illness *causation* (see Table 12–2). To elicit this belief the clinician can ask, "What do you think caused your problem?" and then listen carefully to the answer as it is likely to reveal crucial feelings related to moral failings, discord with significant others, financial and practical challenges in daily life, and whether there is a sense of hope for the future. The clinician should not expect patients to answer questions about causation with simple and mechanistic explanations. Additional probing may also be required. For example, the clinician could follow up with questions such as "What do you think you have? What is the name you give to this condition?" "Why do some people get this illness and not others?" "Who or what is responsible (or to blame) for this problem?" and "Do you ever think that you did (or didn't do) something to bring this on yourself, or that someone else did (or didn't do) something?" Additional questions can allow patients to elaborate on their explanatory model: "What do you think should be done to treat you?" "Do you think a complete cure is possible?" "How long will the problem last?" and "What do you think needs to be done to relieve this problem?" The advantage of such questions is that they are open-ended, are applicable to every patient, and can help to correct or refine initial clinical assumptions or preconceptions. They are also powerful in their ability to provide clues about what the patient will find difficult to understand or accept when it comes to explaining the illness in *biomedical* terms.

Some patients, especially recent immigrants, may be reticent to divulge their explanatory models of illness out of concern that their beliefs will be viewed as ignorant or superstitious. Alternatively, such patients may feel that they have come to hear the doctor's expert opinion, and

Table 12–2. Questions to elicit a patient's explanatory model of illness.

- What do you think caused your problem?
- What do you think you have?
- What is the name you give to this condition?
- Why do some people get this illness but not others?
- What do you think needs to be done to relieve this problem?

that their own perspective is of little consequence. It is sometimes prudent to allow patients' explanatory models to emerge slowly, through gentle probing, over the course of several visits. Inference combined with direct questioning (eg, "other patients believe X, what do you think about this?") and background knowledge of the patient's narrowly defined ethnicity and social location will often be necessary to form a coherent picture.

Fatalism

Members of some groups, including many immigrants, are often said to be fatalistic in their attitudes toward illness. They may be passive about seeking treatment, persist in unhealthful behaviors, or accept misfortune because they believe it is preordained. It is important not to assume that this style of explaining and dealing with illness is indelibly rooted in the culture or religion of the patient's racial or ethnic group. In fact, fatalism is widespread and is common among people who lack education and have little control over the circumstances of their lives. It also emerges out of a kind of valid logic that observes that serious illness can befall even those who have no bad habits and live a "clean" or "virtuous" life. Fatalism does not necessarily imply a lack of interest in preventing or treating disease. Rather, it can be viewed as an idiom for describing a person's perceived powerlessness in the world, lack of hope, and even distrust. The doctor can approach this problem by acknowledging the real challenges the patient faces, but then by being clear about the practical steps the patient can take to resolve or manage the illness.

 CASE ILLUSTRATION 1

A 56-year-old African-American woman who completed a grade-school education declines colon cancer screening. On questioning, she believes that cancer is a "death sentence" and can be caused by something like a bruise. Cancer terrifies her and she therefore sees no point in learning she might have it. The clinician explains that from a medical perspective, cancer is not caused by something as commonplace as a bruise, that it takes many years to develop, and that in people over 50 it can happen in a few individuals out of a hundred. She then tells the patient that the purpose of colon cancer screening—a relatively safe procedure performed thousands of times every year—is not to find a big cancer (which would be extremely unusual) but to save lives by finding a few areas (polyps) where cancer could develop and then snip them out. She provides the patient with an illustrated brochure to look over and consider.

In addition to the patient's beliefs about cancer, the clinician suspects that she distrusts the idea of doctors doing something to her that she, herself, has not requested or previously thought about. Over the course of several appointments, the clinician gently revisits the issue. A year later, the patient agrees. Trust—developed through a continuing relationship, manifest concern on the part of the clinician, and openness in explaining the purpose of medical tests— was a key factor in the patient's decision. Should the patient have continued to decline screening, however, the clinician would have appropriately, and without overt negative judgment, respected her decision.

THE PASSIVE PATIENT

Some immigrants and older patients may be particularly quiet, reserved, or exceptionally deferential in clinical interactions. Some may prefer to avoid direct eye contact. The clinician should guard against assuming that such patients are shy, uninterested, unintelligent, or uneducated simply because they avoid eye contact, agree with everything the doctor says, express a great deal of uncertainty about instructions, or are not forthcoming with information. In these circumstances, the clinician should speak clearly without reverting to a simplistic, commanding, frustrated, or patronizing tone of voice. Further clinic visits and gentle elicitation of questions and concerns by the clinician may be necessary before the patient begins to interact more openly. The patient's behavior may reflect not only cultural norms toward those in authority, but uncertainty, fear, the expression of trust through passivity, or a desire to attain a better impression of the clinician before revealing intimate details.

 CASE ILLUSTRATION 2

An older patient originally from the Philippines arrives for his first primary care visit. He says little, speaks quietly, and seems unable to explain why he has made an appointment. He repeatedly asks for instructions about various laboratory requisitions and forms. Ultimately, it becomes apparent that he is quite intelligent and has understood everything perfectly well. Over the next few visits, he opens up and speaks very articulately about his symptoms and concerns, although he continues to avoid eye contact.

INTERPRETERS

Trained interpreters can greatly facilitate patient–provider communication and improve quality of care. Un-

fortunately, perhaps because of economic constraints and clinicians' beliefs in their own ability to simply "get by," well-trained interpreters are underused in primary care settings, with negative consequences for patient care. For example, although providers with some ability in conversational Spanish may assume they understand a Puerto Rican patient's use of the term "ataque de nervios" (literally a "nervous attack"), the patient is actually referring to a culturally specific syndrome with identifiable precipitants and clear symptoms that has little to do with a "nervous breakdown." Although family members often act as de-facto interpreters, this can also introduce problems. For example, a relative who "already knows" what is wrong with the patient may not wish to bother the physician with the full details of the patient's complaints, thereby omitting important symptoms. Children and adolescents are inappropriate interpreters for many reasons, including an often incomplete mastery of English, insufficient knowledge of the subtleties of translation, and issues of relationship and status.

Good interpreters can provide more than literal paraphrasing: they can interpret patient's illness labels and idioms for the practitioner, and translate biomedical concepts and instructions into the patient's vernacular. Interpreters should be treated as full members of the health care team. Prior to the clinic visit, the provider may want to meet briefly with the interpreter to review the goals for that visit (for example, addressing the patient's understanding of and compliance with a particular medication). In addition, the provider should periodically stop the interview to seek clarification from the interpreter: "The patient has mentioned 'nerves' a few times, I was assuming that she felt nervous, but now I'm not so sure; could you explain to me what she means?" When using an interpreter, it is important to consider the physical arrangement of the participants. The clinician should always face and speak to the patient directly. The interpreter can sit next to the physician (though some patients may find this arrangement threatening), or the patient and interpreter can sit side by side. Some providers prefer the traditional triangular arrangement so that all parties have equal space and symbolic power, but the easy flow of conversation may be lost as patient and provider often cannot resist the impulse to direct their attention toward the interpreter instead of toward each other.

The Clinician

Understanding illness from the patient's perspective— traditionally regarded as the essence of cultural competence—must be balanced by the equally important task of knowing how to communicate *biomedical* explanations about the disease and its treatment to the patient (ie, serving as interpreter of biomedical culture for patients). The desire for such information is usually one of the patient's primary motivations for visiting a doctor. The clinician should offer explanations and education in terms the patient can understand and then gently test this understanding.

NAMING AND EXPLAINING THE DISEASE IN NEUTRAL TERMS

Naming a disease helps to transform a patient's inchoate fears into something that can be perceived and attacked directly. Speaking about disease in neutral and mechanistic ways can also dispel feelings of shame and ideas about etiology that are rooted in personal weakness and social failure. Patients will often seize upon, and benefit from, explanations that appropriately relieve them of personal responsibility for their misfortune. Giving a specific name to a disease and explaining it in neutral terms should be regarded as one of the primary goals of communication. Reaching this point, of course, may depend on an initial period of testing and observation.

 CASE ILLUSTRATION 3

A 65-year-old immigrant is diagnosed as having cancer. The clinician is able to elicit the patient's belief that cancer often occurs in people with "repressed personalities." Believing that he brought his disease upon himself because of such a character flaw, he feels a lack of hope and is less inclined to fight the disease. He benefits from an impersonal biomedical interpretation of cancer that focuses on damaged cellular DNA leading to unchecked cellular proliferation, and treatment aimed at destroying aberrant cells.

MEDICALIZATION

Although reductionistic disease labels and explanations are often helpful, they may contribute to the medicalization of conditions whose etiologies reside in adverse environmental (eg, polluted air and water) or social circumstances (eg, racism, intimate partner violence, sexual abuse, and work-related stress). In other words, defining illness entirely in terms of how it adversely affects the body can direct attention away from other, more proximate causes. It is important to remain mindful of and at times acknowledge the broader context that gives rise to the illness. This is often very difficult for physicians to do, in part because they are not trained to recognize these links and are limited in their ability to resolve problems such as poverty, unemployment, poor housing, and lack of education and opportunity. For example, declaring that a patient's asthma is made worse by living near a factory from which, for economic reasons,

the patient cannot easily move away may imply that nothing can be done about the problem. Nonetheless, awareness of such constraints can help the clinician to better understand and sympathize with the patient and tailor therapies that are realistic and appropriate. In addition, it is extremely common for patients of all backgrounds to believe that illness is caused by breaches in the moral order, social discord, and the failure of one's self or significant others to fulfill expected roles. Purely mechanistic biomedical explanations cannot simply replace these types of beliefs, which tend to be deeply rooted and resistant to change. Educating the patient about disease terms and pathophysiology should complement but not supersede the importance of understanding and acknowledging these other aspects of the patient's explanatory model.

"BLAMING THE VICTIM"

When it is possible to trace the etiology of disease to potentially destructive personal behaviors, such as "risky" sex, smoking, alcoholism, and drug abuse, or the worsening of disease to medical nonadherence, two pitfalls should be avoided. One is emphasizing personal culpability at the expense of helping the patient to understand the nature of the disease itself. Without adequate education, patients may have a difficult time perceiving the relationship between their behavior and the outcomes these generate, and will therefore see less reason to make changes. Although it is important to stress that certain habits are harmful and should be altered or discontinued, this should be done in a straightforward and nonjudgmental manner. The second pitfall is failing to acknowledge the personal situations and social contexts that contribute to or sustain these behaviors. Low self-esteem, depression, chronic pain, social isolation, lack of "legitimate" employment, and a strong desire to experience a sense of social belonging can contribute to many varieties of harmful and risky practices. To the extent possible, clinicians should attempt to determine the factors that perpetuate or encourage harmful behaviors and discuss these with their patients in an open and frank manner. Doing so will demonstrate empathy and concern, and help patients understand how their behavior (arising as it might for understandable reasons) should nonetheless be modified, and how this might be achieved.

COMMUNICATING BAD NEWS

Naming the disease is a cornerstone of communication in the biomedical model. However, a more flexible approach to informing patients of their diagnosis is often appropriate, particularly when the diagnosis is cancer or a terminal illness. The key is knowing how to convey the news of a life-threatening condition in ways that respect patients' and families' preferences for information and their ability to absorb the details, and that preserve a sense of hope. Clinicians sometimes must resolve two competing values: the value of respecting patient autonomy and patients' right to be informed of their illness and the value of respecting traditional patterns of decision making in which certain information, particularly having to do with cancer or other life-threatening diagnoses, may be withheld from the patient by their well-meaning family. Attention must be given to three tasks: (1) assessing patient and family preferences for receiving such information, (2) devising strategies for communicating information regarding the diagnosis, prognosis, etc, and (3) educating the patient and family more completely about the biomedical aspects of the disease while respecting traditional patterns of authority and decision making. As always, assumptions about the patient based on race, ethnicity, and national origin should be avoided. More complete knowledge of the patient's social location and explanatory models of illness (including cancer), as well as in-depth questioning of the patient and family, will provide the best understanding of cultural differences and preferences. If in doubt, err initially on the side of restraint in relating bad news or potential treatment-related complications. Chapter 3 offers a more complete discussion of this topic.

PSYCHIATRIC DIAGNOSES

For patients of many backgrounds, profound stigma is often attached to behavioral and psychiatric diagnoses. Labels such as "depression," referrals to psychiatrists, or prescriptions for "mind-altering" medications may be strongly resisted and, at worst, may be interpreted as insulting and may severely compromise the practitioner–patient relationship. For such patients, somatization is often the most "legitimate" way of expressing distress. Among patients from the former Soviet Union, psychiatry may be resisted because of its history as a coercive mechanism of social control. If there is any doubt regarding the patient's perception of psychiatric labels and referrals, the clinician should carefully explore the meanings that patients and their families attribute to them.

CASE ILLUSTRATION 4

A Mexican immigrant, working-class mother is taken aback by the pediatrician's diagnosis of "attention deficit disorder" in her child and concomitant referral to a child psychiatrist and prescription for Ritalin. She believes these recommendations imply that her child is "crazy" and, by extension, that she, first and foremost, as well as the family as a whole have somehow failed. Her anguish is compounded by the extreme importance she attributes to her role as a mother and homemaker. Furthermore, she holds that psychiatric medicines are "too powerful" for her child who, like all children, is "sensitive and vulnerable." She would have benefited from a discussion that elicited these

beliefs in advance, followed by an approach that acknowledged her fears, reaffirmed her maternal skills and concern, and attempted gently to address her beliefs and misconceptions.

PATIENT INTERPRETATIONS OF ACUTE ILLNESS, CHRONIC ILLNESS, AND PREVENTIVE MEDICINE

Patients, particularly immigrants and those with little formal education, often do not differentiate acute from chronic illness, nor do they make distinctions among curing, managing, and preventing disease. Most commonly, they assume that symptoms or diseases are self-limiting or curative with a single course of therapy. This can frustrate the clinician's ability to provide education and can contribute to poor adherence. Thus, if in doubt, the clinician should determine whether patients believe cure is possible (which is *not* the case with chronic illness) or whether patients believe the absence of current symptoms implies the absence of future disease (suggesting poor understanding of preventive medicine). Gently correcting patients' misconceptions should be viewed as an ongoing process that takes time and bears repetition.

PATIENTS WITH POOR ENGLISH LITERACY

It is estimated that up to 21% of American adults are functionally illiterate and many more are only marginally literate, limiting their ability to understand medical information and engage in meaningful discussions with their providers. Feelings of embarrassment may lead patients to conceal this problem. Strategies for managing such patients include speaking slowly, using simple terms, targeting written materials to at most a fifth-grade reading level, and using clear pictures and diagrams whenever possible. Finally, instruments such as the Test of Functional Health Literacy in Adults (TOFHLA) can provide rapid estimates of the ability to read and comprehend common medical and lay terms. Such tools can assist clinicians in tailoring both written and spoken information, and are probably more accurate at assessing the patient's reading and numerical skills and ability to function effectively in health care settings than subjective clinician impression alone.

In communicating biomedical explanatory models to patients of low literacy, concrete examples in the form of stories and images can be helpful. For example, if the patient does not seem to understand that insulin-dependent diabetes is without definitive cure but requires a lifelong adherence to diet and medication, the clinician might explain that people with diabetes have too much sugar in the blood, that an internal organ (the pancreas) does not produce enough of a substance (insulin) to reduce the amount of sugar in the blood and that it *never* will, and that for this reason diabetics must cut back on the amount of sugar they eat as well as give the body insulin through injections. Furthermore, it is instructive to narrate what will happen if an overabundance of sugar remains in the body for too long a period of time, ie, damage to the eyes, kidneys, heart, blood vessels, etc. Drawing pictures or diagrams brings the message to life.

REVIEWING MEDICATIONS

Failure to discuss medications is one of the most frequent lacunae in practitioner–patient communication. Misunderstandings and fears about medications are extremely common and are often major contributors to nonadherence. Pharmaceuticals, however, are generally the most tangible and therapeutically important products that result from the clinical encounter. Special care should therefore be given to explaining their purpose, mechanism of action, and common side effects. Eliciting patient concerns and questions to uncover erroneous beliefs is also important. This is particularly likely to benefit patients who are reticent or unable to express these concerns on their own.

Sometimes it may be helpful for clinicians to personalize information by acknowledging common challenges they face in educating and treating patients.

CASE ILLUSTRATION 5

A patient has been diagnosed with hypertension. After explaining the benefits and risks of treating hypertension with medication, the physician tries to help the patient see the clinical challenge from her perspective. She explains, "As doctors, we often have difficulty helping patients understand why they should take medicines even when they have no unpleasant symptoms. Understandably, patients often hate to take medicines, especially if they feel perfectly fine. Yet medicines are important for preventing very serious problems down the road."

This kind of approach may help some patients to understand and sympathize with the challenges faced by the clinician, promoting a sense that the two are allies in achieving a common objective.

CONTROVERSIAL AND ALTERNATIVE TREATMENTS

Sometimes there is medical uncertainty about the value of a medical test or intervention [eg, prostate specific antigen (PSA) screening]. Sometimes there may be more than one treatment option, none of which is clearly superior in terms of prevention, cure, or control of symptoms, but each of which differs significantly in terms of cost or in the likeli-

hood of various adverse effects on quality of life (eg, worry over a PSA value of 5). In these instances, before taking action the clinician should attempt to gauge both the patient's desire for information as well as preferences for decision making. Studies have shown that most patients wish to be "maximally" informed about their diseases as well as medical treatments and evaluations, but there is wide variability in their desire to assume or share responsibility for making actual treatment decisions. Only through probing is it possible to determine how much information the patient needs to feel comfortable and whether they want to share in the decision-making process. Providing too much information or attempting to make the patient accept responsibility for a medical decision can be counterproductive; but so can an approach that is reflexively paternalistic. One strategy is for the provider to state that there is a choice and, perhaps, some medical controversy or uncertainty, briefly mention the pros and cons of each option, elicit patient outcome preferences, and then wait for the patient to ask for more details, voice concerns, or express a preference for the provider to make the ultimate decision.

ASSESSING PATIENT UNDERSTANDING

To ensure that biomedical explanations are correctly understood, the clinician should ask patients closed and open-ended questions about their disease process and ask them to repeat instructions. For example, "Tell me what you understand about the cause of your diabetes and what you think will happen if we cannot adequately control your blood sugar. How often should you check your blood sugar? What should you do if you feel light-headed and sweaty?" Such tests help to reinforce knowledge and understanding and identify areas that will benefit from further counseling.

The Clinician as Cultural Broker and Institutional Guide

As described above, cross-cultural communication is enhanced by attention to patients' social location because it allows provisional inferences to be made about how patients, as *individuals,* are likely to interpret and respond to their illness. Initial clinical impressions are then modified by eliciting patients' explanatory models of illness. This information helps to tailor communication regarding the *biomedical* perspective. Finally, communication is further enhanced by understanding how patients perceive key features of the clinical process and by guiding them through its ritual and bureaucratic aspects.

CLINICAL RITUALS

Repetitive and predictable patterns and rules circumscribe patient–clinician interactions. In the ambulatory setting, for example, the nurse measures the patient's blood pressure and then brings the patient to see the physician, who directs the proceedings according to a predefined format of greeting the patient, asking questions in a certain order, examining the patient, and offering explanations and recommendations. The patient is given a specific place to sit and generally knows that the consultation will last a fixed amount of time. The basic format of these rituals is fairly simple and can usually be readily learned.

Such ritual aspects of medicine can both facilitate and impede effective communication. For example, consistency minimizes confusion about what is acceptable and unacceptable and about what will happen. Ritual offers a sense of security when patients are undressed or are sharing personal information. The ground rules and scripts of ritual are translatable from one setting to another and operate even if practitioner and patient have never met. They allow the involved actors to focus greater attention on the *content* of their exchanges and, in themselves, can be comforting and even therapeutic.

On the other hand, rituals can impair communication if patients and practitioners differ in their expectations about how they are supposed to work, or if rituals become inflexible, blind routines that leave little room for digression, variation, and opportunities for patients to express themselves freely and in fully emotional ways. This frequently happens when the clinician is pressed for time and wants the patient to provide the "facts" as tersely as possible, or when the patient yields all spontaneity of self-expression to the perceived all-knowingness and authority of the doctor. Ritual, however, should not become so rigid that its participants behave as mere automatons. Awareness of these pitfalls and the ability to make spontaneous adjustments to unspoken aspects of ritual can do much to enhance communication with the patient. Brief, unexpected, or even surprising disruptions to ritual—such as a joke, a doctor's personal reflection, allowing the patient to shed a tear or relate a piece of medical history during the physical examination, briefly and politely answering a patient's personal question about the doctor or his family—can, when judiciously applied and without breaking the overall structure of the encounter, foster more effective communication and enhance the therapeutic relationship.

For almost all patients, illness is not simply an individual malady, but a social disruption that both affects and requires the involvement of significant others. The paradigmatic private, dyadic nature of biomedicine's doctor–patient relationship can also impair communication when working with patients for whom the involvement of family members is very important. When desired by the patient, and to the extent possible, allowances and arrangements should be made to incorporate the family into diagnostic and treatment plans.

INSTITUTIONAL GUIDE

The provider should be sensitive to immigrants and other vulnerable patients who have a poor understanding of how the health care system works. Providing education about where to report for laboratory work and procedures, when results will be returned and what will be done with these, the roles of various office staff, the hours of operation, rules pertaining to the presence of children, and so on will increase efficiency, improve patient use of resources, and also likely increase patient trust by helping to demystify what seems to be a complex and threatening bureaucracy. Of note, some patients may not wish to fill out forms because of fears of deportation; it is important to be explicit about the purpose and confidentiality of medical information.

"COMPLEMENTARY" & "ALTERNATIVE" HEALERS

Despite its depth of knowledge and undeniable efficacy in many areas, biomedicine is for many patients simply *one* healing option among many others, some of which are employed simultaneously and without apparent contradiction.

 CASE ILLUSTRATION 6

A 65-year-old retired engineer is a Chinese immigrant from Vietnam. He is concerned that his hypertension has worsened because a dispute with a neighbor has thrown his system "out of balance." The patient tells his primary care provider that he has consulted an herbalist who prescribed Ginseng for this problem. He also agrees to follow his provider's recommendation to try stress reduction techniques and a modest increase in his hydrochlorothiazide from 12.5 to 25 mg. He proceeds to follow the advice of both types of healers.

If the patient wishes to discuss or solicit the provider's opinion about other healing modalities, the clinician—unless there are concrete reasons to the contrary—should be willing to acknowledge the beneficial role that nonbiomedical approaches may have for the patient. If there are potential adverse interactions or side effects of "alternative" therapies, or if there is concern that potentially beneficial biomedical therapies might be thwarted by other types of healers, the clinician should express these concerns but should always respect the fact that patients are the ultimate arbiters regarding the healing modalities for which they are best suited (see Chapter 28).

CONCLUSION

Cross-cultural communication can be learned and enhanced through reflection and practice with a variety of patients from different cultures. Biomedicine has its own distinct culture and practices that may be difficult for many patients to comprehend and access. Cultural stereotypes are rarely useful in clinical encounters; instead clinicians should attempt to understand the social location of their patients as reflected in their race and ethnicity, gender, age, immigration status, literacy level, occupation, and other characteristics. As their skills develop, clinicians will find enormous gratification in caring for patients who are in some way different from themselves.

SUGGESTED READINGS

Doak CC, Doak LG, Root JH: *Teaching Patients With Low Literacy Skills.* J.B. Lippincott, 1985.

Fadiman A: *The Spirit Catches You and You Fall Down.* Farrar, Strauss & Giroux, 1998.

Helman C: *Culture, Health, and Illness,* 2nd ed. Butterworth-Heinemann, 1992.

Kaiser Permanente National Diversity Council: *A Provider's Handbook on Culturally Competent Care.* (Available for Latino, African-American, Asian/Pacific-Islander, and Eastern European populations.)

Kleinman A: *Patients and Healers in the Context of Culture.* University of California Press, 1980.

WEB SITE

http://medicine.ucsf.edu/resources/guidelines/culture.html
Provides extensive links to cross-cultural resources in clinical practice.

Lesbian & Gay Patients

13

Jocelyn C. White, MD, FACP

INTRODUCTION

Since the mid-1980s, acquired immunodeficiency syndrome (AIDS) has caused health-care providers to become more aware of the specific health needs of gay men. Similarly, the recent interest in women's health issues has led to a greater awareness of the unique health needs of lesbians. Before this time, the medical literature rarely discussed the health needs of either lesbians or gay men. Consequently, few primary care providers felt competent or comfortable caring for this population. Knowledge and skill are essential for the primary care provider to be able to ascertain the sexual orientation of patients; communicate acceptance and understanding of lesbian, gay, and bisexual health issues; screen for conditions amenable to behavioral medicine; and provide information and resources specific to the needs of lesbian, gay, and bisexual patients. By acquiring and using these skills, primary care providers can give lesbians and gay men access to competent medical care.

Lesbians and gay men make up anywhere from 1 to 10% of the general population—depending on the source quoted and the sampling method used in the study. In most studies, self-identified bisexuals are a small fraction of the lesbian or gay population. Whatever the exact percentage, however, in absolute terms, lesbians and gay men are a large group of patients with unique medical, psychological, and social needs. Many primary care providers currently care for lesbian and gay patients without being aware of the patients' sexual orientation or recognizing or acknowledging their unique needs.

Defining Sexual Orientation

Sexual orientation refers to sexual attraction to another person, including fantasies and the desire for sex, affection, and love. Sexual orientation is not necessarily predictive of sexual behavior, which refers only to sexual activities. Being a lesbian or a gay man involves awareness of a sexual attraction to a person of the same gender and, often, formation of a personal identity influenced by this awareness. This identity is formed by emotions, psychological responses, societal expectations, and the individual's own choices in identity formation. Most self-identified lesbians and gay men are sexually active with a partner of their own gender. In addition, some women and men identify themselves as lesbian or gay, although they are currently celibate or sexually active with a partner of the opposite gender. On the other hand, some men and women, particularly in the African-American and Latino cultures, are sexually active with a partner of their own gender but do not identify themselves as lesbian or gay. Most lesbians and gay men prefer the terms *lesbian* and *gay* to *homosexual,* because such terms refer to emotions, behavior, and a cultural system, as well as sexual orientation, and are nonjudgmental. Patients often see the term *homosexual* as a clinical term and may perceive it as pejorative.

Recent research suggests that a combination of both biological and environmental factors probably determines sexual orientation—heterosexual, homosexual, and bisexual. Studies of neuroanatomy, twins, and genetic markers in the families of gay brothers support a biological basis for homosexuality. The care and treatment of lesbian and gay patients remain the same, however, whether homosexuality is primarily a biological or an environmental phenomenon.

Homophobia

DEFINITION

Homophobia has been defined as an irrational fear of or prejudice against homosexuals. In daily life, lesbians and gay men experience homophobia as interpersonal, workplace, societal, or political bias. In other words, homophobia is prejudice or hatred based solely on a perceived homosexual orientation, and lesbians and gay men often find it difficult to act in accordance with their identity for fear of homophobic responses. They may experience stress and confusion in response to societal attitudes, identity-disclosure conflict, and internalized homophobia from years of living in an intolerant society. Despite the myths to the contrary, however, the potential for positive self-esteem in lesbians and gay men is generally similar to that of heterosexuals.

PROVIDER HOMOPHOBIA

Gay men and lesbians report frequent and often detrimental experiences of homophobia from health-care providers. The manifestations of discomfort with homosexuality in health-care providers cover a wide range. Some providers assume the patient is heterosexual and fail to allow opportunities for disclosure of sexual orientation. Others make frankly homophobic comments or jokes about the fact that the patient is lesbian or gay. Patients and physicians have reported observing substandard patient care because a provider failed to recognize a lesbian or gay sexual orientation or became overtly hostile to a lesbian or gay patient. A man with a perirectal abscess, for example, was lectured about being gay and was denied treatment. He sought care elsewhere and was hospitalized. In another instance, a woman visiting her partner in the recovery room after surgery for breast cancer called her "lover" and "honey." A nursing assistant walked by, shoving her a bit, and said "queer."

Health-care providers must recognize that patients of all sexual orientations are likely to be encountered in the daily practice of medicine (see the discussion of doctor–patient interactions below). Providers can do several things to project a nonjudgmental attitude to all patients. Most important, they can communicate with a patient in a way that does not assume heterosexuality. They can also ensure that office forms, support staff, and environment all convey an accepting attitude to patients—whatever their sexual orientation. Any health-care provider who feels uncomfortable in treating gay or lesbian patients should explain this to the patient and refer him or her to another competent provider.

DOCTOR–PATIENT INTERACTIONS

The doctor–patient relationship is the key to providing primary care to gay and lesbian patients. Without a good provider–patient relationship, patients may avoid medical care, especially primary care screening. Providers who are uncomfortable working with lesbian and gay patients, or who fail to recognize the sexual orientation of a patient, will manage patients incorrectly. They will fail to obtain pertinent information or to recognize important elements of the evaluation and treatment of these patients. Patients who do not obtain competent primary care services, including screening and health-risk and psychosocial counseling, are likely to have a lower health status than their heterosexual counterparts. Providers can develop a good relationship with gay, lesbian, and bisexual patients by showing an understanding of their health needs and communicating a nonjudgmental attitude.

CASE ILLUSTRATION 1

Robert, a middle-aged high school teacher, comes to the doctor's office. This is his first visit, and he hasn't completed the intake history form. After the introductions, the physician looks at the form and prepares to take a social history.

Overcoming Barriers to Communication

Many lesbians and gay men are reluctant to share their sexual orientation with health-care providers for fear of negative judgments and homophobic responses. Some fail to share this information even when asked directly. Unpleasant experiences with health-care providers have made lesbians and gay men more likely to avoid health-care and routine screening. Even sympathetic health-care providers are often uncomfortable with the interaction. They may lack experience with lesbian, gay, and bisexual health issues or feel unsure as to what language to use to elicit information respectfully from these patients. When both patient and provider are uncomfortable, important information is not shared.

THE SEXUAL HISTORY

Gathering information about a patient's gay or lesbian sexual orientation, or sexual practices, is often the first stumbling block encountered by health-care providers. Asking about orientation only while taking a sexual history and not at other times can limit the opportunity to learn whether the patient is gay or lesbian. In addition, the most commonly used questions set up barriers between the provider and patient, and can lead to inaccurate or incomplete information: "What form of birth control do you use?" "Are you married, single, widowed, or divorced?" "When was the last time you had intercourse?" When lesbians or gay men hear these questions, they may not know how to answer because these questions are based on the assumption that the patient is heterosexual. Because the options given do not necessarily pertain to a lesbian or gay patient, the patient must either provide false information or awkwardly stop and explain. Needing to give such explanations can make obtaining an already challenging sexual history even more difficult for both parties. To avoid this awkwardness, patients may play along with the assumption of heterosexuality, which can significantly affect the diagnosis and treatment of any illnesses of the patient.

THE SOCIAL HISTORY

This is a more comfortable part of the interview in which to raise issues of sexual orientation. By using questions with no heterosexual assumptions in taking the social history, the provider can increase the opportunities for, and comfort level in, discussing these issues. In asking about spouses, partners, children, and support systems, providers and patients explore how patients are most likely to cope with difficult situations. Providers learn about the patient's family structure, any stressors the patient might have, and personal and community resources on which patients would be likely to draw (see Chapter 8). Thus, the social history can be a more appropriate and comfortable place for exploring the sexual orientation of all patients and how it affects their health.

SENSITIVE COMMUNICATION

Sensitive questions make no assumptions about sexual orientation and are easily phrased: "Are you single, partnered, married, widowed, or divorced?" "Who is in your immediate family?" "Over your lifetime, have your sexual partners been men, women, or both?" "If you become ill, is there someone important whom I should involve in your care?" "How do you feel about my documenting your sexual orientation on the chart?" "What percentage of the time do you use safer sex?"

Because lesbians and gay men come in all shapes, sizes, ages, and colors, providers need to use questions such as these with all men and women, not just those they suspect of being lesbian or gay. In taking a sensitive sexual history, it is often helpful for providers to explain that they need information on sexual practices to make an accurate diagnosis or provide appropriate education.

In the initial visit with the patient, it is important to discuss explicitly the documentation of sexual orientation in the chart. Many lesbians and gay men are forced to keep their sexual orientation hidden for legal, employment, or child-custody reasons. When a lesbian or gay patient does not want sexual orientation documented, providers may use a coded entry and inform the patient that this is being done. The code serves to remind providers of the patient's sexual orientation for medical purposes but will prevent inadvertent breaches of confidentiality.

CASE ILLUSTRATION 1 (CONT.)

The doctor starts the social history:

Doctor: Are you single, partnered, married, widowed, or divorced?

Robert: I'm divorced, with a 20-year-old son, and I'm partnered now. His name is Tim.

Doctor: How long have you been together? How's the relationship?

Robert: Six years, and there's some tension now.

Further questioning reveals that Tim is younger than Robert—and openly gay. Robert is uncomfortable being that open; he is afraid of a scandal at school and the loss of his job. As the history-taking continues, the physician asks how Robert feels about having the fact that he is gay documented in the chart. After some discussion, the two decide on a coded entry of the information. At the end of the visit, Robert thanks the doctor for being so understanding; the doctor is also happy with the visit because he has been able to screen the patient appropriately and provide him with his first physical examination in 6 years.

Enhancing the Relationship

Providers who show a nonjudgmental attitude are much more likely to develop trusting relationships with gay and lesbian patients. Providers can improve the relationship in several simple ways: offering to include a partner in the discussions, ensuring that a gay or lesbian patient's partner is treated as a spouse in the office and the hospital, including partners in discussions of next-of-kin policies and advance directives, and using office and hospital forms with words that do not assume a heterosexual family structure.

GAY AND LESBIAN PROVIDERS

Gay and lesbian patients often prefer working with gay and lesbian health-care providers because of the presumed absence of homophobia in the relationship. Unfortunately, however, like their heterosexual colleagues, many gay and lesbian providers have learned communication skills without recognizing heterosexual bias. Medical schools and the literature are just beginning to provide information about lesbian and gay health issues. In learning to take care of these patients, providers—current and future—need to learn new language habits for bias-free communication.

Lesbian and gay providers may find themselves in a situation in which the question of whether to disclose their own sexual orientation to their patients arises. As in any other situation, the question is whether disclosure of sexual orientation is in the best interest of the patient. In many cases, such disclosure may be beneficial. When a patient clearly needs to understand that there will be no overt homophobia in the interaction before agreeing to remain in care, it may be reassuring to know that the provider is lesbian or gay. As patient–provider relationships develop, patients often want more personal information about the provider. Gay and lesbian providers must weigh for themselves the therapeutic benefit to the patient, the patient's need for information, and their own level of comfort in self-disclosure. Although many gay and lesbian physicians have reported ostracism, harassment, and professional discrimination from colleagues, teachers, administrators, and health plans, others report being open about their sexual orientation without experiencing any negative consequences.

PROBLEMS
Coming Out

The process of discovering one's sexual orientation and revealing it to others is known as *coming out* and can occur at any age. Stage theories for coming out have been well described and have been summarized as a four-step process:

1. Awareness of homosexual feelings
2. Testing and exploration

3. Identity acceptance
4. Identity integration and self-disclosure

The process of coming out involves a shift in core identity that can be associated with significant emotional distress, especially if family and peers respond negatively. Prevailing social attitudes also influence the experience. Societal and internalized homophobia often causes lesbians and gay men to perform a fatiguing cost–benefit analysis for each situation in which they consider coming out. If the costs of self-disclosure are repeatedly high, an individual may ultimately become socially isolated or revert to denying their gay or lesbian identity.

ADOLESCENTS

Lesbian and gay adolescents are particularly vulnerable to the emotional distress of coming out, and this distress can make adolescent development even more difficult (see Chapter 10). Parental acceptance of the adolescent during the coming out process may be the primary determinant of healthy self-esteem. Primary care providers need to screen for signs of sexual-orientation confusion in their adolescent patients. These signs may include depression, diminished school performance, alcohol and substance abuse, acting out, and suicidal ideation. Providers noting these signs need to consider sexual-orientation confusion in the differential diagnosis, along with depression and substance abuse.

OLDER ADULTS

Coming out, as noted previously, can occur at any age, even among older patients. Because there are varying degrees of disclosure, older individuals may be "out" to themselves and a partner or close friends but no one else beyond that trusted circle. Older lesbians and gay men are vulnerable to social isolation, and primary care providers are often among the primary support resources for older individuals. In exploring the social support network for their older patients, primary care providers need to be alert to the possibility of a lesbian or gay identity and the needs this engenders.

Relationships

COMMUNITY

A gay or lesbian individual's support network may not include the family, as many families have difficulties accepting a lesbian or gay relative's sexual orientation. Lesbian and gay individuals have reported receiving support mostly from partners, friends, and lesbian and gay community organizations. Primary care providers should be aware of a few useful resources in the lesbian and gay community to which they can direct patients (some resources are listed at the end of this chapter). For many gay men and lesbians, the gay and lesbian community serves as an extended family. Discussion groups, activity clubs, gay and lesbian religious organizations, and book stores often serve as a focal point for activities and the means of constructing and maintaining a support network. Lesbian and gay community organizations, newspapers, and book stores are usually the most useful and most commonly available.

PARTNERS

Like most heterosexuals, the majority of lesbians and gay men express a desire to find a partner and develop a relationship. And just like heterosexuals, lesbians and gay men can form and maintain long-lasting primary relationships. Lesbians and gay men may have commitment ceremonies, own homes together, share finances, and raise children.

Because of potential isolation from family, co-workers, and religious organizations, the relationship with a partner can be particularly important to a lesbian's or gay man's psychological well-being. As a result, discord in the relationship may be even more stressful than it might be for a heterosexual couple. In times of relationship stress, an individual may have limited resources for help in coping with the situation. Primary care providers should screen for relationship stress and be able to provide referrals for lesbian- and gay-sensitive couple therapy when appropriate.

PARENTHOOD

Parenthood plays a role in the lives of many lesbians and gay men, and the decision to become parents is usually deliberate and carefully made. Gay men and lesbians may have children from previous heterosexual relationships or through adoption, artificial insemination, heterosexual intercourse, or serving as foster parents. Occasionally, a lesbian couple and a gay couple will agree to have and bring up a child together.

Some members of society oppose parenthood for lesbian and gay men because of concerns about the psychological development and sexual orientation of the children. Studies have shown that there are no demonstrated differences between children raised by lesbians and gay men and those raised by heterosexuals. Open communication with children about their parents' sexual orientation appears to benefit family function, and the children themselves appreciate such openness.

A pregnant lesbian may find it difficult to get support for her pregnancy. The development of her identity as a mother may also be more complex. A primary care provider can support a pregnant lesbian by showing nonjudgmental attitudes and encouraging acceptance of lesbian motherhood among members of the delivery team and childbearing classes. Providers should encourage patients' partners and donor fathers, when appropriate, to participate in all phases of the fertility assessment, preconception and prenatal care, and delivery. It should be noted that partners and donor fathers may also need emotional support after delivery.

Loss

1. Grief—Grieving the loss of a partner may be more difficult for a lesbian or gay man if a support system is not available. Lesbians grieve the loss of partners and friends to breast cancer and other illnesses. Gay men and lesbians are particularly affected by deaths of partners and many friends from AIDS. Some gay men and lesbians report losing 10 or more friends or family members in a single year. In cases such as this, grief becomes a life constant. When a partner dies, the survivor, in effect, loses a spouse. This fact often goes unrecognized in the survivor's own social network. Frequently, the family of the deceased partner excludes the survivor or will not allow him or her to take part as a spouse in the funeral. A close-knit network of surviving friends is often neglected when a grieving family takes over funeral plans.

Occasionally, parents and family of the deceased are shocked and embarrassed to learn of the individual's sexual orientation or AIDS diagnosis. In such cases, the family may feel intense guilt or the need to hide their grief, unable to share it with their support network because of embarrassment. Family members of gay or lesbian individuals can find information and support for this and other issues by contacting the National Federation of Parents and Friends of Lesbians and Gays, a national organization with local chapters (see the list of resources at the end of this chapter).

Primary care providers can assist surviving partners and friends in the grieving process in several ways. Providers can assist the survivor in talking about the loss and expressing his or her feelings, identify and interpret normal grieving behavior and timelines, provide on-going support throughout the grief process, encourage the survivor to develop new relationships and support structures, and help the survivor adapt to new roles and patterns of living. In some cases, the health-care provider may be the only individual in whom the survivor can completely confide (see Chapters 3 and 35).

2. Advance directives—The durable power of attorney for health care is particularly important for lesbians and gay men. Because they are unable to marry legally, lesbians and gay men need to execute these documents to appoint their partners as surrogate health decision makers. Without such a document, the next of kin is considered the surrogate decision maker. Completing this document is the best way to avoid tragic decision-making conflicts between a partner and the estranged family members of seriously ill patients in time of crisis. As with all patients, a discussion of advance directives should be included in the preventive medicine check-up (see Chapter 35).

CLINICAL ISSUES

The American Psychiatric Association removed homosexuality from its list of mental illnesses in 1973. Psychiatric and behavioral interventions used in the past to "cure" patients of homosexuality have proven neither effective nor necessary. Overall, mental illness is no more common in lesbians or gay men than in the heterosexual population. Nonetheless, primary care providers must be aware of the unique psychosocial issues that some lesbians and gay men face.

Depression & Suicide

Some reports have suggested that lesbians and gay men are at higher risk for depression and suicide than the general population. As noted earlier, lesbians and gay men have unique psychosocial stressors, including societal bias, that can put them at risk for depression. African-American lesbians and gay men are particularly vulnerable to depressive distress in the United States, presumably from the pressures of being members of two minority populations that face pervasive discrimination.

Adolescents are particularly vulnerable to depression and suicide. One report suggests that approximately one-third of adolescent suicides are gay adolescents. This number is an alarmingly high proportion of youth suicides in a population that has few resources for counseling on sexual orientation issues. Further studies on depression and suicide in adolescent and adult gay men and lesbians are needed to confirm and update information on risk and prevalence. As part of a comprehensive clinical evaluation, primary care providers should screen all patients, including their lesbian and gay patients, for depression and suicidal ideation. Treatment of these conditions should be nonjudgmental with regard to sexual orientation and sensitive to the needs of specific individuals.

Substance Abuse

As part of the social history with any patient, including gay and lesbian patients, it is important to ask about drug and alcohol use (see Chapter 20). A provider should specifically explore the types of substances, the frequency and quantity, and whether patients use them during or preceding sexual activity. Many substances have a disinhibiting effect on the user and may make individuals more likely to engage in unsafe sex practices than they otherwise would.

There is controversy about the extent of drug and alcohol use in the gay and lesbian community. Older studies are flawed, but methodologically sound studies now exist. Based on some of these latter studies, alcohol and drug use among gay men is probably the same as or slightly more prevalent than among heterosexual men, and gay male drug users may use drugs more heavily than their heterosexual counterparts. According to a comparison of a population-based sample of lesbians in the San Francisco Bay area with a control group, alcohol use appears to be no more prevalent among lesbians than among heterosexual women. There are no population-based studies of drug use among lesbians compared with heterosexual women, but such use does occur.

Treatment for alcohol and other substance addiction can be challenging for both provider and patient. Homophobia, both societal and internalized, compounds the challenges. In many communities, there may be no treatment programs or counselors who are gay sensitive or gay affirmative. Although there are gay and lesbian 12-step meetings in many communities, many people have not come out publicly or do not feel comfortable in such meetings.

Domestic Violence

Contrary to some popular beliefs, battery of lesbians and gay men by their partners exists. The prevalence of battery in gay and lesbian relationships is not known; it often appears to be related to alcohol or drug use. Lesbians perceive that interpersonal power imbalances contribute to battery. They also report that many women's shelters are not responsive to their specific needs. Gay men may find it even more difficult to obtain services related to battery. Primary care providers should screen their gay and lesbian patients—and all patients—for the possibility of domestic violence and be able to give referrals to lesbian- and gay-sensitive resources, including shelters and counselors (see Chapter 33).

Hate Crimes

Also known as bias crimes, these are words or actions directed at an individual because of membership in a minority group. The U.S. Department of Justice reports that gay men and lesbians may be the most victimized group in the nation. Many studies report crimes ranging from verbal abuse and threats of violence to property damage, physical violence, and murder. The number of hate crimes reported by gay men and lesbians is increasing every year. Lesbians at universities, for example, report being victims of sexual assault twice as often as heterosexual women.

Perpetrators of hate crimes often include family members and community authorities. Many gay and lesbian adolescents leave home because of an abusive family member, and homeless gay and lesbian youths are of increasing social concern. When patients present with symptoms of depression or anxiety, providers should consider violence, including hate crimes, as a possible correlate.

EDUCATION, REFERRALS, & RESOURCES

Patient Education

This is a cornerstone of primary care. Providers who care for lesbian and gay patients must know how to advise pa-

tients in health issues, refer them to appropriate educational and community resources, and provide appropriate reference materials to hand out at visits.

Instruction

Instruction in preventing the spread of HIV and other sexually transmitted diseases should be clear and specific to lesbian and gay sexual practices. Physicians should be able to educate lesbians and gay men about risks and screening for sexually transmitted diseases and cancers. They also should be able to counsel patients, or refer them for counseling, about issues such as safer sex, parenting, coming out, battery, drug and alcohol use, depression, and hate crimes.

Referrals

Referrals should include other providers and community-based resources sensitive to the needs of lesbians and gay men. Hot lines, book stores, and bibliographies can help educate. Youth groups, senior groups, community centers, lesbian and gay religious organizations, retirement centers, and counselors who deal with lesbian and gay issues can all provide support. Gay and lesbian 12-step programs and substance-abuse support groups are also available. In areas in which such local resources are not available, a central hot line, book store, or gay and lesbian newspaper elsewhere in the state usually can provide referrals or information.

Provider Education

Health care providers can obtain additional information dealing with health issues and communicating with lesbian and gay patients through textbooks, review articles, teaching videos, and workshops at both national and regional medical conferences. Further information and educational materials are available from the Gay and Lesbian Medical Association (Internet address: GayLesMed@aol.com). Other resources include the following:

- National AIDS Hotline
  (800) 342-AIDS
  www.ashastd.org/nah
- National Center for Lesbian Rights
  Lesbian Health Project
  (415) 392-6257
  www.nclrights.org
- PFLAG—Parents, Families and Friends of Lesbians and Gays (National Federation of Parents and Friends of Lesbians and Gays, Inc.)
  (202) 467-8180
  www.pflag.org
- National Gay and Lesbian Task Force
  (202) 332-6483
  www.ngltf.org

- National Women's Health Network Resource packet on lesbian health issues
(202) 347-1140
www.womenshealthnetwork.org

Caring for lesbian and gay patients can be an educational and rewarding experience. For those providers who, for whatever reason, feel unable to care for lesbian or gay patients, making a referral to another provider is appropriate. Hospital physician referral services may have listings for lesbian- and gay-sensitive providers. Local community organizations may keep lists of providers willing to work with lesbian and gay patients. Polling colleagues to find those educated about lesbian and gay health issues can be fruitful. When referring a lesbian or gay patient to another provider for this reason, a brief but open discussion about the reason for the referral is both appropriate and respectful of the patient.

SUGGESTED READINGS

Aaron DJ et al: Behavioral risk factors for disease preventive health practices among lesbians. Am J Public Health 2001;91(6):972.

Byne W, Parsons B: Human sexual orientation: the biologic theories reappraised. Arch Gen Psychiatry 1993;50:228.

Cabaj RP: AIDS and chemical dependency: special issues and treatment barriers for gay and bisexual men. J Psychoactive Drugs 1989;21(4):387.

Dean L et al: Lesbian, gay, bisexual, and transgender health findings and concerns. J Gay Lesbian Med Assoc 2000;4(3):101.

Diamond M: Homosexuality and bisexuality in different populations. Arch Sex Behav 1993;22(4):291.

Fawzy FI, Fawzy NW, Pasnau RO: Bereavement in AIDS. Psychiatr Med 1991;9(3):469.

Herek GM et al: Correlates of internalized homophobia in a community sample of lesbian and gay men. J Gay Lesbian Med Assoc 1998;2(1):17.

Lock J, Steiner H: Relationships between sexual orientation and coping styles of gay, lesbian, and bisexual adolescents from a community high school. J Gay Lesbian Med Assoc 1999;3(3):77.

Mays VM, Cochran SD: Mental health correlates of perceived discrimination among lesbian, gay, and bisexual adults in the United States. Am J Public Health 2001;91(11):1869.

National Gay and Lesbian Task Force: *Anti-Gay Violence: Causes, Consequences, Responses.* National Gay and Lesbian Task Force, 1986.

O'Neill JF, Shalit P: Healthcare of the gay male patient. Prim Care 1992;19(1):191.

Patterson CJ: Children of lesbian and gay parents. Child Dev 1992;63:1025.

Quam JK, Whitford G: Adaptation and age-related expectations of older gay and lesbian adults. Gerontologist 1992;32(3):367.

Schatz B, O'Hanlan K: *Anti-Gay Discrimination in Medicine: Results of a National Survey of Lesbian, Gay and Bisexual Physicians.* American Association of Physicians for Human Rights (AAPHR), May 1994.

Scout BJ, Fields C: Removing the barriers: improving practitioners' skills in providing health care to lesbians and women who partner with women. Am J Public Health 2001;91(6):989.

Shernoff M: Gay widowers: grieving in relation to trauma and social supports. J Gay Lesbian Med Assoc 1998;2(1):27.

Solarz AL (editor): *Lesbian Health: Current Assessment and Directions for the Future.* National Academy Press, 1999.

van Dam MAA, Koh AS, Dibble SL: Lesbian disclosure to health care providers and delay of care. J Gay Lesbian Med Assoc 2001;5(1):11.

White J, Levinson W: Primary care of lesbian patients. J Gen Intern Med 1993;8:41.

Wismount JM, Reame NE: The lesbian childbearing experience: assessing development tasks. Image: J Nurs School 1989;21(3):137.

Women

Martina J. Jelley, MD, MSPH, E. Montez Mutzig, MD, MPH, FACP & Judith Walsh, MD, MPH

INTRODUCTION

Women and men can present with different problems and often require different approaches to the same disease. Using an evidence-based approach, we will focus on issues unique to women and also on conditions and interventions that may affect women differently. The primary care practitioner should be well informed regarding these areas specific to the overall health of women.

MEDICAL CONDITIONS WITH PSYCHOSOCIAL COMPONENTS

Women are more likely to present for health care because of vague symptoms such as fatigue and pain for which no identified pathology can be found. They are also more likely to present with a functional syndrome such as chronic fatigue syndrome (CFS), fibromyalgia (FM), irritable bowel syndrome (IBS), and chronic pelvic pain (CPP). Research has shown that medically unexplained symptoms and functional syndromes share many biological, clinical, and psychosocial characteristics. In addition to being more common in women, they are associated with significant suffering and disability, symptoms that cannot be explained by objective findings, and psychosocial stressors that worsen or exacerbate their condition. Psychiatric disorders, particularly anxiety, panic, and depressive disorders, and a history of sexual and physical abuse are common with these disorders.

The cause and pathology of these syndromes is not clearly understood and is most likely multifactorial with environmental, cultural, biological, psychosocial, and genetic factors all playing a complex role. Historically, these disorders have been labeled as "psychosomatic," implying that the symptoms were "psychogenic," because an organic cause could not be identified. However, research in the areas of immunology, neuroendocrinology, and neuropsychiatry has made significant contributions to our understanding of the connection between the mind and body. Numerous changes have been identified in the central nervous system that lead to an abnormal processing of nociceptive stimuli, thereby resulting in the patient having a heightened perception and an exaggerated response to pain. The mechanism underlying these changes has not been clearly delineated, but it appears to vary among the different disorders.

The relationship between stress and illness is complicated and heavily influenced by psychological, biological, and cultural factors (see Chapter 29). Research has shown that stress has a profound effect on the patient's functional status. Psychosocial stressors contribute to higher levels of psychological distress and are associated with a worsening of symptoms, an increase in the number of symptoms, a lower threshold for pain, an increased utilization of health care, and an increased degree of disability. The impact of stress on the patient's disability and function is much greater for patients who have a functional syndrome than for those with a chronic medical illness such as diabetes mellitus. This effect is magnified even further when a functional syndrome and a psychiatric disorder coexist.

Patients with functional syndromes have a higher likelihood of having concurrent and lifetime episodes of psychiatric disorders, particularly anxiety, panic, and depression. Patients with a functional syndrome and a co-morbid psychiatric disorder have more unexplained symptoms, worsening of symptoms, and more disability compared with patients who have only a functional syndrome.

Because of the high prevalence of a psychiatric illness coexisting with a functional syndrome, all patients should be screened for a psychiatric disorder. Screening tools such as the PRIME MD (Primary Care Evaluation of Mental Disorders) and the MINI (Mini International Neuropsychiatric Interview) are sensitive, reliable, and valid instruments for use in a primary care setting.

Depression frequently presents as an unexplained medical symptom or as a cluster of unexplained symptoms (see Chapter 21). Depression is five times more likely to occur in patients who experience pain at two or more body sites and pain at multiple sites increases the risk of depression eight-fold. The likelihood of a psychiatric diagnosis increases linearly with the number of symptoms reported and is highly predictive of an underlying psychiatric disorder. Patients who present with more than four unexplained physical symptoms or more than four symptoms on the PRIME MD symptom check list should be screened for a psychiatric illness.

Many patients have more than one functional syndrome and overlap is common. For example, it has been estimated that as many as 70% of patients with FM meet the criteria for CFS; conversely as many as 35–70% of patients with CFS also have FM. IBS is frequently found to overlap with CFS (92%), FM (77%), and CPP (50%). Patients who have two or more syndromes experience a higher degree of psychological distress than patients who have only one syndrome.

Caring for patients with functional syndromes can be challenging and is often difficult. Because of the similarities and significant overlap among these syndromes many of the same management strategies can be applied. Treatments that are specific to each syndrome will be discussed individually in greater detail. A stepwise approach to medical management is recommended. First, it is important to exclude an unrecognized medical disease. Second, all patients should be screened for the presence of a psychiatric disorder. Treating the underlying psychiatric illness will often lead to significant improvement of the patient's symptoms.

Establishing a therapeutic doctor–patient relationship using a patient-centered approach has been shown to be highly effective and should be the primary goal of treatment (see Chapter 1). A therapeutic relationship leads to improved patient satisfaction, fewer patient follow-up visits, and less hospitalizations. The healing effects of the doctor–patient relationship cannot be overemphasized, especially as conventional medical therapies are often ineffective. Special care should be taken to recognize, identify, and validate the patient's symptoms and suffering. This technique alone can be extremely therapeutic. Do not fall into the trap of arguing with patients as to the etiology or the severity of their symptoms.

Education of the patient is paramount. Identifying and understanding patients' stressors and triggers can help them cope with their illness and thereby improve their overall function and quality of life. Most patients when asked will acknowledge that their life stressors exacerbate their symptoms. Significant resistance to psychosocial questions may be a potential clue that the patient has undiagnosed somatization disorder (see Chapter 23).

It is important to establish realistic and well-defined goals for the patient. In doing so, this can diminish or eliminate much of the frustration that surrounds the encounter. It is important to keep in mind that the goal of treatment should focus on helping patients "cope" with their disease and not in trying to "cure" patients. Regularly scheduled appointments give patients the opportunity to express their concerns and reinforce your commitment to helping them. Cognitive-behavioral therapies and exercise have been found to be effective in the treatment of the functional syndromes. These interventions aid in the ability of patients to cope with their illness by reducing somatic symptoms, generalized distress, and disability.

Chronic Fatigue

Fatigue is the most common complaint voiced by women in a primary care setting, with an estimated prevalence of 21–33%. Most patients seek medical care for chronic fatigue that persists for more than 6 months. Fatigue is often described as a lack of energy, a sensation of exhaustion, or being too tired to participate in family, work, or even leisure activities.

The syndrome of chronic fatigue (CFS) is relatively uncommon and will be discussed briefly. CFS is an ill-defined disease that occurs in young to middle-aged women and is characterized by persistent or relapsing fatigue. The terms chronic fatigue and CFS are often used inappropriately and interchangeably. In an attempt to clarify the distinction between the two entities the Centers for Disease Control (CDC) established specific diagnostic criteria for CFS (see Table 14–1).

One-fourth of patients will experience fatigue that lasts for more than 6 months. The cause of the fatigue can be identified as a medical or a psychiatric disease in two-thirds of patients. Twenty-five percent of cases are labeled as idiopathic, as no etiology can be determined and there is insufficient evidence to establish a diagnosis of CFS.

Chronic fatigue is frequently the only manifestation of an undiagnosed psychiatric disorder. Major depression has been found to present as fatigue in 58% of patients. Panic and somatization disorder are the causative agents in 10% of patients with chronic fatigue. A thorough history and physical examination along with basic laboratory tests will identify the cause of the fatigue in most patients. Be-

Table 14–1. Revised CDC criteria for chronic fatigue syndrome.[1]

A case of chronic fatigue syndrome is defined by the presence of the following:

1. Clinically evaluated, unexplained, persistent, or relapsing fatigue that is of new or definite onset; is not the result of ongoing exertion; is not alleviated by rest; and results in substantial reduction in previous levels of occupational, educational, social, or personal activities and
2. Four or more of the following symptoms that persist or recur during 6 or more consecutive months of illness and that do not predate the fatigue:
   - Self-reported impairment in short-term memory or concentration
   - Sore throat
   - Tender cervical or axillary nodes
   - Muscle pain
   - Multijoint pain without redness or swelling
   - Headaches of a new pattern or severity
   - Unrefreshing sleep
   - Postexertional malaise lasting 24 or more hours

[1] Adapted from Fukuda K et al: The chronic fatigue syndrome: a comprehensive approach to its definition and study. Ann Intern Med 1994;121:953.

cause of the high prevalence of a psychiatric illness all patients should be screened for major depression, anxiety, and somatization disorders.

Pharmacological therapy has not been shown to be beneficial in the treatment of chronic fatigue. Antidepressants are frequently used based on their efficacy in the treatment of other functional syndromes. Behavioral therapies such as weekly counseling sessions and relaxation techniques combined with exercise programs are the only treatments that have been found to be effective in patients with chronic fatigue.

Fibromyalgia

Fibromyalgia (FM) is a complex disorder that is characterized by chronic and diffuse pain. The estimated prevalence of FM in women is 3.4% and increases with age, reaching 8% in women 80 years of age. FM is the most common cause of pain and disability reported in women between the ages of 30 and 55.

The exact cause and pathology of FM are unknown. A precipitating illness or exposure to certain stressors such as trauma and emotional distress is known to trigger FM in most patients. Frequently patients are not diagnosed until 5–7 years after the onset of their symptoms.

Widespread chronic pain in the absence of inflammation, fatigue, disturbances in sleep, and stiffness are highly characteristic of this disorder (see Figure 14–1). Fatigue is

present in more than 90% of cases and often is the predominate complaint. Disturbances in sleep patterns and stiffness occur in 73–85% of patients diagnosed with FM. Additional symptoms experienced may include dizziness, palpitations, paresthesias, vulvodynia, night sweats, weakness, and "allergy" symptoms.

Exertion, stress, inadequate sleep, and weather changes are psychosocial stressors known to exacerbate the symptoms of FM. The symptoms wax and wane but tend to remain constant over time. The majority of patients remain functional despite continuing to experience moderate to severe pain, fatigue, and sleep disturbances.

FM commonly coexists with other medical disorders including systemic lupus erythematous (SLE), rheumatoid arthritis, osteoarthritis, Raynaud's phenomena, CFS, and other functional syndromes such as migraine headaches, IBS, CPP, and premenstrual disorders. Approximately one-fourth of patients with FM have a concurrent depression and their lifetime risk of developing depression is increased by 50–70%.

Systemic illnesses that are most likely to be confused with FM include polymyalgia rheumatica, SLE, Lyme disease, autoimmune disorders, and hypothyroidism. In the majority of cases a thorough history and physical examination and a few simple laboratory tests are adequate to rule out these diseases. More extensive testing is usually not necessary.

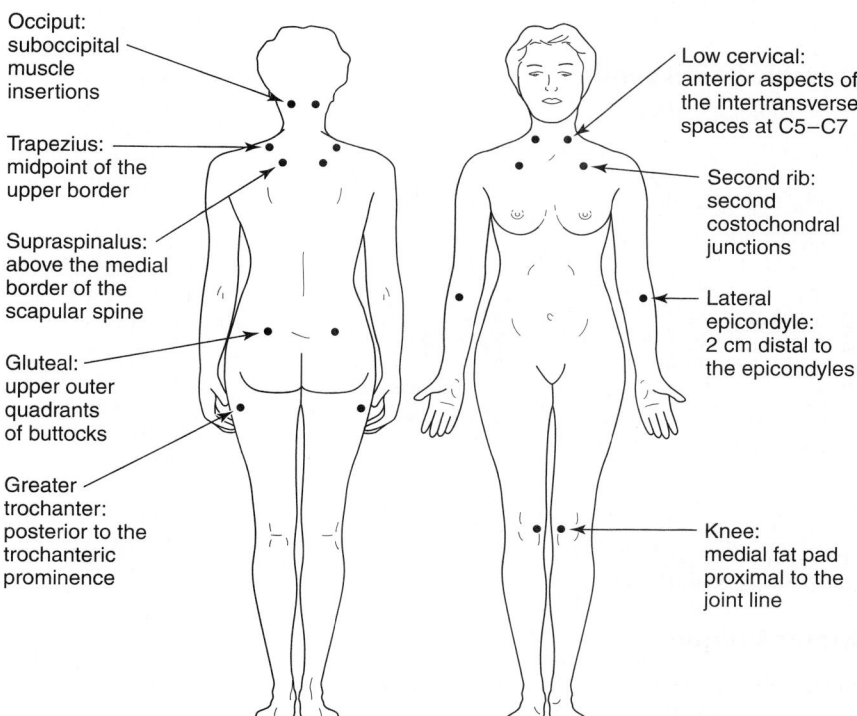

Occiput: suboccipital muscle insertions

Trapezius: midpoint of the upper border

Supraspinalus: above the medial border of the scapular spine

Gluteal: upper outer quadrants of buttocks

Greater trochanter: posterior to the trochanteric prominence

Low cervical: anterior aspects of the intertransverse spaces at C5–C7

Second rib: second costochondral junctions

Lateral epicondyle: 2 cm distal to the epicondyles

Knee: medial fat pad proximal to the joint line

Figure 14–1. Trigger point examination for the diagnosis of fibromyalgia.

The diagnosis of FM can be confirmed by a trigger point examination conducted at predefined anatomical sites (see Figure 14–1). This is best done by applying enough pressure to blanch the examiner's fingernail for a few seconds. A trigger point is positive if it elicits mild pain or causes the patient greater tenderness. The presence of more than 11 of 18 trigger points is highly diagnostic of FM with a sensitivity of 88% and specificity of 81%. An increase in the number of tender points has been associated with worsening depression, fatigue, and anxiety, and a higher number of somatic complaints.

Effective treatment for FM is limited. Tricyclic antidepressants, the most widely used and studied medications, are effective in only 25–45% of patients, and long-term benefits have not been proven. Low dose amitriptyline and cyclobenzaprine at bedtime improve pain, global well-being, and sleep-related problems. Fluoxetine is equally as effective as amitriptyline and the combination of the fluoxetine and amitriptyline is significantly superior to individual therapy. Nonsteroidal antiinflammatory drugs (NSAIDs) are widely used although their efficacy is supported by only one trial that used the combination of naproxen and amitriptyline. A few studies have shown some efficacy with venlafaxine, benzodiazepines, tramadol, S-adenosyl-L-methionine (SAMe), and lidocaine injections of tender points. Randomized clinical trials have demonstrated some improvement of FM symptoms with the use of cardiovascular fitness training, cognitive-behavioral therapy, biofeedback, hypnotherapy, and acupuncture.

Irritable Bowel Syndrome

Irritable Bowel Syndrome (IBS) is the most common gastrointestinal disorder seen in a primary care setting. It is characterized by chronic abdominal pain and altered bowel habits in the absence of an organic cause. IBS has been found in approximately 20% of the population with a female-to-male predominance of 2:1.

Patients typically experience the onset of symptoms in their late teens or early twenties and onset after the age of 50 is rare. In the majority of patients the gastrointestinal symptoms are mild and most never seek medical care. Patients with more severe forms of the disease are two times more likely to present for health care and are three times more likely to miss work than patients with milder symptoms.

Extensive research has yet to reveal the cause of IBS. It is thought to be a disorder of gastrointestinal motility and an increased visceral sensitivity of the gut. Studies show that patients with IBS experience more stressful life experiences and that psychosocial stressors have been shown to both precipitate and exacerbate symptoms. Psychosocial stressors have been associated with the patients experiencing more pain, physician visits, medications, and alternative medical care. Patients with more severe forms of IBS are more likely to report a history of sexual and physical abuse, a major loss (death of a loved one or divorce), or exposure to major trauma. A history of sexual and physical abuse has been identified in approximately one-third of patients. Patients with a history of abuse have poorer health outcomes as manifested by an increase in pain, physician visits, and surgical procedures than patients without a history of abuse.

Chronic abdominal pain that is associated with bowel dysfunction is the hallmark of IBS. Patients typically alternate between constipation and diarrhea with either symptom predominating. The abdominal pain is usually described as a cramping sensation that varies in intensity and frequency and is often precipitated by meals and relieved with defecation. Most patients complain of abdominal bloating and excessive gas production causing flatulence or belching. Other common gastrointestinal symptoms include dysphagia, dyspepsia, nausea, vomiting, and acid reflux. Extraintestinal complaints frequently associated with IBS include sexual dysfunction, dyspareunia, dysmenorrhea, urinary frequency, and urgency. Menstruation has been shown to exacerbate the patient's symptoms.

Patients with IBS have a higher frequency of a coexisting medical illness such as FM, CFS, and chronic pain syndromes. Depression, anxiety, and panic attacks are also common.

The diagnosis of IBS is made predominantly on the patient's history and normal physical examination. Symptoms that require further evaluation include gastrointestinal bleeding, fever, anorexia, weight loss, malnutrition, progressive pain, and pain that awakens the patient or interferes with the patient's sleep.

Effective treatment for IBS involves an integrated pharmacological and behavioral stepwise approach based on the patient's major symptom. Treatment for mild disease generally requires only education and reassurance and the occasional use of over-the-counter medications. Bulk agents are generally recommended in all patients and have been found to improve the satisfaction of bowel movements, ease stool passage, and relieve constipation. Antispasmodics are highly effective for the treatment of abdominal pain and are somewhat helpful for abdominal bloating. Loperamide is beneficial for the treatment of diarrhea. The tricyclic antidepressants appear to be effective for patients who have a coexisting psychiatric disorder and in the treatment of chronic refractory symptoms. Psychological treatments including dynamic psychotherapy, cognitive-behavioral treatment, hypnosis, relaxation, and biofeedback have been shown to be effective treatment for abdominal pain and diarrhea but not for constipation. The data supporting the use of peppermint oil are inconclusive.

Chronic Pelvic Pain

Chronic pelvic pain (CPP) is defined as persistent pain in the pelvis for greater than 6 months. It is reported in 15% of young women, and yet only one-third of patients seek medical care. CPP is usually associated with numerous other symptoms including headache, low back pain, dizziness, shortness of breath, fatigue, and weakness.

Women diagnosed with CPP are more likely to experience depression, anxiety, somatization disorders, sexual dysfunction, and substance abuse. A history of sexual and physical abuse, particularly during childhood, has been identified in over 50% of patients. Medically unexplained symptoms and other functional syndromes, specifically IBS and FM, are frequently associated with CPP.

The cause of CPP is extensive, and in 50% of cases psychopathology is the only identifiable diagnosis. The scientific data to guide treatment for CPP are limited. NSAIDs are usually recommended as emperic therapy for all patients. The tricylic antidepressants have been shown to be somewhat effective in the treatment of other chronic pain syndromes and are commonly used despite lack of supportive data. One study found no benefit using sertraline. Medroxyprogesterone acetate has good evidence to support its use for reducing pain. Cognitive-behavioral therapy and counseling are effective for reducing pain and improving mood. A multidisciplinary approach using pharmacological and cognitive-behavioral therapy has been found to be the most effective treatment for CPP.

ISSUES FOR WOMEN ACROSS THE LIFE SPAN

Adolescents

ISSUES AROUND FOOD/EATING DISORDERS

Eating disorders are common in young women and the primary care physician plays an important role in their detection. The primary care physician also manages the medical complications, determines the need for hospitalization, and coordinates care. In addition, for patients with milder forms of disordered eating who may not be seeing a mental health specialist regularly, the primary care physician may have responsibility for ongoing care, including exacerbations that may mandate coordination with mental health and/or nutritional support. Eating disorders are described in detail in Chapter 19. In this chapter, we will briefly discuss detection of eating disorders in young women.

The American Psychiatric Association *Diagnostic and Statistical Manual of Mental Disorders,* 4th edition, *Text Revision* (*DSM-IV-TR*) diagnostic criteria for anorexia nervosa, bulimia nervosa, and binge eating disorder are listed in Chapter 19. Two groups at high risk for eating disorders include female athletes and females with diabetes.

Screening for Eating Disorders

Because many women will not seek care for an eating disorder, the clinician must remain alert for clues, such as amenorrhea, concern about weight loss by a family member, abdominal bloating, and cold intolerance. Questions that are useful in ascertaining eating habits include: "Are you trying to lose weight?" "What did you eat yesterday?" and "Do you ever binge eat (eat more than you want) or use laxatives, diuretics, or diet pills?" Two questions have been shown to be useful in screening for bulimia nervosa in the primary care setting: "Do you ever eat in secret?" and "How satisfied are you with your eating habits?" Another screening tool, the SCOFF questionnaire, may prove to be useful in screening for eating disorders. The questions included the following: (1) Do you make yourself **S**ick because you feel uncomfortably full? (2) Do you worry you have lost **C**ontrol over how much you eat? (3) Have you recently lost more than **O**ne stone (fourteen pounds) in a three-month period? (4) Do you believe yourself to be **F**at when others say you are too thin? (5) Would you say **F**ood dominates your life? A "yes" answer to any question is worth one point and a score of two is highly predictive of anorexia nervosa or bulimia nervosa; however this test has yet to be validated prospectively in a broader population.

TREATMENT OF EATING DISORDERS[1]

The various treatments for eating disorders are described in full in Chapter 19. A theoretical framework for treating patients with eating disorders is described below.

During the precontemplation and contemplation stages, a patient may not be willing to accept full multidisciplinary treatment for an "eating disorder." She may, however, agree to work with one member of the treatment team, for example a nutritionist, without acknowledging that seriously disordered eating is present. Similarly, counseling for developmental or family issues, or treatment for depression, may be acceptable, again without acknowledgment of the presence of an eating disorder. Whether or not referral to a nutritionist or psychologist is accepted, periodic medical visits to follow the presenting symptom(s), for example, amenorrhea, low heart rate, or loss of weight, allow the primary care clinician to monitor the severity of symptoms (particularly cardiac status or other indications for hospitalization) while gently informing a patient of the medical risks of her condition. Evidence of associated medical risks, such as osteopenia, or concerns about fertility (particularly when the patient has low weight or is estrogen deficient) may encourage a patient to acknowledge the diagnosis and begin full treatment.

---

[1] The authors would like to acknowledge Dr. Polly Wheat for her insight into the theoretical framework for treating patients with eating disorders.

In summary, the first role of the primary care doctor is to detect an eating disorder, which may require maintaining a high index of suspicion. The clinician then must work as a member of a multidisciplinary team, including a mental health professional and a nutritionist, to ensure that the patient gains weight as appropriate, modifies her eating habits, and receives appropriate psychological and or medical therapies.

APPROACH TO THE GYNECOLOGICAL EXAMINATION

Clinicians should ask about any problems with sexual dysfunction before performing the pelvic examination. Sexual dysfunction problems include dyspareunia, vaginismus, and disorders of sexual desire. Problems with sexual desire can sometimes be related to underlying conditions such as hypothyroidism or depression, which should be screened for as deemed necessary. During the pelvic examination, potential causes of dyspareunia and vaginismus such as vaginal lesions, infection, and dryness or atrophy can be ruled out. The approach to sexual dysfunction is discussed in detail in Chapter 27.

Many women fear a pelvic examination, especially when they are undergoing it for the first time. Little research has been done on what strategies are best in performing a pelvic examination, but several techniques have frequently been found to be helpful in clinical practice.

First, it is useful for the clinician to describe exactly what is being done before and during the examination. When the examiner is male, it is appropriate for a nurse or chaperone to be present. Although many women prefer a female provider for a pelvic examination, a recent study done in a emergency room setting concluded that women found a pelvic examination done by a man to be more embarrassing than a pelvic examination done by a woman.

Other techniques that seem to be useful include appropriate draping, using a warm speculum, using the narrowest speculum that will allow adequate visualization of the cervix, and encouraging the patient to use relaxation techniques including deep breathing and use of mental imagery. Deep breathing is suggested when the patient feels uncomfortable, and mental imagery (encouraging the patient to form and talk about a mental image) can be used to help further relax the pelvic muscles, and may be particularly useful for young women and for those who have experienced sexual abuse or rape.

Research has shown that the experience of the first pelvic examination strongly influences attitudes about subsequent examinations. Therefore it is important for clinicians to focus on making the first pelvic examination as positive an experience as possible. In a study describing experiences of the first pelvic examination, a negative evaluation of the examination was associated with pain, embarrassment, and having insufficient knowledge about the examination and what the doctor was doing. Spending time at the first examination providing knowledge and encouraging realistic expectations of the examination may be useful in shaping attitudes about subsequent examinations.

Medical education must continue to focus on training students and residents in techniques of pelvic examination, as research has suggested that residents may receive inadequate training in these skills. Optimal strategies for teaching these important skills are still being developed. Recent research has shown that laywomen (nonphysicians) serving as both teachers and patients may be more effective than attending physicians in teaching the interpersonal skills needed while performing a pelvic examination.

Issues for Reproductive Aged Women

PREMENSTRUAL SYNDROME AND PREMENSTRUAL DYSPHORIC DISORDER

Premenstrual syndrome (PMS) is common in menstruating women and is characterized by cyclic occurrences of a variety of somatic, affective, and behavioral symptoms. As many as 150 symptoms have been attributed to PMS. The most common signs and symptoms are fatigue, irritability, bloating, anxiety or tension, breast tenderness, mood lability, depression, and food cravings. Manifestation of symptoms typically occurs 7–10 days prior to menstruation and usually resolves within a few days after the onset of menses. The International Classification of Diseases (ICD-10) diagnosis of PMS requires only a history of a physical or mood symptom occurring in a cyclic fashion. This patient population probably includes patients with PMS, patients with premenstrual dysphoric disorder (PMDD), and a substantial percentage of patients not meeting criteria for either diagnosis.

Approximately 80% of women experience either emotional or physical changes prior to menstruation. This is a normal sign of ovulatory cycles and not a diagnosis of PMS. PMS occurs in only about one-third of women. These women tend to experience symptoms that are problematic but not severe enough to interfere with daily activities. Three to eight percent of women experience significant impairment in work, school, relationships, or some other aspect of daily living and may be diagnosed with PMDD as classified by the *DSM-IV-TR*. The diagnostic criteria for PMDD specifically exclude premenstrual exacerbation of a known underlying psychiatric disorder. Therefore it is important to evaluate and treat any underlying psychiatric disorder if it is present in this group of patients.

The most important tool that a clinician can use in making the diagnosis of PMS is a prospective daily symptom scale or PMS calendar. Several calendars have been widely used and validated, including the Calendar of Premenstrual Experiences (COPE), which includes a four-point Likert scale for each of the 10 most commonly reported physical symptoms and 12 most commonly reported behavioral symptoms rated daily throughout the menstrual cycle (see Figure 14–2). A total score on this inventory of less than 40 during Days 3–9 of the cycle combined with a score greater than 42 during the last 7 days of the menstrual cycle has been shown to be an excellent pre-dictor of women who meet inclusion criteria for PMDD. The timing of the onset of symptoms around the time of ovulation and a symptom-free period are crucial to the diagnosis. The calendar is helpful as a diagnostic aid and can also be therapeutic to the patient.

Name _____ Month/Year _____ Age _____ Unit # _____

Begin your calendar on the *first* day of your menstrual cycle. Enter the calendar date below the cycle day. Day 1 is your *first* day of bleeding. Shade the box above the cycle day if you have bleeding. Put an X for spotting.

If more than one symptom is listed in a category, i.e., nausea, diarrhea, constipation, you do not need to experience all of these. Rate the most disturbing of the symptoms on the 1–3 scale.

Weight: Weigh yourself before breakfast. Record weight on the box below date.

Symptoms: Indicate the severity of your symptoms by using the scale below. Rate each symptom at about the same time each evening.

0 = None (symptom not present)   2 = Moderate (interferes with normal activities)
1 = Mild (noticeable but not troublesome)   3 = Severe (intolerable, unable to perform normal activities)

Other Symptoms: If there are other symptoms you experience, list and indicate severity.
Medications: List any medications taken. Put an X on the corresponding day(s).

Bleeding																																								
Cycle Day	1	2	3	4	5	6	7	8	9	10	11	12	13	14	15	16	17	18	19	20	21	22	23	24	25	26	27	28	29	30	31	32	33	34	35	36	37	38	39	40
Date																																								
Weight																																								
SYMPTOMS																																								
Acne																																								
Bloatedness																																								
Breast tenderness																																								
Dizziness																																								
Fatigue																																								
Headache																																								
Hot flashes																																								
Nausea, diarrhea, constipation																																								
Palpitations																																								
Swelling (hands, ankles, breast)																																								
Angry outbursts, arguments, violent tendencies																																								
Anxiety, tension, nervousness																																								
Confusion, difficulty concentrating																																								
Crying easily																																								
Depression																																								
Food cravings (sweets, salts)																																								
Forgetfulness																																								
Irritability																																								
Increased appetite																																								
Mood swings																																								
Overly sensitive																																								
Wish to be alone																																								
Other Symptoms																																								
1. _____																																								
2. _____																																								
Medications																																								
1. _____																																								
2. _____																																								

Figure 14–2. Calendar of premenstrual experiences.

The definite underlying etiology of PMS is unknown. The available evidence suggest that PMS results from the interaction of cyclic changes in ovarian steroids with central neurotransmitters. The neurotransmitter most implicated is serotonin. Numerous studies have attempted to identify various stressors in the exacerbation or maintenance of premenstrual symptoms. Life-styles, stressful life events, general stress levels, family dynamics, and work environment have all been found to increase the symptoms of PMS.

Many women with PMS often feel misunderstood by their friends, family, and health care provider. They are frequently told that their symptoms are "all in their head" or "it is just something that you have to live with." Therefore it is critical that primary care providers educate patients that this is a legitimate chronic medical disorder and that treatment can either alleviate or improve symptoms.

Treatment for PMS is approached in a stepwise fashion. For less severe cases, a set of behavioral changes is recommended before pharmacotherapy is begun. Encouraging the patient to exercise regularly, limit salt and caffeine intake, and keep a regular sleeping schedule may be beneficial. These recommendations arise from retrospective studies of risk factors for PMS. Because these recommendations are low risk and part of an overall healthy life-style, they can continue to be suggested as a first step. As mentioned earlier, the prospective daily symptom scale may be therapeutic. It helps patients identify their symptoms and how they relate to the menstrual cycle, and allows them to be proactive in anticipating, managing, and avoiding symptoms. Stress reduction through relaxation exercise, counseling, developing appropriate coping strategies, and psychotherapy may be helpful. There is some evidence from controlled trials that women with PMS may benefit from individual cognitive therapy or coping skills training. Cognitive-behavioral therapy may be beneficial in certain patients.

Most patients with PMDD require pharmacological therapy for significant improvement. The selective serotonin reuptake inhibitors (SSRIs) have led to dramatic improvements in the symptoms of PMDD. Compared with a placebo fluoxetine, given in a daily dose of 20 mg, resulted in a significant reduction in symptoms of tension, irritability, and dysphoria. Although not yet approved for this use, other drugs that inhibit serotonin reuptake, such as clomipramine, nefazadone, sertraline, paroxetine, and citalopram, have been shown to be effective. Recently, several trials have shown benefit from SSRI use only during the luteal phase. This approach can reduce cost and side effects.

The benzodiazepine alprazolam (0.25 mg three or four times a day) and buspirone (25 to 60 mg/d) can be used in the luteal phase to reduce symptoms, but the reduction is smaller than with SSRIs. Patients who do not respond to SSRIs or anxiolytics are candidates for ovulation suppression agents. Because these agents cause a "chemical menopause," several types of steroid "add-back" regimens have been developed. A gonadotropin-releasing hormone agonist is preferable to danazol because of fewer side effects. Early results of retrospective studies of the use of oral contraceptives showed milder symptoms among users but more recent prospective studies have not shown differences from placebo. Oral contraceptive pills may be considered if symptoms are mostly physical, but are probably not effective if mood liability is a primary symptom. Various diuretics have been proposed as treatment for PMS, but only spironolactone has shown efficacy in a double-blind trial.

A variety of complementary or alternative therapies have been tried in the treatment of PMS. A recent systematic review found no compelling evidence to recommend any of these therapies. Evening primrose oil has been tested in a controlled trial in a variety of dosages and preparations, with no benefit found except for relieving breast discomfort. Chaste tree (*Vitex agnus*) is often recommended, but two randomized control trials did not show significant benefit over placebo. One large, well-designed, multicenter trial found that 1200 mg of elemental calcium per day was effective in reducing depression, water retention, pain, food cravings, fatigue, and insomnia in women with PMS. Vitamin B_6, vitamin E, and magnesium have all shown some efficacy in small trials. Another small study of a carbohydrate-rich beverage designed to increase levels of tryptophan was effective in reducing symptoms. More research is needed before any of these therapies can be routinely recommended for patients with PMS (see Chapter 28).

HORMONAL CONTRACEPTION AND MOOD

It is widely accepted that hormonal contraception may affect a woman's mood. Surprisingly, there are few data to support this. Many authorities list depression as a potential side effect of the progestin component of the oral contraceptives. This appears to be quite variable from patient to patient. Because depression is quite prevalent among young females, the symptoms may be falsely attributed to the contraceptive. If progestins were a serious cause of depression, women using progestin-only methods would be expected to have increased rates of depressive symptoms. However, a review of 400 published clinical studies involving 55,000 users of implantable levonorgestrel concluded that reports of mood disturbances, anxiety, and depression were similar to reports by women using hormonal methods containing estrogen. Lacking evidence that use of progestin-only methods is associated with increased risk for developing depression or for worsening preexisting symptoms, the World Health Organization review committee did not include a history of depression in the eligibility criteria as a caution or reason to withhold these contraceptives. Clinicians need to be aware of the possibility of a relationship between mood disturbance and contraceptives, although evidence reveals this is less likely than generally assumed.

Issues for Perimenopausal and Menopausal Women

MENOPAUSE AND DEPRESSION

In the past, it was accepted that menopause increases the risk of depression. More recently, this assumption has been questioned. Most longitudinal population-based studies have not found increased rates of depressive symptoms in menopausal women. Women in the perimenopause may have more depressive symptoms, but this has been shown to be related to vasomotor symptoms associated with changing estrogen levels. Hot flashes often cause disruption of sleep and a continuing sleep disturbance is most likely the cause of increased psychological symptoms. Several small treatment trials have shown reduction in depressive symptoms with hormone replacement therapy (HRT). This improvement may be due to reduction in menopausal physical symptoms. If progestin is used in addition to estrogen, the effect may be blunted. If a perimenopausal woman with vasomotor symptoms also has psychological symptoms, it is reasonable to treat her with a trial of HRT prior to any other drug treatment. If these symptoms do not respond to HRT, or the initial depression is severe, antidepressant medication should be considered. Studies using SSRIs have also shown reduction of vasomotor symptoms in nondepressed women.

URINARY INCONTINENCE

Although urinary incontinence does affect men, it occurs in women at much higher rates. Among women living in the community, between 15 and 30% are incontinent. The rate for women in long-term care facilities is greater than 50%. Many women do not tell their health care provider about this problem and just try to live with it. The psychological morbidity from this "hidden" problem can be high. Problems may include social withdrawal, depression, and sexual dysfunction. Urinary incontinence has been shown to affect several quality of life issues for women. The effect is greatest in the area of coping with embarrassment and interfering with daily activities. Although some women may find incontinence personally and socially overwhelming, others may have very few life-style or emotional problems with it. Only thorough history taking and counseling can uncover these problems with women patients.

Several behavioral treatments have been found helpful in the treatment of urinary incontinence. For stress incontinence, avoiding overfilling of the bladder and regular muscle contraction exercises (Kegel exercises) are beneficial. In urge incontinence, bladder retraining in cognitively intact women can decrease episodes of incontinence by 50%. Biofeedback has also proven to be effective for some women with urge incontinence.

LIFE-STYLE MODIFICATION

Principles of Behavior Change

Maintaining or achieving good health often requires life-style modification. Changing behaviors is often a complex process. Examples of important life-style modifications that result in positive health benefits include smoking cessation, moderation of alcohol intake, engaging in regular exercise, and dietary modifications to achieve weight loss, if necessary, and to ensure adequate nutrient intake.

Many factors influence whether a woman changes her behavior or adopts a new health habit. A woman who has never changed her target behavior, may never have thought of changing, may still be thinking about changing, may intend to change but has not yet done so, or may not want to change. The Stages of Change Model divides individuals into stages of change based on their level of readiness to engage in a behavior (see Chapter 15). This theory has been successfully applied to a number of women's health behavior activities including mammography screening and smoking cessation.

In the Stages of Change Model *precontemplators* are individuals who are presently not engaging in the desired behavior and do not intend to start in a given time period. *Contemplators* are thinking about changing the behavior, but have not yet done so. Those in the *action* stage have initiated a change for a specified period of time. Those in the *maintenance* stage have sustained the change beyond the action period, indicating long-term commitment. *Relapsers* have changed their behavior in the past but are not presently engaging in the desired behavior.

Although physicians often realize the importance of behavior change counseling, many do not feel competent to provide such counseling. Chapter 15 provides a roadmap for physician behaviors appropriate to each stage of change. Careful attention to the indicators of the patient's stage of change, combined with use of the recommended approaches, can help women move through these stages of modifying their life-styles in the following areas.

Smoking Cessation

Cigarette smoking continues to be epidemic among women; in 1998 22% of all U.S. women smoked, and in 2000, 29.7% of high school senior girls reported smoking in the past 30 days. Recent data suggest that lesbian and bisexual women may have higher smoking rates than the general population. A recent report by the Surgeon General entitled *Women and Smoking: A Report of the Surgeon General* summarizes the current status of smoking and smoking-related disease among women. Although many smoking-related diseases such as cancer, pulmonary disease, and heart disease are seen in both men and women, there are also issues of particular importance to women. Lung cancer has surpassed breast cancer as the leading cause of cancer death in women. Exposure to environmental tobacco smoke is a cause of lung cancer and heart disease among women who are lifetime nonsmokers. Smoking during pregnancy continues to be a major public health problem, and even among women who do quit when pregnant, two-thirds of them resume smoking within a year after delivery. Smoking is associated with increased risks of cervical cancer, osteoporosis, early menopause, depression, and infertility.

In general the effectiveness of interventions for smoking cessation are similar in men and women. Psychosocial issues associated with smoking cessation in women include pregnancy, fear of weight gain (which women fear more than men), depression, and the need for social support (which may be greater in women). Exercise as an adjunct may be particularly useful in helping women with short-term and longer term smoking cessation by mitigating withdrawal symptoms and weight gain and improving mood. Most studies of pharmacological interventions for smoking cessation (eg, bupropion, nicotine replacement) have either not focused on differences in outcome by gender or have not found any.

Exercise

Regular exercise is associated with many health benefits in women including decreased mortality due to all causes and specifically coronary heart disease (CHD) and a lower risk of breast cancer.

The typical sedentary patient is less interested in knowing that 20–60 minutes of moderate to high-intensity physical activity three or more times a week is beneficial than she is in knowing "What is the minimum amount of exercise that I have to do?" Moderate intensity physical activity such as brisk walking (even as little as an hour a week) also seems to have significant health benefits.

The current recommendations by the CDC and the American College of Sports Medicine (directed at the large number of U.S. adults who engage in no leisure time physical activity) are that each U.S. adult should engage in 30 minutes or more of moderate intensity physical activity on most if not all days of the week.

How should exercise counseling be provided? Physician counseling is important, but other strategies may provide additional benefit, especially to women. In the Activity Counseling Trial, women who received additional assistance and counseling from a health educator (including behavioral counseling sessions, telephone follow-up, and periodic feedback on their levels of physical activity) had improved physical fitness at 2-year follow-up compared with women who received physician advice alone. Interestingly, the intervention had no effect in men.

Because many physicians do not have access to health educators who provide exercise counseling, physician counseling remains important. Rates of physician counseling about exercise are disappointingly low, particularly among physicians who do not feel successful in their ability to effect changes in behavior. In one recent study, only 28% of patients reported receiving physician advice to increase their level of physical activity, and among those who did receive advice, only 38% received help in formulating a specific plan. Important factors for physicians to consider in exercise counseling include the patient's stage of change with respect to exercise, what the patient enjoys doing, what she sees as potential barriers to behavior change, and the fact that simple interventions (eg, encouraging 30 minutes of walking a day) are more likely to be achievable and are likely to be associated with significant health benefits.

Dietary Modification

OBESITY

Approximately one-third of U.S. women weigh at least 20% more than desirable levels. Increased body weight is associated with increased incidence of CHD and mortality in women. In addition, a weight gain of even 10 kg since age 18 is associated with an increased risk of CHD events. Other diseases caused by or related to obesity include diabetes, hypertension, osteoarthritis, and uterine cancer.

Physician advice is important in helping patients achieve weight loss, yet it is often not given. In one study of obese adults, only 42% reported being advised by a health professional to lose weight. However, those who were told to lose weight were more likely to report actually trying to do so.

Strategies to aid patients in weight loss are described in detail in Chapter 18. Unfortunately, because the majority of overweight women who lose weight gain it back, we do not know whether weight loss will decrease CHD risk. Therefore it is probably prudent to focus our efforts on preventing weight gain in the first place.

OTHER DIETARY MODIFICATIONS

Some dietary modifications should be considered for all women, even those who are not overweight. First, for prevention of osteoporosis, all women should ensure adequate intake of calcium (at least 1200 mg/d) and vitamin D (400–800 IU for individuals at risk for deficiency). Recent evidence from the DASH (Dietary Approaches to Stop Hypertension) study concluded that individuals who ate a diet that emphasized fruit, vegetables, low-fat dairy products, whole grains, poultry, fish, and nuts, and included smaller amounts of red meat, sweets, and sugar-containing beverages, had lower blood pressures independent of sodium intake. In addition to the beneficial effects on hypertension, this type of diet has been associated with a reduction in CHD and possibly colon cancer. All women should be advised to consume a diet that emphasizes low fat, high fiber, and adequate fruit and vegetable intake.

Fall Prevention

Osteoporosis is a major cause of morbidity and mortality in women, and prevention of fractures is an important public health concern. Although much recent focus has been on the use of drugs to prevent and treat osteoporosis, important life-style modifications can also affect risk of fracture and should be emphasized by clinicians as well.

Because most osteoporotic fractures are the result of a fall, interventions to reduce the risk of falling are likely to reduce the risk of fracture. Regular lifelong weight-bearing and muscle-strengthening exercise is recommended to reduce the risk of falls and fractures. As described above, adequate calcium intake, smoking cessation, and moderation of alcohol intake are all important in preventing osteoporosis. Factors that have been associated with an increased risk of falling include use of sedatives and medications such as antihypertensives that have dizziness as a side effect, impaired vision, and environmental hazards such as throw rugs, loose wires, and lack of grab bars and nonskid tape in the tub or shower.

In addition to considering whether patients are candidates for drug therapies for osteoporosis, clinicians should counsel patients about life-style modifications such as regular exercise, household safety, and avoidance of drugs that increase the risk of falling.

Alcohol Use

One complication of heavy alcohol use unique to women is the increased risk of breast cancer. Women who drink 30–60 g of alcohol per day (two to five drinks) have a relative risk of breast cancer 1.4 times that of nondrinkers.

In contrast, moderate alcohol intake appears to be beneficial in both men and women. Women who drink one to nine glasses of alcohol per week have a lower risk of death from CHD than nondrinkers. Women who drink in moderation should be informed that this may be beneficial with respect to reduction of risk of CHD. However, because of the potential risks associated with alcohol abuse, women who do not drink should not be encouraged to start primarily to prevent heart disease.

Problems with alcohol are common in women presenting to primary care settings, and are often unrecognized. In addition, women with alcohol-related problems are less likely than men to have received any alcohol-related treatment.

Screening for alcohol abuse is an effective way of identifying women with alcohol-related problems, however many alcohol screening questionnaires have either not included women or have not included gender-specific analyses. Although most clinicians are familiar with and use the CAGE questionnaire, the TWEAK questionnaire may be more useful in women (see Table 14–2).

Women with a positive result on an alcohol screening questionnaire should undergo additional questioning

Table 14–2. Screening questionnaires for alcohol abuse.

CAGE
- **C** Have you ever thought that you ought to **C**ut down on your drinking?
- **A** Have people **A**nnoyed you by criticizing your drinking?
- **G** Have you ever felt bad or **G**uilty about your drinking?
- **E** Have you ever had a drink in the morning (**E**ye-opener) to steady your nerves or get rid of a hangover?

TWEAK
- **T** **T**olerance: How many drinks can you hold ("hold" version: six or more drinks indicate tolerance) or how many drinks does it take before you begin to feel the first effects of the alcohol ("high" version: three or more drinks indicate tolerance)?
- **W** **W**orried: Have close friends worried or complained about your drinking in the past year?
- **E** **E**ye-openers: Do you sometimes take a drink in the morning when you first get up?
- **A** **A**mnesia: Has a friend or family member ever told you about things you said or did while you were drinking that you could not remember?
- **K** **K**ut down: Do you sometimes feel the need to cut down on your drinking?

about their use of alcohol and potential complications they may have had. Women who are identified as problem drinkers should be referred to an alcohol treatment program and/or should receive brief feedback and advice (see Chapter 20).

Most studies of outcomes of alcohol treatment have not addressed differences between men and women, although it has been suggested that an empathic and nonconfrontational approach addressing specific barriers to women may be useful. Women who were enrolled in all female treatment programs may have improved outcomes, and some evidence suggests that multiple brief primary care interventions may be efficacious in women compared with men.

SUMMARY

The knowledge and treatment of diseases in women are evolving rapidly. It is important that clinicians understand the diseases and behavioral issues that are unique to women or that may affect women differently than men. Only by understanding the illness in the context of the patient's life can providers begin to provide evidence-based health care that is complete and comprehensive to all of their female patients.

SUGGESTED READINGS

Functional Syndromes

Aaron LA, Buchwald D: A review of the evidence for overlap among unexplained clinical conditions. Ann Intern Med 2001;134:868.

Barsky AJ, Borus JF: Functional somatic syndromes. Ann Intern Med 1999;130:910.

Katon W, Sullivan M, Walker E: Medical symptoms without identified pathology: relationship to psychiatric disorders, childhood and adult trauma, and personality traits. Ann Intern Med 2001;134:917.

Chronic Fatigue

Natelson BH: Chronic fatigue syndrome. JAMA 2001;285:20.

Whiting P et al: Interventions for the treatment or management of chronic fatigue syndrome: a systematic review. JAMA 2001; 286:11.

Fibromyalgia

Goldenberg DL: Fibromyalgia syndrome a decade later. Arch Intern Med 1999;159:777.

Hadhazy VA et al: Mind-body therapies for the treatment of fibromyalgia: a systematic review. J Rheumatol 2000;27:2911.

Leventhal LJ: Management of fibromyalgia. Ann Intern Med 1999; 131:850.

Irritable Bowel Syndrome

Drossman DA, Whitehead WE, Camiller M: Irritable bowel syndrome: a technical review for practice guideline development. Gastroenterology 1997;112:120.

Jailwala J, Imperiale TF, Kroenke K: Pharmacological treatment of the irritable bowel syndrome: a systematic review of randomized, controlled trials. Ann Intern Med 2000;133:136.

Chronic Pelvic Pain

Barbieri RL: Chronic pelvic pain. Up to Date (www.uptodate.com). 2001;9:3.

Scialli AR: Evaluating chronic pelvic pain: a consensus recommendation of the pelvic pain working group. J Reprod Med 1999; 44(11):945.

Approach to the Gynecological Examination

Heiligman RM, Pinto K: Proficiency of PG-1 internal medicine residents in performing the pelvic examination. Acad Med 1998;73(3):347.

Kleinman DE et al: Pelvic examination instruction and experience: a comparison of laywomen-trained and physician-trained students. Acad Med 1996;71(11):1239.

Larsen SB, Kragstrup J: Experiences of the first pelvic examination in a random sample of Danish teenagers. Acta Obstet Gynecol Scand 1995;74:137.

Moettus A, Sklar D, Tandberg D: The effect of physical gender on women's perceived pain and embarrassment during pelvic examination. Am J Emerg Med 1999;17(7):635.

Wijma B, Gullberg M, Kjessler B: Attitudes towards pelvic examination in a random sample of Swedish women. Acta Obstet Gynecol Scand 1998;77:422.

Principles of Behavior Change

Prochaska JO, DiClemente CC: Transtheoretical therapy: toward a more intergrative model of change. Psychother Theory Res Pract 1982;19:276.

Prochaska JO, DiClemente CC: Stages and processes of self-change of smoking: toward an integrative model of change. J Consult Clin Psychol 1983;51:390.

Prochaska JO, DiClemente CC: Stages of change in the modification of problem behaviors. In: Hersen M, Eisler RM, Miller PE (editors): *Progress in Behavior Modification,* Vol. 28. Sage, 1992. Psychologist 1992;47:1102.

Rakowski W et al: Increasing mammography among women aged 40–74 by use of a stage-matched, tailored intervention. Prevent Med 1998;27:1.

Smoking Cessation

Brock BC et al: Exercise effects on withdrawal and mood among women attempting smoking cessation. Addict Behav 1999;24(3):399.

Marcus BH et al: The efficacy of exercise as an aid for smoking cessation in women: a randomized controlled trial. Arch Intern Med 1999;159:1229.

Ryan H et al: Smoking among lesbians, gays, and bisexuals. A review of the literature. Am J Prevent Med 2001;21(2):142.

U.S. Department of Public Health. Women and Smoking: A Report of the Surgeon General. Centers for Disease Control and Prevention, National Center for Chronic Disease Prevention and Health Promotion Office on Smoking and Health, 2001.

Alcohol Use

Bradley KA et al: Alcohol screening questionnaires in women: a critical review. JAMA 1998;280:166.

Buchsbaum DG et al: Physician detection of drinking problems in patients attending a general medicine practice. J Gen Intern Med 1992;153:1573.

Cullen K, Stenhouse NS, Wearne KL: Alcohol and mortality in the Busselton Study. Int J Epidemiol 1982;11:67.

Dahlgren L, Willander A: Are special treatment facilities for female alcoholics needed? A controlled 2-year follow-up study from a specialized treatment unit (EWA) versus a mixed male/female treatment facility. Alcohol Clin Exp Res 1989;13:499.

Fuchs CS et al: Alcohol consumption and mortality among women. N Engl J Med 1995;332:1245.

Gordon T, Kannel, WB: Drinking habits and cardiovascular disease: the Framingham Study. Am Heart J 1983;105:667.

Klatsky AL, Armstron, MA, Friedman GD: Red wine, white wine, liquor, beer and risk for coronary artery disease hospitalization. Am J Cardiol 1997;80:416.

Poikolainen K: Effectiveness of brief interventions to reduce alcohol intake in primary health care populations: a meta-analysis. Prevent Med 1999(5):503.

Samet JH, Rollnick S, Barnes H: Beyond CAGE: a brief clinical approach after detection of substance abuse. Arch Intern Med 1996;156:2287.

Smith-Warner SA et al: Alcohol and breast cancer in women: a pooled analysis of cohort studies. JAMA 1998;279:535.

Stason, WB et al: Alcohol consumption and nonfatal myocardial infarction. Am J Epidemiol 1976;104:603.

Wallace P, Culter S, Haines A: Randomized controlled trial of general practitioner intervention in patients with excessive alcohol consumption. BMJ 1988;297:663.

Weisner C, Schmidt L: Gender disparities in treatment for alcohol problems. JAMA 1992;268:1872.

Exercise

Albanes D, Blair A, Taylor PR: Physical activity and risk of cancer in the NHANES I population. Am J Public Health 1989;79:744.

Bernstein L et al: Physical exercise and reduced risk of breast cancer in young women. J Cancer Inst 1994;86:1403.

Blair SN et al: Influences of cardiorespiratory fitness and other precursors on cardiovascular disease and all-cause mortality in men and women. JAMA 1996;276:205.

Frisch RE et al: Lower prevalence of breast cancer and cancers of the reproductive system among former college athletes compared to non-athletes. Br J Cancer 1985;52:885.

Glasgow RE et al: Physician advice and support for physical activity: results from a national survey. Am J Prevent Med 2001;21(3): 189.

Kushi LH et al: Physical activity and mortality in postmenopausal women. JAMA 1997;277:1287.

Lapidus L, Bengtsson C: Socioeconomic factors and physical activity in relation to cardiovascular disease and death: a 12 year follow-up of participants in a population study of women in Gothenberg, Sweden. Br Heart J 1986;55:295.

Lee IM et al: Physical activity and coronary heart disease in women: is "No Pain, No Gain" passe? JAMA 2001;285:1447.

Manson JE et al: A prospective study of walking as compared with vigorous exercise in the prevention of coronary heart disease in women. N Engl J Med 1999;341:650.

Sherman SE et al: Physical activity and mortality in women in the Framingham Heart Study. Am Heart J 1994;128:879.

Simons-Morton DG: Effects of physical activity counseling in primary care: the activity counseling trial: a randomized controlled trial. JAMA 2001;286(6):677.

Vena JE et al: Occupational exercise and risk of cancer. Am J Clin Nutr 1987;45:318.

Vihko VJ et al: Risk of breast cancer among female teachers of physical education and languages. Acta Oncol 1992;31:201.

Walsh JME, Swangard DM, McPhee SJ: Exercise counseling by primary care physicians in the era of managed care. Am J Prevent Med 1999;16:307.

Wee CC et al: Physician counseling about exercise. JAMA 1999; 282:1583.

Dietary Modification

Galuska DA et al: Are health care professionals advising obese patients to lose weight? JAMA 1999;282(16):1576.

Manson JE et al: Body weight and mortality among women. N Engl J Med 1995;333:677.

Michels KB et al: Prospective study of fruit and vegetable consumption and incidence of colon and rectal cancers. J Natl Cancer Inst 2000;92(21):1740.

Sacks FM et al: Effects on blood pressure of reduced dietary sodium and dietary approaches to stop hypertension (DASH) diet. N Engl J Med 2001;344(1):3.

Willett WC et al: Weight, weight change and coronary heart disease in women. JAMA 1995;273:461.

Fall Prevention

National Osteoporosis Foundation, 2000; NIH Consensus Development Panel, 2001.

Physician's Guide to Prevention and Treatment of Osteoporosis. National Osteoporosis Foundation, 1998.

Screening for Eating Disorders

Freund, KM et al: Detection of bulimia in a primary care setting. J Intern Med 1993;8:243.

Mogran JF, Lacey JH: The SCOFF questionnaire: assessment of a new screening tool for eating disorders. Br J Med 1993;319:1467.

Walsh JME, Wheat ME, Freund K: Detection, evaluation and treatment of eating disorders: the role of the primary care physician. J Gen Intern Med 2000;15:577.

Premenstrual Syndrome & Premenstrual Dysphoric Disorder

American College of Obstetricians and Gynecologists. Premenstrual Syndrome: Clinical management guidelines for obstetrician-gynecologists. ACOG Pract Bull 2000;15:1.

Fraser IS et al: Norplant consensus statement and background review. Contraception 1998;57:1.

Kessel B: Premenstrual syndrome: advances in diagnosis and treatment. Obstet Gynecol Clin 2000;27:625.

Steiner M, Born L: Diagnosis and treatment of premenstrual dysphoric disorder: an update. Int Clin Psychopharmacol 2000; 15(Suppl 3):S5.

Steiner M et al: Fluoxetine in the treatment of premenstrual syndrome. N Engl J Med 1995;332:1529.

Stevinson C, Ernst E: Complementary/alternative therapies for premenstrual syndrome: a systematic review of randomized controlled trials. Am J Obstet Gynecol 2001;185:227.

Hormones & Mood

Pearlstein T, Rosen K, Stone AB: Mood disorders and menopause. Endocrinol Metab Clin North Am 1997;26:279.

Schechter D: Estrogen, progesterone, and mood. J Gender-Specific Med 1999;2:29.

Soares C et al: Efficacy of estradiol for the treatment of depressive disorders in peri menopausal women: a double-blind, randomized, placebo-controlled trial. Arch Gen Psychiatry 2001;58:529.

Urinary Incontinence

DuBeau CE et al: The impact of urge urinary incontinence on quality of life: importance of patients' perspective and explanatory style. J Am Geriatr Soc 1998;46:683.

WEB SITES

American Academy of Family Physicians
www.aafp.org/healthinfo

American Psychiatric Association
www.medem.com

Arthritis Foundation
www.arthritis.org

Centers for Disease Control and Prevention (CDC)
www.cdc.gov/ncidod/diseases/cfs

Chronic Fatigue and Immune Dysfunction Syndrome Association of America
http://www.cfids.org

National Institute of Arthritis, Musculoskeletal, and Skin Diseases
www.nih.gov/niams/hi/topics/fibromyalgia/fibroofs.htm

National Institute of Diabetes and Digestive and Kidney Diseases
www.niddk.nih.gov/health/digest/pubs/irrbowel/irrbowel.htm

Section III
Health-Related Behavior

Behavior Change

Daniel O'Connell, PhD

INTRODUCTION

Despite advances in medical technology and evidence-based guidelines, most efforts to improve health require some change in behavior on the part of patients. These changes in behavior might involve reduction or elimination of destructive behaviors (eg, smoking and alcohol dependence), promotion of healthier life-styles (eg, regular exercise, safer sex), and adherence to medical regimens intended to treat acute or chronic illness (eg, taking medications, checking blood glucose). Most clinicians, however, feel more confident in their diagnostic and treatment skills than they do in their ability to ensure that patients will follow these recommendations.

Fortunately work done in the field of behavioral medicine in the past 25 years has great practical application to the routine doctor–patient encounter. In this chapter we will describe and integrate three of the most researched approaches to behavior change: the Stages of Change Model of James Prochaska and Carlo DiClemente, the Motivational Interviewing Model of William Miller and Stephen Rollnick, and the Self-efficacy Model of Albert Bandura. Our goal is to outline a practical approach to influencing patients that respects the complexity of human behavior while breaking clinician interventions into manageable steps.

SUMMARY OF BEHAVIOR CHANGE MODELS

Stages of Change

The Stages of Change Model introduced the idea that people move through a succession of six relatively distinguishable stages in making changes in behavior.

1. *Precontemplation* stage: There is little thought about the problem or its solution.
2. *Contemplation* stage: The problem and the potential methods, costs, and benefits involved in trying to address it are evaluated.
3. *Preparation/Dermination* stage: The focus is on a specific course of action and timetable around which to commit energies to change.
4. *Action* stage: Steps are taken on a regular basis to make the change in behavior (eg, following a diet and exercise program).
5. *Maintenance* stage: Successful changers begin to incorporate Action stage behaviors into a "new normal" way of living.
6. *Relapse:* There is a return to an earlier stage.

In the Relapse stage people may start thinking about change but drift back to a precontemplation mode as other issues take precedence. They may promise to commit to a course of action but lose enthusiasm and stall. They may have started to take action on a daily basis but are unready to overcome obstacles and so fail to follow through. Finally they may have had initial success, but through a series of slips that were not corrected, now find they have relapsed into former patterns. They may now be feeling discouraged and unable to contemplate another attempt at change or perhaps are still committed and are regrouping for another try. (See Table 15–1 for a summary of these stages.)

Relapse is the norm for the majority of efforts to change behavior. Much of the pessimism that exists about change grows from this realization. We fail to appreciate that multiple starts at behavior change often lead to eventual success. Once the problem reaches the contemplation

Table 15–1. Stages of change and patient characteristics.

Stage	Patient Characteristics
Precontemplation	The problem exists, but the patient minimizes or denies it.
Contemplation	The patient is thinking about the problem and the costs and benefits of continuing with the problem or trying to change.
Preparation	The patient commits to a time and plan for resolving the problem.
Action	The patient makes daily efforts to overcome the problem.
Maintenance	The patient has overcome the problem and remains vigilant to prevent backsliding.
Relapse	The patient has gone back to the problem behavior on a regular basis after a period of successful resolution.

stage it is difficult to completely ignore it again. As commitment for taking some regular action increases, we further bolster our assessment of the pros for changing over the cons. Each time we take some action we learn more about what will be necessary for eventual maintenance of the desired behaviors and move closer to the desired benefits. For example, it takes an average of seven quit attempts before smoking cessation is maintained. As we will see, the clinician has a useful role to play in helping patients understand the natural history of personal change and in influencing them to navigate the stages toward eventual success.

Motivational Interviewing

Miller and Rollnick's Motivational Interviewing Model challenged the existing assumption that people change primarily when they are pressured from outside. They realized that many attempts to influence patients were limited to "pushing" types of interactions in which the clinician lectured, explained, exhorted, criticized, inspired, or threatened the patient with dire consequences if change did not occur. They saw little support in the research for the effectiveness of this heavy- handed, coercive approach. On the contrary, they respected the psychological theory of **reactance,** which posits that individuals are strongly motivated to maintain a sense of autonomy and to resist coercion by others. Reactance creates its own logic, and patients who might otherwise have admitted their concern over a problem may instead feel compelled to defend their behavior. Miller and Rollnick demonstrated that the best way to influence patients' behavior is to build on their own motivation to change. This is accomplished through an interview style that emphasizes empathy, curiosity, self-determination, acceptance, and exploration of ambivalence and rolls with resistance rather than fighting resistance with attempts to persuade and coerce.

Self-efficacy

Albert Bandura is a leading figure in the development of Social Learning theory. Social Learning theory is an extension of cognitive and behavioral models into the analysis of how people learn social behaviors, evaluate the desirability of behaviors, and are influenced to adopt behaviors and beliefs. A wide body of research has looked at many types of social influence. Examples include modeling (motivating by example) and social reinforcement (providing a reward following the desired behavior). This research has helped explain how these interactions impact individuals' internal self-assessments about both the desirability of change and the confidence in their capacity to successfully enact a new behavior. We have learned that motivation to try new behavior comes from an interaction of two forces: a conviction that the behavior is necessary/valuable and the self-efficacy/confidence that there will be success in carrying it out.

Conviction emerges from a rational as well as emotional appraisal in which the individual weighs the pros and cons of the behavior and decides upon the value of the outcome at this time. Self-efficacy represents a separate dimension in which the individual blends rational and emotional data to arrive at a level of confidence that trying new behavior will lead to success. Conviction and self-efficacy are continuous rather than dichotomous dimensions, ie, the individual is more or less convinced and more or less confident about the behavior. Utilizing Bandura's model, the clinician asks patients to rate themselves now on these dimensions and to imagine what would help them to be even more convinced and confident in their ability to change. This is a very helpful diagnostic and planning metric for the clinician. If the patient has little conviction that the change is valuable, then increasing conviction is the place to start. If the patient is already convinced that the change would be very valuable (eg, "I know that smoking is killing me."), then the clinician's time is best spent enhancing confidence that it can be achieved. For instance, we know that using nicotine replacement doubles the likelihood of success in an effort to quit smoking. Here is an example of questions to assess conviction and confidence:

Doctor: How convinced are you that cigarette smoking is damaging to your health and that smoking cessation should be a priority for you now?

Doctor: How confident are you that you could stop smoking with the help that we might be able to offer?

In this chapter we will describe the most effective ways in which a clinician can enhance patients' conviction and confidence to promote their movement through the stages of change.

INFLUENCE VERSUS CONTROL

Clinicians are not more effective when they take too much responsibility for the patient's behavior. Nor are clinicians maximimally effective when they limit their role to that of medical advisor, leaving it entirely up to the patient to choose when and if to adhere to medical treatments. Clinicians erroneously believe that patients are making progress only when they are taking observable actions on a daily basis. Research suggests that fewer than 20% of patients report that they are expecting to take that kind of regular action on a change in health behavior in the next 30 days (Preparation/Determination stage). Therefore much of the clinician's work involves increasing patients' readiness to prepare for and take regular action. Rather than attempting to *control* the patient's behavior, which the patient predictably will resist, the clinician exerts an *influence,* which, when combined with other factors internal and external to the patient, may lead to the desired change.

Fortunately clinicians are not alone in this effort. Friends, family, media, employers, laws and law enforcement, commercial enterprises (eg, health clubs, for-profit weight loss centers), and self-help groups all serve to generate motivation and provide resources for behavior change. Clinicians can take comfort in knowing that the responsibility for promoting healthier behaviors is not theirs alone.

PROMOTING BEHAVIOR CHANGE

The Clinician's Demeanor: Empathy & Curiosity

Research has consistently demonstrated the power of an empathic and involved supporter in promoting growth and change (see Chapter 2). It is best to adopt an attitude of respectful curiosity whenever patients behave in ways that seem illogical or counterproductive (eg, failure to stop smoking despite related illnesses). Dismissing such behavior as stupidity, dependency, irresponsibility, or the result of a personality disorder blocks a more helpful conversation. For example, the clinician can inoffensively question nonadherence to an agreed upon plan without provoking defensiveness. The most productive questions are those that convey respectful curiosity and that focus the patient on identifying and overcoming specific obstacles to change.

Here is how that might be done.

Doctor: I'm curious as to why you didn't start the exercise program we discussed at your last visit. (Pause for a

response). What do you think is the most important thing you must do or overcome in order to get an exercise program started?

Clinicians who are aware of the theory of reactance do not try to force change on patients because of their own sense of urgency. For example, a clinician who is concerned about the pregnancy of a teenager who smokes cigarettes and drinks alcohol will have no more influence over this behavior than the strength of the clinician–patient relationship at that moment allows. When patients feel shame or embarrassment they are as likely to become defensive and avoid the topic and the clinician as they are to be spurred into action. Forgetting that most people strive to be self-directed and resist coercion frustrates the clinician and impairs the clinician–patient relationship. Paradoxically, although the clinician may feel momentarily more effective through this confrontation/exhortation behavior, research indicates that the empathic clinician promotes changes in behavior more successfully over time.

Ambivalence

An important contribution of the Motivational Interviewing Model is its emphasis on understanding and exploring ambivalence. People almost always feel two ways about behavior change. They see discomfort and disruption in the short term and the hope of desirable outcomes in the longer term. Starting an exercise regimen certainly fits this mold, but ambivalence is almost universal. For example, the hassle of the diabetic's daily finger sticks to test blood sugars and adjust diet and insulin is offset by the reduced likelihood of complications later. The depressed patient's taking steps to find a psychotherapist now will lead to better interpersonal and emotional functioning later. A patient with hypercholesterolemia tolerates medication expense and side effects now in trade for lowered risk of stroke and heart disease in the future.

Conversely, most addictive behavior has the quality of supplying short-term pleasure at the expense of longer term cost. In the short term smoking cigarettes brings smokers pleasure and not smoking brings them discomfort. It is only because the costs mount up that a smoker considers quitting (as over 45 million Americans have).

The effective promoter of behavior change empathically brings up this ambivalence in the conversation and asks the patient to consider the resulting stalemate and its effects. This can be done in brief exchanges rather than with rhetorical questions (eg, "Don't you think that . . . ?" or more prolonged interrogations).

Doctor: It sounds like you are weighing the disruption of starting to exercise regularly against being upset with yourself for not doing more to reduce your risk of another heart attack. How are you seeing that now and what could you do to resolve the impasse?

The clinician can express concern that, although ambivalent, patients who do not make a choice will not ultimately feel better about problems that brought them to the medical encounter. Using the language of "I am concerned" emphasizes the desire to be helpful in resolving the concerns that trouble the patient.

> **Doctor:** I am just concerned that you will become more and more of an invalid unless you can get yourself out of the house for some activity every day.

> **Doctor:** I am just concerned that without going back to physical therapy and starting the home stretching program again, you will continue to feel this back pain and be limited in your activities.

Apply the Model to Yourself First

Because behavior change is an area of practice that many clinicians find frustrating, it is important to guard against feeling either irritation or apathy. Take a moment to first apply these behavior change models to your own life. Most of us can readily bring to mind behaviors that we have been contemplating, or even promising to change for years without consistent success (eg, regular exercise or getting sufficient sleep). This self-reflection helps us to appreciate the timespan, false starts, achievements, and relapses that are normal in the process of change.

What Makes a Successful Encounter?

Success occurs in an encounter in which patients view themselves as engaged in the process of changing a problem behavior. The key is recognizing that change is a process, not an event. Each encounter provides an opportunity to promote movement through all of the stages leading up to the patient taking daily action. Rather than waiting for the patient to become ready to change, the clinician helps make that process more efficient by focusing on those questions and ideas that match the patient's present stage and anticipate the work of the next stage. Understanding the stages and the process involved also relieves clinicians of some of the burden that comes with unrealistic expectations and increases both parties' feelings of hopefulness about eventual success. If the average smoker (as reported in one study) took 7 years to move from precontemplation to maintenance of smoking cessation, then accelerating that progression to take only 3 years is a significant improvement.

One of the most valuable contributions of the Stages of Change Model has been to understand the natural history of behavior change and allow patient and clinician to map their present location in the process and to anticipate the work of the next stage.

Clinicians' Reluctance to Utilize These Models

Many clinicians fear that they will appear too permissive if they do not take a forceful, persuasive stance in pressing for patients to change potentially harmful behaviors. Others react with frustration and anger rather than strategize how to be more effective in a conversation with a patient who appears resistant. It is natural to imagine that greater force will overcome greater resistance. The recommendations that we are making here come from a large body of research that has consistently demonstrated that this belief is untrue when it comes to changes in health behavior. Let's look instead at how these models might be applied by clinicians at each stage in the process of behavior change. The clinician with a roadmap often finds it easier to remain strategic rather than irritated when talking about behavior change. The effort begins with the clinician assessing the patient's current stage of change.

ASSESSING STAGES OF CHANGE

Assessing the patient's stage of change starts most naturally with a question.

> **Doctor:** What do you think about your smoking?

> **Doctor:** How much of a problem do you believe your drinking is causing?

> **Doctor:** How convinced are you that stretching and strengthening exercises will reduce your back pain?

> **Doctor:** How confident are you that you can follow this regimen?

> **Doctor:** What are you doing now to control your weight?

> **Doctor:** The last time you were in we were talking about dietary changes to reduce your cholesterol. How much have you been able to change your diet since our last visit?

> **Doctor:** There are a number of behavior changes that can be very helpful after a heart attack. Let me list some and then tell me which ones you want to focus on more in today's visit.

> **Doctor:** Now that you are in for a physical, tell me about some of the things you are doing to get and stay healthy?

> **Doctor:** Is there anything you are doing now that you think may be undermining your health/recovery?

Research suggests that it is best to think of behavior change as having specific rather than general targets. The following list of behavior changes would be advised for a patient at high risk for a heart attack: exercise, diet, medication adherence, smoking cessation, alcohol moderation, and stress reduction. Each of these is a different behavior. The patient may have already succeeded in smoking cessation, but done little to change diet and exercise, perhaps even putting on a few pounds while quitting smoking. As we will see next, the patient will eventually need to work through the stages in changing each of these behaviors.

Once the clinician has established the patient's current stage of change for a specific behavior the next step is to focus on brief interventions that identify and target specific obstacles to the patient's movement to the next stage (Table 15–2). The goal is to induct and maintain the patient in the change process until long-term success is achieved and to shorten the amount of time required to accomplish a sustained change in behavior. Each conversation is in furtherance of this goal, yet the patient dictates how much movement is possible in any period. We now look at each stage and identify its main characteristics and strategies to promote movement to the next stage.

Precontemplation

In this stage patients minimize or deny the existence of problem behavior. The problem has typically been identified by others—spouses, clinicians, employers, etc. They try not to think about or talk about it much in any setting. The topic was probably not on their agenda for the visit. Much of their resistance can be understood from reactance theory as patients resist being pressed to discuss a topic about which they may feel somewhat embarrassed, criticized, and blindsided.

It is important for clinicians to differentiate between true Precontemplation stage behavior (true denial and minimization) and the reluctance to discuss uncomfortable issues that stems from other dynamics such as shame, demoralization, or a lack of trust in the clinician. Some patients are only too well aware of the problem and its costs to them and others (Contemplation stage awareness); they may feel overwhelmed by it and powerless to succeed in its resolution. They are often afraid of being put on the spot by the clinician. The clinician's interview style will greatly influence the patient's willingness to discuss the problem. Without empathic curiosity, arguments, frustration, and antagonism on the part of both patient and clinician are highly likely.

Drug and alcohol addiction are often described as diseases of denial. How can someone appear oblivious to the damage this behavior is causing? Yet closer examination often reveals that abusing or addicted individuals may spend considerable effort trying to figure out and manage their addictive behavior. Cocaine addicts may try to restrict their use to the weekend or alcoholics may switch from hard liquor to beer and wine or make repeated promises to restrict their number of drinks in hopes of preventing the worst of their binges. In the right situation, these individuals may be willing to contemplate more effective ways to manage their problem, even if they are unwilling to commit to abstinence at this moment.

Overweight people are similarly often misjudged to be in the Pre-contemplation stage. We mistakenly assume that overweight individuals must be oblivious to the problems their weight causes if they do not raise this concern in a medical encounter. A sensitive interviewing style often makes the patient comfortable enough to reveal the demoralization and self-recrimination that may lie just under the surface. Again, embarrassment and fear of judgment will sometimes make individuals appear to be in the Precontemplation stage when they are actually stuck further along in the process of change.

CASE ILLUSTRATION 1

Jack is 50 years old and is being seen by his internist. The appointment was made by Jack's wife Clara, ostensibly for follow-up of treatment for persistent high blood pressure. The actual reason, as explained to the nurse-receptionist, is Clara's concern about her husband's drinking and his failure to follow the clinician's latest recommendations for blood pressure control. During the appointment, Jack does not mention any problems with alcohol or any difficulty following the recommended regimen. When the doctor presses Jack for more details about the amount of alcohol he is consuming, Jack becomes evasive and irritated. The physician backs off and ends the visit with only a change in medication—and a feeling of frustration.

Strategies for the Precontemplation Stage

Defensiveness can often be defused if practitioners ask the precontemplator for permission to talk about the problem.

> **Doctor:** Would it be all right if we talk a little more about how your drinking might be contributing to some of the problems you mentioned today?

The clinician explores the patient's degree of awareness as a way to move the conversation further into contemplation.

> **Doctor:** What do you already know about the risks of sustained high blood pressure?

Questions of this kind, asking patients to *contemplate* the possible connections between the physical symptoms that bother them and the behaviors that may be provoking those symptoms, are among the most helpful to precontemplators.

As much as possible, the physician's agenda should be linked to concerns the patient has already expressed. If a female patient asks for birth control, the clinician can use her concern about pregnancy as a basis for asking how else she had been protecting herself when having sex. This may lead naturally to a discussion about using condoms with new partners, an issue that was not on her agenda for this visit.

Table 15–2. Stages of change and clinician strategies.

Stage of Change	Patient Characteristics	Clinician Strategies
Precontemplation	Denies problem and its importance. Is reluctant to discuss problem. Problem is identified by others. Shows reactance when pressured. High risk of argument.	Ask permission to discuss problem. Inquire about patient's thoughts. Gently point out discrepancies. Express concern. Ask patient to think, talk, or read about situation between visits.
Contemplation	Shows openness to talk, read, and think about problem. Weighs pros and cons. Dabbles in action. Can be obsessive about problem and can prolong stage.	Elicit patient's perspective first. Help identify pros and cons of change. Ask what would promote commitment. Suggest trials.
Preparation/Determination	Understands that change is needed. Begins to form commitment to specific goals, methods, and timetables. Can picture overcoming obstacles. May procrastinate about setting start date for change.	Summarize patient's reasons for change. Negotiate a start date to begin some or all change activities. Encourage patient to announce publicly. Arrange a follow-up contact at or shortly after start date.
Action	Follows a plan of regular activity to change problem. Can describe plan in detail (unlike dabbling in action of contemplator). Shows commitment in facing obstacles. Resists slips. Is particularly vulnerable to abandoning effort impulsively.	Show interest in specifics of plan. Discuss difference between slip and relapse. Help anticipate how to handle a slip. Support and reemphasize pros of changing. Help to modify action plan if aspects are not working well. Arrange follow-up contact for support.
Maintenance	Has accomplished change or improvement through focused action. Has varying levels of awareness regarding importance of long-term vigilance. May already be losing ground through slips or wavering commitment. Has feelings about how much the change has actually improved life. May be developing life-style that precludes relapse into former problem.	Show support and admiration. Inquire about feelings and expectations and how well they were met. Ask about slips, any signs of wavering commitment. Help create plan for intensifying activity should slips occur. Support life-style and personal redefinition that reduce risk of relapse. Reflect on the long-term—and possibly permanent—nature of this stage as opposed to the more immediate gratification of initial success.
Relapse	Consistent return to problem behavior after period of resolution. Begins as slips that are not effectively resisted. May have cycled back to precontemplation, contemplation, or determination stages. Lessening time spent in this stage is a key to making greater progress toward fully integrated, successful, long-term change.	Frame relapse as a learning opportunity in preparation for next action stage. Ask about specifics of change and relapse. Remind patient that contemplation work is still valid (reasons for changing). Use "when," rather than "if," in describing next change attempt. Normalize relapse as the common experience on the path to successful long-term change.

Some patients are in the Precontemplation stage with regard to understanding the interaction between their emotional and their physical health (eg, anxiety and somatic preoccupation). Often the clinician first considers all the "legitimate" medical causes of symptoms before enquiring about emotional involvement. A negative work-up may lead to an awkward conversation in which the physician implies "It is all in your head" and suggests mental health referral or medication and the patient insists on more medical tests and referrals. Adherence is unlikely until the patient has been helped to contemplate and think through obstacles to the revised treatment plan. An alternative is to ask early in the history about psychosocial contributors to the somatic symptom.

Doctor: Tell me about anything that is going on in your life that could be affecting the frequency or intensity of the headaches. Let's think about how we can take that into account in understanding and treating your symptoms.

Discrepancies between the patient's present behavior and the expressed goal of feeling better should be pointed out empathically. Physicians can also express their concern that the patient may not achieve the desired improvement without addressing the behavior that contributes to it.

Doctor: I'm concerned that you'll always worry about another heart attack unless you know that you've changed your life-style and lowered the risk.

Doctor: I'm concerned that none of these medicines will be able to relieve your stomach discomfort as long as you drink alcohol and caffeine.

The goal with precontemplators is to increase their willingness to contemplate the connections between behavioral health and physical health as the next step toward change. Much of the actual work of contemplation is done between visits. Clinicians can ask the patient to think about, keep track of, and read about the problem and potential solutions—or talk to someone else about them—before the next appointment. The clinician notes the patient's response and mentions it at the next visit.

Doctor: Sounds like you and your wife disagree about how much and how often you are drinking. You could resolve that if you are willing to make a note on the calendar each day how much alcohol you had to drink. Then it would be more clear to the two of you how much of an issue there actually is.

Doctor: What would you look at to tell you whether your drinking was causing trouble in your life?

Doctor: I am curious. Why do you think that I place so much emphasis on your stopping smoking?

In the Motivational Interviewing framework, the clinician is looking for self-motivational statements from the patient. For the precontemplator most of the motivational statements are being made by others. "Honey, you are embarrassing the children with your drinking. Why won't you stop?" We want the patient to begin reflecting on these situations more often without relying on pressure from others.

Doctor: How do the people at home feel about your drinking? (pause for response) How important are their feelings to you?

At some point the precontemplator begins to think about the problem and how it might be solved. Movement in this direction could have been prompted by threats from others, developmental pressures (eg, "Now that I'm a father, I don't feel as much like partying"), a compelling example in real life or fiction, or a skillful interaction that makes the person aware of the negative consequences of the behavior without increasing defensiveness. The patient then moves into the Contemplation stage of change for that behavior.

Contemplation

In this stage the patient demonstrates some of the following characteristics:

- The patient is open to thinking about and discussing the problem with little prompting and may even have initiated the discussion of the problem.
- The patient appears interested, may ask for additional information, and weighs the pros and cons of changing or not changing the problem behavior.
- Unless the patient is pushed to make a specific commitment to take action, there is less risk of irritation and argument than with the precontemplator.
- The contemplation stage can be prolonged or obsessive. Patients request more convincing data and look for an ideal time and situation in which to initiate change.
- Patients may seem to be dabbling in action without a commitment to overcome obstacles that arise. They may, for example, decline an occasional dessert, not drink on weekdays, or make early-morning promises not to smoke—and break them by midafternoon.
- Contemplators may be thinking about obstacles from too limited a framework, for example, doubting that they have sufficient "will power" to follow through.

Some contemplation behavior is necessary for later successful resolution of the problem. Patients must anticipate costs and obstacles, identify their motivations, assess how easy or difficult the behavior change might be, and feel that they are making informed and independent decisions, rather than being coerced by others. Although some people claim that they impulsively threw away their cigarettes, or that they quit drinking suddenly and never once looked back, research suggests that even these people may have been quietly doing contemplation work in the years and months leading up to the presumably impulsive action.

CASE ILLUSTRATION 2

Joanna is 44 years old and has been smoking a pack of cigarettes a day since she was 17. When prompted by her primary care provider she is very willing to discuss the pros and cons of smoking. Joanna tells her doctor that she is being pressured by her children about secondary smoke and that she agrees with their position. She thinks that the habit is both expensive and stupid. On the other hand, she believes that smoking is one of the few things that relax her throughout the day at work and at home. One of her friends quit smoking and gained 25 pounds; this possibility is frightening to Joanna, who is already concerned about her weight. She wonders whether medication or a nicotine patch or gum would make quitting easier and perhaps keep her from gaining weight. By the end of the discussion, Joanna has promised her doctor to think even more seriously about quitting.

Strategies for the Contemplation Stage

The clinician's goal is to help patients resolve their ambivalence to a point sufficient to enable them to commit to a specific plan and timetable for starting the Action stage of change.

To accomplish this the clinician should ask for the patient's perspective before offering advice, asking questions that elicit self-motivational statements.

Doctor: What are your thoughts about your cigarette smoking and what you might be able to do about it?

Patients can be helped to identify the pros and cons of change and to examine the current pleasures and ultimate consequences of the problem behavior. It is axiomatic that people engage in unhealthful behavior because they desire the pleasures such acts bring. Many patients already believe that they would be better off if they ate differently, exercised more, drank less, stopped or cut down on drug use, lost weight, reduced stress, and so on.

Contemplators may remain ambivalent because of the possibility that the change process itself will be psychologically or physically unpleasant, costly, and likely to fail. They may need help identifying and working their way through these anticipated obstacles. The time-efficient clinician can ask the patient what has been the greatest obstacle to taking action to resolve or ameliorate the problem, and then focus the conversation on curiosity about this obstacle.

Patients often claim that because of insufficient will power they are powerless to stop smoking, quit drug or al-

cohol abuse, or change any other behavior. They can be asked questions that reframe will power as an energy that rises and falls in relation to how convinced they are that change is valuable and the size of the step that they are asking themselves to take.

Doctor: If you were to become convinced that your life depended on your not smoking for 3 months, do you think you could resist temptation that long? Where would the will power to do it come from?

Doctor: Let's think about an amount and type of physical activity that you would be able to fit into your week now.

Doctor: Will power can be thought of like money. It goes a lot farther when we spend it wisely. Let's think about taking smaller steps that do not involve using so much will power.

Similarly, patients can be asked what they think would bring about a commitment to change the behavior:

Doctor: If I were to meet you years from now and find that you had completely stopped using crack cocaine, what do you think you would tell me was the reason you finally quit? (Pause for response) How do you imagine you would have accomplished this?

Depending on the answer, these questions might follow:

Doctor: Knowing that such an unpleasant event (eg, relationship or health problem, arrest, etc) is likely to come about, what do think about trying to resolve the problem before that happens?

Doctor: What approach do you think you would use to overcome the problems if you believed you really had to? (Pause for response) What obstacles would you encounter if you were to start using that approach now?

Clinicians can encourage patients to think about an upcoming time in which taking action to resolve or improve the problem situation would be least taxing. Because self-efficacy is related to the size of the step to be taken, suggestions for limited trials of smaller steps can build the patient's confidence and willingness to commit to some action:

Doctor: Would you be willing to cut down from 20 to 15 cigarettes a day and make a note of how hard or easy this is for you?

Patients in the Contemplation stage usually need to evaluate not only the pros and cons of the problem, but also the advantages and disadvantages of different means of overcoming the problem. The clinician can sometimes be most helpful by assisting patients in contemplating the many ways that change can be accomplished in order to increase their readiness to commit to a plan of action.

Doctor: There are a number of over-the-counter and prescription medications that reduce the craving that nicotine withdrawal can cause when you first stop smoking. Let me briefly describe them to you.

Sometimes the clinician asks the contemplator to do something now that will make effective action more possible at a later date.

> **Doctor:** Would you be willing to always carry a condom with you so that it's available the next time you have intercourse?

> **Doctor:** Before our next appointment, would you be willing to check with your health plan about your options for getting alcohol treatment in the evening? That way, if you should decide to start treatment, you wouldn't miss work and no one there would have to know about the problem.

Often the clinician helps the contemplator confront the ambivalence that can, unless resolved, stalemate change. Short summaries serve to sharpen the focus, clarifying and reinforcing the contemplation work that is being done while hinting at resolution to the ambivalence.

> **Doctor:** It sounds as though you realize that changing your behavior—not smoking—will be best for you in the long term, and you're also trying to anticipate the short-term sacrifices and decide how you'll cope with them.

Due to limited time or unfamiliarity with the best way to approach a behavior problem, the clinician should often choose to delegate the contemplation work to another resource with more time and expertise. This may reduce the number of medical appointments that run overtime because the clinician is trying to provide advice about complex problems, or, conversely, reduce the possibility that because the clinician is busy, important psychosocial and behavioral contributors to somatic problems are not identified and addressed.

> **Doctor:** There is so much valuable information about diet changes for diabetes and weight control that I think we should give you a chance to sit down with our nutritionist and think this through. Should we arrange that next?

> **Doctor:** It sounds to me that stresses at home are a big part of your depression. I am afraid that we would be too rushed here to fully understand the problem and discuss how best you could overcome it. What do you think about sitting down with a counselor and giving yourself the time to understand and address this better?

Following a period of contemplation—which can range from a few days or several years—many people move toward a greater resolve and sense of urgency about changing the problem behavior. Energy to move ahead may come from salient information, threat or pressure (eg, the alcoholic husband whose wife threatens divorce, the smoker who learns she is pregnant), an inspiring model, encouragement or an opportunity to join a program, or a change in setting or circumstance, such as a job transfer, a move, or a new health plan that covers behavioral health better. Many things move quickly when they first get "unstuck." For example, a patient with a new diagnosis of heart disease may be energized to move rapidly through contemplation to a willingness to take recommended actions (at least initially). Such changes lead to the Preparation/Determination stage.

Preparation/Determination

In this stage the patient experiences a mounting sense of urgency and commitment to change.

- The patient talks about having made the decision to change, in contrast with the contemplator's desire or hope for change.
- The patient has chosen a specific goal: "I am going to stop smoking completely." "I will exercise three times a week."
- The patient mentions a specific time to begin the activity: "Next month. . . ." "After my surgery. . . ." "When the kids start school in September. . . ."
- The patient has chosen a specific course of action, such as joining a commercial weight-loss program or Alcoholics or Narcotics Anonymous (AA, NA), or is asking for a referral so the health plan will cover treatment.
- The patient anticipates and is ready to pay the costs of change, including out-of-pocket expenses, the time required for the change, physical discomfort, embarrassment, and public exposure.
- The patient considers the potential reactions of important people who may resist or be threatened by the change. A spouse or partner who smokes or drinks or is overweight, for example, may react negatively to the patient's plans to overcome the problem. Sometimes this occurs because such individuals anticipate pressure to face their own problems. In other cases, spouses, partners, and friends may resist the patient's decision to change because of some anticipated personal inconvenience (eg, the husband who must watch the children while his wife goes to an aerobics class) or embarrassment over the possibility of exposing a weakness to friends or neighbors (a teenager entering a drug treatment program).
- The patient can now envision overcoming obstacles that lie ahead. This is the combination of conviction and confidence that builds motivation to take action.

 CASE ILLUSTRATION 3

Mike is a 15-year-old boy who has been doing poorly in school for several years. Although he has been diagnosed with attention deficit hyperactivity disorder

(ADHD), his parents, teachers, and pediatrician have been unable to convince him that he should take a medication that could help. Now he has asked for an appointment with his pediatrician to discuss the situation. During the visit, Mike confesses that he is tired of his problem behavior and poor school performance. Further questioning by the physician reveals that one of Mike's friends admitted to being treated with medication for ADHD. Mike noticed and envied his friend's success; he asks the physician to prescribe "whatever it will take to get me out of this." The parents are invited into the examining room, and all agree on a plan that will begin with a trial of stimulant medicine. The effects of the medication will be reassessed in a month, based on questionnaires filled out by Mike and his parents and teachers.

Strategies for the Preparation/ Determination Stage

In this stage patients should be encouraged to set a date to start action on the problem. They should be helped to choose a specific approach and to understand more clearly the program they are planning to follow, including structured activities or referrals. Summaries can be helpful for clarification and reinforcement of what the patient is preparing to do:

> **Doctor:** So you're planning to start Weight Watchers at work next month with the goal of losing 35 pounds this year?

> **Doctor:** You've committed yourself to getting 30 minutes of aerobic exercise four times a week.

These commitments can be noted on the chart in the patient's presence, and the patient can be told that the clinician is looking forward to hearing about what happens next.

Patients should be supported with reassurance that initiating action to change problem behavior is always the right thing to do. Even when the attempt is not fully successful, the experience will yield helpful information about how to succeed eventually. It is important not to appear so enthusiastic and hopeful that patients who are unsuccessful want to avoid you. Because public commitments are more likely to be kept than private ones, patients should be encouraged to tell others about their intention to change.

Follow-up is also helpful, either by scheduling an appointment, sending a postcard, or requesting a note or phone message soon after the proposed start date. Clinicians should warmly reinforce the patient's commitment as being an important step toward accomplishing a valuable health behavior change.

Now the day finally arrives when the individual begins to put the chosen plan into action. Some people may move back and forth between Preparation/Determination and Contemplation a few times before taking action. The clinician helps patients in the Determination stage to intensify their commitment to start a specific course of action at a specific time.

Action

In the Action stage, patients regularly engage in activities intended to achieve the goals they have set. The clinician may not always fully agree with the patient's initial action plan, for example, a patient's diet and exercise regimen may be too limited to produce the desirable weight loss. Yet it is easier to make adjustments to a plan in Action than to overcome the inertia of getting a plan started. Characteristics of the Action stage include the following:

- The patient has begun a set of actions intended to solve the problem. He or she has joined and is attending a weight-reduction group, has started going to AA and cut down or stopped drinking, has recently quit or cut down on smoking and may be wearing a nicotine patch, or is exercising regularly, or recording daily glucometer readings.

- The patient may be focusing on one day at a time or trying to look past the initial discomfort by focusing on the long-term benefits.

- The patient recognizes and deals with the obstacles that arise before they can derail the program. The work done previously in the Contemplation and Preparation/ Determination stages is evident in the patient's comments during discussions with the clinician (eg, the patient makes self-motivational statements).

- Unlike the Contemplation stage, this is not experimental dabbling in change to see what it might be like. The patient has already decided that the discomfort of changing will be worthwhile. It remains to be seen whether the actual experience will be more difficult than expected and whether the action plan can be maintained.

- By frequent reminders of the motivations for change, the patient reinforces the commitment to overcome discomforts and obstacles.

This is a time of maximum focus and effort. When Action first begins the patient suffers most of the discomfort and realizes little of the desired benefit. The greatest risk is that second thoughts may plague the patient. Unexpected discomfort, resistance from others, or temptations that were neither anticipated nor planned may overwhelm the patient's commitment to change. The action plan may then be abandoned precipitously.

CASE ILLUSTRATION 4

Martha is a 45-year-old diabetic patient. Over the past few years, her doctor has encouraged her to lose weight and exercise regularly, without much success. Martha comes in today and proudly reports that she has joined a weight-loss group that is held at her work site. Two colleagues have also joined, and they have all been attending faithfully and following the dietary recommendations for the past 3 weeks. The doctor encourages Martha to talk about her efforts. She is eager to talk; she reports feeling a great sense of pride and satisfaction. She admits that although she had been disgusted with herself for getting so heavy, she never before felt ready and able to tackle the problem. When her friends suggested that they join the group together she understood that this was the situation she had been hoping for, one that could provide support in making a difficult change.

Martha also admits to some anxiety, since many people now know that she is trying to lose weight, and she does not want to fail publicly. Although she has been tempted to cheat on the diet, she has resisted the urge. She tells the doctor that she had felt somewhat discouraged when she did not lose as much weight as she had hoped the previous week. She asks the doctor to look over the program's dietary recommendations to be sure that they are safe in light of her diabetes.

While checking the weight-loss program's recommendations, Martha's doctor asks open-ended questions about what Martha is doing and how the effort is going. The doctor warmly reinforces the effort at change. Given enough time during the visit, the doctor can make additional helpful suggestions to reduce the risk of early relapse and orient Martha more firmly toward long-term maintenance. The doctor's warm, curious, and engaged demeanor has reverberations beyond the visit. Martha can use the pleasant memory of the encounter to further internalize the value of the effort toward change. "One more important person is rooting for me."

Strategies for the Action Stage

In this stage the clinician and patient anticipate what might be needed to maintain the initial changes in behavior. This involves problem-solving obstacles that are already emerging as well as planning ahead for how slips will be checked before a full-blown relapse can set in.

As in the above example, warm inquiry about the specifics of the patient's activities to promote change adds

the support and encouragement of a professional person to the patient's other social supports.

Clinicians should also ask about any obstacles the patients encounter (obstacles and second thoughts are to be expected) and how they are handling the problems.

The clinician can suggest that patients write out the advantages of making the change and post them prominently as an aid to maintaining their motivation.

Patients should be asked for permission to consult with other professionals involved in the program. A brief contact with a chemical-dependency counselor, diabetic educator, smoking-cessation group leader, psychotherapist, and so on demonstrates that the physician values and supports the patient's efforts during the most vulnerable period of active change.

It is important to help patients prepare for recovery from slips—smoking a cigarette, having a drink, missing an exercise session or AA meeting, or having seconds at a meal. A slip need not become a relapse if patients anticipate the possibility, prepare for it, and react once it is recognized by throwing out the rest of the cigarette pack, pouring out the remainder of the bottle, adding another exercise session or AA meeting, eating a smaller-than-usual portion at the next meal, and reaffirming the commitment to conquer this problem.

Some type of follow-up (eg, a note or call, an appointment) can be scheduled both to obtain a progress report and to reassure and show support for the patient. Making a note on the chart will remind the physician and office staff to inquire about the effort at change at the next patient contact.

The Action stage is a time of concerted effort to change a behavior. Once change has begun, however, many individuals are surprised to find that their resolution fades, and all the ground gained during the Action stage may be lost in relapse. Long-term vigilance and occasional (or even frequent and prolonged) activities are necessary to prevent backsliding into a full relapse. This period of sustained vigilance and activity is known as the Maintenance stage of change. For people who must control their weight, this stage may last a lifetime. In one study, former smokers reported some temptation to smoke 18 months after quitting. Problem drinkers may continue in AA for many years before they feel comfortable that their risk of relapse is low. Clinicians should be concerned about patients who have made good progress on resolving health-behavior problems but cannot describe their long-term plans to prevent relapse. Helping patients anticipate and find answers to the questions addressed in the next section is an important way in which clinicians can promote ultimate success.

Maintenance

The Maintenance stage is the period of sustained vigilance and activity needed to preserve the improvements achieved during the Action stage. It is where initial success is transformed into the new "normal."

- The patient has achieved a period of success—as he or she has defined it—in overcoming the problem. The patient may have cut down or stopped drinking, reduced to the desired weight, or gone without cigarettes for several months. He or she may be managing time and commitments better so that stress is no longer overwhelming, may have gained consistent control over a short temper, or may have accomplished other desired outcomes.
- Some patients assume a positive identity as people who have overcome a problem. Patients who begin an exercise and diet program to lose weight, for example, may become avid hikers whose leisure time is devoted to rigorous outdoor adventures. These people have made a life-style and identity change in which the former problem behavior has no place.

  To maintain these improvements, the patient must be able to handle both predictable and unpredictable obstacles and may have to accept the constraints of abstinence. This requires dealing appropriately with the temptations and frustrations that inevitably arise in the months and years following successful action.

- Some patients may feel frustrated that success in dealing with one problem has not brought about hoped-for changes in other areas. For example, although the weight loss may produce a slimmer, healthier body, it does not necessarily lead to an idealized slenderness and attractiveness. Abstinence from crack cocaine may not be enough to end all marital, job, and financial problems. Patients who reduce their workaholic schedules to spend more time with their families may find they've traded more admiration at home for less at work. They must first take satisfaction in accomplishing their stated goals and then be ready to go to work on other dissatisfactions.
- The initial intensity of effort may be tapering off. Attendance at support-group meetings, for example, may have become erratic. The patient may be wondering whether it is now safe to quit the group or treatment program or to end a diet. It is hard to know when one is "out of the woods" and the problem is resolved; successful maintenance requires both accurate self-appraisal and ongoing vigilance.
- Slips into the problem behavior may begin to be tolerated or justified: "I'll have just one glass of wine when I'm out with friends." "I'll only have a cigarette if I'm feeling really tense." These seductive thoughts must be resisted if successful maintenance is to continue; it may be necessary to renew the intense efforts of the Action stage to do so (eg, rejoin Weight Watch-

ers, return to a 12-Step Support Group, go back to psychotherapy and/ or anitdepressant medication).

CASE ILLUSTRATION 5

At 55 years of age, Bill is overall doing very well, seeing his internist periodically for health maintenance. Bill had been a very heavy drinker for 20 years. Five years ago a citation for driving under the influence of alcohol and the threat of divorce by his second wife pushed him into an alcohol treatment program. He achieved abstinence while attending the formal, court-mandated, 2-year outpatient treatment program. Since that time he has continued in AA, attending at least two meetings a week and occasional weekend conferences and workshops. Bill also sponsors a younger man in the AA group. In his conversations with his doctor, Bill describes himself as a recovering alcoholic. He schedules an appointment to discuss his distress over problems his son is experiencing—for which he holds himself partly responsible. The doctor thinks antidepressant medicine might be helpful, particularly in light of Bill's disturbed sleep and preoccupied demeanor. Bill questions the internist closely about the risk of addiction and explains his reluctance to use "another crutch" to control his moods.

Bill's doctor can recognize that because Bill is consciously in maintenance he is extremely vigilant about anything he sees as a threat to his sobriety. The doctor asks directly and respectfully how Bill believes antidepressant medication might undermine his sobriety or stimulate a new addiction. Bill says that he is basically afraid of becoming dependent on the medication. The physician explains that antidepressant medications are not addictive and that individual psychotherapy is also an effective treatment, and advises Bill to think about the recommendation, to speak with other AA members and confidants about the two alternatives, and to give him a call when he decides how to proceed.

Strategies for the Maintenance Stage

Inquiring about how well the patient is maintaining the improvements achieved in the Action stage is an important first step:

Doctor: What have you been doing to keep your weight down?

Doctor: Have you been going to your support-group meetings regularly?

Doctor: How well have you been doing with your exercise program?

Doctor: Patients sometimes have trouble keeping up with multiple daily medications. What problems with confusion or missed doses have you been having?

Successful maintenance often involves making life-style changes that turn out to have significant positive effects beyond controlling the original problem. The sedentary patient who starts a program of physical activity for cardiovascular conditioning may find, as a bonus, both long-term weight control and unexpected skill on the tennis court. In addition, clinicians who have successfully stopped smoking, lost weight, or become more physically active can sometimes use themselves as examples of making and maintaining change. The key here is to emphasize that the new behavior can become an integral part of a more healthful and satisfying life-style.

Patients should be asked about slips that have already occurred and how they responded. It is important to emphasize the difference between a slip and a full relapse. Patients should be prepared for the likelihood of a slip and have a plan for how to deal with it at once. They may protest that the clinician is being too pessimistic. Explaining to patients that such preparation is a way of protecting their newly achieved change can provide a more positive tone.

Patients can also be asked what they have learned so far about the change process as well as how confident they are that they will maintain the improvement over the next time period. They can also be asked to describe situations in which the risk of a slip or relapse is high—such as going to a party or experiencing emotions such as anger, sadness, or exuberance—and how prepared they feel to handle these high-risk situations without a slip.

Each of these recommendations involves showing interest, support, and curiosity and suggesting that anticipation and vigilance are the keys to successful maintenance. Although busy clinicians may not be taking a leading role in the change (eg, counselors, diabetic educators, and support group members may be much more actively involved), their empathic curiosity and focused advice can still be very useful.

Clinicians should be alert for any signs of waning enthusiasm and express empathic curiosity about the cause. As noted earlier, patients often become discouraged when improvement in one area does not resolve other life dissatisfactions. They may feel that others do not recognize and appreciate the effort that they have made to change. A sincere compliment from a clinician accompanied by a message that "I am rooting for you" creates a memory that can be recalled during moments of discouragement.

Unfortunately, the odds favor relapse over any other outcome for a single attempt at health-behavior change. Clinicians know from both research and experience that patients' attempts to lose weight, stop alcohol or drug abuse, change their life-styles to reduce stress, alter their diets in a more healthful direction, and even to floss their teeth daily often end in relapse. The false starts, failed promises, and pounds promptly regained tend to obscure the reality that persistent effort often does result in successful resolution of the problem. Although any single effort to change may get derailed before the patient achieves successful long-term maintenance, repeated efforts tend to yield the desired result eventually (this is borne out by Schacter's classic 1982 study). It is worth noting that more than 45 million Americans have now quit smoking, many on their third or fourth serious try.

Relapse

All relapse begins with a "slip," a deviation from the action plan. In a slip, the patient has an episode of problem behavior after a period of self-defined success in having overcome the problem. A slip might constitute engaging in an undesirable behavior such as smoking or not engaging in a desirable behavior such as exercising. In the Relapse stage, patients return to consistent problem behavior. With prompting by the clinician, patients may be able to describe the circumstances that led to the slips and eventually to relapse. They can learn how to anticipate and correct these vulnerabilities when they take action again.

- The typical patient in relapse may have regained lost weight, begun drinking heavily again, started smoking cigarettes again, or stopped using condoms during sexual intercourse with new partners.

- The patient may now talk or act like a person in an earlier stage of change. He or she may have entered a period of resistance and avoidance that is characteristic of the Precontemplation stage. Alternatively, the patient may be contemplating change again, possibly even considering action in the near future.

- The stories of patients who have relapsed are more complex than those of patients who have never relapsed. The reasons offered for the relapse provide many clues to the steps that must be taken to reinvigorate the patient's willingness to tackle the problem again. One patient may think: "I did it once, I can do it again!" whereas another patient may think: "I guess I don't have the will power to do this."

The time the patient spends in relapse before initiating the next Action stage of change accounts for much of the observed slowness in achieving final success for many health-behavior problems.

Even in professional treatment, as many as two-thirds of the participants are likely to have relapsed within a year after achieving initial alcohol or drug sobriety. Success in smoking cessation, weight control, or alcohol and drug sobriety is usually achieved after a number of separate, unsuccessful attempts at change. In one study of smoking cessation, it took an average of 7 years to move from the Precontemplation to the Maintenance stage. The typical participant had three or more relapses during which regular smoking was not resumed.

If handled empathically, patients in this stage are usually not too entrenched in denial or resistance. They had already concluded at least once that change was needed and can often recount the costs of continuing the problem behavior. It is the uneasiness they feel in anticipation of again trying to change that often has them stuck.

CASE ILLUSTRATION 6

Barbara is a 28-year-old woman who is being seen 2 months after the birth of her second child for renewal of her birth control prescription. Her physician is delighted to see Barbara again. As the interview evolves, Barbara sheepishly reveals that she is back to smoking a pack of cigarettes a day. The clinician is both disappointed and surprised, since Barbara had been quite proud of the fact that she stopped smoking during the pregnancy. The doctor takes a deep breath and calmly asks Barbara how this happened so quickly. Barbara talks about how frazzled she has felt taking care of both her baby and her 3-year-old son. She explains how, at first, she found it relaxing to smoke a cigarette or two after dinner with her husband (who is also a smoker); she had not pictured herself smoking a pack a day again. Soon, however, she was smoking with a friend who stopped in to visit. Now she has begun looking forward to a cigarette whenever she has a break from the immediate demands of her family. She tells her doctor that although she tries never to smoke when the baby is up, even this control is starting to erode.

The doctor's first challenge is to manage her own frustration and not leave Barbara feeling judged and ashamed. She points out Barbara's success in caring for her (then) 2-year-old child and dealing with the mood swings and physical discomforts of pregnancy without smoking. She also expresses her support and encouragement for Barbara's recommitment to abstinence. Reaffirming the health benefits of not smoking—for both the patient and her children—helps reinforce the commitment. As a further step, the clinician reenforces Barbara's no-smoking rule in the house and encourages her to talk with her husband about this as well. (Harm reduction is a legitimate goal for behavior change.) She recognizes that Barbara has relapsed back into the Contemplation stage of change and so focuses her questions and comments on wondering how she can help Barbara reestablish smoking cessation or at least reduced smoking for now.

Strategies for the Relapse Stage

The key to dealing with relapse is to reframe it as a valuable learning experience that will shed light on how best to go about the next attempt at change. It is therefore helpful that clinicians express their interest in the last attempt at change and ask the patient to describe exactly how initial success was achieved and how slips led to a full-blown relapse. If there is not enough time in the visit to have this discussion, the patient can be encouraged to sketch out a timeline at home, noting successes, slips, progression to full relapse, and what forces were operating at each juncture. The intention of the "homework" is to assist the patient in learning from the relapse and guide you both toward more effective action in the future.

Some patients promptly—and erroneously—conclude, "I tried it and it didn't work; therefore, it never will work." This is too global a statement; it obscures the successful components that could be used in the next effort at change. The physician's response might be:

> **Doctor:** It sounds as though you were very successful in quitting smoking using the action strategies you described, and they might work well again. Where you fell down was in thinking that you could have one cigarette and not recognizing how dangerous this could be for you. What do you think about that?

The next attempt at change should be discussed as inevitable—*when* rather than *if*. Patients should be reminded that all the analysis and conclusions that led to deciding to change last time remain valid. The question the relapser must answer is "What next step will enable you to move again toward change?"

CONCLUSION

One of the most helpful aspects of using the Stages of Change Model is the optimism it generates for both clinician and patient. The concept that pursuing the change process knowledgeably and persistently over time brings about the desired change is a welcome counter to the frustration and pessimism so often reported by clinicians and patients alike. Although clinicians usually are convinced that behavior change would be helpful, they often report low self-efficacy about their ability to influence behavior in the brief medical interview. Although they often feel responsibility and frustration, they may actually do very little during visits to help with behavior change. The goal of this chapter has been to map out pragmatic approaches that the clinician can utilize in even the briefest encounters (eg, "I just want to encourage you to do anything you can to cut down or stop smoking until this bronchitis clears up.") or to offer guidance for how longer discussions could be conducted should time allow. Perhaps this chapter will help clinicians make addressing behavior change a part of their "new normal" clinical style.

SUGGESTED READINGS

DiClemente CC: Motivational interviewing and the stages of change. In: Miller WR, Rollnick S (editors): *Motivational Interviewing: Preparing People to Change Addictive Behavior.* Guilford, 1991.

Prochaska JO, Norcross JC, DiClemente CC: *Changing for Good.* Guilford, 1994.

Rollnick S: Readiness, importance and confidence: critical conditions of change in treatment. In: Miller WR, Heather N (editors): *Treating Addictive Behaviour,* 2nd ed. Plenum, 1998.

Rollnick S, Mason P, Butler C: *Health Behavior Change: A Guide for Practitioners.* Churchill Livingstone, 1999.

Schacter S: Recidivism and self-cure of smoking and obesity. Am Psychol 1982;37:436.

WEB SITES

Transtheoretical Model Cancer Prevention Resource Center University of Rhode Island
http://www.uri.edu/research/crpc/TTM/detailedoverview.htm

The Motivational Interviewing Page
http://www.motivationalinterview.org/

Patient Adherence

M. Robin DiMatteo, PhD

INTRODUCTION

When patients fail to follow treatment recommendations made by their physicians, problems in clinical care can result. **Nonadherence** (also called **noncompliance**) typically involves patients who take antibiotics incorrectly (eg, only until the symptoms abate) or do not take them at all, who forget or refuse to take longer term medications (such as for hypertension), and who persist in activities that jeopardize their health (such as smoking and high-risk sexual activity). As a result of their failure to adhere to recommended treatments, patients might become more seriously ill and treatment-resistant pathogens may develop. Physicians might then incorrectly adjust the treatment (such as increasing medication dosages) and may be misled about the correct diagnosis. Both practitioners and patients become frustrated by nonadherence, and the time and money spent on the medical visit can be wasted.

Considerable research on this topic suggests that an average of 4 of 10 patients do not follow the treatment recommended during medical visits. Rates of nonadherence vary with the type of regimen that is prescribed. Approximately 20% of patients fail to follow short-term treatments for acute conditions (such as taking an antibiotic correctly), about 40–50% are nonadherent to longer term regimens (such as taking regular medication for a chronic disease), and more than 75% of patients fail to adhere to recommended life-style changes such as limiting the consumption of alcohol and dietary fat, exercising, or ceasing to use tobacco products. Adherence to treatment is even more problematic when patients have serious medical conditions (for example, HIV disease, cardiovascular diseases, cancer, or glaucoma) and their lives or quality of life depend upon following treatment recommendations.

It is important that primary care providers recognize the potential for nonadherence among all patients, and avoid being judgmental toward them. Following medical treatments correctly can interfere with patients' quality of life, and can serve as a constant and disturbing reminder of the illness. Patients need emotional and practical support, as well as information and guidance, to be adherent. Research on patient adherence shows that patients do only what they believe in and are able to do. The most important ingredients in achieving patient adherence are effective communication and patients' informed collaboration with the physician.

AWARENESS OF NONADHERENCE

Nonadherence is often difficult to recognize (Table 16–1). Patients rarely admit to having difficulties following their treatment regimens and few are willing to tell their providers that they have no intention of following recommendations. Patients may weigh their physician's recommendations against their own beliefs and what they have learned from other sources, and may reject recommendations if the benefits of adhering do not appear to outweigh the costs in terms of interference in their quality of life.

Patients who are passive and uninvolved and appear to be unquestioningly obedient are often the least adherent. Passive patients are more likely to disregard medical directives than are patients who ask questions, offer opinions, and even attempt to negotiate a more acceptable regimen. Any hints of patient depression should be considered "red flags" regarding adherence. Nonadherence should always be considered whenever a patient is inconsistently responsive—or remains unresponsive—to treatment, and when the clinical picture is confusing or does not appear to make sense.

CASE ILLUSTRATION

Shirley is a 46-year-old attorney in an urban law firm. She has moderate essential hypertension. She is about 40 pounds overweight, rarely exercises, and describes herself as being under considerable stress. Despite recommendations to follow a low-fat diet and an exercise program, Shirley remains overweight and is completely sedentary. Antihypertensive medication has been prescribed for 4 months, with little or no reduction in blood pressure. After returning several times for scheduled office visits, Shirley cancels several appointments.

Eventually Shirley returns for a follow-up visit, but her clinical parameters remain unchanged. The physician's tasks are threefold: (1) to begin a dialogue with the patient about the stressful factors in her life that affect her health behavior (including assessing her for depression), (2) to educate Shirley about the very real dangers of excessive weight and hypertension, and (3) to develop a treatment regimen that she can

Table 16–1. Typical clues to nonadherence.

Patient passivity and lack of involvement
Appearance of unquestioning obedience
Patient depression
Lack of response or inconsistent response to treatment
Confusing or indistinct clinical picture

believe in and integrate into her life. These tasks must be accomplished while maintaining Shirly's trust and commitment to improving her health. Once a therapeutic alliance is established, the patient's emotional experience is understood, and support is provided, Shirley can begin to accept that her continued noncompliance could result in her having a stroke or heart attack. The physician can then work with the patient to negotiate an acceptable treatment regimen. At the very least, this will involve recognition (and if necessary treatment) of depression. It will also involve establishment and monitoring of a graduated regimen of physical activity that Shirley enjoys and that may help to reduce her stress, and a gradual modification of her diet—most likely with support from nutritional counseling or a self-help group. It will also involve education about and negotiation of drug-treatment choices, with regular assessment of the medications' effects on her quality of life. These goals should be expected to be achieved over the course of regular office visits.

UNDERSTANDING ADHERENCE PROBLEMS

The most important step in dealing with adherence problems is to talk openly with the patient about the illness and its treatment while maintaining respect for the patient's beliefs. In doing this, Shirley's physician discovers that although she is a highly educated person, she does not fully understand the meaning of hypertension, the risks of leaving it untreated, or the role of medication and life-style changes in lowering blood pressure. The physician is surprised to learn, for example, that Shirley takes medication only when she feels "hyper" or "tense." Shirley does not understand or believe in the efficacy of taking medication regularly; in fact, she thinks it might be dangerous. Shirley is embarrassed by being "the kind of person who has to take medicine," and she believes that the antihypertensive medication makes her feel tired and interferes with her job and with her ability to care for her family. Shirley works extremely hard at her profession, claiming that she does not have time to devote to exercise and nutritious meals.

Psychological Mechanisms

Problems with adherence are not caused by patient personality type, gender, ethnicity, class, or educational attainment. Very affluent and highly educated patients can be as nonadherent as those who are poor and uneducated. The primary causes of nonadherence (Table 16–2) are poor provider–patient communication, lack of understanding of the treatment regimen and the reasons for its importance, lack of trust and mutual caring, and provider behavior that is controlling and paternalistic. Nonadherence occurs when patients do not understand the costs, benefits, and efficacy of the recommended regimen, when patients do not believe the regimen is valuable and worthy of commitment, and when physicians fail to anticipate and help patients overcome barriers to adherence (such as feelings of hopelessness and depression, the inability to afford costly medication, lack of social support, and a hectic or irregular daily schedule).

Nonadherence can sometimes be the patient's way of equalizing the balance of power in the physician–patient relationship. When patients feel they cannot assert their preferences, they often make private plans for their own medical well-being. Nonadherence might be thought of as a strategy for restoring a lost sense of control felt in the face of illness and medical treatment. A patient's apparent passive acceptance of the regimen is likely to be interpreted by the physician as a sign of commitment instead of as a warning of nonadherence. Although the patient may be agreeing verbally, body language—crossed arms, stiff posture, lack of eye contact, depressed affect—may indicate the opposite. Without further persuasion and support, the patient might fail to follow the prescribed treatment regimen.

Assessing Adherence in Practice

Studies show that physicians are consistently poor at recognizing problems with adherence. Some physicians

Table 16–2. Causes of nonadherence.

Poor provider–patient communication about the regimen
Lack of trust and mutual caring in provider–patient
    relationship
Controlling, paternalistic provider behavior
Patient's failure to understand costs, benefits, and efficacy
    of regimen
Patient's lack of commitment to regimen
Patient depression and hopelessness
Patient's lack of social support
Provider's failure to anticipate and overcome practical barriers
    to adherence

assume higher levels of adherence among their patients than actually occur, and many cannot identify which of their patients have difficulties with adherence. Problems with adherence can be particularly challenging to detect if they are viewed as aberrant behavior rather than as rational choices. It should be assumed that every patient is potentially nonadherent, often for good reasons. Physicians might think back to their own personal instances of nonadherence to gain perspective on how reasonable such a choice might sometimes seem to be. When patients attempt to hide difficulties with adherence, it is often to avoid disappointing their physicians and because of the social and normative pressures to be a "good patient." Patients are especially circumspect if they anticipate any criticism from their providers or negation of their right to make choices. Conversely, providers might be reluctant to inquire about nonadherence for fear that such revelation would be awkward and frustrating and require additional time trying to gain patients' cooperation. The goal in questioning patients about their adherence is not to assert the authority of the physician or to reprimand patients for failures in adherence, but rather to improve patients' health and quality of life. Patients must be helped to make collaborative decisions with their physicians instead of unilateral choices that might jeopardize their well-being.

The most effective approach to assessing patient adherence is to recognize and accept that patients are autonomous and that they appropriately make personal choices to maximize their quality of life *as they see it*. Patients are experts about their own values, preferences, and capabilities, just as physicians are experts in medical diagnosis and treatment. The provider's task is to be a sensitive, supportive advocate, not an authoritarian adversary. The patient is a complex individual, psychologically and socially, and has unique values, life-style, and beliefs about quality of life that must be incorporated into decisions about medical treatment.

Patient responsibility for adherence requires effective practitioner–patient communication and collaboration toward the goal of self-management. Without efforts toward collaboration, with their inevitable but manageable conflicts, providers and patients create relationships in which their expectations are never discussed. When patients are not informed about and involved in their care, they provide less adequate histories and they tend to delay reporting important symptoms to their physicians. Patients who are uninformed typically remain uninvolved, and the responsibility they must assume for adherence to treatment may never be achieved.

MANAGING NONADHERENCE

What the Primary Care Physician Can Do

Whether medical intervention improves patient outcomes depends, to an appreciable extent, on patient adherence.

Thus, the health outcomes the care physicians deliver depend on their mastery of the elements listed in Table 16–3.

EFFECTIVE, ACCURATE COMMUNICATION OF INFORMATION

The provider must build the two essential elements of provider–patient communication: accurate transmittal of information between physician and patient and emotional support and understanding of the patient's unique emotional needs and personal experiences. Unfortunately, such communication is not the norm in medical practice; close to 50% of all patients leave their doctors' offices not knowing what they have been told and what they are supposed to do to take care of themselves. Physicians regularly use medical terms that patients do not understand, and patients are usually unwilling or lack sufficient skill to articulate their questions. Although the vast majority of patients greatly value obtaining as much information about their conditions as possible, including various treatment alternatives, such information is rarely provided to them. Physicians often unwittingly discourage patients from voicing their concerns and requests for information by exhibiting rushed behaviors, such as looking at their wristwatches and interrupting patients' questions. Despite their confusion about technical terms and medical jargon used by their physicians, patients typically do not ask for clarification. Educating patients and answering their questions may initially take a few extra minutes, but that time is very well spent in the long run.

EMOTIONAL ASPECTS OF CARE

The second element of provider–patient communication involves empathy and the building of interpersonal trust in the physician–patient relationship (see Chapter 2). This aspect of care has traditionally been a source of some discomfort for health professionals because it is often perceived as taking too much time, and as something for which physicians feel they have not been trained. However if

Table 16–3. Essential elements of achieving patient adherence.

Accurate transmission of information between patient and provider

Emotional support and understanding of patient

Awareness and modification of patient's beliefs

Help in choosing an acceptable course of action to which a commitment can be made

Help in overcoming barriers to adherence

Acceptance of the value of provider–patient negotiation

Focus on the overall quality of life of the patient

Development of a specific plan to implement the regimen

Recognition and treatment of patient's depression and hopelessness providers attend only to diseases, and ignore their patients' suffering, they are likely to fail to support their patients' adjustment and healing.

Physicians' behavior and communication style during office visits directly affect patients' trust in and satisfaction with their providers, their recall of medical information, and their subsequent adherence to prescribed treatment regimens. Emotional support of patients appears to enhance positive expectations for healing and patients' fulfillment of those expectations. Providers who are more sensitive to and emotionally expressive with nonverbal communication have patients who are more satisfied and who are more likely to adhere to the recommended treatments. Physicians can contribute a great deal to their patients simply by giving them their full attention and genuinely listening to their concerns. Providers who make patients feel rushed or ignored, devalue patients' views, fail to respect and listen to them, and fail to understand their perspectives invite a host of problems including patient dissatisfaction, nonadherence, and, if the outcome of care is less than satisfactory, malpractice litigation. It is important to note that there is empiric evidence that technical skill is not sacrificed in developing the capacity to respond to patients' feelings. In fact, studies show that the provision of good psychosocial care for patients is correlated with better treatment outcomes.

PATIENTS' BELIEFS AND AN ACCEPTABLE COURSE OF ACTION

The physician should assess and, if necessary, modify the patient's beliefs about the regimen. Patient adherence depends on commitment to what may be a disruptive, difficult course of action. Commitment depends on the patient's clear understanding of the regimen and on the belief that it is worth following; that it is likely to be effective; and that the benefits outweigh the costs in time, money, discomfort, possible embarrassment, and life-style adjustment. Such a commitment by the patient requires detailed discussion about the recommendation, including its value compared with other courses of action and any potential risks or problems that might be encountered. Discussion of any possible disadvantage of a regimen should take place before the choice is made, so that the patient is able to be involved in the choice of the regimen and so that any adverse effects do not result in abandonment of the regimen.

IMPROVING PATIENTS' QUALITY OF LIFE

In choosing and reinforcing a treatment regimen, it is essential to focus on the patient's overall quality of life. Striving for patient adherence to precisely what the physician has chosen is a problematic strategy. The goal of treatment should not be to achieve the provider's agenda, but rather to recognize that the patient knows more about himself or herself than the clinician. The patient is the one whose quality of life will be affected by the results of the medical

decisions that are made, the one who will benefit if the regimen is a success, and the one who must live with the results if the treatment fails. Therefore, the physician and patient should explore together the chances of achieving the goals that they have jointly chosen, and various alternatives for the future for the patient that may result from different courses of action, including the possibility of no treatment at all.

NEGOTIATING THE TREATMENT REGIMEN

The physician must accept the inevitability—and the value—of disagreements with the patient. For example, patients tend to be more risk averse than their physicians, and they usually favor more conservative interventions. Choosing the best course of action to enhance a patient's quality of life and solve a medical problem should be expected to take some time and effort. The mutual exploration of alternatives can help physician and patient learn to work together despite their likely differing perspectives on the clinical situation. Because patient involvement in the decision process is likely to lead to more satisfactory outcomes, physicians should actively pursue with patients any possible conflict and work to unearth patients' objections in the process of negotiation and collaborative decision making. It is important that the clinician accept the possibility that the patient has a different definition of the problem, different goals, and a different idea of what methods are acceptable for achieving those goals. There must be a recognition that the most effective interaction occurs if each party fully understands the objectives and preferences of the other.

When a patient's perspective is not known to the clinician, continuity of conflict rather than resolution is inevitable. Thus, physicians should explore patients' assessments and feelings about all proposed actions and lead therapeutic conversations to legitimate expressions of conflict, making it clear that the encounter is one in which differences can be resolved through negotiation. Steps to effective negotiation include stating principles and goals on which doctor and patient agree, eliciting the patient's feelings and concerns about alternative methods, respectfully acknowledging physician–patient differences, and compromising whenever possible.

Helping Patients Overcome Barriers to Adherence

After the patient has truly come to understand and believe in the value of the regimen, and to make a commitment to following it, the clinician should work with the patient to incorporate the plan into the patient's life. Physician and patient must identify ways to overcome practical problems that may serve as barriers to adherence. For example, many patients are likely to have difficulty taking medication four times a day but find that two times a day is much easier.

A clinical regimen that can be associated with regular activities such as eating meals or brushing teeth, or one that can be paired with a wristwatch alarm or a medication schedule posted on the refrigerator, should improve adherence. At this stage, advancement in adherence requires working with the patient to determine precisely how the regimen can be implemented for maximum clinical effectiveness.

It is important to develop—with the patient—methods for follow-up and continued maintenance, such as regular telephone calls and office visits to check on progress, to solve inevitable problems, or to modify the regimen when necessary. Some physicians write out brief contracts with their patients, specifying what the patient is to do (the details of the treatment regimen) and what the physician is to do in return (eg, regular telephone contact for encouragement). The involvement of an encouraging and supportive family member of the patient's choosing can also help to enhance adherence to treatment.

Patients who are involved in both choosing and planning the implementation of their treatment regimens are much more involved in their own care, ask more questions, and express greater satisfaction with their care than those who are not. Involved patients also have greater alleviation of their symptoms and better control of their chronic conditions, less distress and concern about their illnesses, and better responses to surgery and invasive diagnostic procedures. Patients who are involved in their care also feel a greater sense of control over their health and their lives, and demonstrate better adherence to the treatment they have helped to choose.

Indications for Referral

In many cases, primary care providers may find it difficult or impossible to devote extended time to patient counseling, education, follow-up, and maintenance. Written materials can be helpful for information, but only if those materials are used to supplement what has been discussed with the patient. Although office nurses or health educators can provide valuable adjunctive care to patients, their role in education and supportive care should never fully take the place of the physician's. Patients often need additional referrals, such as to a nutritionist for dietary modification or an exercise counselor/personal trainer for fitness education and training. The primary provider should always remain involved, consulting with these ancillary providers and monitoring the patient's own views of progress. The primary provider should be familiar with and believe in the methods used by referral providers; his or her enthusiasm for these referrals affects patient adherence to their recommendations as well.

Considerable recent research shows a substantial negative correlation between patient adherence and mild to moderate patient depression. Although severe depression might be easily recognized as a clear indication for referral, milder depression including feelings of sadness and hopelessness, withdrawal from social support, and/or impairment in constructive thinking can seriously limit adherence and should be examined. If necessary, the patient should be referred for cognitive- behavioral therapy (with or without antidepressant medication). In addition, although the clinician must avoid overinterpreting nonadherence as a behavioral or mental disorder, there are cases in which a patient's seemingly irrational noncompliance should be evaluated by a mental health professional, particularly if that noncompliance is life-threatening. Finally, many patients with chronic diseases are likely to do well with a support group, in which ideas for coping as well as practical help may be provided by others with the same illness experience.

SUGGESTED READINGS

Brody H. The placebo response. Recent research and implications for family medicine. J Fam Pract 2000;49:649.

Cassell EJ: *Talking with Patients,* Vol. 1: *The Theory of Doctor-Patient Communication.* MIT, 1985.

DiMatteo MR: The role of the physician in the emerging health care environment. Western J Med 1998;168:328.

DiMatteo MR, DiNicola DD: *Achieving Patient Compliance.* Pergamon, 1982.

DiMatteo MR, Lepper HS, Croghan TW: Depression is a risk factor for noncompliance with medical treatment: meta-analysis of the effects of anxiety and depression on patient adherence. Arch Intern Med 2000;160:2101.

Levinson W: Physician-patient communication: a key to malpractice prevention. JAMA 1994;272:1619.

Myers L, Midence K: *Adherence to Treatment in Medical Conditions.* Harwood, 1998.

Roter DL, Hall JA: *Doctors Talking with Patients/Patients Talking with Doctors.* Auburn House, 1992.

Roter DL et al: Effectiveness of interventions to improve patient compliance: a meta-analysis. Med Care 1998;36:1138.

Shumaker S et al (editors): *The Handbook of Health Behavior Change,* 2nd ed. Springer, 1998.

Smoking

17

Nancy A. Rigotti, MD

INTRODUCTION

Cigarette smoking is the leading preventable cause of death in the United States, responsible for an estimated 419,000 deaths per year, or one in every five deaths. Physicians must take care of the health consequences of their patients' tobacco use. It is equally important for them to prevent smoking-related disease by treating their patients' smoking habits.

■ PATTERNS OF TOBACCO USE

The prevalence of cigarette smoking in the United States rose rapidly in the first half of the twentieth century and peaked in 1965, when 40% of adult Americans smoked cigarettes. Since then, smoking rates have declined, reflecting growing public awareness of the health risks of tobacco use and public health efforts to discourage tobacco use. By 1999, adult smoking prevalence had fallen to 23.5%. Smoking starts during childhood and adolescence; 90% of smokers begin to smoke before the age of 20. The rates of tobacco use in men and women, once very different, are converging. In 1999, 21.5% of adult women and 25.7% of men smoked cigarettes.

In the United States, smoking is more closely linked to education than it is to age, race, occupation, or any other sociodemographic factor. Educational attainment is a marker for socioeconomic status, and these data indicate that smoking is a problem that is becoming concentrated in lower socioeconomic groups.

■ HEALTH CONSEQUENCES OF TOBACCO USE

Cigarette smoking increases overall mortality and morbidity rates and is a cause of cardiovascular disease (including myocardial infarction and sudden death); cerebrovascular disease; peripheral vascular disease; chronic obstructive pulmonary disease; and cancers of the lung, larynx, oral cavity, and esophagus.

Lung cancer, once a rare disease, has increased dramatically. It has been the leading cause of cancer death in men since 1955 and in women since 1986. Cigarette smokers also have higher rates of cancers of the bladder, pancreas, kidney, stomach, and uterine cervix. Smoking interacts with alcohol to increase the risk of laryngeal, oral cavity, and esophageal cancers. Tobacco also interacts with occupational exposures such as from asbestos to greatly increase cancer risk.

Smoking is associated with many pregnancy complications, especially low birth weight (<2500 g). This is primarily attributable to intrauterine growth retardation (IUGR), although smoking in pregnancy also increases the risk of preterm delivery. Other adverse pregnancy outcomes linked to smoking are miscarriage (spontaneous abortion), stillbirth, and neonatal death. Smoking during pregnancy affects children even after birth. Sudden infant death syndrome is two to four times more common in infants born to mothers who smoked during pregnancy. Cognitive deficits and developmental problems in childhood are also linked to maternal smoking during pregnancy.

Cigarette smoking also increases a woman's risk of postmenopausal osteoporosis and fracture. Smokers have higher rates of upper and lower respiratory infections, peptic ulcer disease, cataracts, macular degeneration, and sensorineural hearing loss than nonsmokers. Smokers have more prominent skin wrinkling than nonsmokers, independent of sun exposure. The majority of residential fire deaths are caused by smoking.

There is no safe level of tobacco use. Smoking as few as one to four cigarettes per day increases the risk of myocardial infarction and cardiovascular mortality. Smoking cigarettes with reduced tar and nicotine content does not protect against the health hazards of smoking.

The health hazards of smoking are not limited to those suffered by smokers. Nonsmokers are harmed by chronic exposure to environmental tobacco smoke (ETS). The children of parents who smoke have more serious respiratory infections during infancy and childhood, more respiratory symptoms, and a higher rate of chronic otitis media and asthma than the children of nonsmokers. Nonsmoking women whose husbands smoke have a higher risk of lung cancer than nonsmoking women whose husbands do not smoke. A 1993 Environmental Protection Agency report identified ETS as a source of carcinogens, responsible for approximately 3000 lung cancer deaths per year in U.S. nonsmokers. Passive smoke exposure also increases nonsmokers' risk of coronary heart disease.

HEALTH BENEFITS OF SMOKING CESSATION

Epidemiological data demonstrate that smoking cessation has health benefits for men and women of all ages. Even those who stop smoking after the age of 65 or who quit after the development of a smoking-related disease derive benefit. Smoking cessation decreases the risk of lung cancer and other cancers, heart attack, stroke, chronic lung disease, and peptic ulcer disease. After 10–15 years of abstinence, overall mortality rates for smokers approach rates of those who never smoked. The risk reduction for cardiovascular disease occurs more rapidly than the risk reduction for lung cancer or overall mortality. Half of the excess risk of cardiovascular mortality is eliminated in the first year of quitting, whereas for lung cancer, 30–50% of the excess risk is still evident 10 years after quitting and some excess risk remains after 15 years.

The benefits of stopping smoking translate into a longer life expectancy for former smokers compared with continuing smokers. The degree to which former smokers benefit from cessation depends on their previous lifetime dose of tobacco, their health status at the time of quitting, and the elapsed time since quitting. Smokers who benefit the most are those who quit when they are younger, have fewer pack-years of tobacco exposure, and are free of smoking-related disease. The health benefits of smoking cessation far exceed any risks from the small weight gain that occurs with cessation.

SMOKING BEHAVIOR

Cigarettes and other tobacco products are addicting. Nicotine is capable of creating tolerance, physical dependence, and a withdrawal syndrome in habitual users. Nicotine withdrawal symptoms include (1) cravings for a cigarette, (2) irritability, (3) restlessness, (4) anger and impatience, (5) difficulty concentrating, (6) anxiety, (7) depressed mood, (8) excessive hunger, and (9) sleep disturbance. These symptoms begin within a few hours of the last cigarette, are strongest during the first 2–3 days after quitting, and gradually diminish over a month or more. Other than craving for a cigarette, the symptoms are nonspecific, and many smokers fail to recognize them as nicotine withdrawal. The severity of nicotine withdrawal is variable and related to the level of prior nicotine intake. Smokers who smoke more than 25 cigarettes daily, have their first cigarette within 30 minutes of awakening, or are uncomfortable when forced to refrain from smoking for more than a few hours are likely to suffer nicotine withdrawal symptoms when they try to quit.

The discomfort of nicotine withdrawal is one reason smokers fail in their efforts to stop. However, the attractiveness of smoking is attributable to more than nicotine dependence. Smoking is also a habit, a behavior that has become an integral part of a daily routine. Smokers come to associate cigarettes with enjoyable activities, such as finishing a meal or having a cup of coffee. These actions trigger the desire for a cigarette in smokers who are trying to quit. Smokers also use cigarettes to cope with stress and negative emotions such as anger, anxiety, loneliness, or frustration. Quitting smoking represents the loss of a valuable coping tool.

SMOKING CESSATION

Approximately half of living Americans who ever smoked have quit smoking. According to surveys, a majority of the remaining smokers would like to stop smoking and have made at least one serious attempt to do so.

Surveys of former smokers reveal how and why smokers stop smoking. The reason most often cited by former smokers for stopping smoking is fear of illness. Awareness of health risks is not sufficient to motivate smoking cessation, however. Over 90% of current smokers know that smoking is harmful to their health, yet they continue to smoke. Many smokers rationalize that they are immune to the health risks of smoking until these risks become personally salient. Current symptoms (eg, cough, breathlessness, chest pain), even if they represent minor illness rather than the onset of a smoking-related disease, stimulate change in smoking behavior more powerfully than does fear of future disease. Illness in a family member may also motivate smoking cessation. Another frequently cited reason for quitting is growing social pressure from work, family, and friends not to smoke.

The majority of former smokers did not succeed in stopping on their first try. About 30% of smokers who attend formal programs are not smoking 1 year later; most resume smoking within 3 months. Behavioral scientists relate smoking cessation to a learning process rather than to a discrete episode of will power. Smokers learn from mistakes made during a prior attempt at quitting, thereby increasing the likelihood that the next attempt will succeed. Psychologists have identified a series of cognitive stages through which smokers pass as they move toward nonsmoking: (1) initial disinterest in quitting; (2) thinking about health risks and contemplating quitting; (3) preparing to quit within the next month; (4) currently taking action to stop smoking; and (5) maintained nonsmoking (see Chapter 15).

In surveys, 80% of former smokers say that they quit on their own. Most quit abruptly ("cold turkey"), although smokers can progressively reduce daily cigarette intake in preparation for quitting. However, smokers who seek assistance with stopping smoking achieve higher rates of success.

SMOKING CESSATION METHODS

Evidence-based clinical guidelines for smoking cessation were released by the U.S. Public Health Service in 2000 (www.surgeongeneral.gov/tobacco). This document identified two methods with strong evidence of efficacy: cognitive-behavioral counseling and pharmacotherapy.

Their impact is synergistic. There is little evidence to support the efficacy of hypnosis for smoking cessation, and acupuncture is not effective.

PSYCHOSOCIAL COUNSELING

Cognitive-behavioral treatment methods address the barriers to quitting smoking that are rooted in habit. These methods are effective in aiding smoking cessation. Counseling can occur in person in individual or group settings or can be provided by telephone. In a typical program, smokers monitor their cigarette intake to identify cues to smoking, change their habits to break the link between the trigger and smoking, and learn to anticipate and handle the urges to smoke that do occur. The counselor also provides social support to bolster the smoker's confidence in his or her ability to stop smoking. Cognitive-behavioral treatment techniques can be also be packaged into booklets or videotapes for individuals to use at home.

PHARMACOLOGICAL TREATMENT

Five products have been approved by the U.S. Food and Drug Administration (FDA) as smoking cessation aids and all are considered first-line drugs by the U.S. Public Health Service tobacco treatment guidelines (Table 17–1). Four are nicotine replacement products. The fifth is bupropion, initially approved as an antidepressant. Two other drugs, nortriptyline and clonidine, have shown efficacy for smoking cessation in clinical trials but are not approved by the FDA for this indication and are considered second-line drugs by the U.S. Public Health Service guidelines.

Nicotine Replacement Therapy

The rationale of nicotine replacement is to supply nicotine in a form other than tobacco to block the symptoms of nicotine withdrawal. Nicotine replacement permits the smoker to break the smoking habit first and taper off nicotine later. Four forms of nicotine replacement are currently approved for use in the United States. Nicotine polacrilex (a gum) and a transdermal skin patch are sold without prescription. A nicotine nasal spray and an oral vapor inhaler are prescription-only products. The nicotine patch produces a relatively constant blood level of nicotine, a substantially different pattern from the fluctuating nicotine levels produced by cigarette smoking. The gum, inhaler, and nasal spray produce nicotine levels that vary and offer the individual more control over nicotine level. The nicotine supplied by the gum, patch, or nasal spray is sufficient to block nicotine withdrawal symptoms but not to reproduce the pleasures of smoking.

Randomized placebo-controlled trials demonstrate that nicotine gum, patch, inhaler, and nasal spray all reduce symptoms of nicotine withdrawal and double the rates of smoking cessation compared with placebo. Combinations of the patch with the gum, inhaler, or nasal spray are safe and, in most studies, produce higher rates of cessation than single agents. The effectiveness of all products depends on what instruction and counseling accompany it. This is particularly true for the gum, nasal spray, and inhaler, which require careful instruction for proper use. Compliance is less of a problem with the nicotine patch. The most effective use of any product, however, requires that the physician provide the smoker with concurrent behav-

Table 17–1. Pharmacotherapy for smoking cessation.[1]

Name	Dosage per Day	Recommended Duration of Use
Nicotine Replacement Products		
Transdermal nicotine patch		
24 hour	21 mg/24 h	8 weeks
	14 mg/24 h	
	7 mg/24 h	
16 hour	15 mg/16 h	8 weeks
Nicotine gum		
2 mg	9–12 pieces/day[2] (maximum 30)	2–3 months (maximum 6)
4 mg	9–12 pieces/day[2] (maximum 20)	2–3 months (maximum 6)
Nicotine nasal spray	1–2 doses/h (maximum 8/day)	3 months
Nicotine inhaler	6 cartridges/day	3–6 months
Nonnicotine Agents		
Bupropion SR	150–300 mg/day[3]	3 months

[1] Products approved by U.S. Food and Drug Administration as smoking cessation aid.
[2] Chew as needed or 1 piece every 1–2 h while awake.
[3] Start 1 week before quit day. Use 150 mg/day for 3–5 days then 150 mg twice a day.

ioral counseling of some type that teaches how to break the cigarette habit.

Nicotine replacement is safe to use in smokers with stable coronary artery disease, but it is contraindicated in smokers with unstable cardiovascular disease (myocardial infarction in the past 2 weeks, unstable angina, or life-threatening ventricular arrhythmias).

TRANSDERMAL NICOTINE PATCH

The nicotine patch contains a reservoir of nicotine that is released at a fixed dose and is absorbed through the skin. The most common side effect is local skin irritation, which rarely requires discontinuation of treatment and can often be managed with topical steroids. Vivid dreams, insomnia, and nervousness have also been reported; they can be managed by removing the patch at bedtime or using a lower-dose patch.

The smoker applies the first patch on the morning of the quit day and applies a new patch to rotating skin sites each morning afterward. One product is intended for 24-hour use, whereas a second is removed after 16 hours (eg, at bedtime). The 24-hour patch is available in three sizes to permit tapering, whereas the 16-hour patch is sold in a single dose. Data suggest that patch use continue for 2 months. Lower starting doses are recommended for patients weighing under 100 lb. or smoking fewer than 10 cigarettes/day. Long-term dependence on the nicotine patch is rare.

NICOTINE GUM

Nicotine gum is available without prescription in 2-mg and 4-mg strengths. Careful instruction in proper chewing technique is essential for it to be effective and to avoid side effects. The gum should not be chewed like regular gum. A piece is chewed only long enough to release the nicotine, producing a peppery taste, then placed between the gums and buccal mucosa to allow for nicotine absorption. When the taste disappears, the gum is chewed again until the taste reappears, then "parked" again. After 30 minutes, it is discarded. No liquid should be drunk while the gum is in the mouth, and acidic beverages (eg, coffee) should be avoided for 1–2 h before gum use. Side effects are common but minor; they include those related to nicotine (nausea, dyspepsia, hiccups, dizziness) and to chewing (sore jaw, mouth ulcers). The product is approved for use as needed to handle urges to smoke; however, its onset of action is slower than smoking. Most patients chew fewer than the recommended 9–12 pieces daily. Consequently, many experts use fixed-dose schedules (eg, chewing one piece for the first 30 minutes of every hour) to achieve blood nicotine levels adequate to prevent withdrawal. Long-term dependence on the gum is uncommon.

NICOTINE INHALER

The nicotine inhaler, sold by prescription only, is a hand-held device containing nicotine in a plug that is vaporized when the smoker inhales. The nicotine is absorbed by the oral mucosa rather than in the lungs. Therefore, the bioavailability of the inhaler resembles that of nicotine gum, with peak nicotine levels reached 20 minutes after start of use. The inhaler mimics the hand-to-mouth behavior of cigarette smoking, a feature that may appeal to some smokers. The inhaler doubles the cessation rate compared to placebo in randomized trials. Side effects are minimal; throat irritation and cough are the most common.

NICOTINE NASAL SPRAY

A nicotine nasal spray is sold only by prescription. Nicotine in the spray is rapidly absorbed from the nasal mucosa, reaching a peak within 15 minutes. The variable pattern of nicotine exposure produced from repeated use of the nasal spray resembles that produced by smoking cigarettes. It doubles the cessation rate compared with a placebo spray in randomized controlled trials, but has a high incidence of side effects (nose and throat irritation, watery eyes, sneezing, and cough). Careful instruction is required for its proper use. The dose is one spray in each nostril; this delivers a dose of 1 mg of nicotine.

Bupropion

Bupropion is an antidepressant with dopaminergic and noradrenergic activity. In its sustained-release form (Zyban, Wellbutrin SR), bupropion has doubled smoking cessation rates, and it is FDA approved for smoking cessation. The most serious side effect is to reduce the threshold for seizure. The risk of seizure is 1 in 1000 patients or less, but the drug is contraindicated in patients with a seizure disorder or predisposition. Common side effects are insomnia, agitation, headache, and dry mouth. Doses of 150–300 mg/day are effective for smoking cessation and double rates of cessation compared with placebo.

Other Pharmacological Agents

Clonidine, a centrally acting α-adrenergic agonist, is used to treat craving for psychoactive drugs other than nicotine. In randomized, placebo-controlled trials, both oral and transdermal clonidine reduced withdrawal symptoms and increased rates of cessation. Clonidine is not FDA approved for smoking cessation and side effects (sedation, dizziness, and dry mouth) generally limit its use.

Nortriptyline, a trycyclic antidepressant, has demonstrated efficacy for smoking cessation in two randomized trials. It is not FDA approved as a smoking cessation aid. Hypotension and dry mouth are the most common side effects.

There is no evidence to support the use of any other antidepressants or any antianxiety agents for smoking cessation.

■ BARRIERS TO SMOKING CESSATION

WEIGHT & SMOKING CESSATION

Smokers weigh 5–10 lb. less than nonsmokers of comparable age and height. When smokers quit, 80% of them gain weight. The average weight gain of 10 lb. (4.6 kg) poses a minimal health risk, especially when compared with the benefits of smoking cessation. Though many smokers fear large weight gains, only about 10% gain more than 25 lb. after cessation. Heavier smokers (>25 cigarettes/day) gain more than lighter smokers. The mechanism is incompletely understood, but a nicotine-related decrease in metabolic rate and possibly increases in food intake appear to be largely responsible. Although weight gain has been considered a trigger to relapse, some studies show that successful abstainers gain more weight than relapsers. The best approach to the problem may be to help smokers to accept a small weight gain and reassure them that the expected amount is less than they may fear. A vigorous exercise program reduces postcessation weight gain and promotes cessation. Smokers who use nicotine gum or bupropion gain less weight than those who quit with a placebo, although weight gain may just be delayed until after drug treatment stops. However, this may help weight-concerned smokers to quit.

SOCIAL SUPPORT

Smokers with nonsmoking spouses are more likely to quit than smokers whose partners smoke. Smokers whose efforts to stop are supported by partners, family, and friends are more likely to succeed than smokers without this support. This is especially true for women smokers. Those who live with smokers can ask them to restrict smoking to outdoor areas or to limited areas of the home in order to provide a smoke-free area in the home. Formal cessation programs provide an additional source of social support.

MOOD DISORDERS

Stopping smoking represents a loss for many smokers. Cigarettes have been reliable "companions" as well as coping tools. Transient sadness is common and requires no special treatment. Acknowledgment that this is normal can be helpful. There is, however, a strong association between smoking and mood disorders. Smokers have more depressive symptoms than nonsmokers and are more likely to have a history of major depression. Depressed smokers are less likely to stop smoking than nondepressed smokers. Clinicians should be alert to the possibility of depression in smokers. If present, it should be treated before cessation is attempted. Smokers with a history of depression should be watched for the reemergence of symptoms during smoking cessation.

SUBSTANCE ABUSE

There is a high rate of smoking among abusers of alcohol, cocaine, and heroin. Depression and substance abuse should be considered as potential comorbid disorders in smokers who repeatedly try and fail to quit. Even among smokers who do not abuse alcohol, drinking is frequently an ingredient in relapse situations. Smokers attempting to quit are commonly advised to avoid alcohol temporarily after quitting.

■ THE PHYSICIAN'S ROLE

Because smoking behavior begins early in life, preventing young people from starting to smoke is a task for physicians who care for children and adolescents. The challenge for physicians taking care of adults is smoking cessation. Physicians have the opportunity to intervene with smokers, because each year they see an estimated 70% of the smokers in the United States. They have the additional opportunity of seeing smokers at times when symptoms have made them concerned about their health and therefore more likely to change their smoking behavior. For example, one-third of smokers stop smoking after a myocardial infarction, and this proportion can be increased with brief counseling delivered by a physician or nurse. For women, pregnancy encourages smoking cessation. Approximately 25% of female smokers stop smoking while pregnant, although many resume smoking after delivery. Other smoking-related conditions may also provide "teachable moments" when smokers are more receptive to advice to stop smoking.

Providing brief advice to stop smoking to all patients seen in the office increases patients' rates of smoking cessation, as was demonstrated in a randomized controlled trial of British general practitioners. Although advice alone is effective, randomized controlled trials in general medicine and family practices have demonstrated that supplementing advice with brief counseling is more effective. Counseling smokers in office practice is as or more cost effective than other accepted medical practices, and counseling smokers as part of prenatal care is cost saving.

SMOKING CESSATION COUNSELING STRATEGY FOR OFFICE PRACTICE

Evidence-based clinical guidelines for smoking cessation treatment by primary care providers were released by the U.S. Public Health Service in 2000. These guidelines recommend that the primary care of adults should include a routine assessment of smoking status in all patients, strong advice to all smokers to quit, assessment of a smoker's readiness to quit, assistance for those smokers who are ready to stop, and follow-up for all smokers. The guidelines have been organized into a five-step protocol for use in office practice (Table 17–2).

1. **ASK:** Physicians should routinely ask all patients at every visit whether they smoke cigarettes.

2. **ADVISE:** Regardless of a smoker's degree of interest in quitting, it is the physician's responsibility to deliver clear advice to each smoker about the importance of stopping smoking. The message should be strong and unequivocal; for example, "Quitting smoking now is the most important health advice I can give you." If appropriate, advice should be tailored to the clinical situation, either current symptoms or family history. For example, smokers can be informed that they will have fewer colds or less asthma if they stop smoking. Advice is more effective when phrased in a positive way; for instance, emphasizing the benefits to be gained from quitting rather than the harms of continuing to smoke.

3. **ASSESS:** The third step is to assess a smoker's interest in stopping smoking. Categorizing smokers in this way is a clinically useful approach that helps the physician to determine what counseling strategy is appropriate and to set achievable goals for that encounter. Although the clinician's overall goal is to assist the smoker to stop permanently, a realistic goal for a single office visit is to move the smoker to the next stage of readiness to stop smoking.

4. **ASSIST:** The fourth step is to assist the smoker in quitting smoking. The physician's approach should vary according to the smoker's readiness to stop smoking.

   If the smokers are interested in quitting smoking, the physician should ask whether they are ready to set a "quit date," a date within the next 4 weeks when they will stop smoking. If so, the date should be recorded in the chart and on material given to them to take home. The physician should discuss with the patient what approach is most likely to be successful based on the smoker's level of nicotine dependence and past experience trying to quit. Both behavioral treatment and pharmacotherapy should be offered. Behavioral treatment can be provided by a take-home booklet containing standard behavioral modification strategies or by referring the smoker for group, individual, or telephone counseling for smoking cessation. The physician should be prepared to discuss management of barriers to cessation if the smokers ask.

Table 17–2. Smoking cessation counseling protocol for physicians.

1. **ASK**—about smoking at every visit: "Do you smoke?"
2. **ADVISE**—every smoker to stop.
   a. Make advice clear: "Stopping smoking now is the most important action you can take to stay healthy."
   b. Tailor advice to the patient's clinical situation (symptoms or family history).
3. **ASSESS**—readiness to quit: "Are you interested in quitting?"
4. **ASSIST**—the smoker in stopping smoking.
   a. For smokers ready to quit
      (1) Ask smoker to set a "quit date."
      (2) Provide self-help material to take home.
      (3) Offer pharmacotherapy.
      (4) Consider referral to a formal cessation program for smokers with other substance use, depression, poor social support for nonsmoking, or low self-confidence in the ability to quit.
   b. For smokers not ready to quit
      (1) Discuss advantages and barriers to cessation, from smoker's viewpoint.
      (2) Provide motivational booklet to take home.
      (3) Advise smoker to avoid exposing family members to passive smoke.
      (4) Indicate willingness to help when the smoker is ready.
      (5) Ask again about smoking at the next visit.
5. **ARRANGE**—follow-up visits.
   a. Make follow-up appointment 1 week after quit date.
   b. At follow-up, ask about smoking status.
   c. For smokers who have quit:
      (1) Congratulate!
      (2) Ask smoker to identify future high-risk situations.
      (3) Rehearse coping strategies for future high-risk situations.
   d. For smokers who have not quit:
      (1) Ask: "What were you doing when you had that first cigarette?"
      (2) Ask: "What did you learn from the experience?"
      (3) Ask smoker to set a new "quit date."

Source: Adapted from U.S. Public Health Service Guideline Treating Tobacco Use and Dependence (www.surgeongeneral.gov/tobacco).

Pharmacological therapy should also be offered unless medically contraindicated. More intensive treatment is indicated for smokers who have been unsuccessful in previous attempts to quit. The options include referral to a formal smoking cessation program and consideration of combination pharmacotherapy. Smoking cessation programs provide intensive training in behavioral smoking cessation skills combined with social support from the counselor and other group members. Combinations of pharmacotherapy and behavioral counseling are more effective than either one alone.

For smokers not interested in quitting or not ready to set a quit date, the physician should ask what they consider to be the benefits and harms of smoking. From an understanding of the patients' perspective, the physician can provide missing information about health risks and correct misconceptions about the process of smoking cessation. The discussion should focus on short-term benefits rather than distant risks, and the physician should be prepared to discuss common barriers to smoking cessation. The clinician should advise the smokers not to expose family members to passive smoke (eg, not to smoke inside the home if nonsmokers are present), and indicate future availability of help when they are ready to quit.

5. **ARRANGE:** Randomized trials have demonstrated that arranging follow-up visits to discuss smoking increases the success of physician counseling. Smokers should be asked to return shortly after the quit date to monitor progress; this is especially important for smokers using nicotine replacement.

If smokers are not smoking at the follow-up visit, they should be congratulated but warned that continued vigilance is necessary to maintain abstinence. The level of nicotine withdrawal symptoms should be assessed, and if indicated, treated by starting or increasing pharmacological treatment. To prevent relapse to smoking, patients should be asked to identify future situations in which they anticipate difficulty remaining abstinent. The physician can help to plan and rehearse coping strategies for these times. Further follow-up visits or telephone calls should be offered.

If smokers have not been able to remain abstinent, the physician's role is to redefine an experience that the smokers consider a failure into a partial success. They can be told that even 1 day without cigarettes is the first step toward quitting and be reminded that it takes time to learn to quit, just as it took time to learn to smoke. To help smokers learn from the experience, the physician should ask in detail about the circumstances surrounding the first cigarette smoked after the quit date. They should be asked what they learned from the experience that can be used for the next attempt to quit. Finally, these smokers should be asked whether they are ready to set a new quit date.

Office Organization

Smoking counseling in an office need not and should not be limited to the physician's actions. A system-wide approach is at least as effective as a physician-focused model, and it reduces the burden on a busy physician. In this model, the patients' smoking status is assessed before the physician sees them. The staff member who checks weight or blood pressure also asks about smoking and labels the chart to remind the physician to discuss smoking. Simple reminder systems such as this increase the amount of time physicians spend counseling smokers. The physician's prime role is to provide advice to stop smoking and ask the patient to set a quit date. Office personnel build on physician advice to provide counseling, medication instruction, or referrals to outside programs.

SUGGESTED READINGS

Curry SJ et al: Use and cost-effectiveness of smoking cessation services under four insurance plans in a health maintenance organization. N Engl J Med 1998;339:673.

Hajek P et al: Randomized comparative trial of nicotine polacrilex, a transdermal patch, nasal spray, and an inhaler. Arch Intern Med 1999;159:2033.

Hughes JR et al: Recent advances in the pharmacotherapy of smoking cessation. JAMA 1999;281:72.

Jorenby DE et al: A controlled trial of sustained-release bupropion, a nicotine patch, or both for smoking cessation. N Engl J Med 1999;340:685.

Lancaster T et al: Effectiveness of interventions to help people stop smoking: findings from the Cochrane Library. Br Med J 2000; 321:355.

Lasser K et al: Smoking and mental illness: a population-based prevalence study. JAMA 2000;284:2606.

Marcus BH et al: The efficacy of exercise as an aid for smoking cessation in women. Arch Intern Med 1999;159:1229.

Prochazka AV et al: A randomized trial of nortriptyline for smoking cessation. Arch Intern Med 1998;158:2035.

Rigotti NA: Clinical crossroads: a 36-year-old woman who smokes cigarettes. JAMA 2000;284:741.

Rigotti NA: Clinical practice: treatment of tobacco use and dependence. N Engl J Med 2002;346:506.

Russell MAH et al: Effect of a general practitioner's advice against smoking. Br Med J 1979;2:231.

Tobacco Use and Dependence Clinical Practice Guideline Panel: A clinical practice guideline for treating tobacco use and dependence. JAMA 2000;283:3244. (Full text of guidelines available at www.surgeongeneral.gov/tobacco)

Williamson DF et al: Smoking cessation and severity of weight gain in a national cohort. N Engl J Med 1991;324:739.

WEB SITES

Healthfinder Smoking Cessation Resources
http://www.healthfinder.gov/scripts/SearchContext/asp?topic=801

National Women's Health Information Center Smoking Cessation Guidelines
http://www.4woman.gov/QuitSmoking/index.cfm

Surgeon General's Report on Women and Smoking
http://www.surgeongeneral.gov/library/womenandtobacco/

Surgeon General's Report on Reducing Tobacco Use
http://www.surgeongeneral.gov/library/tobacco_use/

U.S. Public Health Service Tobacco Cessation Guideline
http://www.surgeongeneral.gov/tobacco/

Obesity

Robert B. Baron, MD, MS

INTRODUCTION

Obesity is one of the most common problems in clinical practice. Defined as a body mass index >30 kg/m², 20% of adult Americans are obese. Because obesity is at the center of chronic disease risk and psychosocial disability for millions of Americans, its prevention and treatment offer unique patient care and public health opportunities. If all Americans were to achieve a normal body weight, it has been estimated that the prevalence of diabetes would decrease by 57%, hypertension by 17%, coronary artery disease by 17%, and various cancers by 11%.

Unfortunately, obesity is often one of the most difficult and frustrating problems in primary care for both patients and physicians. Considerable effort is expended by primary care providers and patients with little benefit. Weight-loss diets, for example, even in the best treatment centers, result in an average 8% reduction in body weight. This lack of clinical success has created a never-ending demand for new weight-loss treatments. Approximately 45% of women and 25% of men are "dieting" at any one time, spending billions of dollars each year on diet books, diet meals, weight-loss classes, diet drugs, exercise tapes, "fat farms," and other weight-loss aids. The challenge for health care providers is to identify those patients with obesity who are most likely to benefit medically from treatment and most likely to maintain weight loss, and to provide them with sound advice, skills for long-term life-style change, and support. For patients not motivated to attempt a weight-loss program, health providers must continue to be respectful and empathic and focus on other health concerns (see Chapter 15). Whenever possible, health providers should emphasize prevention of obesity and further weight gain and the importance of physical fitness independent of body size.

DEFINITIONS

Obesity is defined as an excess of body fat. Body fat can be measured by several methods including total body water, total body potassium, bioelectrical impedance, and dual-energy x-ray absorptiometry. In clinical practice, however, obesity is best defined by the body mass index (BMI)—body weight divided by height squared (kilograms per square meter). The BMI correlates closely with measures of body fat and with obesity-related disease outcomes. According to the National Institutes of Health, an individual with a BMI <18.5 kg/m² is classified as underweight, 18.5–24.9 kg/m² as normal, 25.0–29.9 kg/m² as overweight, and ≥30.0 kg/m² as obese.

HEALTH CONSEQUENCES OF OBESITY

The relationship between body weight and mortality is curvilinear, similar to other cardiovascular risk factors. Most studies have demonstrated a J-shaped or U-shaped relationship, suggesting that the thinnest portion of the population also has an excess mortality. This is primarily due to the higher rate of cigarette smoking in the thinnest group, except in the elderly, in whom malnutrition is predictive of excess mortality independent of cigarette use.

The increase in total mortality related to obesity results predominantly from coronary heart disease (CHD). Although it is not fully established that obesity is an "independent" risk factor for CHD, obesity is clearly an important risk factor for the development of many other CHD risk factors. Obese individuals aged 20–44, for example, have a 3- to 4-fold greater risk for type II diabetes, a 5- to 6-fold greater risk for hypertension, and twice the risk for hypercholesterolemia. The obese also have an increased risk for some cancers, including those of the colon, pancreas, prostate, uterus, and breast.

As a result of these conditions, mortality from all causes for persons with a BMI of 30 kg/m² or above is 50–100% greater than for those with a normal BMI. Individuals with extreme obesity, BMI ≥40 kg/m², have a 3- to 5-fold increase in mortality from all causes.

Obesity is also associated with a variety of other medical disorders, including degenerative joint disease of both weight-bearing and non-weight-bearing joints, diseases of the digestive tract (gallstones, reflux esophagitis), thromboembolic disorders, heart failure (both systolic and diastolic), respiratory impairment, and skin disorders. Obese patients also have a greater incidence of surgical and obstetric complications, are more prone to accidents, and are at increased risk of social discrimination. Several studies have also shown a rate of depression higher in the obese than in normal weight subjects and a very high rate (approximately 30%) of binge eating disorder.

In addition to the total amount of excess body fat, the location of the excess body fat (regional fat distribution) is a major determinant of the degree of excess morbidity and mortality due to obesity. Increased upper body fat (abdomen and flank) is independently associated with increased cardiovascular and total mortality. Body fat distribution can be assessed by a number of measurement techniques. Measurements of skin folds (subscapular and triceps) reflect subcutaneous fat. Measurement of circumferences (waist and hip) reflect both abdominal and visceral fat. Computed tomography (CT) and magnetic resonance imaging (MRI) scans measure subcutaneous and visceral fat. Clinically, measurement of the waist and hip circumference is most useful, especially in individuals with BMI 25–35 kg/m². A circumference in men >102 cm (>40 inches) and in women >88 cm (>35 inches) can be used to identify individuals at increased risk of developing obesity-related health problems.

ETIOLOGY OF OBESITY

Numerous lines of evidence, including both epidemiological studies of adoptees and twins and animal studies, suggest strong genetic influences on the development of obesity. In a study of 800 Danish adoptees, for example, there was no relationship between the body weight of adoptees and their adopting parents but a close correlation with the body weights of their biological parents. In a study of approximately 4000 twins, a much closer correlation between body weights was found in monozygotic than in dizygotic twins. In this study, genetic factors accounted for approximately two-thirds of the variation in weights. Studies of twins reared apart and the response of twins to overfeeding showed similar results. Studies of regional fat distribution in twins has also shown a significant (but not complete) genetic influence.

Recent genetic studies have confirmed a clear relationship between genetics and obesity in both animals and humans. Over 250 genes, markers, and chromosomal regions of the human genome have been linked or associated with obesity and 25 Mendelian disorders exhibiting obesity as a clinical manifestation have been mapped. Studies suggest that genetic influences may impact both energy intake (control of appetite and eating behavior) and energy expenditure.

Differences in the resting metabolic expenditure (RME), for example, could easily result in considerable differences in body weight as RME accounts for approximately 60–75% of total energy expenditure. The RME can vary by as much as 20% between individuals of the same age, sex, and body build; such differences could account for approximately 400 kcal of energy expenditure per day. Recent evidence suggests that the metabolic rate is similar in family members, and, as expected, individuals with lower metabolic rates are more likely to gain weight. Differences in the thermic effect of food, the amount of energy expended following a meal, may also contribute to obesity. Although some investigators have shown a decreased thermic effect of food in the obese, others have not.

Environmental factors are also clearly important in the development of obesity. Decreased physical activity and food choices that result in increased energy intake also clearly contribute to the development of obesity. Medical illness and some medications can also result in obesity, but such instances account for less than 1% of cases. Hypothyroidism and Cushing's syndrome are the most common. Diseases of the hypothalamus can also result in obesity, but these are quite rare. Major depression, which more typically results in weight loss, can also present with weight gain. Consideration of these causes is particularly important when evaluating unexplained, recent weight gain.

PATIENT SELECTION FOR WEIGHT LOSS

Weight loss is indicated to assist in the management of obesity-related conditions, particularly hypertension, diabetes mellitus (type II), and hyperlipidemia, in any patient who is obese (BMI >30 kg/m²). Many patients with BMI 25–30 kg/m² who have one of these conditions (particularly hypertension, diabetes, lipid disorders, or significant psychosocial disability) also often dramatically benefit from weight reduction.

Weight loss to prevent complications of obesity in patients without current medical, metabolic, or behavioral consequences of obesity is more controversial. In young and middle-aged individuals, particularly those with a family history of obesity-related disorders, treatment should be based on the degree of obesity (BMI 25–30 kg/m²) and body fat distribution. Such individuals with upper body obesity (increased waist circumference) should be considered for treatment; those individuals with lower body obesity and no significant consequences of obesity can be reassured and followed for development of additional upper body obesity and its metabolic consequences. Many such patients, however, desire weight loss for psychological, social, and cosmetic reasons. A careful discussion of the risks and benefits of weight loss in such instances helps patients make informed decisions about various weight-loss strategies.

A medical or psychosocial indication for weight loss is necessary but not sufficient to begin treatment. Only motivated patients should be treated. Considerable effort should be made to assess the patient's motivation for significant diet and exercise changes. Questions should focus on how the current attempt compares with previous attempts; a realistic assessment of the patient's goals for the amount and rate of weight loss; the extent to which outside stresses, mood disorders, or substance abuse might impair the attempt; and the degree to which others can provide support. Patient motivation can be further assessed by requiring the patient to complete specific pretreatment assignments. For example, patients can be asked to complete a 3-day diet record and to submit an exercise plan that includes both the type of aerobic exercise the patient plans to begin and how the patient plans to fit it into his or her schedule. When obesity coexists with other significant psychiatric disorders, particularly depression, binge eating disorder, and substance abuse, treatment should initially be directed at the concurrent disorder. (See Chapter 15 for further discussion of assessment of patients' readiness to change.)

DIET THERAPY

Standard dietary treatment of obesity should use the same nutritional principles as diet recommendations for healthy people. Total fat intake should be limited to 30% or less of total calories, protein to 15%, and carbohydrate (primarily complex carbohydrates) to 55% or greater. For most patients a low-calorie diet (LCD) of 800–1500 kcal/day will result in an energy deficit of 500–1000 kcal/day. Because 1 pound of fat equals approximately 3500 kcal, these deficits should result in a 1–2 pound weight loss per week. LCDs comprised of different percentages of macronutrients (eg, low carbohydrate diets, etc) can also be designed to create daily energy deficits. Such diets may result in greater initial weight loss due to greater initial sodium and water losses and may result in improved adherence for some patients. There is no evidence that such diets are more effective than standard diets for weight loss at 6–12 months or for long-term weight maintenance. LCDs can easily be designed in medical settings with the assistance of clinical dietitians or other health professionals, or patients can be referred to well-established community resources that follow these principles. Clinical trials of LCDs demonstrate an average 8% weight loss at 6- to 12-month follow-up.

A major development in the dietary treatment of obesity is the use of safe and effective very-low-calorie diets (VLCDs). Previously known as protein-sparing modified fasts and protein-formula liquid diets, these diets restrict calorie intake to 400–800 kcal/day. Patients ingest only preformulated, usually liquid, food that provides adequate protein, vitamins, and minerals. Additional intake is limited to 2–3 quarts of calorie-free beverages per day. The major advantage of these diets is the "complete removal of patients from the food environment" to facilitate adherence. In addition, the significant energy deficit results in rapid weight loss, usually 2–4 pounds/week, encouraging the patient to continue. Ongoing concerns about these diets include their cost, side effects, and long-term results. Recent studies suggest that the use of 800-kcal VLCDs can lower cost and prevent most of the significant side effects associated with the lower-calorie (400–600) VLCDs, including gallstones and fluid and electrolyte disorders, with equal long-term efficacy.

As with standard diet therapy of obesity, VLCDs require adherence during the diet, and long-term nutritional and behavioral changes to maintain weight loss. Well-planned programs that combine VLCDs with behavior modification, exercise, and social support report improved long-term results. For example, an average weight loss of 55 pounds with 75% and 52% of the loss maintained at 1- and 2½-year follow-up, respectively, and maintenance of an average of 24 pounds after 2- to 3-year follow-up have been reported. Other systematic reviews demonstrate more modest long-term weight loss and it is not clearly established that VLCDs result in better long-term outcomes than standard LCDs. VLCDs do, however, result in more rapid weight loss than LCDs and may be useful in selected clinical settings in which the pace of weight loss is important (eg, prior to joint replacement surgery, for patients with type II diabetes severely out of control, etc).

HEALTH CONSEQUENCES OF DIETING & WEIGHT LOSS

Surprisingly few studies have examined the effects of weight loss on morbidity and mortality. Studies examining the effect of weight loss on cardiovascular risk factors generally show beneficial changes with weight loss as predicted. Descriptive studies on mortality, however, show inconsistent results. Such descriptive studies are unable to clarify if changes in mortality are caused by the weight change, if disease or other factors that contribute to disease, such as cigarette smoking, cause weight loss, or if both are related to a third factor. No randomized trials of long-term effects of voluntary weight loss on mortality have been published.

Because so many Americans are dieting at any one time, and having so little long-term success, considerable interest has been focused on the potential adverse effects of weight cycling ("yo-yo" dieting). Numerous adverse effects of weight cycling have been hypothesized, primarily from animal studies. These include making further weight loss more difficult, increasing total body fat and central obesity, increasing subsequent calorie intake, increasing food efficiency, decreasing energy expenditure, increasing levels of adipose-tissue lipolytic enzymes and liver lipogenic enzymes, increasing insulin resistance, increasing blood pressure, and increasing blood cholesterol and triglyceride levels. Most experts currently feel that these phenomena occur inconsistently, if at all. Descriptive studies that have addressed this question by looking at the impact of weight fluctuations on CHD incidence, CHD mortality, and total mortality have shown mixed results.

There is also debate over whether weight loss diets cause eating disorders or binge eating. Although a history of dieting often precedes the development of eating disorders, there is no evidence proving a causal link. In addition, approximately 50% of individuals with binge eating disorder report that binging preceded dieting. There is also some evidence to suggest that successful weight loss may reduce binge eating in the obese (see Chapter 19).

Thus, there is only indirect evidence suggesting that dieting has negative health effects. This remains an important question, however, and reinforces the idea that casual attempts at quick weight loss should be avoided. At present, however, committed attempts at long-term weight loss should not be discouraged because of adverse health effects or the potential of regaining weight.

Dieting also has a significant effect on energy balance both during and after weight loss. As every successful dieter has observed, the rate of weight loss slows during the course of dieting. Because this can be quite discouraging to the unwary patient (or uninformed health care provider), it is important to inform the patient prior to initiating a weight-loss diet that this is likely to occur. Weight loss is most rapid during the initial days of hypocaloric feeding due to changes in sodium and water balance caused by early loss of glycogen and protein (both contain water) and, depending on the degree of calorie deficit and type of diet, loss of sodium associated with ketonuria. Following this initial phase, weight loss depends on the extent of energy deficit. With time, however, the rate of weight loss slows again as the body's metabolic rate decreases and the energy deficit becomes smaller. This change in metabolic rate can be two to three times greater than that predicted from changes in body weight. The lower the energy content of the diet, the lower the metabolic rate. Although it was initially suggested that exercise occurring during a period of hypocaloric feeding could prevent this decrease in metabolic rate, recent studies have suggested that it has no direct effect during hypocaloric feeding (but exercise does increase the postdiet metabolic rate by preserving lean body mass).

Following the period of hypocaloric feeding (resumption of normal energy intakes), the resting metabolic rate increases, but to a level below that observed before beginning the diet. This reduction is in part a reflection of the loss of lean body mass and in part due to additional, poorly understood effects on energy metabolism. Overall energy expenditure is further reduced due to a decrease in the thermic effect of food (the individual eats less) and in differences in physical activity (it takes less energy to perform the same amount of activity for a smaller person). Thus, to maintain weight loss, individuals need to consume less energy than before dieting (and increase energy expenditure by increasing the amount of physical activity).

EXERCISE

Exercise offers a number of significant advantages to patients attempting to achieve long-term weight loss. First and foremost, exercise increases energy expenditure, helping to create the energy deficit necessary for weight loss. Unfortunately, the amount of energy expended during most aerobic exercises (walking, jogging, swimming, etc) for the typical periods performed (20–30 minutes four to five times per week) is modest, approximately 500–1000 kcal/week. Thus, exercise can be predicted to have little effect on short-term weight loss. Clinical trials reflect this modest effect: some studies demonstrate weight loss with exercise alone or extra weight loss when exercise plus diet is compared with diet alone, but other studies do not show such an effect.

The importance of exercise for successful maintenance of weight loss is more clearly established. In addition to the cumulative effect of increased energy expenditure (500–1000 kcal/week × 52 weeks = 7–15 pounds/year), exercise affects the composition of the body substance lost during weight loss. When exercise is directly compared with diet, or when exercise plus diet is compared with diet alone, exercise results in greater preservation of lean body mass. That is, for each pound of weight lost, less fat and more muscle are lost during weight-loss programs without exercise. This is particularly important as the body's resting metabolic expenditure (a major portion of the total daily energy expenditure) is closely correlated with lean body mass.

The observation that much of the long-term effect of exercise is through preservation of lean body mass has resulted in an increased interest in the potential role of resistance training (weight lifting, circuit training, etc). Preliminary results suggest that resistance training during dieting does result in maintenance of lean body mass compared with the result from dieting alone. Thus, highly motivated patients can be instructed to add resistance training to their aerobic exercise program.

Regular aerobic exercise results in a number of other benefits to the obese patient, including improved cardiovascular training effect (increased exercise tolerance), decreased appetite (per calorie expended), a general sense of well-being, decreased blood pressure (in hypertensives), improved glucose metabolism and insulin action (in diabetics), improved blood lipids (in lipid disorders), and, in the long term, decreased mortality from cardiovascular disease and all other causes.

Young patients with mild-to-moderate obesity can be started directly on a regular aerobic exercise program. Patients are commonly instructed to select two exercises and to perform either one of them four to five times per week for 30 minutes/day. Patients are taught to take their pulse and to generate a sustained tachycardia at 70–80% of their maximum predicted heart rate. Sedentary patients, older patients, and patients with severe obesity are instructed to begin walking programs without initial concern about meeting target heart rates. As weight loss proceeds, and patients become used to exercising regularly, they can be advanced to formal aerobic programs.

BEHAVIOR MODIFICATION & SOCIAL SUPPORT

Sustained weight loss requires long-term changes in eating behavior. Patients must learn specific skills to facilitate decreased calorie intake and increased energy expenditure. Although formal behavior modification programs are available, most patients can be taught basic behavioral strategies in the office.

The most useful behavioral skills are planning and recordkeeping. Patients can be taught to plan both menus and exercise programs in advance. Patients are instructed to record actual food intake and exercise behaviors. The act of recordkeeping itself aids in behavioral change, and the availability of records also helps the health care provider assess progress and make specific suggestions for additional problem solving. Specific reward systems are also useful for many patients. Refundable financial contracts have been shown to be effective in a number of small studies. Additional behavioral strategies include breaking behaviors into identifiable parts (antecedents, consequences, etc) and specific techniques for stimulus control. Methods for slowing eating may also be effective. Efforts to identify and understand lapses and to prevent relapses are particularly important for long-term weight maintenance.

Social support is an additional essential component for any successful weight-loss program. Most successful programs use peer group support. Diet partnerships are effective for some patients. Involvement of family members is also important. A comprehensive review of published results of weight-loss programs strongly suggests that close provider–patient contact is a better predictor of success than the particular weight-loss intervention.

MEDICATIONS FOR TREATMENT OF OBESITY

Medications for the treatment of obesity are widely available over the counter, via the Internet, and by physician prescription. A recent Centers for Disease Control survey suggested that 7% of Americans used nonprescription weight-loss drugs. Among young obese women and among those on prescription weight-loss medications the use of nonprescription weight-loss medications was 28.4% and 33.8%, respectively.

A variety of weight-loss medications are currently available by prescription in the United States. These include various amphetamines (Drug Enforcement Administration schedule II), benzphetamine and phendimetrazine (schedule III) and phentermine, diethylproprion, mazindol, sibutramine, and orlistat. Most obesity experts agree that there is no current role for the schedule II or III drugs. Only sibutramine and orlistat are approved by the Food and Drug Administration (FDA) for long-term use (1 year). Fluoxetine and sertraline have also been studied for long-term weight loss but neither drug received FDA approval.

Considerable controversy exists about the efficacy of and indications for these medications. Numerous clinical trials, some up to 2 years in duration, demonstrate statistically significant weight loss in subjects who take an obesity medication compared with placebo. Total weight loss is modest, approximately 4 kg greater than placebo. There is no convincing evidence that any one of these medications results in more weight loss than others. Although some studies also show improvement in obesity-related metabolic abnormalities (eg, blood sugar, blood pressure, lipids, etc), these reductions are also small and are substantially less than those achieved with hypoglycemic, antihypertensive, or lipid-lowering medications. In addition, no studies have yet demonstrated that weight loss achieved with medications results in reductions in obesity-related mortality or cardiovascular disease outcomes.

A recent National Institutes of Health (NIH) guideline suggested that based on limited data, weight loss drugs that were approved by the FDA for long-term weight loss may be useful as an adjunct to diet and physical activity for patients with BMI ≥ 27 kg/m^2 and obesity-related risk factors or diseases, and for any patient with BMI ≥ 30 kg/m^2. Based on the modest efficacy noted above, however, these guidelines have not been widely implemented. Prescriptions for weight-loss drugs should be limited to patients adhering to weight-loss diets and physical activity. In addition, weight loss in the first month of use correlates highly with weight loss at 12 months. Thus, for patients in whom no weight loss is achieved within the first month of use, weight-loss medications should be discontinued.

SURGERY FOR WEIGHT LOSS

Surgery for weight loss is typically considered the last resort for patients with severe obesity. Current operations primarily modify the stomach to reduce food intake. Recent studies suggest the roux-en-y gastric bypass is the most effective technique. In some centers gastric bypass can be done laparoscopically. These procedures have replaced intestinal bypass procedures designed to create malabsorption. Case series report weight loss of up to 60% of excess weight with gastric procedures, results much greater than those reported with diets or medication. Reports of long-term maintenance of weight loss of up to 55% of excess weight at 10-year follow-up are also highly superior to results published for diets or drugs. Complications of surgery, including incisional hernia, wound infections, staple line failure, anastomotic problems, depression, and nutritional deficiencies, occur in up to 40% of patients. Perioperative mortality occurs in 0.5%.

The NIH currently states that weight loss surgery may be an option for carefully selected patients with BMI ≥40 or ≥35 kg/m² with comorbid conditions. Such patients must be at high risk for obesity-related morbidity and mortality, must have failed medical therapy, must have stable psychiatric status, and must be fully committed to lifetime life-style changes

SUMMARY

No specific behavioral technique serves as the magic bullet for the very challenging, but medically important task of weight loss. Although many of the most common problems encountered in medical practice can be treated by weight loss alone, only motivated patients should be started on weight-loss programs. Weight-loss treatments vary considerably in terms of risk, cost, and efficacy. For most patients with mild or moderate obesity, a multifactorial approach, including diet, exercise, behavior modification, and social support, can be prescribed. Close patient–provider contact and long-term follow-up with emphasis on exercise are key ingredients for success. Motivated patients with severe obesity should be considered for supervised VLCDs, again emphasizing long-term dietary change, exercise, behavior modification, and social support. The role of medications and surgery for the treatment of obesity is increasing but should still be limited to selected, highly informed patients.

SUGGESTED READINGS

Anderson JW et al: Long-term weight-loss maintenance: a meta-analysis of US studies. Am J Clin Nutr 2001;74(5):579.

Blanck HM, Khan LK, Serdula MK: Use of nonprescription weight loss products: results from a multistate survey. JAMA 2001; 286(8):930.

Bray GA, Ryan DH: Clinical evaluation of the overweight patient. Endocrine 2000;13(2):167.

Davidoff R et al: Echocardiographic examination of women previously treated with fenfluramine: long-term follow-up of a randomized, double blind placebo-controlled trial. Arch Intern Med 2001;161:1429.

Expert Panel Executive summary of the clinical guidelines on the identification, evaluation, and treatment of overweight and obesity in adults. Arch Intern Med 1998;158:1855.

Glazer G: Long-term pharmacotherapy of obesity 2000. A review of safety and efficacy. Arch Intern Med 2001;161:1814.

Hauptman J et al: Orlistat in the long-term treatment of obesity in primary care settings. Arch Fam Med 2000;9(2):160.

Jakicic JM et al: American College of Sports Medicine position stand. Appropriate intervention strategies for weight loss and prevention of weight regain for adults. Med Sci Sports Exerc 2001; 33(12):2145.

James WP et al: Effect of sibutramine on weight maintenance after weight loss: a randomised trial. STORM Study Group. Sibutramine Trial of Obesity Reduction and Maintenance. Lancet 2000;356(9248):2119.

Mokdad AH et al: The continuing epidemics of obesity and diabetes in the United States. JAMA 2001;286:1195.

Nawaz H, Katz DL: American College of Preventive Medicine Practice Policy statement. Weight management counseling of overweight adults. Am J Prevent Med 2001;21(1):73.

Poston WS et al: Where do diets, exercise, and behavior modification fit in the treatment of obesity? Endocrine 2000;13(2):187.

Rankinen T et al: The human obesity gene map: the 2001 update. Obesity Res 2002;10(3):196.

Straus RSS, Pollack HA: Epidemic increase in childhood overweight 1986–1998. JAMA 2001;286:2845.

Wei M et al: Relationship between low cardiorespiratory fitness and mortality in normal-weight, overweight, and obese men. JAMA 1999;282:1547.

Wirth A, Krause J: Long-term weight loss with sibutramine. A randomized controlled trial. JAMA 2001;286:1331.

Yanovski SZ, Yanovski JA: Drug therapy: obesity. N Engl J Med 2002;346:591.

WEB SITES

American Dietetic Association
http://www.eatright.org/

American Society for Clinical Nutrition
http://www.faseb.org/ascn/

Center for Food Safety and Applied Nutrition
http://vm.cfsan.fda.gov/

Center for Nutrition Policy and Promotion, USDA
http://www.usda.gov/cnpp

Children's Nutrition Research Center
http://www.bcm.tmc.edu/cnrc/

Food and Drug Administration
http://www.fda.gov/

Food and Nutrition Information Center
http://www.nal.usda.gov/fnic/

NHLBI Obesity Education Initiative, Aim for a Healthy Weight
http://www.nhlbi.nih.gov/health/public/heart/obesity/

Nutrition Analysis Tool
http://www.ag.uiuc.edu/~food-lab/nat/

Nutrition.Gov
http://www.nutrition.gov/home/index.php3

Nutrition Navigator
http://navigator.tufts.edu/

United States Department of Agriculture: Center for Nutrition Policy and Promotion
http://www.usda.gov/cnpp

Eating Disorders

Steven J. Romano, MD, & Katherine A. Halmi, MD

INTRODUCTION

The eating disorders, including anorexia nervosa and bulimia nervosa, are receiving more clinical and research attention than ever before, paralleling an increase in their prevalence over the past few decades. Such disturbances in eating behavior are, of course, not new. Historical documentation of anorexia nervosa dates back to the early Christian saints. Binging and purging, although distinct from our current concept of bulimia nervosa, took place in the lives of ancient Romans.

The eating disorders are best viewed as clinical syndromes rather than specific diseases, as they do not result from a single cause or follow a single course. As psychiatric syndromes, they are defined largely by a constellation of behaviors and attitudes that persists over time and produces characteristic complications contributing to physical and psychosocial dysfunction. Because of the complexity and breadth of contributing factors, as well as the extent of comorbid psychopathology, knowledge of the behavioral characteristics of the eating disorders can lead to improved recognition and implementation of effective treatment strategies. In light of the complicated interplay of psychiatric, psychosocial, and medical consequences, treatment beyond initial medical stabilization generally requires referral to specialists.

MULTIDIMENSIONAL MODEL

A comprehensive multidimensional model best illustrates the role various factors play in the genesis of clinically significant eating disturbances. In this schema, also referred to as a stress diathesis model, psychological, biological, and sociocultural stressors contribute to the development of symptomatic expression.

Psychological factors include personality features, such as the anorectic's obsessive-compulsive qualities, constrained affect, and sense of ineffectiveness, and the bulimic's impulsivity. They also include the influence of developmental stressors and family dynamics.

Biological factors are most often due to the adverse effects of starvation, malnutrition, and purging behaviors, including vomiting and the misuse of laxatives and diuretics. Restrictive dieting and subsequent malnourishment may contribute to the development of comorbid psychiatric conditions, such as anxiety and depression. A preexisting biological vulnerability may exist and is supported by preliminary findings of neurophysiological investigations showing dysfunction of serotonin, dopamine, and norepinephrine neuromodulators; a small number of patients with anorexia develop amenorrhea preceding significant weight loss.

Sociocultural factors figure prominently in the etiology of the eating disorders. The idealization of thinness contributes to dieting behavior, often beginning in early adolescence. Of note, dieting is almost always present as a precipitant to the development of an eating disorder. Other precipitants include periods of illness leading to weight loss; in vulnerable individuals this may be followed by willful dieting.

THEORETICAL CONSIDERATIONS

Conceptual models aid in understanding the etiology and possible sustaining factors involved in the genesis and persistence of eating-disordered behavior. Important models include those derived from learning theory and neurophysiological abnormality or dysfunction.

Cognitive-behavioral theory, which is derived from learning theory, states that cognition influences behavior in a predictable manner. Cues, both internal and external, can provoke behavioral outcomes through activation of cognitive sets. A change in negative cognition therefore influences a change from dysfunctional to healthy behavior. Thoughts that overvalue weight, food, and diet, especially the idealization of thinness, lead to the perpetuation of compromising responses, such as heroic dietary measures and abuses of substances believed effective for weight reduction. The coupling of such cognitions and behaviors affects self-esteem and may severely impair an individual's psychological state. Cognitive-behavioral therapy has been effective in achieving symptom reduction and improvement in both medical and psychological status.

The search for specific biological markers that may help identify patients with eating disorders has focused increasingly on neurotransmitters and other neuromodulators. Research findings suggest that dysfunction in various neurotransmitter systems, including serotonin, dopamine, and norepinephrine, as well as opioids and cholecystokinin (CCK), might play a role in the development and maintenance of the eating disorders. Rationale for the examination of these hormones and other substances derives from our understanding of the pathways modulating appetitive behavior, including hypothalamic regulation and the known connection between the gastrointestinal tract and the central nervous system. The complexity of these disorders, including the stress of eating-disordered behavior on physiology, however, makes it unlikely that a neurophysiological hypothesis alone can explain the etiology and maintenance of these complex syndromes.

ANOREXIA NERVOSA

Description

Anorexia nervosa is a relatively rare disorder affecting less than 1% of young women and a much smaller percentage of young men. Its most striking behavioral manifestation is the willful restriction of caloric intake secondary to an irrational fear of becoming fat, frequently in concert with a grossly distorted view of one's self as overweight, even in the presence of severe emaciation. Patients often exhibit a phobic response to food, particularly to fatty and other calorically dense items. They develop an obsessive preoccupation with food, eating, dieting, weight, and body shape and frequently exhibit ritualistic behaviors involving choosing, preparing, and ingesting meals (eg, cutting food into very small pieces or chewing each bite a specific number of times).

Early in the course of the illness, patients begin to restrict many food items, as is typical of most dieters. As the disorder progresses, although, the anorectic's menu becomes grossly constricted and she demonstrates greater rigidity. Minor variations in meal content can produce tremendous anxiety. Unlike the average dieter, the anorectic continues her pursuit of thinness to an extreme and becomes dependent on the daily registration of weight loss. This fuels even more restrictive dieting. Extreme dieting is often complicated by other weight-reducing behaviors. Exercise is frequently compulsive, and hyperactivity in underweight patients is a curious but often-encountered concomitant. Weakness, muscle aches, sleep disturbances, and gastrointestinal complaints, including constipation and postprandial bloating, are common physical findings. Amenorrhea, reflecting endocrine dysfunction secondary to malnourishment, is generally present.

Some anorectics engage in bulimic behaviors, including binging and purging. This binge–purge subtype of anorexia nervosa contrasts with the purely restricting subtype described earlier. Often, purging behavior, such as self-induced vomiting or the misuse of laxatives and diuretics, is seen in the absence of binging. The coupling of purging with self-starvation compounds the medical consequences of the disorder. Furthermore, anorectics, particularly adolescents, generally minimize their symptoms and the negative consequences of their disorder and are thus rarely motivated for treatment. The characteristics of the illness, both medical and psychological, are intensified with weight loss, further frustrating attempts at engaging the patient in a meaningful therapeutic process. Family and friends be-

come increasingly anxious, angry, and at times alienated, as their loved one regresses. Superficial compliance, as is sometimes seen, belies a profound resistance. Anorectic patients can be challenging to treat as they cling tenaciously to their beliefs and behaviors.

Psychosocial dysfunction is common in patients with anorexia. Although educational performance may not be affected in adolescent patients, social relations become increasingly constricted, and sexual interest is generally diminished or absent.

Differential Diagnosis

The pathognomonic features of anorexia nervosa, namely the intense fear of becoming fat coupled with the relentless pursuit of thinness, are generally absent in other medical and psychiatric conditions. The term *anorexia,* which itself refers to absence of appetite, is a misnomer in the case of the syndrome of anorexia nervosa. True anorexia, such as encountered in many medical conditions or diseases, would be accompanied by other signs or symptoms of those illnesses (as in gastrointestinal disease or many cancers).

Lack of appetite or decreased intake, with or without subsequent weight loss, is encountered in a number of psychiatric disorders. These include depression, hysterical conversion and other psychosomatic disorders, schizophrenia, and certain delusional disorders, but each of these is associated with a cluster of other substantiating symptomatology. Some patients with obsessive-compulsive disorder (OCD) may exhibit what appears to be bizarre behaviors around food, eating, or meal preparation, but, on further exploration, their behavior is in response to obsessional ideation, for example, the fear of contamination. Such patients, in contrast to those with anorexia nervosa, generally admit their discomfort with the need to perform such compelling and often excessive or senseless acts.

In summary, although comorbid psychopathology may be encountered in patients with anorexia nervosa, including symptoms of depression or OCD, the hallmark of anorexia nervosa (the morbid fear of becoming fat and the relentless pursuit of thinness) is absent in the other psychiatric syndromes. In none of these syndromes does the goal of weight loss drive the behavior.

Medical Complications & Treatment

Treatment of anorexia nervosa is initially directed at correcting the acute medical complications and is followed by supportive nutritional rehabilitation. Most medical consequences resolve with nutritional rehabilitation and the discontinuation of purging behaviors. Exceptions include persistent osteopenic changes in those who have experienced extended periods of malnourishment and suppression of growth in severe cases of adolescent anorexia.

In most cases of anorexia associated with significant weight loss (15–20% or more of ideal body weight) a structured inpatient facility is necessary to maintain an adequate level of medical surveillance and sustain a steady rate of weight gain. On admission to an inpatient treatment facility, laboratory screening should include tests for electrolytes, liver function, amylase (elevated in patients who purge), thyroid function, a complete blood count with differential, and a urinalysis. Common laboratory findings include leukopenia with a relative lymphocytosis, metabolic alkalosis with associated hypokalemia, hypochloremia and elevated serum bicarbonate levels, and, occasionally, metabolic acidosis in patients who abuse large amounts of stimulant-type laxatives. An electrocardiogram should also be obtained since emaciation and associated electrolyte disturbances can contribute to significant cardiac abnormalities, especially in those who purge. Hypokalemia can lead to arrhythmia and the risk of cardiac arrest.

Acute medical conditions generally requiring immediate attention include electrolyte disturbances and dehydration, both of which are readily reversible. In most cases, initiating oral intake of fluids and food reverses minor disturbances in electrolytes and establishes adequate hydration. More severe cases, eg, patients with significant hypokalemia, may require intravenous hydration and parenteral replacement of depleted electrolytes, with daily electrolyte checks until the patient's condition stabilizes. Care should be taken to avoid overhydration and the consequences of excess fluid retention in vulnerable individuals. Importantly, treatment must ensure prevention of purging behaviors in patients with this history, as persistence of purging will alter electrolyte and fluid balance.

In patients who are significantly underweight, use of a liquid supplement, initially as replacement for solid food, helps ensure necessary caloric intake. When given in divided feedings throughout the day, it may decrease the patient's sense of postprandial discomfort and early satiety, both frequent consequences of extended caloric restriction and semistarvation. Further, this approach to refeeding decreases the inevitable manipulations around food choices. Replacement of solid food with a liquid supplement may also lessen the patient's phobic avoidance of food and the subsequent anxiety around meal choices.

Psychotherapeutic Interventions

Given the lack of motivation and strong resistance to treatment exhibited by the majority of patients with anorexia, it is helpful to initiate behavioral strategies as soon as any acute medical condition is stabilized. Initial behavioral interventions, tied to daily weight gain in increments of no less than 0.25 lb. or 0.1 kg, include obtaining visits from family or friends, lessening physical restrictions, and increasing involvement in activities on and off the unit. It is important that all contingencies be tied to daily weight gain, which is measured each morning at the same time and in like manner, as this is a quantifiable observation not open to argument or discussion. A milieu supportive of such interventions helps to motivate the patient and exerts pressure toward positive change.

As the patient reaches a target weight range and establishes some degree of commitment to treatment, solid food can replace the liquid supplement. The ability of the patient to maintain weight through normalization of intake marks a transition to less structured treatment, such as a partial hospitalization program or outpatient follow-up.

Other treatments applicable to both inpatient and outpatient settings include individual psychotherapy and family intervention. The initial focus in family therapy should be on psychoeducation and obtaining the support of family members. The dynamics that may be contributing to the patient's eating disorder should be identified and, when possible, resolved. Such treatment often requires extensive contact beyond any acute interventions.

Individual psychotherapy is of limited value in the early stages of treatment, as the anorectic individual is generally unmotivated and, due to cognitive disturbances secondary to self-starvation, not capable of meaningful therapeutic work. Supportive therapy during this acute stage is often helpful in allaying anxiety and encouraging compliance. The more focused cognitive-behavioral and interpersonal therapies are generally more effective when the patient has begun to gain weight and is beyond acute medical risk. Cognitive-behavioral therapy focuses on the particular disturbing or distorted thoughts that contribute to the patient's maladaptive behaviors and helps the patient establish more effective behavioral alternatives. It may also be effective in dealing with the central psychological features of anorexia nervosa, such as disturbance in body image. Interpersonal therapy may also be helpful. It focuses on interpersonal conflicts rather than specific eating disturbances. Following stabilization and resolution of the acute crisis, including achievement of weight restoration, patients often require longer term psychotherapeutic interventions.

Pharmacotherapy

Pharmacological therapy can play an adjunctive role in the management of both primary eating symptoms and their comorbid psychiatric features, including anxiety and depression. Such treatments should focus on particular target symptoms or behaviors. No single medication is consistently effective in managing the primary psychiatric disturbances of anorexia nervosa. Antidepressants, especially the selective serotonin-reuptake inhibitors, can alleviate depressive symptoms and, due to their ability to regulate obsessive-compulsive symptomatology, may help reduce the preoccupations and ritualistic behaviors encountered in most anorectics. Low doses of antipsychotics may sometimes be employed in severely obsessional or agitated patients. Anxiolytics in general should not be given to anorectics as they are prone to develop addictions.

BULIMIA NERVOSA

Description

Bulimia nervosa affects approximately 2–3% of young women and 0.2% of young men, although bulimic behaviors may be encountered in many more patients. Bulimia nervosa is generally precipitated by periods of restrictive dieting. Bulimic individuals engage in regular episodes of binge eating, followed by compensatory behaviors to counteract the weight gain from ingested calories. Binge eating is characterized by the rapid consumption of large amounts of food over a short time, usually 1–2 hours. It is associated with a sense of being out of control and is often followed by feelings of guilt or shame and other dysphoric affective states, such as depression or anxiety. Some patients report alleviation of dysphoria or even emotional numbing during or immediately following the episode, although this is short-lived. During a binge, a few thousand to as many as 15,000 kcal or more may be consumed. Sometimes trigger foods, often a fattening sweet such as chocolate, precipitate a binge, although the overall content of food consumed, by macroanalysis of nutritional content, varies. The bulimic individual generally binges in private; grossly overeating is humiliating. Embarrassment can lead to varying degrees of social avoidance or isolation.

Contributing further to avoidance behavior is the need to compensate for eating, frequently by purging. Most bulimic individuals induce vomiting during or after a binge, and some also use laxatives or diuretics. A minority of patients employ laxatives or diuretics alone. Nonpurging compensatory behaviors include compulsive exercising and restrictive dieting or fasting between binges.

Another characteristic of bulimia nervosa is patient dissatisfaction with body shape or weight. This may evolve into a significant degree of obsessional preoccupation, with self-evaluation overly influenced by these physical concerns. It can have a profound effect on self-esteem and is evidenced in part by comorbid depressive symptomatology in the majority of patients. Impulsive behavior is encountered in many individuals with bulimia nervosa and at times leads to substance abuse, sexual promiscuity, and theft.

Differential Diagnosis

Few medical or psychiatric disorders can be confused with bulimia nervosa. More frequently, signs of self-induced vomiting or use of diuretics or laxatives in a young woman who does not admit to binging or purging behaviors lead the primary care clinician to search for another primary medical diagnosis. Signs and symptoms associated with gastritis, esophagitis, dehydration, or electrolyte disturbances lead to primary care or emergency room visits, postponing psychiatric consultation. If the patient is underweight, amenorrheic, and is binging and purging, she has anorexia nervosa, of the binge–purge subtype, rather than bulimia nervosa.

Medical Complications & Treatment

The majority of medical complications due to bulimia nervosa are consequences of purging behaviors. Self-induced vomiting can lead to gastritis, esophagitis, periodontal disease, and dental caries. Gastric dilatation and gastric or esophageal rupture are rare medical emergencies. Metabolic alkalosis with the development of clinically significant hypokalemia in patients who vomit is not unusual, and serum electrolytes show typical indices. When present, electrocardiographic changes are significant. Arrhythmias can lead to cardiac arrest if hypokalemia and related disturbances are not effectively corrected. Use of diuretics causes similar disturbances. Metabolic acidosis can develop in patients who use a significant number of stimulant-type laxatives. Dehydration, sometimes requiring intravenous hydration, can accompany each of the aforementioned purging behaviors. More often associated with bulimic behaviors are general physical complaints such as fatigue and muscle aches. Long-term use of the emetic ipecac can lead to myopathies, including cardiomyopathy, the latter a rare cause of death in patients with bulimia.

Most patients with bulimia nervosa can be treated as outpatients or in more structured partial hospitalization programs. An individual with an acute medical condition, however, such as dehydration or symptomatic hypokalemia accompanied by electrocardiographic changes, requires hospitalization for medical stabilization. Patients who have failed outpatient treatment and continue to binge and purge frequently, and those with significant depression and associated suicidal ideation, may require inpatient treatment.

Psychotherapeutic Interventions

Helping patients recognize the negative consequences of their behavior and dispelling myths about the efficacy of many of their dietary maneuvers, especially the usefulness of laxatives, diuretics, and self-induced vomiting, may be enough to motivate them to decrease the frequency of bulimic behaviors. Similarly, self-monitory intake with the use of food diaries and normalization of meal patterns can lead to short-term gains in control of bulimic symptoms. Time-limited psychotherapy, focused specifically on the disturbed eating patterns, can be conducted in an individual or group format and is often useful. More traditional exploratory psychotherapies, which are generally not time limited, do not predictably affect outcome but may play a role in the treatment of underlying or persistent difficulties following improvement or resolution of bulimia.

Cognitive-behavioral therapy is an established treatment for bulimia nervosa and can lead to both acute reduction in symptoms of binging and purging and longer term maintenance of gains. It targets the behavioral manifestations and challenges the cognitive distortions typically encountered in these patients. In cognitive-behavioral therapy, identifying disordered behaviors is the first step toward productive intervention, because behavioral consequences follow specific cues. To intervene, one must recognize the various cues and respond to them deliberately rather than automatically. Cues affecting eating-disordered patients are either internal or external. Internal cues include physiological ones, most significantly hunger, as well as emotions and thoughts. External cues encompass a broad array of experiences from sensual, such as sight or smell, to situational. Cues lead to consequences that are either positive or negative; both can be reinforcing.

Following the identification of cues, associated responses can be addressed more specifically and in greater detail. Responses consist of thoughts, feelings, and behaviors. Helping the patient understand that thoughts and feelings affect behavioral responses to a cue is of great significance because both thoughts and feelings can be altered through cognitive-behavioral techniques. For each cue identified, patients are taught to delineate the various response components and to evaluate the appropriateness of each. Although schematically simple, many eating-associated responses are automatic, and learning to identify the cues and various responses requires much practice.

During cognitive-behavioral therapy patients are taught to recognize that behaviors follow cues and responses to cues can be broken down into thoughts, feelings, and behaviors. What a patient thinks and feels about a cue dictates whether her response is adaptive or maladaptive. How she feels is influenced by how she thinks, therefore the restructuring of thoughts is of primary importance. Eating-disordered patients manifest certain patterns of distorted thinking; these patterns negatively influence feelings and fuel the maladaptive behaviors. These various styles of thinking are identified, and strategies to challenge and ultimately to alter the distortions are developed.

A simple example helps illustrate the applicability of cognitive-behavioral therapy. A common cue that frequently leads to a bulimic response is the normal sense of fullness. Rather than recognizing satiety as a normal physiological response, the eating-disordered patient often misinterprets this cue, stating instead, "I feel fat." This distorted thought, unchallenged, is associated with negative feelings and often leads to dysfunctional behaviors. Rather than the appropriate response to fullness, understanding that it is temporary and will pass, the patient believes she must compensate for being "fat" and rids herself of the meal through purging or compensates for the caloric intake through exercise. Such a response causes the cycle to reassert itself.

Pharmacotherapy

Pharmacological management may play a significant role in treatment and, unlike its effect in anorexia, can more predictably affect outcome. Many antidepressants, including monoamine oxidase inhibitors (MAOIs), tricyclic antidepressants (TCAs), and selective serotonin-reuptake inhibitors (SSRIs; most notably fluoxetine), have been effective in treating bulimia. (Dietary proscriptions limit the usefulness of MAOIs and lethality in overdose limits treatment with TCAs.) They reduce symptoms of depression and anxiety as well as the frequency of binging and purging. Bupropion is the only antidepressant that is contraindicated, as the metabolic imbalances precipitated by purging can make the patient more prone to seizures.

SUMMARY

Eating disorders represent a broad spectrum of psychopathological features. They are best understood in terms of multiple etiological factors influencing the development of clinical syndromes. Understanding the complexity of these disorders, the behaviors associated with them, and their comorbid psychiatric features aids in the recognition of clinically significant cases. Focusing initially on control of these primary eating disorder behaviors helps reduce the likelihood of psychological morbidity. It also limits the medical complications that frequently develop in these conditions. Interventions to control behavior range from response prevention (for patients placed on special inpatient wards) to cognitive-behavioral therapies for more motivated patients. Behavioral control may be augmented through pharmacological management as well as other psychotherapies (psychoeductional and interpersonal) that help reduce the role that sustaining factors play in the maintenance of these disorders.

SUGGESTED READINGS

Fairburn CG, Wilson GT (editors): *Binge Eating: Nature, Assessment, Treatment.* Guilford Press, 1993.

Halmi KA (editor): *Psychobiology and Treatment of Anorexia Nervosa and Bulimia Nervosa.* American Psychiatric Association Press, 1992.

Halmi KA: Eating disorders. Pages 857–875 in: Hales KE, Yudofsky SC, Talbott J (editors): *American Psychiatric Press Textbook of Psychiatry,* 2nd ed. American Psychiatric Association Press, 1994.

Hsu LKG: *Eating Disorders.* Guilford Press, 1990.

Mitchell JE: *Bulimia Nervosa.* University of Minnesota Press, 1990.

Walsh BT, Devlin MJ: Psychopharmacology of anorexia nervosa, bulimia nervosa, and binge eating. Pages 1581–1589 in: Bloom FE, Kuffer DJ (editors): *Psychopharmacology: The Fourth Generation of Progress.* Raven Press, 1995.

WEB SITES

American Psychiatric Association
www.psych.org
Harvard Eating Disorders Center
http://www.hedc.org/
Academy for Eating Disorders
http://www.aedweb.org/
American Psychological Association
http://www.apa.org/

Alcohol & Substance Use

20

William D. Clark, MD

INTRODUCTION

CASE ILLUSTRATION

Jim is a 50-year-old factory worker with high blood pressure. He has a follow-up visit with the doctor who has been his primary care physician for the past decade. He mentions that he recently received his second DUI/OUI/DWI and considers it unfair. His probation officer ordered Jim to undergo alcohol counseling at the local alcohol treatment center. Jim has no interest in counseling but he thinks he must attend to keep his driver's license, needed to get to his job.

In this chapter, we will discuss identification and management of substance use problems, and how Jim's success in coping with his problems will be affected by his physician's interactions with him.

Physicians are well aware of the harm that the use of drugs and alcohol brings to their patients and families. The prevalence of substance-use disorders exceeds 20% in ambulatory care practices, involving everyone from adolescents, teachers, and shipyard workers, to doctors themselves. Physicians report that conversations with patients about drinking are stressful and conflict laden, and that patients are unmotivated to change their behavior. Physicians' negative feelings derive from family experiences or from encounters with intoxicated patients who are hostile, uncooperative, and often violent. Anyone entangled in the web of substance abuse is likely to act irresponsibly—driving while intoxicated, attempting suicide, engaging in high-risk sexual behavior, and sharing, dealing, and stealing illegal drugs—despite legal, moral, and family sanctions. These dynamics, combined with the sense that substance abuse may not really be a "medical" issue, tend to keep physicians from speaking up and prevent them from helping their patients.

Strong evidence from many sources provides reason for optimism, however, and shows that doctors who take a few moments to thoughtfully structure their interventions with patients succeed in reducing harm. In so doing, physicians

not only lower medical care costs and morbidity for patients and their family members, they also strengthen family and social relationships, self-esteem, and emotional stability. Indeed the recovery rate from substance abuse, 30–40% of treated patients, exceeds that from most chronic illnesses. Recovering patients often credit their clinicians with being a primary factor in their recovery and with literally saving their lives. For physicians, participating in the reversal of substance abuse can be as gratifying as helping patients recover from leukemia, pneumonia, or other life-threatening illnesses. Of course, caring for patients with these problems is more like helping patients with depression, dysthymia, elevated cholesterol, or arthritis than patients with acute problems that respond to pharmacotherapy or surgery.

NEW INTERVIEW CONCEPTS

Research into life-style change by many investigators with different interests and hypotheses has allowed development and description of strategies and skills that can be effectively used in primary care. Researchers label the ideas based on their orientation, and the major new concepts include *brief intervention, motivational interviewing, shared decision making, relationship-centered care,* and *autonomy support.* This brief summary will describe application of these principles to the task of promoting change, whether the patient's diagnosis is "at-risk use," "drug abuse," or "drug dependence."

The fundamental **principles** derived from this research that are most relevant to primary care interviews around substance use and abuse are as follows (some might call these attitudes or values):

- Generally speaking, the physician takes responsibility for calibrating and adjusting interventions to prepare patients to hear information and feedback that create or amplify differences between the way life is now and the goals and values patients espouse. Using an empathic and caring style, the physician shows that discrepancies between the actual and the potential might be minimized if patients change their drug-use patterns.

- Patients will not change until they are ready, and ambivalence about change and/or resistance to change is universal. Physicians can promote change by adjusting interventions to meet the patient's current readiness.

- Physicians can best promote change by maintaining an empathic and relationship-centered style. Taking a strongly persuasive stand usually fails to promote change.
- Only the patient can take responsibility for change and effect change. Physicians can promote change by providing information (both feedback about the patient's health and problems and information about resources), by showing attentiveness and listening carefully to the patient's ideas about both the pros and the cons of possible changes, and by helping boost the patient's self-confidence about change.

The fundamental **content messages** physicians should include in interviews are as follows:

- I am concerned that your drug use is hurting you and others you care about (or has the potential to hurt you).
- Most people use a lot less than you, or abstain.
- For better health, you should curb (or cease) your drug use.
- The key choices are up to you, you are the person who will decide what to do.
- I will give you my best advice, which is based on ideas from the experts and my experience with other patients with similar problems.
- Changing drug-use habits may turn out to be difficult and scary.
- I want to collaborate with you, even if progress is slow or intermittent.

The fundamental **process strategies** physicians should include in interviews are as follows:

- Maintain dialogue when giving information and recommendations.
- Make clear recommendations, but do not try to persuade patients.
- Calibrate recommendations to keep them consistent with the patient's *stage of change* (see Chapter 15).
  1. Suggest that patients in the *precontemplation* stage **think** it over.
  2. Help patients in the *contemplation* stage **examine** the pros and cons of change before they make a decision.
  3. Help patients in the *preparation* stage explore the various **options** available.
  4. Ensure that patients in the *action* stage make a **plan** that is likely to succeed.
  5. Remind patients in the *maintenance* stage to attend to their **weak spots.**

- State explicitly that you will advise, but that the patient decides.
- Establish clearly the patient's commitment to any plans on which you agree.
- Never argue with patients and do not try to overcome resistance, reluctance, rebellion, or rationalization. Learn how to "roll with resistance."
- Support the patient's self-confidence.

We will describe some of the process strategies, and then illustrate how they might be used to deliver content messages to patients who have problems of varying severity and who are in different stages of change. Physicians should then understand the rationale for the content messages and be able to deliver them using some of the process skills that will be described and illustrated in this chapter.

SUBSTANCE USE PROBLEMS

Etiology & Pathophysiology

No one seeks to develop these problems, nor is any person immune to nervous tissue actions of alcohol and other drugs. People use alcohol or drugs to have good times in the company of others. People modulate use according to feedback from internal states such as shame or hangover, and external cues such as reprimands, criticism, and sanctions. People succeed or fail in limiting use because of the interplay of physiological (genetic), psychological, and social/cultural factors.

 CASE ILLUSTRATION (CONT.)

Jim cannot remember his father, but knows he had serious drinking problems and left the family when Jim was 4.

When people do not limit their drug or alcohol use, the predictable, inevitable, and multitudinous brain effects of heavy use facilitate a vicious circle of using more, developing problems, and discounting the role of drugs. The insidious development of tolerance to intoxication and the cognitive deficits and the dysphoric aspects of related states (hangover, for example) engender unhealthy social dynamics. These relationship problems are exaggerated because friends and family resent the (apparently) voluntary "having fun and being irresponsible" nature of overindulgence. People become adept at ignoring reality and suppressing negative feelings. Longer times spent in brain-altered states result in the dramatic neurophysiological changes of addiction and withdrawal. Further, emotional isolation develops because people make excuses for their behavior, direct blame onto others, and show hostility whenever sensible limits are discussed. They select friends and partners who tolerate heavy use and tacitly agree to overlook the consequences.

CASE ILLUSTRATION (CONT.)

Jim began drinking as a teenager and got up to a 12-pack per day. He cut back once he got out of his 20s since "that was going nowhere" but still drinks four to six beers daily—at his club or playing pool or cards with his buddies, and up to two six-packs per day on the weekend. (Based on his self-report and national survey data, only 3% of American men drink more than Jim.)

WORKING WITH SUBSTANCE-ABUSING PATIENTS

Two key steps can assist physicians in doing a better job with substance-abusing patients. The first is to intervene when any clue suggests that a drug-use problem might be present—do not wait for "better data." Physicians can better limit serious consequences of drug use by broadening their focus from the detection of dependence or addiction to include the detection of use and risk.

The second key step is to conduct those interventions using techniques specifically structured for this purpose. For patients who are compelled to hide symptoms, lie about shameful behaviors, or behave in hostile or attacking ways with their doctors, there are tools of proven value. These techniques are clearly more effective than supportive or persuasive strategies in use by most practicing physicians. We will discuss first the process of deciding which patients require interventions, and then discuss the principles, content, and strategies of physician interventions. Physicians should intervene as early as possible, whether they have found a clear diagnosis or not.

You are clear that this is a time to intervene with Jim, and we will return to that dialogue after some preliminary discussion of diagnosis and management.

DIAGNOSTIC CATEGORIES

Drug and alcohol problems exist on a continuum (Table 20–1), and in an individual case diagnosis may be elusive because of scant or imprecise information. Nevertheless, experts agree on an evidence-based classification

Table 20–1. Descriptors for the continuum of drug and alcohol use.[1]

"Hazardous use" has approximately the same meaning as "at-risk" use.[2]

"Abuse" of alcohol or drugs is a maladaptive use pattern leading to impairment or distress

"Dependence" on alcohol or other drugs is a maladaptive use pattern leading to impairment or distress, more pervasive and persistent than for abuse, and often (but not necessarily) including physical dependence and withdrawal symptoms.

[1] See Fiellin et al (2000).
[2] See Table 20–4 for alcohol amounts; any use of illicit drugs is "at risk;" see text for prescription drug use.

system that is useful in guiding physician actions. People on the severely afflicted end of the continuum, with the prototype syndrome, *alcohol or drug dependence* (often called "alcoholism," or "drug addiction"), suffer medical and social consequences from uncontrolled use. A striking 5–10% of adults develop this syndrome. People with dependence are recognizable across cultures and nationalities (for example, women or men, Hispanic or Anglo, in France, the United States, or Russia) because a distinctive, defensive interactive style develops in parallel with typical medical and social complications. People hide important facts, defend their "right" to use, and respond with hostility and reticence to attempts to talk about drinking or drug use. **Physical dependence** and **withdrawal syndromes** mean *drug dependence* virtually 100% of the time.

People toward the center of the continuum, with problems of modest severity, have *drug abuse,* a "maladaptive pattern which leads to impairment or distress" (American Psychiatric Association *Diagnostic and Statistical Manual of Mental Disorders,* 4th edition, *DSM-IV*) Note that what distinguishes the patient with drug abuse from the patient with drug dependence is not the **nature** of the problems, but the **frequency, persistence, and pervasiveness** of the problems. Thus, both *drug abuse* and *drug dependence* may include health problems (eg, stroke from cocaine use, hypertension from alcohol use, oversedation from benzodiazepines), legal problems (eg, arrests for driving under the influence or violence), family dysfunction, and performance problems at school or work.

On the mild end of the continuum are *"at-risk,"* or *"hazardous,"* users. These people use too much, but do not yet have important negative consequences. Physicians should intervene with them on the basis of the quantity of intake—in contrast, intervention with patients with "abuse" or "dependence" is made because of negative consequences and high quantity of use. Most, but not all people who experience serious life consequences use very excessive amounts, but the decision about how vigorous to be with interventions is made on the severity of problems, not on the amount consumed. The need to know about the amount to determine whether a patient is on the mild end and the need to know about consequences to determine whether a patient is on the severe end cause confusion for physicians. Data about both amounts and consequences should be sought, but the full meaning of the data about amount remains unclear until the physician obtains a clear picture of adverse consequences or lack thereof.

Regarding alcohol, expert consensus is that *"moderate drinking"* is defined by low quantity of intake (fewer than 14 drinks per week for men and fewer than seven for women), a social setting for drinking, and little intoxication (not more than four drinks per occasion for men and three for women). Drinking above these limits is variously called *"at risk"* or *"hazardous,"* and is likely to cause harm, according to long-term studies.

"At-risk" prescription drug use includes patients on mood-altering drugs or prescription pain medications for more than 3 months. The majority of patients using long-term sedative drugs to manage insomnia, anxiety, depression, and other disorders, as well as those using narcotics to treat chronic pain, develop neither problems nor dependence. Similar to drinkers and users of illicit drugs, however, 10–20% do experience problems such as falls, oversedation, drug interactions, drug overdoses, or symptoms of dependence, such as taking more medication than prescribed.

Any use of an illicit drug (or tobacco) is *"at-risk"* use.

IDENTIFYING SUBSTANCE-USE PROBLEMS

In the past, clinicians were urged to look for dependence, but this prior focus is too narrow and ignores hazardous and at-risk users, according to research and consensus panels. New studies on the effectiveness of brief interventions demonstrate that physicians can help at-risk users and drug abusers to avoid serious negative consequences of overindulgence. This is analogous to working with the patient with angina or high cholesterol, rather than waiting for the heart attack. Current recommendations urge physicians to expand their interventions to all users.

We suggest simple strategies that separate healthy users from potentially problematic ones. Subsequent sections advise physicians what to do in each case.

History

Because drinking or drug use is not an illness, but a behavior that carries with it societal myths and stigmas, talking about this behavior is always a sensitive matter. The physician's history-taking style and techniques strongly affect patients' subsequent willingness to participate in treatment activities. Many studies suggest that a structured,

stepped approach is both efficient in practice and effective with patients.

STEP ONE

Step one is to **ask about alcohol or drug use in the past year.** Closed rather than open-ended questions are helpful here, because if patients answer open-ended questions vaguely, forcing the clinician to ask clarifying questions, they quickly feel accused of lying and become defensive. Questions might include "When was your last drink of alcohol?" "When was your last use of marijuana or other nonprescription medication?" "When was your last use of a prescription medication for pain or emotional problems?" If the patient had no alcohol or drug use in the past year, nothing else need be done. The abstinent subgroup with past problems often discloses this spontaneously.

STEP TWO

Step two seeks to identify current or recent users who deserve substantial attention. Because the typical defensive interactive style of people with dependence or serious abuse promotes minimization and cover-up rather than exposure, there may be no discernible clue unless a structured screening strategy is used. We favor **a short screen for dependence** as the next step. At present, physicians miss 60–80% of cases, and lives can be saved by screening, just as in the case of hypertension or cervical cancer. *Consistent use of any validated strategy* is a far more powerful determinant of clinical effectiveness than which strategy a physician chooses for routine use.

We like the two **TICS** (two-item screen) questions: "In the last year, have you ever drunk or used drugs more than you meant to?" and "Have you felt you wanted or needed to cut down on your drinking or drug use in the last year?" They are effective, efficient, and straightforward. The **CAGE** test (Table 20–2) is a more thoroughly studied simple screen. It is less accurate for women and African-Americans. Studies show that substituting "alcohol or drug" for "alcohol" in the screen is effective. Any positive response to TICS or CAGE means that the physician needs to intervene, usually beginning with a further search for specific adverse effects.

Table 20–2. **CAGE** screening test for dependence symptoms.

Have you ever felt that you should **Cut down** on your drinking?
Have people **Annoyed** you by criticizing your drinking?
Have you ever felt bad or **Guilty** about your drinking?
Have you ever had a drink first thing in the morning to steady your nerves or get rid of a hangover? (**Eye-opener**)

We recommend that clinicians avoid using the natural question "How much do you drink/use?" as **Step two.** Not only is "How much?" a reminder to people of shameful overindulgence, but it invites vague answers and subsequent defensiveness (see above). Further, it fails to encourage reflection, and research demonstrates that asking "How much?" may limit patients' responses to subsequent questioning.

Screening questions to search for specific illicit drug dependence have not been widely tested in primary care settings. One question—"Have you used marijuana more than five times in your life?" (chosen from the National Institutes of Mental Health's diagnostic interview schedule)—can be repeated for narcotics, amphetamines, and other drugs of interest.

STEP THREE

If Step two is negative, ask the National Institute on Alcohol and Alcoholism (NIAAA)'s recommended **questions about quantity and frequency** (Table 20–3). The NIAAA expert panel declares that "safe limits" are (for men) 14 or fewer drinks a week, and never more than four drinks on one occasion. They suggest limits of seven drinks per week and three per occasion for women (Table 20–4). If a person drinks below these limits, **and** Step two shows no positive response, **and** no other hints exist that the patient has alcohol problems, no urgent intervention is needed.

Of course, when withdrawal symptoms are apparent, or liver disease is accompanied by odor of alcohol, or the patient has signs of injection drug use, or the spouse confides about problems, clinicians do not need screening strategies.

STEPS TWO AND THREE

If any dependency screen (eg, the CAGE) is positive, or if intake exceeds safe limits, or if another clue from examination or the family suggests a drinking or drug problem, the clinician needs more detail to clarify the extent of the problems. A search for characteristic negative consequences is warranted and not time consuming if thoughtfully structured. The physician decides when to conduct this inquiry based on priorities for the present encounter; however, because alcohol and drug use produce many symptoms and affect many other illness conditions, at least a brief inventory when the issue initially surfaces is usually imperative.

Table 20–3. NIAAA questions on quantity and frequency of drinking.

On average, how many days per week do you drink?
On a typical day when you drink, how many drinks do you have?
What is the maximum number of drinks you had on any given occasion during the past month?

Table 20–4. "Hazardous" or "at-risk" alcohol intake limits.

Men: more than 14 drinks[1] per week, or more than four drinks per occasion.
Women: more than seven drinks[1] per week, or more than three drinks per occasion.

[1]A drink is 12 oz beer, 5 oz wine, or 1.5 oz (bar shot) of hard liquor.

Asking the questions in Table 20–5 provides ample data for the primary care assessment. Protocols for drug-use assessment are less well developed than those for alcohol, perhaps in part because so many drugs of interest are illicit that research on them is particularly complex. Patients can be assessed further by inquiring how much money they spend a week on drugs, the frequency of use, and how many days or weeks they abstained in the past 12 months.

Interviews with others, including family, nurses, or social workers, enlarge the inquiry if the patient furnishes insufficient data. Records from other physicians or hospitals may contain unanticipated information that establishes a diagnosis.

Obtaining a thorough evaluation allows the physician to discuss impressions in a compassionate manner. In fact, experimental data show that thoughtful diagnostic conversation itself produces beneficial therapeutic effects.

 CASE ILLUSTRATION (CONT.)

*You have asked Jim the **CAGE** questions in the past, and at that time he said that when he was a lot younger he needed to **cut down,** and he drank **eye-openers** in the morning, again in the distant past. He said he was not **annoyed** because of criticism of his drinking, and that he never felt **guilty** or remorseful after drinking.*

Table 20–5. Symptoms of alcohol abuse or dependence.

Somatic: gastritis, trauma, hypertension, liver function disorder, or new-onset seizure
Psychosocial: symptoms of anxiety, depression, insomnia, overdose, or a request for psychotropic medications
Alcohol-specific: any spontaneous mention of drinking behavior, such as "partying" or hangover, family history, AA attendance, arrests for driving while intoxicated, withdrawal symptoms, tolerance, blackouts

Responding Effectively to Challenge, Resistance, & Ambivalence; Learning to "Roll with Resistance"

We introduce this process strategy in this section on identification of problems because patients usually show their initial resistance and challenge as the physician asks a few more questions, seeking to determine whether to intervene. Of course, asking the questions is an intervention of sorts, and physicians can improve the quality of the data as well as minimize tension by responding effectively in this situation.

On the one hand, to learn and use science well physicians must think and act logically, learn to argue a point, and be persistently persuasive. On the other hand, it is normal for people to resist change and to resist any attempts to persuade them before they are ready. Research suggests that using the interview skill of "reflection" (sometimes called active listening) helps increase motivation and engagement, reduces tension, and is a response that helps avoid argument (see Chapter 1). Doctors more often prefer familiar skills such as asking questions (getting more data), giving advice, persuading or arguing the point, or shifting the interview focus. With a little effort, physicians can respond helpfully to expressions of ambivalence, resistance, or challenge.

Reflection, or paraphrasing the patient's message or meaning (Table 20–6), especially when the patient seems negative or hostile, is not an intuitive response. Physicians who can gently reflect back the resistance, ambivalence, or challenge they receive from patients can generate an atmosphere of alliance and partnership. This is so because reflection shows a desire to fully understand the speaker, and gives the speaker full choice over where to go next (unlike questions, advice, agreement or disagreement, or statements of values, etc). Reflection demonstrates acceptance of the person and a willingness to listen more. Because it is neither aggressive nor defensive, it helps minimize arguing, fighting, hostility, and negativity. In fact, studies demonstrate that doctors who reflect negative, resistant, or reluctant (and so on) statements help patients to voice the more positive view.

Table 20–6. Reflection.

Description: Tell the patient the message you heard (or perceived nonverbally). Always statements, not questions, agreement or disagreement, judgment, etc. Always brief: reflector may have to choose among several messages to be brief.
Examples: "I see, you think that none of your problems is related to drug use." "Alcohol really helps you to sleep." "That I think these abnormal liver tests are from alcohol is confusing to you, because you drink so little." "You seem irritated with my continuing to discuss drug use."

Patient: I drink a lot because of the neuropathy and pain in my feet, so that I can sleep.

Doctor: So, alcohol helps you a lot.

Patient: Well, it's probably not so good for my liver.

This is one aspect of helping patients recognize discrepancies between their current status and what they might desire. Physicians can equally well reflect a person's statements about feeling, thinking, attribute, choice, action, or behavior.

Reflection helps the physician by encouraging patients to share more of their perspectives, feelings, and thoughts, and reflection thus engenders more trust and a feeling of safety in both persons. As patients who initially show disinterest, hostility, a sullen demeanor, or confusion reveal more of themselves, physicians become less judgmental and critical, more inclined to join patients and to support them in their struggles with life. Patients who feel joined become better able to listen to their doctors, and have more strength to take responsibility for attempting change that might at first seem unimaginable. Reflection is useful in all interview stages, whether the physician seeks more information about drug use and its consequences, additional psychosocial information, or wishes to develop sensible management strategies for a patient.

 CASE ILLUSTRATION (CONT.)

You decide to begin your assessment of Jim's current situation by asking him the CAGE questions again. You ask about cutting down:

Jim: Look, doc, my father may have been alcoholic, and many of my buddies drink a lot more than me, but I'm not an alcoholic, and I can take it or leave it.

Rather than confronting him with the considerable evidence already available to you that indicates his situation qualifies as at least alcohol abuse and possibly dependence, you decide to use an empathic style and reflect his apparent feeling state as well as the content of his declaration.

Doctor: Jim, I see this is a sensitive topic, as it is for most people, and I get it that you are convinced that drinking is not a problem for you.

Jim: I quit several times when my wife complained, no problem. But two years ago she took the kids and left, saying that I was unreliable and that they couldn't live with me unless I quit drinking. I don't understand women!

You have important new data about drinking and about Jim's life, and Jim feels understood rather than interrogated.

Physical Examination & Laboratory Studies

Physical and laboratory examinations are useful adjuncts to structured interviewing and help doctors set priorities for the pacing and vigor of subsequent discussions. *Odor of alcohol* is alarming, and distinctly abnormal in medical encounters. If alcohol is easily smelled in the room, the blood alcohol level (BAL) is likely greater than 0.125 g/dL, and a less dramatic odor indicates a BAL between 0.075 and 0.125 g/dL. The nose is a good breath analyzer. Alcohol on the breath is a convincing sign, and always signals a serious alcohol disorder.

Intoxication in any encounter is worrisome, and means a high likelihood of drug or alcohol disorder, even in the emergency situation. To underscore this important point, assume that the alcohol- or drug-dependent 10% of the population are intoxicated once a week (it is often more than once), and assume that the 60% who are not abusers or dependent are intoxicated once yearly (it is often less than once). Thus, in a year, from a population of 100, 30 abstainers yield no episodes of intoxication, 60 users (not in trouble) yield 60, and 10 dependent people yield 520! Further, moderate users seldom become as intoxicated and are more likely to use in controlled environments (eg, where someone else can drive). Intoxicated people in the emergency situation are not healthy users or drinkers who "have had one too many."

Further, with respect to alcohol, if the odor of alcohol is apparent, and if the patient manifests no evidence of intoxication (slurred speech, incoordination, and emotional lability), *tolerance* to alcohol effect is present. Tolerance indicates brain adaptation to intoxicating alcohol levels, which is caused by heavy drinking, is inevitably toxic, and means alcohol dependence is present. Withdrawal syndromes (see the next section) indicate additional brain dysfunction, and are easier to discern than tolerance. The same reasoning holds for other drugs, but our ability to quantify use or blood levels, as well as our ability to detect intoxication (except for sedatives or opiates), is limited, so tolerance must be inferred less directly from the patient's history.

Other physical and laboratory findings (see general medicine textbooks for the multitudinous possibilities) are poor screening tests (low sensitivity and specificity). Once again, more data are available about alcohol than for other drugs. Because of alcohol's broad toxicity, an abnormality may prove useful in context. First, an unexplained finding may begin a fruitful investigative process. For example, despite a negative CAGE test, the concerned physician of a young woman with palmar erythema continued the assessment, allowing the patient to reveal her alcohol problem. Second, in the presence of a clue, physical or laboratory findings substantially raise the posttest probability, and physicians should order appropriate tests, such as mean corpuscular volume (MCV) and liver enzymes [include a γ-glutamyltransferase (GGT), the most sensitive to alcohol intake]. For example, a 55-year-old man with chronic pulmonary disease was admitted for atrial fibrillation. His wife complained about his drinking, and elevated MCV and aspartate aminotransferase (AST) confirmed not only alcoholism, but also "holiday heart" (alcohol-induced arrythmia after binge drinking). In a sedated patient with few clues, a response to naloxone confirms opiate intoxication.

Illicit drugs are readily detectable in urine; however, the ability to identify certain drugs varies with the technique used. Oxycodone is not detected with current methods, but this is likely to change because of the magnitude of recent problems with Oxycontin. Other drugs that may not be included in routine panels are methadone, anabolic steroids, and short-acting designer drugs. Marijuana can be detected for up to 30 days in the urine of daily smokers (for 1–3 days in intermittent smokers), but all other illicit drugs are cleared within 72 hours; for example, a positive test for cocaine indicates use within the past 2–3 days. Simply being near a marijuana smoker never produces a positive urine test (it can be detected by mass spectroscopy, but levels are well below the cut-off levels of routine urine testing).

CASE ILLUSTRATION (CONT.)

On repeated checks over the past couple of years, Jim has had an elevated MCV, but the rest of his complete blood count, metabolic panel, and liver function panel are repeatedly normal. He tells you his blood alcohol concentration was 0.22 (220 mg/dL, 100 is the "legal limit" in most states; some have lowered this to 80) when he was cited.

MANAGEMENT OF WITHDRAWAL

Treatment of alcohol or drug withdrawal is of special concern to the primary care physician. Other urgent complications such as arrhythmia, alcohol or viral hepatitis, bleeding, gastritis, pancreatitis, skin abscess, sepsis, and overdose are covered in appropriate medical textbooks. Alcohol and opiate withdrawal are the most common withdrawal disorders, and physicians can manage many patients in outpatient settings if the withdrawal syndrome is of mild to moderate severity. Important parameters that patients should meet for adequate treatment in the outpatient setting include a commitment to abstaining from all mood-altering drugs during withdrawal (except as prescribed for withdrawal) and an expressed willingness to engage in continuing treatment. Homeless people or others not living with someone who can help monitor medication and symptoms in case of adverse events, those with important polysubstance use, and those with important or unstable medical or psychiatric illness should not be treated as outpatients.

With regard to alcohol, as physical dependence develops, initial manifestations of anxiety, sleep disorder, tremor, and vague discomforts are mild, sometimes not attributed to alcohol, but easily relieved by drinking. As months pass, however, alcohol less reliably controls symptoms, and intoxication is fleeting, occurring only at high BAL (greater than 250 mg/dL). Withdrawal is not an all-or-nothing state, and addicted patients experience symptoms whenever their BAL falls. The altered neurophysiology in the brain perceives a drop in BAL as disruptive to the new steady-state condition of addiction, and expresses the disruption through withdrawal symptoms. Soon, the person drinks steadily to alleviate withdrawal, but relief is brief. The range of BAL at which the person feels "not sick" diminishes, and severe symptoms, even delirium tremens, may develop despite a BAL of 300 mg/dL or more.

Outpatient treatment is sensible in mild withdrawal, but inpatient support is required for severe cases. Physicians should hospitalize patients with clouded sensorium, fever, hyperventilation, or a concomitant medical problem (hepatic failure, pancreatitis, etc). In addition, the presence of three risk factors (Table 20–7) suggests that inpatient management would be appropriate. Degree of tremor, anxiety, tachycardia, and stomach symptoms are poor predictors of need for inpatient care. When outpatient management is feasible, pharmacological support helps with symptom relief (Table 20–8) and should be integrated with patient education and referral options designed to help patients change entrenched behaviors.

With regard to opiate withdrawal, physicians can be helpful. Unfortunately, patients who use high doses of opiates, particularly those who inject heroin, experience intolerable craving during withdrawal and few patients succeed in outpatient settings. People using opiate drugs should never be given other opiates for treatment. First,

federal law prohibits the prescription of opiates for treatment, and second, in this case the strictness of the law is clinically helpful, because provision of opiates by well-meaning clinicians is never successful. People who are ready to stop abusing oral opiates (especially prescription pain medications) can sometimes avoid hospitalization if treated with clonidine, benzodiazepines, and antiemetics for a few days to a week or two (see Table 20–9 for a suggested regimen). Patients should check with the physician face to face every 2–3 days until symptoms are minimal, and during the withdrawal process make initial contact with a professional treatment program, as treatment of withdrawal never eliminates drug dependence. The dependence pattern develops over months to years, and always involves the patient's friends, family, and a network of supply sources. The patient will relapse unless support in coping with other aspects of the dependence cycle is available.

Patients with a high tolerance who are taking the equivalent of more than 60 mg of diazepam a day are not candidates for outpatient treatment. Equivalent doses for other benzodiazepines are 300 mg chlordiazepoxide, 12 mg lorazepam, and 5 mg alprazolam. Sedative or tranquilizer dependence is best managed by addiction professionals, as pharmacological treatment must be individualized and closely monitored as an inpatient.

Table 20–7. Risk factors for severe alcohol withdrawal.

Drinking around the clock
Daily consumption of a fifth of liquor, a case of beer, or more than a half-gallon of wine
Heavy drinking for more than 5 years (on most days)
Poor nutrition
Concomitant heavy sedative, cocaine, or opiate use
History of severe withdrawal within the past 2 years

Table 20–8. Medication for outpatient alcohol withdrawal.

Day 1: Give 25–75 mg chlordiazepoxide initially, then 25–50 mg every 4–6 hours, if needed.
Day 2: Give 25 mg chlordiazepoxide every 4–6 hours.
Day 3: Give 25 mg chlordiazepoxide every 6–8 hours.
Anticipate 400 mg for worst case (16 doses of 25 mg): 200 mg Day 1, 125 mg Day 2, 75 mg Day 3. Admit for inpatient withdrawal treatment if the patient drinks or uses other drugs.

Table 20–9. Medication for outpatient opiate withdrawal.

Day 1: Give 0.1 mg clonidine every 1 or 2 hours until dizzy or maximum of 0.6 mg is given; give 5–10 mg diazepam up to four times daily, including at bedtime.
Day 2: Give 0.1 or 0.2 mg clonidine three times daily, and repeat the diazepam regimen.
Days 3–5: Repeat Day 2.
Do not go higher as an outpatient. Suppository of prochloperazine or equivalent may help if nausea/emesis is severe, and lomotil or equivalent if diarrhea is prominent.

OFFICE INTERVENTION STRATEGIES

Physicians should initiate dialogue whenever they perceive a potential problem with drugs or alcohol. Early intervention is more important than certainty about diagnosis or having "all the facts." All patients will have high levels of ambivalence and resistance, and the physician's initial office interventions will address universal dynamics about the change process. During any one interview, and over multiple encounters, physicians will obtain more data, improve the accuracy of their diagnoses, and fine-tune their interventions. Studies show that recurrent brief encounters using the style and skills listed above and discussed in the following sections are more critical to success than getting any one encounter "exactly right." People and life-styles are too complex and entrenched to expect that one "right answer" or "correct" conversation can accomplish the goals of change.

Life-Style Change: Changing Drinking & Drug-Use Patterns

Prochaska and colleagues have found that people progress through a series of stages on the way to successful life-style change (see Chapter 15). This is true across studies of at least a dozen behaviors. In the first stage, "precontemplation," a person does not think that the behavior (drinking, for example) is a problem, and naturally has no interest in changing. People thinking about changing are in "contemplation." Ambivalence is the hallmark of this stage, and people find reasons to stay the same as well as reasons to change. As the balance tips toward change, people enter "preparation" and imagine change strategies or new behaviors (such as wondering how to avoid their drug suppliers, or where to find an AA meeting). In the "action" stage, people take action and try out new behaviors (such as changing from liquor to beer, or quitting for a time). When persistently successful and no longer sliding back to old behaviors, people are in the "maintenance" stage.

Experienced clinicians find the concept of stages intuitively useful. Tracking whether a preponderance of patient conversation suggests progression through stages is useful for physicians, as they evaluate readiness to change and consider potential interventions.

Because only the patient can effect change, the doctor's task is to trigger change. The general mechanism is to create or amplify a discrepancy between patients' perceptions of their current status and their desired short-term or long-term goals. The specific strategies and skills vary according to patients' readiness to address important questions. Evidence shows that empathic, trusted physicians who are willing to intervene and strive to build a sense of autonomy, optimism, and confidence will help trigger change.

Giving Information & Recommendations

The section on pathophysiology emphasizes the deep roots of drug dependence. It is sustained by drug-induced brain changes, unhealthy social dynamics, and emotional isolation, as well as the intense feeling that the "devil you know" must be better than changing. Change seems unimaginable, like jumping into a black, featureless abyss. This illness dynamic ensures that patients will ignore reality, suppress negative feelings, and so flawlessly, as if by second nature, reject sound advice. The challenge for physicians is correspondingly great.

Patients' behaviors are negative, confusing, and hurtful. Often, roles are reversed, and the physician, directly or unwittingly, rejects and humiliates the patient. This fundamental distortion in physicians' experience of caring for patients is painful and profoundly unsatisfying. So, it is no surprise that physicians fail to intervene, and mirror patients' lack of awareness, reluctance, and often hopelessness. Clinicians come to believe that any intervention is unwarranted interference in the patient's life. The situation becomes framed as, "Shall I now confront Jim and waste valuable time for unlikely gain, or simply address Jim's high blood pressure?" Substance abuse remains unaddressed.

Studies of successful interventions show that effective interviewers give information and advice in dialogue, calibrate the advice to the stage of change, and make recommendations clearly, but without persuasion or pressure. They roll with resistance by using reflection frequently, and remain consistently relationship centered by responding to feelings empathically.

CREATE DIALOGUE

True dialogue is difficult in conversations that involve substantial differentials in perspectives, expertise, and/or power. Patients tend either to defend a point of view or to be passive and silent. Clinicians can encourage dialogue by consciously employing a format of "tell, ask, tell, ask," which supports taking turns and results in a dialogue. Briefly provide bits of information or advice, and then ask patients what they think about it, or how it feels to hear it, or what they intend to do about it. Keeping the "telling" brief helps clarity, and "asking" allows the patient to choose a "change-enhancing" or "change-obstructing" response. The manner in which patients respond to being asked also suggests to the clinician which next steps are likely to be helpful. Generally, "change-enhancing" responses include statements of agreement, commitment, or optimism, and they suggest that exploring the facts might be helpful. Generally, "change-obstructing" responses, such as statements of disagreement, reservation, pessimism, defensiveness, noncommittal statements, and all questions that do not ask for clarification of meaning, suggest that the clinician should reflect back the response as the next step in the conversation. Reflection invites patients to look inside themselves, and encourages motivation and discrepancy. "Asking" thus fosters exploration and choice.

 CASE ILLUSTRATION (CONT.)

Your physical examination shows Jim's blood pressure is controlled, and you find no evidence for new medical problems or active withdrawal from alcohol. You agree to continue the lisinopril:

Doctor: We have talked about alcohol quite a bit today, Jim. What are you thinking about this, now?

Jim: I'm quitting until I get my license back, no problem.

Doctor: You feel you are in full control of your alcohol intake.

Jim: I'm fine, doc, and thanks for checking.

Doctor: It would be a mistake for me to not share my concerns with you, Jim; I'd like to give you some information before you go—can we take just 3 minutes more?

CREATE AN OBJECTIVE, SCIENTIFIC CLIMATE FOR EDUCATING AND ADVISING PATIENTS

Create a climate of fact, not opinion, by giving all information, feedback, and advice/recommendations in an "objective" or "scientific" way. In short, start with the facts, not conclusions or opinions about meaning. Physicians who display arrogance, or an "I absolutely know what is right for you" posture about the meaning of the facts, without regard to the usual cautions that apply to science (today's truth is tomorrow's fiction, and every case is unique), make patients defensive, and encourage arguments. Then, after exploration of some of the facts, give advice tentatively, as part of a search for options or alternatives. "Wagging one's finger," actually or figuratively, tends to push patients into a corner, highlights any feelings of shame or stigma, and generally inhibits discussion. The following give examples as well as more details.

Give *information* about what is known about alcohol problems in an impersonal way: "Research shows that treatment helps;" or "Steady drug use changes brain function;" or "Having a high tolerance for alcohol means that a person is deprived of the early warning system that tells him to stop drinking before the alcohol level gets so high as to be dangerous;" or "95% of men drink less than 35 drinks per week;" or "Many people are terrified to imagine stopping drug use;" or "Generally, being sick in the morning until after a drink means a person's brain has become hooked on alcohol." Next, ask what the patient thinks of this information.

Doctor: Guidelines from extensive research show that drinking more than 14 drinks a week is risky. (You ask Jim what he thinks of that.) Most people who like drinking and do so regularly are reluctant to consider changing their patterns, especially if they are pressured to do so. (You ask Jim what he thinks of that.) Men with any close relative with drinking problems have an almost 50% chance of developing serious problems themselves. (You ask Jim what he thinks of that.)

Give *feedback* about the patient's situation as a fact, a number, or score, rather than a conclusion: "Three of your liver tests are abnormal," rather than "alcohol has damaged your liver;" or "Your alcohol level when you arrived in the emergency room was 0.160," rather than "You were drinking heavily before you came into the emergency room;" or "You have a serious infection in your arm," rather than "You got this infection because you were injecting;" or "You mentioned three important things—that your relationship with your wife is going poorly, that you are having a lot of stomach trouble, and that you lost your license to drive," rather than "Alcohol is wrecking your marriage, your career, and your body;" or "You are very shaky and sick to your stomach until you can get another pill," rather than "You are addicted to tranquilizers." Next, ask what the patient thinks of this information. The patient's response to the "ask" indicates whether motivation and/or discrepancy is enhanced, and gives the physician ideas about next steps.

Doctor: Jim, your red blood cells are too big, 109 units instead of less than 94. (You ask Jim what he thinks of that.) Your alcohol level of 0.22 is high. (You ask Jim what he thinks of that.) Jim, this is your second arrest. (You ask Jim what he thinks of that.) Jim, you have quit drinking several times. (You ask Jim what he thinks of that.)

Give *advice and explicit recommendations* with three characteristics. First, give an objective rationale derived from a broader database than simply this case; second, give advice as a possible option; and finally, make your advice consistent with your assessment of your patient's stage of change. Examples include the following: "One option that I recommend, based on data in the medical literature, and my experience with experts who have advised me about similar patients, is that you stop drinking all alcohol. Of course, no one can be certain that this is the right thing for you to do, or that it will work for you;" or "Most people find that talking with people in Alcoholics Anonymous is helpful. AA might or might not be right for you. I recommend you go there;" or "No one asks to get hooked on tranquilizers, it always sneaks up on people. Usually, people in this situation find that talking with an expert is helpful. I recommend that you talk with the person with whom I frequently consult about these problems, Dr. Mack." Next, ask what the patient thinks of this advice.

Patients will not do things that they do not choose themselves to do; commanding or ordering instead of checking the result of giving advice and making recommendations ensures poor adherence. If clinicians push ahead and try persuading patients in spite of reluctance, they foster continued ambivalence, raise resistance to change, and begin an enervating downward spiral in which both participants become further demoralized and discouraged.

> **Doctor:** Jim, one option that I recommend, based on my experience with experts who have advised me about similar patients, is that you take this opportunity to stop drinking all alcohol, and actively participate in the counseling. Of course, no one can be certain that this is the right thing for you to do, or that it will work for you.

Jim responds to your information and feedback in the way that you expect:

> **Jim:** Thanks for your concern, Doc, but I know I'm OK; I'll zoom through the stupid counseling thing and get my license right back.

This confirms *precontemplation*, as you are certain Jim has more trouble than he can see right now. You might end with a reflection that acknowledges his lack of readiness, and just give advice appropriate for a person in *precontemplation*.

> **Doctor:** We clearly have different perspectives right now, Jim. I appreciate that you do not intend to get involved right now. I wonder if you would be willing to think more about why I'm so concerned before your next check with me, which I will schedule for about 6 weeks from now?

Jim may respond to your information and feedback in a way that suggests he is willing to look more closely at the facts:

> **Jim:** Thanks for your concern, Doc; you know me pretty well, so I suppose there is some truth in what you say (suggesting he is *contemplating* your perspective).

> **Doctor:** Jim, I appreciate that you are thinking about this matter, but are not interested in making that kind of commitment right now. Before your next check with me, which I will schedule for about 6 weeks, I wonder if you would be willing to take careful note of both the *good* things about drinking and the *not-so-good* things about drinking? Think a bit about the *good* things and the *not-so-good* things about NOT drinking, too. Then, I'd value the chance to seek a deeper understanding of the total picture, and help you make the best decision you can for yourself, as time goes by.

Jim's response might surprise you:

> **Jim:** You know, a fellow at work has been pushing me to go to AA, and I almost went with him after I got my OUI (suggesting that a part of Jim is actually in *preparation*).

You might act on this hypothesis:

> **Doctor:** It seems to me that we agree that it might be good to do something differently right now. In fact, from a medical and health point of view, my recommendation is that you quit or dramatically curb your drinking. Many

people learn a lot about themselves when they go to a few AA meetings with an open mind. Would you be willing to go to one meeting a week until I see you again in a month or so?

CREATE COMMITMENT AND CONFIDENCE ABOUT CHANGE

Patients most reliably make commitments and decisions in an atmosphere that genuinely tolerates and respects the full expression of ambivalence, resistance, and uncertainty, with respect to both facts and feelings. Physicians create such an atmosphere when they use reflection and explicitly emphasize the patient's autonomy, while simultaneously offering their own expertise and support. Physicians augment patients' confidence about change when they witness out loud patients' special and unique strengths.

When feeling supportive physicians should remind patients that they are in charge of all the important decisions, and free to choose whatever action (or inaction) they want.

In Jim's *precontemplation* dialogue above, instead of saying, "I appreciate that you do not intend to do that right now," you could say:

> **Doctor:** It is your choice whether you wish to make any change in your drinking. I will always give you my best advice, and you make the final decisions.

At a suitable time when the conversation is going well (a true dialogue and not argumentative or discouraging) tell patients why they have a chance of success, based on facts the doctor knows about their unique characteristics, past successes, attitude, and other attributes. "You've told me how independent, even stubborn, you can be, and that may mean that when you decide to do something difficult, you can stick to it." "You quit using drugs for 5 years once before, so you know it is possible." "You said you are pretty depressed, and I also hear/see that you have come through similar moments in the past by getting involved with people in AA." Psychologists call this action "supporting self-efficacy." People do not attempt difficult change unless they think success is somehow possible.

In Jim's *contemplation* dialogue above, you might continue your opening phrase, "Jim, I appreciate that you are thinking about this matter" differently. You could see if it strengthens his commitment:

> **Doctor:** I know you have been able to take your blood pressure medicine very steadily over the years, so you can accomplish what you put your mind to. I wonder if you would be willing to take careful note of both the good and the not-so-good things about drinking and also about not drinking in the next few weeks?

Another method is to help people express their own commitment, especially if they can do so emphatically. Again, find a suitable moment when the conversation is going well (a true dialogue and not argumentative or discouraging). Then, when the patient makes a statement that is positive, or hopeful, or promises success, the clinician expresses the patient's previously stated skepticism or ambivalence. This reminder (actually, a *reflection* of prior patient statements) encourages patients to take the "healthful" side in the dialogue, perhaps even to claim strength, or give a new reason for hope.

For example, consider the *preparation* dialogue above, after Jim says "and I almost went to AA with him after I got my OUI." You could calibrate his commitment:

Doctor: From what you said about not having any problems, it does not seem to me that you are quite ready to go to AA, yet.

Jim: I feel my only good choice is to get to AA!

You can then build on this discrepancy between prior and current expectations.

Doctor: Would you be willing to share what you learn at AA with me when I see you again in a month or so?

Prochaska and DiClemente conceptualize life-style change as a continuum of psychological processes that includes noticing, contemplating, imagining, and deciding to take action. Research shows that moving one stage toward change increases the likelihood of ultimate success in adopting new behaviors. Clinicians can therefore be justifiably optimistic when patients progress from one stage to the next, rather than discouraged when patients don't take action and accomplish permanent changes as soon as they would like.

MANAGEMENT STRATEGIES FOR SPECIAL SITUATIONS

Which Patients Should the Primary Care Physician Refer to a Specialized Treatment Program?

Treatment programs provide patients with specialized care, and physicians should refer any patients who do not make good progress on changing substance-use patterns. Whether patients are making progress is more important to the need for referral than the apparent level of problem or the specific diagnosis of at-risk use, abusive use, or dependent use. Substance-dependent patients may benefit from access to detoxification services and multidisciplinary counseling opportunities. Treatment programs can help patients initiate contact with community-based self-help organizations, halfway houses, and intensive counseling, sometimes in an inpatient setting. Programs with dual-diagnosis treatment capabilities are able to serve patients with additional psychiatric problems (40–60% of all referrals in most programs) more comprehensively than any physician's office. Physicians in treatment programs are better prepared to prescribe and monitor medications of specific utility, such as disulfiram, naltrexone, and clonidine.

How Can Physicians Increase the Likelihood That Patients Will Follow Through on Referrals?

The foremost strategy is to confirm the patient's intention and commitment to follow through, as discussed in the sections above on making choices, supporting autonomy, and giving advice. An additional strategy is to emphasize your need for a second opinion from a specialist, just as might be the case with referral to a cardiologist. Set up the appointment before the patient leaves the office. Tell the patient you will send a referral letter summarizing your views and asking for advice from the specialist. Let the patient know that you will speak with the specialist after the assessment, and that you would like to participate in the treatment plan and provide follow-up with visits to your office, if everyone agrees to this.

Many communities have programs for patients with special needs, such as adolescents, women, abusers of particular drugs (methadone treatment for opiate abuse is the best-known example), and patients with severe psychiatric problems. Self-help alternatives to Alcoholics Anonymous exist in many communities; Rational Recovery is one example and Women for Sobriety is another.

PHARMACOLOGICAL CONSIDERATIONS IN PRIMARY CARE PRACTICE

One option that a primary care physician might suggest is disulfiram or naltrexone. Each has been shown to be effective in certain circumstances. Disulfiram provokes acetaldehyde accumulation after the ingestion of alcohol, producing a toxic state manifest by nausea, headache, unpleasant flushing, and respiratory distress. Severity depends on dose of alcohol and blood level of disulfiram. Patients must take several doses of disulfiram to achieve an adequate blood level, and similarly, a patient must go 4–7 days without medication to avoid the reaction to alcohol. Randomized studies of disulfiram use are negative, and of uncertain generalizability. Clinicians who present disulfiram as one option to patients not doing well, using the skills discussed above, find patients who clearly benefit from it. The recommended prescription is two 250 mg tablets daily for 4 days, then one daily. Have patients commit to use in 3-month blocks, so as to avoid undermining their commitment to abstinence by frequently asking the question, "Have I used this long enough; can I stop now?"

Disulfiram and naltrexone can be useful adjuncts. Although randomized treatment studies are mostly negative, they usually involve selected populations. Many addiction specialists agree that each drug can be helpful for patients who commit to abstinence, and cannot remain sober. Because patients may imagine that these medications will provide a miraculous cure, the physician should promote this additional step towards abstinence, and also steer the patient towards an improved recovery regimen. The PCP should refuse to prescribe unless the patient undertakes additional action steps, for example towards more involvement with addiction professionals or self-help groups.

Disulfiram provokes acetaldehye accumulation after alcohol ingestion, producing a toxic state manifest by nausea, headache, flushing, and respiratory distress. Severity depends on dose of alcohol and blood level of disulfiram. Achievement of adequate blood levels requires several doses of disulfiram, and one must wait 4–7 days after discontinuation to avoid the alcohol reaction. We recommend two 250 mg tablets daily for 4 days, then one daily. Naltrexone diminishes craving, and treated patients who do drink usually have shorter drinking episodes. Because of possible nausea and other side effects, start naltrexone at half-dose, 25 mg daily for 4 days, then increase to 50 mg. Monitoring of liver function tests is suggested. Patients should commit to use in 3-month blocks to avoid undermining the commitment to abstinence by frequently asking, "Have I used this long enough; can I stop now?"

SUGGESTED READINGS

Brown R et al: A two-item screening test for alcohol and other drug problems. J Fam Pract 1997;44:151.

Fiellin D, Reid C, O'Connor P: Outpatient management of patients with alcohol problems. Ann Intern Med 2000;133:815.

Fleming MF et al: Brief physician advice for alcohol problems in older adults. A randomized community-based trial. J Fam Pract 1999;48:378.

Friedman P, Saitz R, Samet J: Management of adults recovering from alcohol or other drug problems: relapse prevention in primary care JAMA 1998;279:1227.

Garbutt J et al: Pharmacological treatment of alcohol dependence: a review of the evidence. JAMA 1999;281:1318.

Krystal JH, Cramer JA, Krol WF, Kirk GF, Rosenheck RA, the Veterans Affairs Naltrexone Cooperative Study 425 Group: Naltrexone in the Treatment of Alcohol Dependence. N Engl J Med 2001;345: 1734–1739

Mayo-Smith M: Pharmacological management of alcohol withdrawal: a meta-analysis and evidence-based practice guideline. JAMA 1997;278:144.

Miller W: Motivational interviewing: research, practice, and puzzles. Addict Behav 1996;21:838.

Miller WR, Benefield RG, Tonigan JS: Enhancing motivation for change in problem drinking: a controlled comparison of two therapist styles. J Consult Clin Psychol 1993;61:455.

Miller WR, Rollnick S: *Motivational Interviewing: Preparing People to Change Addictive Behavior.* Guilford Press, 1991.

NIAAA: The physicians' guide to helping patients with alcohol problems. Government Printing Office, 1995 (NIH publication #95-3769).

O'Connor P, Schottenfeld R: Patients with alcohol problems. N Engl J Med 1998:338:592.

Prochaska JO, DiClemente CC, Norcross JC: In search of how people change. Applications to addictive behaviors. Am Psychol 1992;47:1102.

Sanchez-Craig M, Wilkinson D, Davila R: Empirically based guidelines for moderate drinking: 1-year results from three studies with problem drinkers. Am J Pub Health 1995;85:823.

WEB SITES

www.alcoholmd.com
www.asam.org
www.drugabuse.gov
www.niaaa.nih.gov

Section IV
Mental & Behavioral Disorders

Depression

21

Steven A. Cole, MD, John F. Christensen, PhD, Mary Raju Cole, RN, MSN, FNP,
& Mitchell D. Feldman, MD, MPhil

INTRODUCTION

Depression is common, disabling, and often unrecognized or inadequately treated in general medical practice. This chapter focuses on the diagnosis and management of major depression. Other mood disorders are briefly discussed, including chronic depression (dysthymia), minor depression [adjustment disorder with depressed mood and depression not otherwise specified (NOS)], depression secondary to general medical conditions, and bipolar disorder (Table 21–1).

DEFINITIONS

Major depression (MD), the most severe form of depression, is associated with considerable disability, morbidity, and mortality. Epidemiological studies demonstrate that depression is associated with as much, and often more, physical and social disability as other chronic illnesses, such as diabetes, arthritis, hypertension, and coronary artery disease. The increased risk of death seen in patients with depression is only partially attributable to the increased risk of suicide. Recent studies indicate a 59% increase in mortality among nursing home patients with major depression and a threefold increased risk of mortality among postmyocardial infarction patients with comorbid major depression. Patients with diabetes and depression have decreased adherence, higher glycosolated hemoglobin levels, and higher micro- and macrovascular complications.

Chronic depression, or **dysthymia,** is a milder but chronic form of depressive illness that is associated with significant disability. Dysthymia is diagnosed when depressed mood and at least two other symptoms of depression have been present "most days" during the previous 2 years.

Minor depression, which causes functional impairment but does not meet the criteria for major depression, includes adjustment disorder with depressed mood and depressive disorder not otherwise specified (NOS). **Adjustment disorder with depressed mood** results from an identifiable stressor, such as divorce or job loss. It presents with a level of impairment greater than expected for most individuals and can be diagnosed within the first 6 months after a stressor has occurred. A "normal" reaction to a distressing life event should not be diagnosed as an adjustment disorder. When a stressor precipitates a depressive syndrome that meets the severity criteria for major depression, the diagnosis of major depression is made. **Depressive disorder NOS** is a condition that lasts longer than 6 months after a precipitating stressor. Depression NOS is also used to describe mixed states of anxiety-depression that do not meet criteria for other anxiety or depressive diagnoses.

Mood disorders due to a general medical condition (or substance) refers to a psychiatric syndrome judged to result from the direct physiological consequence of a general medical condition (eg, hypothyroidism), substance use (eg, amphetamine withdrawal), or medication (eg, reserpine). Treatment focuses on resolution of the underlying general medical problem or withdrawal of the offending medication, although specific psychiatric treatment may also be required.

Bipolar disorder (also known as "manic-depressive" illness) is a common and severe mental illness that occurs in about 1% of the population and carries a strong genetic

Table 21–1. Mood disorders.

1. Major depression
2. Chronic depression (dysthymia)
3. Minor depression
   a. Adjustment disorder with depressed mood
   b. Depression NOS (not otherwise specified)
4. Depression secondary to a general medical condition
5. Bipolar disorder

vulnerability. Patients with presumptive diagnoses of depression should always be screened for bipolar disorder.

EPIDEMIOLOGY

Epidemiological studies demonstrate a lifetime prevalence of major depression in 7–12% of men and 20–25% of women. The point prevalence of major depression in a community sample is 2.3–3.2% for men and 4.5–9.3% for women. Reasons for these gender differences have not been fully elucidated, but both biological and sociocultural factors are involved. Numerous studies report a 5–10% prevalence of major depression in primary care settings with a substantially higher rate (20–40%) in patients with coexisting medical problems, particularly in those with diseases associated with strong biological or psychological predispositions to depression (eg, stroke, Parkinson's disease, traumatic brain injury, pancreatic cancer, and other terminal illnesses).

Prevalence of depression varies among age groups. Recent data point to a cohort effect through which current "baby boomers" (age 35–50 years) experience the highest rates of depression of any previous generation. Although the most current epidemiological findings show a surprisingly low 1-year prevalence rate of major depression in the elderly (1–2%), the rate of major or minor depression in elderly patients who seek treatment in primary care practices is 5%, with rates ranging from 15% to 25% in nursing home residents. Major depression is often misdiagnosed in elderly primary care patients as signs of aging, and cognitive impairment may also complicate accurate diagnosis. Some medications commonly prescribed in the elderly population may actually precipitate the onset of depression. Because the usual age of onset of depression is under 40, an apparent first episode of depression in an older patient should prompt a thorough evaluation to exclude other underlying disease and medication effects.

Depression is often mistakenly believed to be an "expected" result of stressful life events. Studies of individuals under stress (eg, terminal cancer or natural disaster) do show rates of major depression above the general population rate, but these rates rarely exceed 50%. Although sad or depressed affect is an expected accompaniment of a stressful event, the full syndrome of major depression does not necessarily emerge. Thus, there may be "good reasons" for sadness, but no good reasons to explain a syndrome of major depression. If such a syndrome emerges following a stressful life situation, the primary care provider should strongly consider the diagnosis of major depression and treat it appropriately.

The term *reactive depression* has historically suggested a mild syndrome without a biological substrate, resulting from a psychological precipitant, and treatable with psychotherapy alone. None of these assumptions is true. A very severe depressive syndrome can result from a stressful event; a biologically predisposed individual may suffer major depression in response to a life event; a major depression resulting from a life stress may develop a biological substrate; and a major depression from a life stress may respond to biological therapy as well as or better than it responds to psychotherapy. *Thus, the presence or absence of identifiable precipitants is irrelevant to the diagnosis of major depression,* which can be treated pharmacologically whether or not the condition resulted in part from psychological stressors.

A comorbid general medical condition (such as cancer or Parkinson's disease) may seemingly "cause" many of the physical symptoms of major depression, such as fatigue, anorexia, or psychomotor retardation. These symptoms may lead clinicians to discount their relevance and thus disregard the possibility of a treatable depression. Emerging data and the revised American Psychiatric Association *Diagnostic and Statistical Manual of Mental Disorders,* 4th edition (*DSM-IV*) criteria for major depression emphasize the importance of including these symptoms in the initial diagnostic approach to depression in the medically ill, and excluding them only if their origin is clearly the result of medication or a physiological condition. Although this "inclusive" approach might seem to result in an overdiagnosis of major depression, studies in stroke, Parkinson's disease, and traumatic brain injury indicate that the problem of overdiagnosis is, if anything, quite low (around 2%).

ETIOLOGY

Major depression represents a heterogeneous group of disorders, most probably arising from a host of etiological determinants. Because no clear anatomic, biochemical, or physiological lesions have been found to explain major depression, most investigators agree that it is a complex psychobiological syndrome that can be diagnosed only on clinical, syndromal criteria. Some promising genetic, biological, and psychosocial studies, however, suggest etiological possibilities as well as therapeutic interventions.

GENETIC FACTORS

Research to date identifies a combination of environmental and biological factors underlying severe mood disorders.

Apparently, genetic and family experiences both play roles, although neither is a determining factor. For example, even for bipolar disorder, which has very strong genetic loading, monozygotic twins may experience a 50% concordance prevalence rate, whereas dizygotic twins show a 10% concordance rate (about the same as siblings). Recent data from twin studies on depression in women indicate that genetic factors play the strongest etiological role in depression, followed by recent (as opposed to early environmental) negative life events. Animal studies, on the other hand, demonstrate that early environmental stress predisposes to biological abnormalities associated with depression that may not emerge until adult life.

BIOLOGICAL FACTORS

Numerous biological "markers" of depression have been identified. Although these factors may underlie major depression, they do not necessarily "cause" it. Environmental stress can lead to psychic distress precipitating a biological cascade eventuating in major depression. Several biological markers reliably and statistically differentiate groups with and without major depression, but no marker is specific enough to be used diagnostically.

Some markers include endocrine factors: elevated cortisol; inability to suppress endogenous cortisol production after receiving exogenous dexamethasone (DST); blunted response of thyroid-stimulating hormone (TSH) to thyroglobulin-releasing factor (TRF); and increased growth hormone response to prolactin. Central nervous system levels of norepinephrine (NE) and serotonin (5-hydroxytryptamine: 5-HT) may be altered, but more likely, NE or 5-HT receptor function (or both) or number is affected by depression. Platelet imipramine and platelet paroxetine binding have been identified as markers of central serotonin activity. Major depression also impairs sleep physiology, with early induction of rapid eye movement (REM) sleep and overall increase of REM density. Positron emission tomography studies point to anatomically specific sites of metabolic differences between depressed individuals and controls.

SOCIAL & PSYCHOLOGICAL FACTORS

Significant psychosocial stressors, especially those involving loss, often trigger depression. The loss of a parent or spouse, the end of a relationship, and events involving loss of self-esteem, such as termination from a job, seem to be especially vulnerable periods for patients. It is important that the primary care provider not overlook a major depression because of having attributed it to the presence of a major life-stressful event. In addition, the absence or perceived lack of social supports increases an individual's vulnerability to depression in the face of life stressors.

Postpartum "blues" typically occurs in 50–80% of women within 1–5 days of childbirth and lasts up to 1 week.

This "normal" reaction should be distinguished from postpartum psychosis, which occurs in 0.5–2.0/1000 deliveries and typically begins 2–3 days after delivery. It is also distinct from nonpsychotic depression, which occurs in 10–15% of women in the first 3–6 months after childbirth.

DIAGNOSIS

DSM-IV criteria for major depression require that five of nine symptoms be present for a 2-week period (Table 21–2). One of these nine symptoms must be either a persistent depressed mood (present most of the day, nearly every day) **or** pervasive anhedonia (loss of interest or pleasure in living).

Thus, clinicians should realize that a depressed mood is not synonymous with major depression. Depressed mood is neither necessary nor sufficient for a diagnosis of major depression. Sadness (or tearfulness) does not constitute major depression (four other symptoms described in the following paragraph are necessary), and, conversely, major depression can be diagnosed without the presence of depressed mood (if pervasive anhedonia is present).

Clinical evaluation can be facilitated by organizing these nine symptoms into clusters of four hallmarks: (1) depressed mood; (2) anhedonia; (3) physical symptoms (sleep disorder, appetite problem, fatigue, psychomotor changes); and (4) psychological symptoms (difficulty concentrating or indecisiveness, guilt or low self-esteem, and hopelessness). Physical symptoms predict a favorable response to biological intervention. For example, when middle insomnia is present (awaking at 3 or 4 AM with an inability to return to sleep) and when a diurnal variation in mood is present (feeling more depressed in the morning), patients are more likely to respond to biological interventions.

Table 21–2. Diagnosis of major depression.

1. Depressed mood
2. Anhedonia (lack of interest or pleasure in almost all activities)
3. Sleep disorder (insomnia or hypersomnia)
4. Appetite loss, weight loss; appetite gain or weight gain
5. Fatigue or loss of energy
6. Psychomotor retardation or agitation
7. Trouble concentrating or trouble making decisions
8. Low self-esteem or guilt
9. Recurrent thoughts of death or suicidal ideation
10. Five symptoms from the preceding list, but depressed mood or anhedonia is required. The symptoms must all have been present most of the day, nearly every day for 2 weeks

THE MEDICAL INTERVIEW

The medical interview is the key to the assessment of major depression. Efficient assessment involves attention to data-gathering as well as rapport-building functions of the interview. Physicians should observe nonverbal cues: for example, a sad mood may be communicated by downcast eyes, slow speech, wrinkled brow, or tearful affect. When a depressed mood is detected or emotional distress is suspected, physicians should use open-ended questions and facilitation techniques to provide patients with the opportunity to discuss the issues that are troubling them (see Chapter 1).

Physicians screening specifically for depression should focus on anhedonia ("What do you do for a good time?") or sleep ("How is your sleep?"). These questions often yield positive responses, despite the patient's focus on physical complaints or tendency to deny depressed mood. The lack of capacity for pleasure is a central hallmark of major depression.

BARRIERS TO DIAGNOSIS

Patient Barriers

SOMATIC PRESENTATIONS

Many patients with major depression present with problems such as pain (headache, backache), fatigue, insomnia, dizziness, or gastrointestinal problems. Such somatizing patients seldom state or even recognize the fact that they may be depressed. In these patients, evaluating both general medical and psychiatric problems simultaneously saves time, expense, and frustration for both physician and patient.

STIGMA

Many patients and families are reluctant to accept the diagnosis of depression because of its associated social stigma. Physicians sometimes also avoid diagnosing depression because of this stigma. Physicians can help overcome this barrier by understanding and explaining to patients and families that depression is a common and treatable illness, like other medical illnesses. Depression represents a chemical imbalance that can, like diabetes and other medical conditions, be corrected or managed with adequate treatment.

Clinician Barriers

In at least 30–70% of patients depression is either undetected or is not adequately treated by primary care providers. Inadequate knowledge and skill, lack of time, reluctance to "open up" new domains of emotional distress, and financial discrimination all operate as barriers to recognition and treatment.

"PANDORA'S BOX"

Physicians often feel reluctant to pursue psychiatric or emotional problems for fear this will open a "Pandora's box" and take an unreasonable amount of time. Attention to emotional issues, however, can be efficient and cost effective when physicians respond to patients' emotions and appropriately manage psychiatric disorders. Time can be conserved, while minimizing the number of extended work-ups for nonspecific physical complaints.

FINANCIAL DISCRIMINATION

Providers may avoid the diagnosis and treatment of mental disorders because coding for counseling or pharmacotherapy of depression may not be reimbursed or may be reimbursed at lower rates than treatment of general medical conditions.

SUICIDE

Suicide is one of the top 10 causes of death in all age groups, one of the top 3 causes in young adults and teenagers, and needs to be evaluated in all patients with symptoms of depression. Risk factors for completed suicide include gender (elderly white males are at highest risk), alcoholism, psychosis, chronic physical illness, and lack of social support. Higher risk of suicide has also been noted among adolescents (see Chapter 10) and among gay and lesbian patients (see Chapter 13). Explicit suicidal intent, hopelessness, and a well-formulated plan indicate high risk. In assessing the risk of a stated plan for suicide, clinicians can use the mnemonic **SAL**. Is the method **S**pecific? Is it **A**vailable? Is it **L**ethal? Many patients who eventually commit suicide visit a primary care physician in the month before they take their lives.

The assessment of suicidal ideation is best approached gradually, with general questions like, "Do you sometimes feel that life is not worth living?" Eventually, the patient needs to be asked directly, "Do you ever feel like hurting yourself, or actually taking your own life?" Other approaches to this issue are summarized in Table 21–3.

Physicians are sometimes reluctant to explore suicidal ideation in the mistaken belief that asking about suicide may actually increase a patient's risk. To the contrary, assessment of suicidal tendencies usually reassures patients, reduces anxiety for both patient and provider, and facilitates partnership in suicide prevention.

Once a patient reveals suicidal ideation, the physician must consider psychiatric consultation and hospitalization. This clinical judgment has no absolute decision rules. The presence of risk factors should be kept in mind, but clinical judgment remains primary. If outpatient management is considered, physicians can rely on a "no suicide contract." Although no data on the effectiveness of this technique exist, it represents one common and useful tool for clinical practice. The no suicide contract involves asking the patient

Table 21–3. Questions for the suicidal patient.

1. How does the future look to you?
2. Do you ever feel that life is not worth living?
3. Do you sometimes feel it doesn't matter whether you live or die?
4. Have you ever considered taking your own life?
5. Have you developed a plan about how you might kill yourself?
6. Are you willing to promise me that you will call me (or this number) if you feel you cannot control an impulse to take your own life?

to promise the physician that he or she will contact the physician (or other appropriate caregiver) if there is a danger of losing control of a suicidal impulse. Clinicians should be cautioned, however, that having obtained a no suicide contract with a patient may give the clinician a false sense of security. Consequently, it is important to continue assessing suicide risk according to the indicators mentioned earlier throughout the course of the patient's depression.

SCREENING & ASSESSMENT TOOLS

Studies in primary care have reported that 30–70% of cases of major depression are not diagnosed. Recognizing the seriousness of undetected and untreated depression in primary care, the U.S. Preventive Services Task Force (USPSTF) now supports the use of primary care screening for depression "in clinical practices that have systems in place to assure accurate diagnosis, effective treatment, and careful followup." Although many tools to screen for depression are available, USPSTF recommends the use of a two-item screener for major depression that is as effective as longer screening instruments. Clinicians should ask, 1. "Over the past 2 weeks, have you ever felt down, depressed, or hopeless?" And 2. "Over the past 2 weeks, have you felt little interest or pleasure in doing things?" A positive answer to either of these two questions requires a full diagnostic assessment for depression.

One of the most important recent advances for the assessment and management of depression in primary care has been the validation of a very brief, patient-administered self-report tool, the Patient Health Questionnaire (PHQ-9). A nine-item instrument, the PHQ-9 has documented high sensitivity and specificity for the diagnosis of major depression. It also can be used as a severity tool to track patients' symptom severity and improvement over time. (The instrument and scoring key are in Appendices 21–A and 21–B. Pfizer holds the copyright for this tool, but it can be used in the public domain for clinical purposes or research. Readers are also referred to the web site of the MacArthur Foundation Initiative on Depression in Primary Care for materials related to the use of this instrument, www.depression-primarycare.org.)

This instrument in now endorsed by the Robert Wood Johnson Foundation, the MacArthur Foundation, the Institute for Healthcare Improvement, and the Bureau of Primary Healthcare for general use throughout primary care. We strongly encourage primary care providers to use the PHQ-9 routinely to assess depression and to monitor severity of depressive symptoms in response to treatment. An experimental item at the end of the instrument also helps clinicians identify patients who may be suffering from dysthymia (chronic depression).

PHYSICAL EXAMINATION

There are no specific diagnostic signs of depression. Some nonverbal cues, however, are suggestive (eg, wrinkled brow, downcast eyes, slow speech, psychomotor retardation or agitation, hand wringing, sighing, or shoulder-shrugging). A careful medical history and physical examination are required for the evaluation of depression at all ages, but especially in the elderly.

LABORATORY STUDIES

No laboratory studies can definitely diagnose major depression. A laboratory screen (complete blood count, chemistry profile, urinalysis, thyroid-stimulating hormone, and vitamin B_{12} levels), however, can rule out other conditions that may mimic or exacerbate depression. In treatment-resistant cases, or when indicated, a computed tomographic (CT) scan, magnetic resonance image (MRI), electroencephalogram (EEG), or lumbar puncture (LP) can be considered, but these studies do not need to be part of the standard work-up. Patients over age 40 usually require an electrocardiogram (EKG) to rule out conduction disturbances or bradycardia, especially if treatment with a tricyclic antidepressant is anticipated.

DIFFERENTIAL DIAGNOSIS
Mental Disorders

Other mental disorders also present with symptoms similar to depression and may, therefore, lead to misdiagnosis. In addition, depression often presents in combination with other mental disorders. Thus, knowledge of the other mental disorders common in primary care is essential. In general, the best way to approach the issue of psychiatric comorbidity is to evaluate the patient for major depression and treat the depression if it is present. Modifications of treatment may be necessary depending on the comorbidity present.

Anxiety Disorders

Anxiety is as common as depression in primary care. Anxiety is present in most cases of major depression, and depressive symptoms are common in anxiety disorders.

The most important anxiety disorders for the primary care physician are generalized anxiety disorder (GAD), panic disorder (PD), and obsessive-compulsive disorder (OCD). Central features of these disorders include pervasive and disabling anxiety (GAD), discrete panic attacks (PD), or the presence of unreasonable and recurrent behaviors or thoughts (OCD). Treatment of major depression by itself, however, often helps to resolve or improve these other co-existing conditions (see Chapter 22).

Somatoform Disorders

Because depression often presents with unexplained bodily complaints, the differentiation between a depressive illness and a somatoform disorder can be difficult (see Chapter 23). Depressive disorders are highly treatable, but somatoform disorders can be more chronic and refractory to treatment. Somatoform disorders are usually managed conservatively with a focus on improved functioning, whereas depression should be treated aggressively with the goal of complete recovery. Any of the somatoform disorders (conversion, somatization, hypochondriasis, body dysmorphic disorder, and somatoform pain disorder) can present comorbidly with major depression. Most patients with somatization disorder experience a major depression sometime in their lives.

Primary care physicians should focus on recognizing the symptoms of major depression. Despite the presence of a somatoform disorder, appropriate treatment of the major depression usually improves the somatoform disorder. With treatment of a comorbid depression, somatoform patients typically feel somewhat better, improve their functioning, and decrease their inappropriate use of general medical services.

Substance Abuse

Patients with alcoholism or other substance abuse problems commonly present with major depression. Physicians should be cautious about treating major depression in the context of substance abuse to avoid further enabling the abuse problem. Rather, the problem of the substance abuse needs aggressive intervention and treatment. Unlike anxiety disorders or somatoform disorders, treatment of major depression comorbid with alcoholism does not usually alleviate the substance abuse problem. Physicians need to evaluate patients for substance abuse and design separate treatment programs whether or not major depression is present. Mental health referral is usually indicated in such cases (see Chapter 20).

Personality Disorders

Personality disorders represent enduring character patterns that are deeply ingrained and are not generally amenable to alteration (see Chapter 24). They often complicate the diagnosis and management of mood disorders. Because patients with personality disorders can be difficult and demanding, physicians often try to minimize contact with them. Unfortunately, this may lead to avoidance of emotional issues and failure to diagnose depression.

Effective treatment of major depression often improves functioning when the depression coexists with a personality disorder, even if the underlying disorder is not fundamentally changed. Thus, physicians should evaluate the basic symptoms of depression in all distressed individuals, whether or not they have a comorbid personality disorder.

Dementia

In its early stages, dementia can be difficult to distinguish from depression. Depression leads to reversible cognitive impairment in the form of decreased concentration, memory difficulties, impaired decision-making ability, difficulty planning and organizing, and difficulty getting started on tasks. These are also impairments that can result from an irreversible dementing process. Likewise the effect of dementia on a person's functioning can lead to depressed mood. When diagnostic uncertainty exists, clinicians can treat the depressive component (with both medication and counseling) and observe for changes in the patient's cognitive symptom cluster.

Depression due to General Medical Conditions or Medications

Approximately 10–15% of all depression is caused by general medical illness. The diagnosis of "depression due to a general medical condition" is recognized by *DSM-IV* as a psychiatric condition and is considered to be the direct physiological result of a medical illness, such as hypothyroidism or hyperthyroidism, pancreatic cancer, Parkinson's disease, or left-sided strokes (Table 21–4). Because there are

Table 21–4. General medical conditions with high prevalence of depression.

Disease/Condition
Alzheimer's disease
End-stage renal failure
Parkinson's disease
Stroke
Cancer or AIDS
Chronic fatigue
General outpatient
Chronic pain

Source: Adapted, with permission, from Cohen-Cole SA, Kaufman K: Major depression in physical illness: diagnosis, prevalence, and antidepressant treatment (a ten-year review: 1982–1992). Depression 1993;9:181.

no clear criteria to help guide clinicians in their evaluation, this diagnosis is ultimately made on clinical inference, considering the timing of the depression in relation to the physical illness. The diagnosis becomes "depression due to a general medical condition, with major depressive episode" when five of nine of the symptoms of major depression are present. Data seem to indicate that standard treatments for major depression are effective in these cases.

Similarly, depression can be caused by exogenous medications (Table 21–5). For example, reserpine has long been known to cause a severe depressive condition in 15% of patients. Of critical importance is the understanding that no medication has been noted to "cause" depression in all patients. It is, therefore, crucial to carefully evaluate the clinical history and link the onset of depressive symptoms to the initiation of new medications or changes in the current regimen.

TREATMENT

Communicating with Depressed Patients

The process of the clinician's communication with a depressed patient should take into account the patient's slower rate of cognitive processing. Because busy primary care providers are used to processing information at a high volume, the mismatch between the provider's and the depressed patient's rate of processing can be equivalent to having a 28,800-baud modem interfacing with one that is operating at 1200 baud or slower. Consequently, it is important to present information in smaller chunks and allow silences for the patient to assimilate the information. Empathy skills appropriate to the relationship-building function of the medical interview (see Chapter 1) are important here. A simple reflection by the clinician of how bad the patient is feeling enhances rapport.

Presenting the Diagnosis

After eliciting symptoms from the patient, the clinician can summarize them as a preface to stating simply that "these symptoms indicate to me that you are suffering

Table 21–5. Medications that can cause depression.

- Antihypertensives
- Hormones
- Anticonvulsants
- Steroids
- Digitalis
- Antiparkinsonian agents
- Antineoplastic agents
- Antibiotics

---

from depression." It can be helpful to then add a couple of additional symptoms not mentioned by the patient, but which are often part of the depressed constellation, such as difficulty concentrating or making decisions. The addition of these symptoms enables the clinician to determine whether they are present or absent in the patient and, if present, enhances the patient's perception of the clinician's knowledge about this disease.

Because some patients may associate depression with a stigma, it is helpful to explain that major depression is a common biological disorder. Drawing a picture of a synapse and neurotransmitters may be helpful for some patients. It is often helpful to name famous people, such as Thomas Jefferson or Abraham Lincoln, who are known to have suffered from depression and yet led productive lives.

A crucial part of presenting the diagnosis is to instill hope that depression is a curable illness. The cure involves mobilizing patient resources (see the section on "Counseling by Physician") and sometimes external resources such as medication. Indicate that painful depressive symptoms can be relieved in time, and note that "others may notice improvements in you before you notice the change yourself" (see Chapter 6). When adverse life circumstances play a role in the cause of major depression, the physician can acknowledge the role played by the stressors, but must also help the patient understand that treatment of the depression can help him or her cope better with life's adversities.

 CASE ILLUSTRATION

A 45-year-old single woman came in to see her primary care physician complaining of abdominal pain and "nervous exhaustion." In the interview her physician noted that her affect was flat and that she spoke with long latencies. She was having trouble sleeping, frequently awakening after 4 hours of sleep with perspiration, heart palpitations, and obsessive worries about her job. She had assumed a new job 4 months earlier as manager of a hospital clinic that was converting to a new data management system. After the physician ascertained that the patient was not suicidal, she summarized the patient's concerns and presented her diagnosis in the following dialogue:

Doctor: It's obvious that these last few weeks have been like torture for you.

Patient: (Tearful) When I go to bed, I dread getting up the next day,... and I know I have to hold it together, because the whole clinic is depending on me.

Doctor: It sounds like you carry a lot of responsibility. Let's talk about what I think is going on, and then I'd like to get your ideas about that. You've said that you have less energy during the day and that you awaken frequently at night, sometimes getting only a few hours of sleep. You tend to judge yourself harshly, and lately you feel guilty that you're not accomplishing more. You've lost interest in things you used to enjoy, and lately all you can think about is your job. You're finding it harder to concentrate, and making simple decisions feels overwhelming. Did I leave out anything?

Patient: No . . . I . . . just don't know what's happening to me.

Doctor: All these symptoms indicate to me that you're suffering from depression. This is an illness that affects our nervous system in ways that rob us of our usual ability to enjoy the pleasures of life and to have confidence in our abilities. Your depressed mood causes you to view yourself through a distorted lens that filters out all recognition of your competence and abilities. (Pauses to check patient's response. After head nod from patient, she proceeds as follows.) Fortunately, depression is a very treatable illness and there are some very effective strategies you and I can work on together. This may be hard for you to believe right now, because of the hopeless feeling that accompanies depression, but I'm quite confident that within a few weeks you'll be feeling much better about yourself and about life.

Choice of Treatment

Research and experience of experts indicate that treatment is effective in approximately 70–90% of cases. Treatment can include medication, counseling by the physician, referral to a mental health specialist (psychiatrist, clinical psychologist, clinical social worker, or psychiatric nurse practitioner) for psychotherapy, pharmacotherapy, and in some cases electroconvulsive therapy (ECT). Patients may need to be reminded that they deserve to feel better. They should also be told that without treatment, they will probably continue to suffer the same symptoms for a long time.

Numerous recent quality improvement studies indicate that systematic implementation of a "chronic illness care" (or "chronic disease management") model of health care adds to the cost effectiveness of care for depression in primary care. Key aspects of the new model include the use of a care manager to help with education and follow-up of patients, as well as structured access to decision support tools or behavioral health specialists in a targeted way to provide collaborative care providers along with primary care providers.

Counseling by the Physician

The importance of the doctor–patient relationship cannot be overemphasized for the recognition and treatment of depression, especially in the presence of suicidal ideation. The physician must convey feelings of concern for patients to discuss personal and distressing aspects of their lives. Thus, the primary care physician should be skilled at the recognition and management of emotional distress.

Office counseling by the primary care physician may be helpful to patients with milder forms of depression, including major depression. The patient, however, should be notified that this interaction is not formal psychotherapy, unless the practitioner is actually trained in such treatment modalities. Psychotherapeutic situations invariably arouse strong emotions in both patients and physicians. When complex interpersonal issues or strong feelings emerge during office counseling, the physician should seek supervision from a trained therapist or consultation from a colleague.

The acronym SPEAK was developed by one of the authors (John F. Christensen) to help primary care physicians offer office counseling to depressed patients (Table 21–6). The five components of **SPEAK** (**S**chedule, **P**leasurable activities, **E**xercise, **A**ssertiveness, and **K**ind thoughts about oneself) are elements in behavioral, interpersonal, and cognitive approaches to psychotherapy. They provide a framework both for patient education and for ongoing supportive counseling by the physician. A one-page handout summarizing the SPEAK approach that can be given to patients is given in Appendix 21–C.

Following a *schedule* counteracts the motivational deficits and anergia that accompany depression. Frontal lobe functions of planning, organizing, and initiating activity are frequently impaired by depression. The physician can advise the patient to plan ahead and fill out a weekly schedule. The instructions are to follow what the schedule says, "whether or not you feel like it," thus making the patient's activities less mood dependent and more time contingent. The physician can present a rationale for the schedule, as well as other elements of SPEAK, perhaps using a metaphor like giving a car battery a "jump start" by getting the car moving.

The schedule should include *pleasurable activities* to counteract anhedonia and the tendency of depressed patients to withdraw from these types of activities. Although initially patients may feel they are "just going through the motions," ultimately involvement in pleasure may operate synergistically with the other elements of SPEAK in mild depression and with antidepressant medication in more severe depression to help restore neurotransmitter/neuroreceptor function. To stimulate patients to plan these activities the physician can administer a brief "Pleasant Event Inventory" (see Appendix 21–D), in which the

Table 21–6. SPEAK approach to physician counseling for depression.

S	Schedule
P	Pleasurable activities
E	Exercise
A	Assertiveness
K	Kind thoughts about oneself

patients are asked to list the 15 activities they find most enjoyable. Patients can be asked to complete this at home and bring it with them to a follow-up appointment.

Exercise, depending on the medical condition and physical capabilities of the patient, is important as a short-term mood enhancer and long-term prophylaxis against depression. Exercise not only involves kinesthetic movement (breaking somatic rigidity, which can play a role in maintaining a depressed mood) but also may release endorphins. The patient should be encouraged to exercise several times a week.

Assertiveness, often difficult for depressed individuals because of low self-esteem and a tendency to doubt their own judgment and opinions, is a key behavior in reversing depression. The physician can help the patient distinguish among nonassertive, assertive, and aggressive behaviors. It is helpful to describe assertiveness as "being direct with others about your feelings, opinions, and intentions." The physician can encourage the patient to make small acts of self-assertion (with significant others, friends, strangers) and to reflect on both their mood and interpersonal outcomes. Self-assertion often mobilizes and discharges affect externally, as opposed to depleting energy by inhibiting affect. It may be helpful to recommend some reading, such as Alberti and Emmons' *Your Perfect Right: Assertiveness and Equality in Your Life and Relationships.*

Kind thoughts about oneself is perhaps the most challenging element of the SPEAK approach for depressed patients. Patients can become more aware of the self-punishing nature of their thoughts. Using an approach developed by Ellis (1977), patients can be taught to trace the origin of a depressed mood to particular recurrent thoughts and to replace the self-punishing thoughts with positive ones, ideally on a three-to-one ratio of positive-to-negative thoughts. The physician can give patients a worksheet, such as the "ABCD Method of Thought Analysis" shown in Appendix 21–E, to review their emotions, activating events, and beliefs about those events, and to dispute irrational non-evidence-based beliefs giving rise to negative feelings.

There are two further considerations about the SPEAK approach to physician counseling of depressed patients. First, it is not meant to be a substitute for psychotherapy or medication when the use of either or both of these is clearly indicated according to the criteria mentioned elsewhere in this chapter. The primary care provider may consider trying it as a first approach, however, with medication or psychotherapy to be initiated if there is no response. More commonly the SPEAK approach works synergistically with appropriate medication. Second, this approach to counseling does not require an excessive time commitment by the physician. Often the SPEAK approach can be explained to the depressed patient in about 10 minutes, with about 5 minutes devoted to reviewing the relevant elements of SPEAK in follow-up visits.

Role of Formal Psychotherapy

Cognitive-behavioral, interpersonal, problem-solving, and psychoanalytical approaches to psychotherapy are all used in the treatment of depression. There is little evidence that psychoanalytical therapies are effective for primary care patients. Cognitive therapy attempts to identify and challenge pessimistic or self-critical thoughts that cause or sustain depression. Behavioral therapy (often combined with cognitive therapy) focuses on increasing involvement with rewarding activities. Problem-solving therapy teaches patients to break down larger life problems into smaller elements and to identify specific steps to address these elements. There is good evidence that cognitive-behavioral therapy is as effective as antidepressant medication in achieving a significant reduction or remission of depression (over 50% response rate) after 10 weeks of treatment. Although the response to treatment with antidepressants is greater in the first 4 weeks, the rate of response to psychotherapy is greater following that time period, and by 12 weeks the efficacy of medication and psychotherapy is similar. The most significant benefit, however, occurs with a combination of antidepressants and cognitive-behavioral therapy (85% of patients experienced remission in one study). The clinical benefits of psychotherapy are usually seen in 6–8 weeks, and the duration of treatment is typically 6–16 sessions.

Considerations for choosing psychotherapy in the acute phase of treatment are shown in Table 21–7. Besides being an adjunct to medication for the treatment of depression, psychotherapy may also have a role in prophylactic maintenance therapy for the prevention or delay of future depressive episodes in patients susceptible to recurrences. Consequently, psychotherapy can be useful for women with major depression who want to become pregnant and bear a child in a drug-free condition or for other patients with major depression who must be medication free for limited periods. In milder depressions, psychotherapy alone may be nearly as effective as psychotherapy combined with antidepressants.

The clinical criteria for referral to a mental health specialist depend a great deal on the experience and expertise of the primary care physician. Primary care physicians should inform patients at an early stage of treatment that consultation with a mental health specialist may be neces-

Table 21–7. Considerations for acute-phase treatment with psychotherapy alone.

- Less severe depression
- Prior response to psychotherapy
- Incomplete response to treatment with medication alone
- Chronic psychosocial problems
- Availability of trained, competent therapist
- Patient preference

sary if the depression does not fully remit. This can make referral at a later stage much more acceptable. Because partial remission is a common occurrence, physicians should make every effort to establish clear indications of pre-depression functioning, and if full return to baseline functioning does not occur, referral to a specialist should be made. In making the referral, the primary care provider should communicate with the mental health specialist and provide the following information: the nature of the depressive symptoms; baseline premorbid functioning; other treatments, including medication, that have been tried previously or are concurrent; and patient understanding and expectations about psychotherapy. Communication should be maintained with the mental health therapist about whether therapy is completed, since premature discontinuation of psychotherapy is even more common than premature discontinuation of pharmacotherapy.

Medication

Evidence demonstrates that antidepressant medications are effective for the treatment of major depression and dysthymia. There is no compelling evidence to date, however, to support the use of antidepressant medication for patients with minor depressive disorders. The initial treatment of choice for patients with minor depression is "watchful waiting," which amounts to physician support, office counseling, and close observation, with repeat assessment to document improvement, remission, lack of improvement, or possible transformation into major depression. Patients with minor depression who do not improve after 3–6 months of watchful waiting can be treated empirically with a trial of antidepressant medication or referred for psychotherapy.

Once a decision is made to initiate therapy, the provider should conceptualize treatment of depression as a three-phase process. The **acute phase** of treatment lasts approximately 6–12 weeks and has as its goal the reduction and removal of signs and symptoms of depression and the return to a premorbid level of functioning. Patients who achieve only a partial response (but not full remission) have a higher risk of relapse into acute depression again. Thus, patients who do not achieve a full remission (which can be defined as a score of less than 5 on the PHQ-9) should have their antidepressant medications adjusted or their psychotherapy intensified appropriately until full remission is attained. Once a remission is reached, the patient enters the continuation phase of therapy.

The **continuation phase** lasts for 4–9 months after the full remission of symptoms with the main goal being prevention of relapse. Medication should be continued at full dose. The **maintenance phase** of treatment, lasting 1 year or longer, aims to prevent recurrence in high-risk patients such as those with two prior episodes of depression or other special circumstances (see AHCPR guidelines).

Regular visits are essential for the proper care of the depressed patient. Follow-up in 2 weeks (or sooner if clinically indicated) by phone contact or formal visit is recommended in the beginning of treatment to evaluate dosage, side effects, and consequential changes in condition. Once the patient has become stabilized on a medication, monthly visits are important for support. Maintenance treatment, at previously prescribed antidepressant dosages, helps prevent recurrence and is recommended for patients who have experienced a total of three episodes of major depression. Quarterly visits are usually adequate during maintenance treatment.

For patients with fewer than three total episodes of major depression, the decision about maintenance treatment should be made in partnership between patient and provider. Approximately 50% of patients with one episode of major depression suffer a recurrence. Most experts recommend that patients should be tapered from antidepressant medications at the end of the continuation phase of a first episode of depression, especially if it has not been particularly severe. Medication can be tapered over a period of 2–8 weeks depending on the class and type of medication, raising the dose only if prodromal symptoms of depression reappear or the patient experiences significant symptoms of withdrawal.

Maintenance treatment with antidepressants, however, may also be warranted for patients with only one prior episode of major depression who also meet the following conditions: (1) a first-degree relative with bipolar disorder or recurrent major depression; (2) history of recurrence within 1 year after previously effective medication was discontinued; (3) early onset (before age 20) of the first episode; and (4) both episodes were severe, sudden, or life-threatening and occurred within the past 3 years. For prophylaxis, full-treatment dosages of antidepressants should be used on a chronic basis. Antidepressants are also effective for the acute, continuation, and maintenance treatment of patients with dysthymia.

CHOOSING AN ANTIDEPRESSANT

Table 21–8 summarizes current antidepressant medications used commonly in primary care. In selecting an antidepressant medication, the patient's concurrent medical or psychiatric illnesses, history of prior response, use of other medications, patient preference, cost, and side effects should all be taken into account. In general, all Food and Drug Administration (FDA)-approved medications are efficacious, so the key is to be aware of side effects and to exploit them clinically if at all possible.

First-line treatment by the primary care provider should generally be initiated with a selective serotonin reuptake inhibitor (SSRI) or one of the "other" first-line agents (see Table 21–8). They are all efficacious, even in more severe depression, but have very different side effect profiles. If a patient fails to respond to the first-line therapy, it is usually preferable to switch to a drug from a different class,

Table 21–8. Antidepressants: side effects, mechanisms of action, dosages.[1]

Antidepressants	Sedation	ACh Blockade	Orthostasis	SRI	NRI	Other Activity	Dosage (mg)
Tricyclics							
Amitriptyline (Elavil)	+++	+++	+++	++	+	0	75–300
Desipramine (Norpramin)	+	+	+	0	+++	0	75–250
Doxepin (Sinequan)	+++	+++	+++	++	+	0	75–300
Imipramine (Tofranil)	++	+++	++	++	+	0	75–300
Nortriptyline (Pamelor)	++	++	++	+	++	0	75–150
SSRIs							
Citalopram (Celexa)	0	0	0	+++	0	0	20–40
Fluoxetine (Prozac)	0	0	0	+++	0	0	20–80
Paroxetine (Paxil)	+	+	0	+++	0	0	20–50
Sertraline (Zoloft)	0	0	0	+++	0	0	50–200
Other new agents							
Bupropion (Wellbutrin)	0	0	0	0	+	DA/NE	150–450
Mirtazapine (Remeron)	+++	0	0	0	0	—[2]	15–45
Nefazodone (Serzone)	++	0	0	+	0/+	5-HT_{2A}[3]	300–600
Venlafaxine (Effexor)	0	0	0	+++	++	0	75–375

[1]0, none; +, slight; ++, moderate; +++, marked. ACh, acetylcholine; SRI, serotonin reuptake inhibition; NRI, norepinephrine reuptake inhibition; DA/NE, dopaminergic/noradrenergic activity.
[2]Blockade of α_2-NE, 5-HT_{2A}, 5-HT_{2C}, and 5-HT_3 receptors.
[3]Blockade of 5-HT_{2A} receptors.

although there are anecdotal reports that suggest that some patients who fail to respond to one SSRI will respond when switched to another.

Because antidepressant medication may initially increase anxiety or insomnia, especially in patients with an underlying anxiety disorder, it is important to inform patients of this possible, but usually time-limited side effect. Such medication-related anxiety or insomnia usually improves rapidly, and adjunctive low-dose sedating medication (eg, hydroxyzine, doxepin, trazodone, clonazepam, or lorazepam) may be used for a short time. Venlafaxine and most SSRIs are now known to be effective long-term antianxiety agents as well (for generalized anxiety disorder, panic disorder, social phobia, and obsessive-compulsive disorder), despite their potential to cause short-term increases in anxiety. Because of these antianxiety effects most patients on antidepressants are able to stop adjunctive anxiolytic medications, but some require continued combination therapy. Care should be exercised in the prolonged use of benzodiazepines, however, because of the possibility of habituation, tolerance, and build-up of drug levels with the use of long-acting agents.

COMMUNICATING WITH PATIENTS ABOUT MEDICATION

Patients initiating antidepressant medication for the first time sometimes are concerned about the stigma associated with their use. Some fear getting "hooked" on the medicine or that it will change their personality in some way. It is important to explain that this is a powerful but nonaddictive medicine that can restore the natural balance of neurotransmitters in the brain. It can be helpful to inform the patient about the possibility of experiencing some of the known side effects of the particular antidepressant and to refer to those side effects as an indicator of the drug's potency to achieve the desired results (see Chapter 6). Finally it is important to build a realistic expectation about the tempo of therapeutic effectiveness by letting the patient know that even though the symptoms of depression may persist for a week or two after starting the antidepressant, the healing process has already begun.

SELECTIVE SEROTONIN REUPTAKE INHIBITORS (SSRIs) AND OTHER FIRST-LINE AGENTS

SSRIs and other newer agents have revolutionized psychiatric practice, especially for treatment of depression in the elderly and in patients with comorbid general medical illnesses. Many patients too physically ill to be safely treated in the 1960s and 1970s can now receive these antidepressants without fear of dangerous side effects. These agents have an extraordinarily low suicide risk from overdose.

The most widely used of these medications include the SSRIs (citalopram, fluoxetine, paroxetine, and sertraline), bupropion, mirtazapine, nefazodone, and ven-lafaxine. These agents are generally safe and well tolerated. Unlike the older antidepressants, they do not cause postural hypotension or cardiac conduction delay. Antihistaminic side effects are minimal or nonexistent, and, with the exception of paroxetine (which has mild anticholinergic effects), none has any appreciable anticholinergic effects.

Four SSRIs are currently available in the United States (see Table 21–8) and are approved for use in depression. SSRIs potently and selectively block the reuptake of serotonin, one of the key neurotransmitters implicated in the symptoms of depression and anxiety.

All of the SSRIs used for depression can be dosed once daily. SSRIs undergo extensive metabolism by cytochrome P-450 (CYP450) enzymes in the liver. In addition, with the possible exception of citalopram and sertraline (at low, but not higher levels), SSRIs have high affinity for different isoenzymes of the CTP450 system and may be subject to numerous drug–drug interactions leading to increased drug levels (for example, anticonvulsants, digitalis, and warfarin). We recommend that providers utilize access to an electronic database (either on a hand-held device or desktop) to ensure that no known serious and potentially dangerous drug interactions are likely to ensue from such antidepressant prescriptions. The starting dose of the SSRIs is often the effective treatment dose. Patients not responding to the starting doses of SSRIs after 1 month should be given increased doses. Elderly patients and patients with liver disease or other general medical illness often require smaller starting doses, for example, one-half of the recommended dose.

The SSRIs may cause side effects such as anxiety, insomnia, gastrointestinal (GI) distress, and agitation. These tend to be mild, occur in less than 20% of patients, and usually do not lead to discontinuation of medication. Increasing attention is now being directed at understanding SSRI-induced sexual difficulties in males and females: decreased libido, difficulty attaining and sustaining arousal, and difficulty achieving orgasm. These sexual side effects may occur in 50% or more of patients using the SSRIs, and providers need to discuss these issues openly with their patients. Sexual side effects can be persistent and troubling.

Antidotes such as yohimbine and cyproheptadine have been tried with limited success as well as the adjunctive use of bupropion SR (up to 150 mg twice a day), but the only treatment with at least limited support from randomized clinical trials has been the use of sildenafil in males. Sexual side effects sometimes necessitates switching patients from SSRIs to an antidepresssant less likely to cause these problems, eg, bupropion.

Adjunctive use of a sedating antihistamine (diphenhydramine or hydroxyzine), sedating antidepressant (trazodone or doxepin), or anxiolytic (eg, clonazepam or lorazepam) can be helpful for patients who experience anxiety with SSRIs. When prescribing a sedating serotonergic antidepressant (such as trazodone) along with an SSRI, low doses of the sedating agent should be used to avoid a possible serotonergic syndrome. These adjunctive agents should usually be discontinued after a short time, but continued treatment with two agents is sometimes indicated. If a long-acting benzodiazepine is used in the elderly, care must be exercised to avoid a build-up of medication that can lead to confusion, sedation, or falls after several weeks of treatment.

Fluoxetine has the longest half-life (24–72 hours) of the SSRIs and has a long-acting metabolite with a half-life of 7 days. A long half-life may be problematic for some patients experiencing side effects or drug interactions, but it has not appeared to be a significant problem in clinical practice. In fact, with a long-acting agent such as fluoxetine, missing doses does not lead to breakthrough depressive symptoms and has led to the development of a once-weekly formulation. When the drug is to be withdrawn, doses can eventually be given once or twice a week, to allow for very smooth tapering. For elderly patients and those with hepatic impairment all SSRIs should be started at no more than half of the usual starting dose. Fluoxetine tends to be the most activating SSRI and may lead to more insomnia, and paroxetine is the most sedating and is often used in patients with concurrent anxiety (see Table 21–9). Patients who find paroxetine too sedating should be advised to take the medication at bedtime. Weight gain and withdrawal symptoms seem to occur more commonly with paroxetine than with other SSRIs.

Table 21–9. Comparative adverse effects of SSRIs.[1]

Drug	Nausea/ GI Upset	Insomnia	Somnolence	Weight Gain	Sexual Dysfunction	Anticholinergic Effects
Fluoxetine	+++	++++	+	+	+++	+/0
Sertraline	+++	++	++	+	+++	+/0
Paroxetine	+++	++	+++	+++	++++	++
Fluvoxamine	++++	+	++++	Unknown	++	+/0
Citalopram	+++	++	++	Unknown	+++	+/0

[1] 0, none; +, minimal; ++, mild; +++, moderate; ++++, severe.

Other first-line agents include bupropion, nefazodone, mirtazapine, and venlafaxine. Bupropion is chemically unrelated to other classes of antidepressants. It may be useful for patients with pronounced fatigue since it tends to be more activating. Unlike the SSRIs, it does not promote sexual dysfunction and in fact can be used with an SSRI to improve sexual function. Use of bupropion in doses above 450 mg/day or more than single doses of 150 mg at one time has been associated with an increased incidence of seizures so is contraindicated in patients with a history of seizure disorder as well as those with eating disorders or other conditions likely to result in electrolyte imbalance, or with a history of head trauma.

Nefazodone is a serotonin-2 agonist/serotonin reuptake inhibitor that is useful for patients with concurrent depression and anxiety. It seems to have little effect on any CYP450 system other than 3A4, which can be a particular problem for use with other drugs metabolized by this system, such as erythromycin, alprazolam, and ketoconazole. Its main side effect is sedation, often quite noticeable in the beginning of treatment, but which is tolerated as treatment continues. Sexual side effects are rare. Nefazodone should be initiated at a dose of 50–100 mg twice a day and titrated to a final dosage of 150–300 mg twice a day. The FDA has recently required a black box warning for nefazodone, however, because of a very rare (perhaps 3/100,000) side effect of liver failure, leading to the necessity for liver transplantation or in a few cases to death.

Mirtazapine is an α_2-receptor blocker that enhances both noradrenergic and serotonergic activity. Dosage is typically 15–30 mg and it is generally taken at night. Like nefazodone, it is especially useful in patients with prominent anxiety and depression and is seldom associated with sexual dysfunction. Common side effects include drowsiness (in up to 50% of patients) and weight gain. A very rare, but potentially fatal, side effect is agranulocytosis.

Venlafaxine is a combined serotonin and norepinephrine reuptake inhibitor that may assist patients who are refractory to other antidepressants. It has also attained a formal FDA indication for the treatment of generalized anxiety disorder. One recent meta-analysis comparing remission rates in multiple head-to-head comparisons of venlafaxine and SSRIs demonstrated that venlafaxine achieved significantly higher rates of remission than all other comparable SSRIs. This increased rate of remission is probably related to its broad range of activity at both serotonin and norepinephrine receptors. Side effects are similar to those of the SSRIs. The extended release (XR) formulation is easier to use and is generally better tolerated. About 3% of patients develop hypertension on this medication at lower doses and up to 10% on doses of 300 mg or above. Other aspects of venlafaxine that increase its usefulness in the medically ill and the elderly include its negligible effect on liver enzymes and its very low protein binding.

HETEROCYCLIC MEDICATIONS AND SIDE EFFECTS

Heterocyclic medications (see Table 21–8) include the tricyclics, which have been available since the 1950s, and several other agents similar in structure including maprotiline, amoxapine, and trazodone. Although the unit costs of these generic medications are usually much lower than brand name SSRIs, additional visits and other medical procedures are sometimes required with the use of heterocyclics making their overall health care costs about equal to that of the SSRIs.

When opting for a heterocyclic antidepressant, it is generally best to use a secondary amine (desipramine or nortriptyline) and to avoid the parent tertiary amines (eg, amitriptyline and imipramine) as they have more severe side effects, namely anticholinergic effects (dry mouth, constipation), antihistaminic effects (sedation), and postural hypotension. Start with a low dosage and gradually titrate up as tolerated. For example, start nortriptyline at 25 mg at night for 3 days and increase by 25-mg increments every 2–3 days until the patient reaches 75–150 mg. Patients can be kept at this dose for about 1 month, at which point the dose should again be raised if the patient has not reached remission. Heterocyclics can be given once a day (generally in the evening) to minimize side effects. There should be some beneficial effects after 2–3 weeks, with a full therapeutic response occurring after 4–6 weeks. If there is little or no response after an appropriate interval on an appropriate dose, check the blood level and increase the dose as indicated. The most common error leading to "treatment failure" with the heterocyclics is inadequate dosing. There is no reason to follow blood levels, however, in patients with an appropriate response and minimal side effects. The heterocyclic antidepressants have varying degrees of problematic side effects, including anticholinergic, antihistaminic, antiadrenergic, and quinidine-like effects.

CASE ILLUSTRATION (CONT.)

In the case of the 45-year-old clinic manager, the physician, after presenting the diagnosis, reviewed the SPEAK approach to the treatment of depression. She gave the patient the handout to read (Appendix 21–C). Discussion revealed that the patient had neglected pleasurable activities and that she engaged in negative self-judgments about her productivity, leading to a compulsive work schedule and failure to attend to the symptoms of fatigue. They decided that the P and K components of SPEAK deserved special attention, and the physician prescribed a long 4-day "strategic retreat" from work so the patient could implement a schedule that included exercise, pleasurable activities, and reflection on her thought processes, using the Pleasant Events Inventory (Appendix 21–D) and the ABCD Method of Thought Analysis (Appendix 21–E). The physician discussed the advisability of antidepres-

sant medication and the possibility of referral to a psychotherapist, but the patient was reluctant at this time to take these steps. The physician then negotiated an agreement that the patient would try the new schedule, that she would come back for an appointment in 2 weeks, and that if there was no improvement in sleep patterns and mood, she would undergo a trial of antidepressant medication.

The patient returned in 2 weeks, having forced herself to schedule in pleasurable activities and exercise, and having limited her work hours to a 40-hour week. Her symptoms of dysphoria and nocturnal awakening persisted. As they had agreed, the patient then began a trial of an SSRI in the morning and trazodone 50 mg at bedtime to aid in sleep. Within 4 days, a phone call to the doctor indicated that her sleep had improved dramatically. At an appointment 2 weeks later the patient showed improved affect and she reported feeling better. She indicated she was interested in pursuing psychotherapy to change her negative self-evaluations. The physician referred her to a psychotherapist for short-term therapy focused on altering these thought processes.

The patient showed complete resolution of symptoms in 6 weeks. Trazodone was discontinued, and she was maintained on the SSRI for 6 months. During that time she underwent eight sessions of psychotherapy, which resulted in increased self-awareness of her thought processes and a method to shift her thinking in a positive direction. She was seen for two additional therapy sessions in the month after discontinuing the SSRI to consolidate the gains she had made and

to monitor her for any recurrence of symptoms. At 9 months she reported to her primary care physician that she remained symptom free and that she was taking a 2-week vacation to the Caribbean.

ANTIDEPRESSANTS IN THE ELDERLY AND MEDICALLY ILL

For many of the reasons enumerated earlier, the new agents have generally become the agents of choice in the elderly and in the medically ill. Among heterocyclic agents, the safest agents are nortriptyline and desipramine, which are still widely used because of their relatively low anticholinergic and antiadrenergic side effects. They are also widely used as second-line treatment choices and play a role in the treatment of refractory depression, either as adjunctive or alternative treatments.

Dosing strategies in the elderly and medically ill are to "start low and go slow." Pharmacokinetically, these agents are metabolized more slowly, resulting in accumulation and toxicity. Increased pharmacodynamic effects in the elderly may result from lower albumin levels, leading to higher levels of unbound drug.

Electroconvulsive Therapy (ECT)

ECT is still the most effective means available for the treatment of refractory depression. It is the treatment of choice for patients with psychotic depression, depression refractory to pharmacotherapy, and for some patients who are

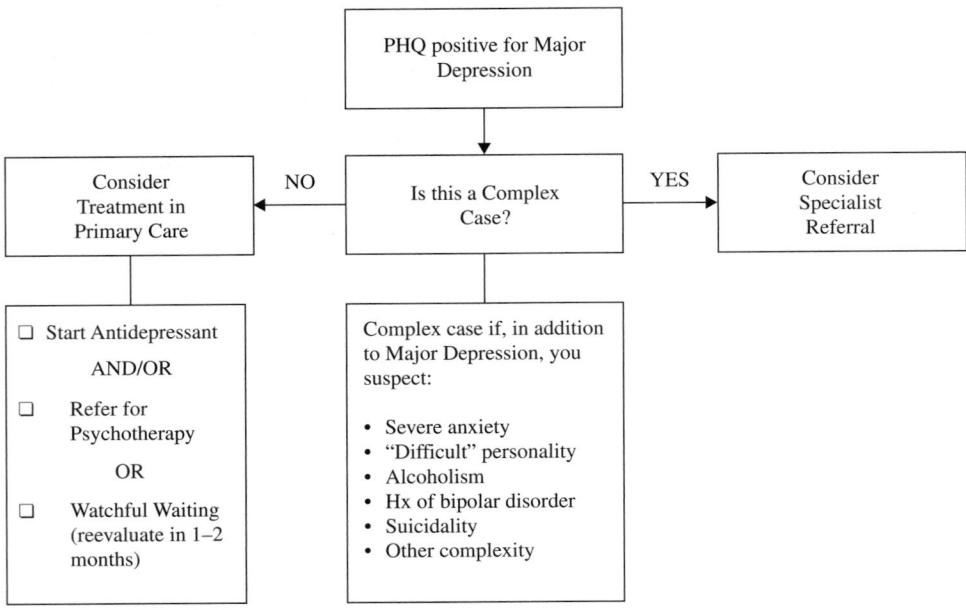

Figure 21–1. Treatment guidelines for major depression.

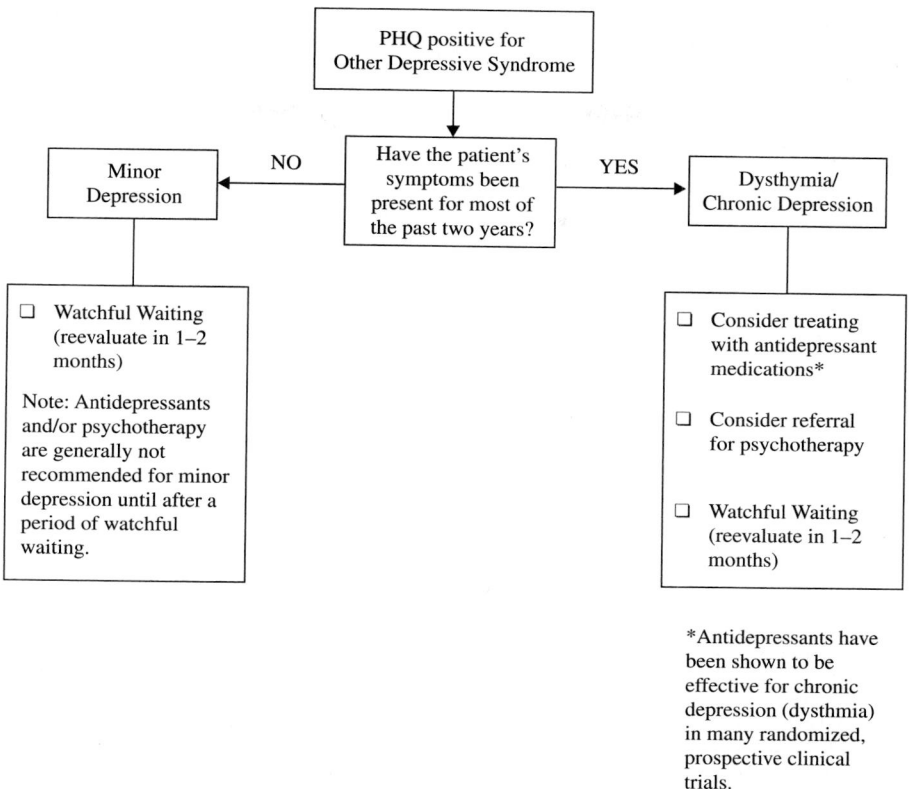

Figure 21–2. Treatment guidelines for other depressive syndromes.

acutely suicidal. Despite prejudices and fears about ECT, new methods of administration have proven it to be a safe and effective treatment modality. In fact, ECT can be safer than antidepressant medication in the elderly. Some short-term memory loss is common, but research indicates that this reverts to normal in virtually all patients. In some cases, ECT can be life-saving and should not be denied to patients because of poor understanding or unrealistic fear. ECT does not lead to permanent remission of depression in patients susceptible to recurrence. Thus, patients with recurrent depression who receive ECT should receive either prophylactic medication after a course of therapy (as an outpatient) or maintenance ECT.

See Figures 21–1 and 21–2 for treatment guidelines for major depression and for other depressive disorders.

MANAGED CARE

The time and organizational pressures of managed care settings may promote even further underdiagnosis and undertreatment of depression in primary care. Health services research indicates that fee-for-service and psychiatric set-tings may be more effective than prepaid settings for both the recognition and the treatment of major depression. With the sustained growth of capitation and managed care, however, new systems need to be developed to align clinical and financial incentives to increase the accurate assessment and optimal management of depression in primary care. Because depression is associated with increased use of health care services, as well as increased morbidity and mortality, attention to improving the assessment and treatment of depression in primary care should become a high priority for adding value to health care and improving the quality of patients' lives. Advances in chronic illness care, as noted above, including the effective use of care managers, hold great promise to broadly improve care for depressed patients in the primary care sector.

SUGGESTED READINGS

American Psychiatric Association: *Diagnostic and Statistical Manual of Mental Disorders,* 4th ed. American Psychiatric Association, 1994.
American Psychiatric Association: *Diagnostic and Statistical Manual of Mental Disorders,* 4th ed. *Primary Care Version* DSM-IV-PC. American Psychiatric Association, 1995.

Brody DS, Larson DB: The role of primary care physicians in managing depression. J Gen Intern Med 1992;7:243.

Brody DS et al: Strategies for counseling depressed patients by primary care physicians. J Gen Intern Med 1994;9:569.

Brown C, Schulberg HC: Diagnosis and treatment of depression in primary medical care practice: the application of research findings to clinical practice. J Clin Psychol 1998;54:303.

Byrne A, Byrne DG: The effect of exercise on depression, anxiety and other mood states: a review. J Psychosom Res 1993;37:565.

Cohen-Cole SA: *The Medical Interview.* Mosby-Year Book, 1991.

Cohen-Cole SA, Kaufman K: Major depression in physical illness: diagnosis, prevalence, and antidepressant treatment (a ten year review: 1982–1992). Depression 1993;1:181.

Davidson JRT et al: Effect of *Hypericum perforatum* (St John's Wort) in major depressive disorder: a randomized controlled trial. JAMA 2002;287.

Ellis A: The basic clinical theory of rational emotive therapy. In Ellis A, Grieger C (editors): *Handbook of Rational Emotive Therapy.* Springer, 1977.

Ernst E, Rand JI, Stevinson C: Complementary therapies for depression: an overview. Arch Gen Psychiatry 1998;55:1026.

Janicak PG et al: *Principles and Practices of Psychopharmacology.* Williams & Wilkins, 1993.

Karasu TB: *Psychotherapy for Depression.* Jason Araonson, 1990.

Keller MB et al: A comparison of nefazodone, the cognitive behavioral-analysis system of psychotherapy, and their combination for the treatment of chronic depression. N Engl J Med 2000;342:1462.

Kendler et al: The prediction of major depression in women: toward an integrated etiologic modal. Am J Psychiatry 1993;150:1139.

Olfson M et al: National trends in the outpatient treatment of depression. JAMA 2000;387:203.

Rush AJ et al: *Depression in Primary Care: Clinical Practice Guideline,* Number 5. U.S. Department of Health and Human Services, Public Health Services, Agency for Health Care Policy and Research, 1993. AHCPR Publication No. 93-0550.

Schulberg HC et al: Best clinical practice: guidelines for managing major depression in primary medical care. J Clin Psychiatry 1999;60(Suppl 7):19.

Simon GE, VonKorff M: Recognition, management, and outcomes of depression in primary care. *Arch Fam Med* 1995;4:99.

Spitzer RL et al: Utility of a new procedure for diagnosing mental disorder in primary care. The PRIME-MD 1000 study. JAMA 1994;272:1749.

Thase ME: Overview of antidepressant therapy. Manag Care 2001; 10(8 Suppl):6.

Thase ME et al: Treatment of major depression with psychotherapy or psychotherapy-pharmacotherapy combinations. Arch Gen Psychiatry 1997;54:1009.

Weismann MM et al: Brief diagnostic interviews (SDDS-PC) for multiple mental disorders in primary care. Arch Fam Med 1995;4: 220.

Whooley MA, Simon G: Managing depression in medical outpatients. N Engl J Med 2000;343:1942.

Whooley MA et al: Case-finding instruments for depression: two questions are as good as many. J Gen Intern Med 1997;12:439.

Williams JW et al: Rational clinical examination. Is this patient clinically depressed? JAMA 2002;287:1160.

PATIENT BIBLIOGRAPHY

Alberti RE, Emmons ML: *Your Perfect Right: Assertiveness and Equality in Your Life and Relationships,* 8th ed. Impact Publishers, 2001.

Lewinsohn et al: *Control Your Depression.* Prentice-Hall, 1978.

Seligman MEP: *Learned Optimism.* Knopf, 1991.

WEB SITES

National Institute of Mental Health Depression Information
http://www.nimh.nih.gov/publicat/depressionmenu.cfm
Agency for Healthcare Research and Quality
http://www.ahcpr.gov/research/mentalix.htm#Depression
The MacArthur Initiative on Depression and Primary Care
http://www.depression-primarycare.org/

Appendix 21–A. Patient Health Questionnaire—PHQ-9.

Name _____ Physician _____ Date _____

Over the *last two weeks,* how often have you been bothered by any of the following problems?

	Not At All (0)	Several Days (1)	More Than Half the Days (2)	Nearly Every Day (3)
1. Feeling down, depressed, or hopeless?	☐	☐	☐	☐
2. Little interest or pleasure in doing things?	☐	☐	☐	☐
3. Trouble falling or staying asleep, or sleeping too much?	☐	☐	☐	☐
4. Feeling tired or having little energy?	☐	☐	☐	☐
5. Poor appetite or overeating?	☐	☐	☐	☐
6. Feeling bad about yourself—or that you are a failure or have let yourself or your family down?	☐	☐	☐	☐
7. Trouble concentrating on things, such as reading the newspaper or watching television?	☐	☐	☐	☐
8. Moving or speaking so slowly that other people could have noticed? Or the opposite—being so fidgety or restless that you have been moving around a lot more than usual?	☐	☐	☐	☐
9. Thoughts that you would be better off dead or of hurting yourself in some way?[1]	☐	☐	☐	☐

10. If you are experiencing any of the problems on this form, how **difficult** have these problems made it for you to do your work, take care of things at home, or get along with other people?
☐ Not difficult at all ☐ Somewhat difficult ☐ Very difficult ☐ Extremely difficult

11. In the past two years, have you felt depressed or sad most days, even if you felt okay sometimes?
☐ Yes ☐ No

Office Use Only
Number of Symptoms: _____ _____ **Severity Score:** _____

[1] *If you have had thoughts that you would be better off dead or of hurting yourself in some way, please discuss this with your doctor, go to a hospital emergency room, or call 911.*

PHQ-9 is adapted from PRIME-MD Today, developed by Spitzer, Williams, Kroenke, and colleagues. Copyright 1999, by Pfizer, Inc. All rights reserved. Reproduction permitted for the purposes of clinical care and research only.

Appendix 21–B. Scoring the Patient Health Questionnaire.

How to Score the Patient Health Questionnaire (PHQ)

The PHQ can assist in diagnosing depression, as well as planning and monitoring depression treatment. There are three steps to scoring the PHQ: Number of Depressive Symptoms, Severity Score, and Functional Assessment. The Number of Depressive Symptoms is used to aid in making the diagnosis of Depression. The PHQ Severity Score and Functional Assessment are measured at initial assessment and regularly after treatment begins to determine the severity of depression and to evaluate patient progress.

Number of Depressive Symptoms (Diagnosis)

1. For questions 1–8, count the number of symptoms the patient checked as "More than half the days" or "Nearly every day." For question 9, count the question positive if the patient checks "Several days," "More than half the days," or "Nearly every day."
2. Use the following interpretation grid to diagnose depression subtypes:
   0–2 PHQ symptoms   Not clinically depressed
   3–4 PHQ symptoms[1]   Other depressive syndrome[2]
   5 or more PHQ symptoms[1]   Major depression

Severity Score

1. Assign a score to each response by the number value under the answer headings (Not at all = 0; Several Days = 1; More than half the days = 2; and Nearly every day = 3).
2. Total the values for each response to obtain the severity score.
3. Use the following interpretation grid:
   0–4   Not clinically depressed
   5–9   Mild depression
   10–14   Moderate depression
   15 or greater   Severe depression

Functional Assessment

The final two questions on the PHQ ask the patient how emotional difficulties or problems impact work, things at home, or relationships with other people and if this has caused difficulty for two years or more. Patient responses can be one of four: "Not difficult at all"; "Somewhat difficult"; "Very difficult"; or "Extremely difficult."

- If the patient selects one of the last two responses, "Very difficult" or "Extremely difficult," his/her functionality at work, at home, or in relationships with other people is significantly impaired.
- If the patient has had difficulty with these problems for two years or more, consider the diagnosis of dysthymia (chronic depression).

---

[1] *PHQ items #1 or #2 must be one of the symptoms checked.*
[2] *See algorithms (Figures 21–1 and 21–2) to differentiate minor vs. chronic depressions, with treatment recommendations.*

Steven Cole, MD, University of Connecticut.

Appendix 21–C. Overcoming your depression: The SPEAK approach.

S Schedule:

Make a weekly schedule for yourself, with columns for each day of the week and rows for the hours of the day. Using a pencil (so you can make changes) make a plan for activities you will do each hour. Some of the times will already be structured for you, eg, at work. Focus especially on the times that are currently unstructured. Start with things you know you usually do, eg, eating meals, preparing meals. Include on the schedule time to do household chores and errands, but also include times for fun activities and exercise. Because temporarily you may not feel the motivation or desire to do any of these things, follow what the schedule says **whether or not you feel like doing it.** Sometimes you might feel like you are just going through the motions. When the time comes to switch to another activity, do so **whether or not you have completed the previous task.** You are making progress by putting in time on all these activities, not by getting through your "to do" list. Proceeding in this way will help you move out of depression by getting yourself moving through the day.

P Pleasurable activities:

Some of the items on your schedule should be activities that previously were fun for you before you became depressed. You might have identified some of these pleasures on the Pleasant Events Inventory. For the time being you may feel you are just going through the motions in these activities. When we are depressed the part of the brain that allows us to feel pleasure is not functioning smoothly, so it is important to have a "jump start." You should plan something each day that would normally be fun and make yourself do it.

E Exercise:

Aerobic exercise increases oxygen and circulation to the brain and counteracts the hormonal changes caused by depression. It helps activate the natural pharmacy in your brain that will work with other parts of your treatment to help you come out of depression. Times for daily exercise should be included on your schedule. Running, swimming, bicycling, aerobic dancing, and walking are all forms of exercise that will help.

A Assertiveness:

This involves being **direct** with other people in your communication. Practice letting others know your feelings, needs, wants, opinions, and choices. This is more difficult when we are depressed, because we tend to doubt our own judgment. Or we might hold back because we are afraid others will think poorly of us. These thoughts are a product of depression, so it is necessary to act as if you were confident, even though inside you don't feel it. It takes more energy to hold in feelings than to express them. You might find that by stating clearly what you need or by saying "No" to what you don't want will help increase your energy and confidence. Read *Your Perfect Right* by Alberti and Emmons.

K Kind thoughts about yourself:

Since depression leads us to think self-punishing thoughts, it is very important to increase your awareness of when this is happening and to replace the negative thoughts with positive ones. Most of the time these negative thoughts are strongly held opinions that are not based on evidence. It is like carrying a negative, opinionated relative with you wherever you go. Once you become aware of this pattern of thoughts, begin to analyze them using the **ABCD** worksheet. You might write the most persistent negative thought on a 3×5 card. Then turn the card over and write three positive thoughts that you could replace it with. Carry this card with you and refer to it frequently. It takes about three positive statements to counteract the effect of one negative statement.

John F. Christensen, PhD.

Appendix 21–D. Pleasant Events Inventory.

Pleasant Event[1]	With Whom[2] A = Alone P = Partner F = Family O = Other People	How Often[3]	Last Time[4]	$ Amount if Costs Money[5]
1.				
2.				
3.				
4.				
5.				
6.				
7.				
8.				
9.				
10.				
11.				
12.				
13.				
14.				
15.				

[1] List the activities or events that have brought you the most pleasure over the years.
[2] Indicate with whom you like to share the pleasure.
[3] Indicate how often you do this activity.
[4] How long has it been since you engaged in this activity? If it has been months or years, perhaps you should schedule time for it soon.
[5] Make a $ sign if the pleasure costs money. You might be surprised at how many of your pleasures are free.

Appendix 21–E. ABCD method of thought analysis.

Activating Event	Belief	Consequence	Dispute
#2	#3	#1	#4
What happened before "C"?	What am I telling myself about "A"?	What am I feeling?	Where's the evidence for "B"?

DIRECTIONS:

1. Start your analysis in the C (*consequence*) column, by writing the negative emotion you have been feeling today. This emotion (eg, sadness) is a consequence of something else.
2. List in the A column the *activating event* that triggered the emotion. Answer the question, "What happened before I started feeling sad?" An example might be that a close friend did not reply when you said hello.
3. Now move to the B column and write down your *belief* about the activating event. This belief is the actual cause of your negative emotion. Answer the question, for example, "What am I telling myself about my friend ignoring me?" This answer will often be an irrational judgment not based on evidence, eg, "He's rejecting me," or more generally, "I'm a rejectable person."
4. The final step is to *dispute* the irrational belief by asking, "Where's the evidence for the statement in B?" Then write down a statement in Column D that is a more appropriate, less self-punishing belief about the activating event. For example, you might write down, "My friend was distracted because he's been under a lot of stress lately."

Anxiety

Jason M. Satterfield, PhD, & Wendy Levinson, MD

INTRODUCTION

Anxiety is a common, normal emotion; most people experience occasional trepidation, fear, nervousness, "jitters," or even panic. Mild anxiety may aid mental sharpness as uncertainty or pressure mounts. For some individuals, however, anxiety occurs as part of an anxiety disorder that is a prominent, persistent, and disruptive aspect of their daily lives. Among the general population in the United States, about 25% will experience an anxiety disorder at some time in their life, making anxiety more common than depressive disorders. At about $50 billion per year, the costs associated with anxiety surpass those of all the other mood disorders combined.

The major anxiety disorders are panic disorder (with or without agoraphobia), generalized anxiety disorder (GAD), adjustment disorder with anxiety, posttraumatic stress disorder (PTSD), acute stress disorder (ASD), specific phobia, social anxiety disorder (formerly social phobia), and obsessive-compulsive disorder (OCD). These disorders are particularly common among patients seeking primary care, as the majority of patients with anxiety disorders are initially seen in general medical settings. Because affected patients tend to complain of the prominent physical symptoms rather than the emotional symptoms of anxiety, providers must be alert and ask carefully worded questions to screen for these common disorders. (Table 22–1 lists some sample screening questions.) Comorbid psychiatric diagnoses are present in a substantial percentage of patients; depression, substance abuse, and another anxiety disorder are the most common of these. Distinguishing among the various anxiety disorders and identifying possible comorbidities are essential because of differences in treatment, complications, and prognoses. Cross-cultural epidemiological research has shown that anxiety disorders are present in all cultures, ethnicities, and age groups. The American Psychiatric Association *Diagnostic and Statistical Manual of Mental Disorders,* 4th edition—*Primary Care Version (DSM-IV-PC)* suggests an algorithm for determining which anxiety disorder may be the problem (Figure 22–1). Table 22–2 summarizes this algorithm. Diagnostic algorithms for depression, substance abuse, or other likely cormorbidities are found in other chapters of this text.

DIAGNOSIS

Careful use of office testing with one of a number of common screening surveys can improve the detection of anxiety and other mental disorders. These tests can also be used to evaluate treatment response or symptom progression in previously diagnosed patients. Before seeing the provider, patients can complete self-report measures, such as the Beck Anxiety Inventory or the anxiety subscale of the Hopkins Symptom Checklist 90 Revised (SCL-90). Brief, semistructured interviews such as the Hamilton Anxiety Rating Scale (HARS) must be administered by a provider but offer the advantage of quantifying the clinical assessment of symptoms of anxiety. However, many studies have shown that screening alone may not improve patient outcomes. Although screening can identify patients most likely to suffer from treatable anxiety disorders, it produces many false-positive results and does not provide guidance on appropriate treatment or improving patient adherence. If screening is used providers should follow positive screening tests with a more careful diagnostic assessment and selection of treatment.

The Primary Care Evaluation of Mental Disorders (PRIME-MD) uses this principle to improve available screening techniques. It uses a time-efficient two-stage assessment: (1) an initial patient-administered questionnaire that screens for anxiety and other mental disorders most common in primary care and (2) a structured interview that provides more detailed diagnostic information about identified problem areas. Published standardization data show that the interview requires an average of 8.4 minutes per patient and need not be administered by a physician.

Symptoms & Signs

Anxiety disorders typically manifest with emotional symptoms (eg, fear, nervousness), cognitive symptoms (eg, worry, a sense of doom, or derealization), and physical symptoms (eg, muscular tension, rapid heart rate, or dizziness). Primary care providers must therefore decide how much diagnostic investigation is both feasible and necessary to rule out other important nonpsychiatric diseases. For example, should a patient with palpitations undergo cardiac monitoring, thyroid function studies, or even cardiac catheterization? Should a patient presenting with nausea and abdominal pain undergo upper and lower en-

Table 22–1. Suggested screening questions for anxiety.

Disorder	Questions
Generalized anxiety disorder	Would you describe yourself generally as a nervous person? Are you a worrier? Do you feel nervous or tense?
Panic disorder	Have you ever had a sudden attack of rapid heartbeat or rush of intense fear, anxiety, or nervousness? Did anything seem to trigger it?
Agoraphobia	Have you ever avoided important activities because you were afraid you would have a sudden attack like the one I just asked you about?
Social anxiety disorder	Some people have strong fears of being watched or evaluated by others. For example, some people don't want to eat, speak, or write in front of people for fear of embarrassing themselves. Is anything like this a problem for you?
Specific phobia	Some people have strong fears or phobias about things like heights, flying, bugs, or snakes? Do you have any strong fears or phobias?
Obsession	Some people are bothered by intrusive, silly, unpleasant, or horrible thoughts that keep repeating over and over. For example, some people have repeated thoughts of hurting some one they love even though they don't want to; that a loved one has been seriously hurt; that they will yell obscenities in public; or that they are contaminated by germs. Has anything like this troubled you?
Compulsion	Some people are bothered by doing something over and over that they can't resist, even when they try. They might wash their hands every few minutes, or repeatedly check to see that the stove is off or the door is locked, or count things excessively. Has anything like this been a problem for you?
Acute stress and posttraumatic stress disorder	Have you ever seen or experienced a traumatic event when you thought your life was in danger? Have you ever seen someone else in grave danger? What happened?

doscopy? Understanding the signs, symptoms, and epidemiological features of the various anxiety disorders can help the physician make an accurate diagnosis and initiate timely, appropriate treatment while avoiding invasive or unnecessary testing. Appropriate diagnosis by the primary care doctor can prevent a series of referrals to specialists—each of whom may investigate the symptoms pertaining to his or her own specialty area. Early recognition of anxiety disorders can reduce patients' discomfort, medical expenses, iatrogenic complications, anxiety-related complications (eg, inability to face others or a fear of leaving home), and mortality (eg, suicide). In addition, an appropriate diagnosis of anxiety can reduce substance abuse, as patients may self-medicate with alcohol, benzodiazepines, or other substances in an effort to ameliorate their symptoms of anxiety.

CASE ILLUSTRATION 1

Gwen is a 28-year-old woman seeking care because of episodes of shortness of breath, racing heartbeat, and

a sensation that she is going to faint. The episodes have been occurring for 4 months, increasing in frequency until she is experiencing as many as four of them per week. She has seen another physician who conducted a number of tests, including thyroid function studies and a Holter monitor. The results are normal. The patient's concerns about her symptoms are escalating, and she is fearful that she may have an attack while driving or when out with her young children. The patient's husband is supportive and has assumed responsibility for routine household chores, such as grocery shopping and transporting the children. More detailed history revealed the patient is reluctant to perform these tasks for fear of having an episode. She is worried about her heart, as her mother had heart disease in her early fifties.

The physician recognizes that the symptoms are consistent with panic disorder. Further historical details eliminate other medical or substance-related illness. The doctor reassures Gwen that her symptoms are not unusual or unique to her and that 2–4% of all people suffer from panic disorder. Sensing that the patient might be embarrassed by a psychological diagnosis, the doctor explains the nature of panic disorder

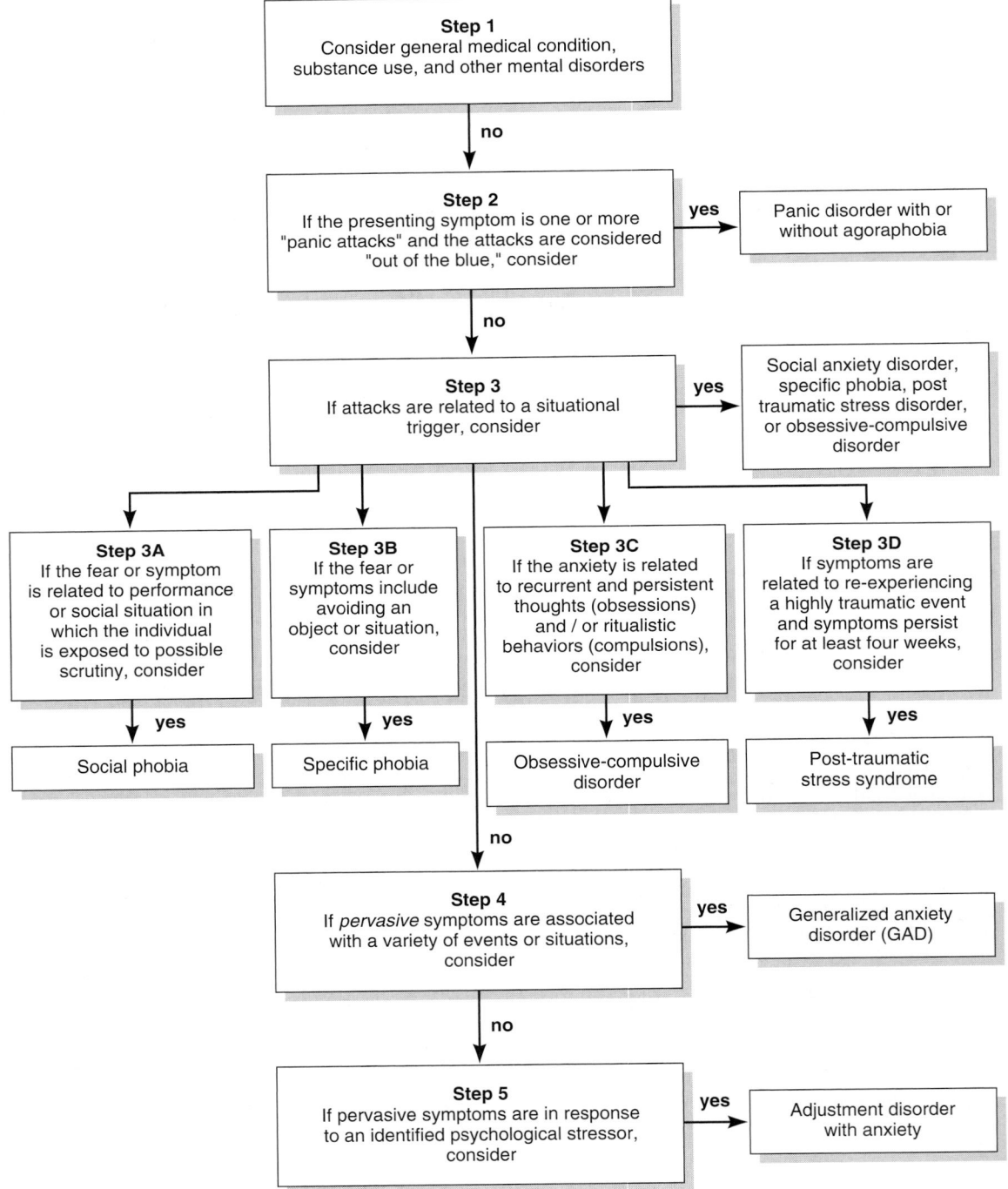

Figure 22–1. Anxiety algorithm. [Modified, with permission, from American Psychiatric Association: Diagnostic and Statistical Manual of Mental Disorders, 4th edition—Primary Care Version (DSM-IV-PC). American Psychiatric Association, 1994.]

Table 22–2. Symptoms associated with panic disorder.

Choking sensation or "lump in the throat"
Skipping, racing, or pounding of the heart
Excessive sweating
Rubbery or "jelly" legs
Nausea or abdominal distress
Trembling or shaking
Difficulty in getting one's breath, smothering sensations, hyperventilating
Chest pain, pressure, discomfort
Faintness, lightheadedness, or dizziness
Feeling off balance or unsteady
Tingling or numbness in parts of the body
Hot flashes or chills
Preoccupation with health concerns
Feeling that things in the environment are strange, unreal, foggy, or detached
Feeling outside or detached from all or part of the body, having a floating feeling
Fear of dying or that something terrible is about to happen
Feeling of losing control or going insane
Agoraphobic avoidance behavior
Feeling frightened suddenly and unexpectedly for no immediate reason

Source: Reproduced, with permission, from McGlynn TJ, Metcalf HL (editors): *Diagnosis and Treatment of Anxiety Disorders: A Physician's Handbook,* 2nd ed. American Psychiatric Press, 1991.

emphasizing its biological basis. Panic symptoms originate in the stem of the brain, the part that controls the fight-or-flight response to a perceived threat. In some people, this brainstem alarm system randomly misfires and causes unanticipated surges of adrenaline, accompanied by sudden fear and troubling (though benign) somatic symptoms. The alarm system can be reset with a combination of medicines, relaxation techniques, and gradual mastery of feared activities and feared somatic symptoms. To help Gwen learn more about panic disorder the doctor gives her a book to read on anxiety (see Suggested Readings). She is started on paroxetine, 10 mg daily, which is later increased to 20 mg daily. After a month of encouraging her to gradually try previously avoided situations and to experience previously feared physical sensations, her symptoms resolve and she returns to full function.

Differential Diagnosis

Substance intoxication from theophylline preparations, over-the-counter cold preparations, caffeine, cocaine, amphetamines, and marijuana or substance withdrawal from alcohol, benzodiazepines, barbiturates, and other central nervous system (CNS) depressants can precipitate serious symptoms of anxiety. *DSM-IV* classifies this as a substance-induced anxiety disorder. Symptoms of anxiety can also occur as a consequence of a medical condition, for example, in a patient who experiences anxiety after a myocardial infarction. Medical problems—including endocrine disorders (such as hypo- and hyperthyroidism, pheochromocytoma, or hypoglycemia), cardiovascular problems, pulmonary embolism, arrhythmias, and neurological conditions (such as vestibular dysfunction)—can also mimic symptoms of anxiety. Historical and examination data suggest that these are substantially less likely than anxiety disorders.

Etiology

The development of anxiety disorders involves multiple factors, including biological abnormalities, past and present psychological stressors, maladaptive cognitions, and environmentally conditioned behaviors. Abnormalities in the central nervous system associated with anxiety disorders relate to the γ-aminobutyric acid (GABA) receptor as well as to the locus ceruleus. Animal studies have shown that stimulation of the locus ceruleus produces hyperarousal states similar to those seen in anxious humans. GABA is an inhibitory neurotransmitter found throughout most of the CNS. It may decrease anxiety by inhibiting locus ceruleus activity and modulating the reticular activating system, another area of the brainstem thought to affect alertness and fear. Benzodiazepines, a class of medications commonly used to treat anxiety, bind to specific sites on the GABA receptor. When the benzodiazepine molecule binds the GABA receptor, the effect of GABA on the GABA receptor is enhanced, reducing anxiety. Two other neurotransmitters, serotonin and norepinephrine, are also under investigation based on therapeutic responses to medications that affect these systems (eg, selective serotonin reuptake inhibitors). Poor regulation of the adrenergic system is also suspected as β-adrenergic agonists induce symptoms of panic and α-adrenergic agonists decrease symptoms of anxiety.

Genetic factors are also likely to play a role in anxiety disorders, as evidenced by twin studies showing a higher concordance for panic disorder and obsessive-compulsive disorder among monozygotic twins than among dizygotic twins.

A frequently discussed approach, called cognitive-behavioral therapy, holds that behavior is driven by underlying beliefs, or *cognitions.* Patients with anxiety typically overestimate danger or threats and underestimate their ability to effectively cope. These patients subsequently feel "stressed" or anxious and select avoidant or other maladaptive coping strategies.

Conditioned learning may also play a pivotal role in the development of anxiety disorders and the resulting avoidance that often seriously compounds patients' anxiety-related functional impairment. For example, patients may notice some unusual autonomic arousal or physical sensation while driving a car. They may catastrophically misinterpret this random and benign sensation as a life-threatening event (eg, "I'm having a heart attack!"), which further intensifies the autonomic response, fuels the misinterpretation, and snowballs into a full-blown panic attack. They may associate the physical sensation and the subsequent attack with the act of driving and feel heightened anxiety—fueled by catastrophic thinking—when they drive or anticipate driving. Initially, the association between driving and panic is coincidental (driving is not the event provoking the initial sensation or the panic attack). Eventually, however, a patient may completely stop driving for fear that another panic attack will occur. This learned relationship between driving and panic may gradually become so strong that driving becomes a precipitant of panic attacks. Thus, the driver mistakenly learns to fear driving.

Stressful or catastrophic life events are also key factors leading to anxiety disorders, particularly posttraumatic stress disorder. Posttraumatic stress disorder and adjustment disorder with anxiety are examples of disorders in which these events play a specific causal role. Other research suggests that childhood trauma can predispose individuals to develop hyperactive physiological responses to everyday stressors, placing them at greater risk for developing anxiety and other mood disorders.

SPECIFIC DISORDERS

Panic Attacks

A panic attack is characterized by a discrete period of intense fear accompanied by the abrupt onset of several cognitive and somatic symptoms (see Table 22–2). Frightening physical symptoms are commonly prominent and scare many patients into seeking urgent medical care. Primary care providers can usually be reassuring, as panic attacks are often infrequent, self-limited, and not related to any serious mental or physical disorder. Panic attacks are categorized as follows:

- Unexpected (untriggered or uncued)
- Situationally bound (always environmentally or psychologically cued), or
- Situationally predisposed (sometimes, but not invariably, cued).

Panic attacks can occur in a number of anxiety disorders other than panic disorder, including social and specific phobias, OCD, and PTSD. The presence and type of a panic trigger help clinicians make a correct diagnosis. Uncued panic attacks are characteristic of panic disorder, whereas cued attacks suggest other psychiatric conditions such as the following:

- Social phobia (attack triggered by fear of embarrassment in social situations),
- Specific phobia (fear of places or things),
- OCD (triggered by exposure to the object of an obsession, such as contamination), or
- PTSD (triggered by an event resembling the original trauma).

Panic attacks are quite common; most people experience a subclinical, or limited-symptom, attack at some time. Only about 9% of people, however, ever experience a full-blown panic attack.

Panic Disorder

DIAGNOSIS

Panic disorder is diagnosed when panic attacks are uncued and recurrent and are followed by a month or more of persistent fear of another attack or avoidance of situations because of fear of having another attack. Only about 2–4% of the population has ever had panic disorder, and about 7% of primary care patients suffer with it. The dilemma for the primary care physician is whether to evaluate the patient's specific symptoms, as patients with panic disorder often focus on the bodily symptoms of the disorder, presenting to primary care providers with chest pain, dizziness, and other unexplained complaints. Because panic disorder is so frequently misdiagnosed by physicians, unnecessary procedures and treatments aimed at alleviating the physical symptoms can cause iatrogenic illnesses. A sound clinical strategy is to evaluate conservatively those symptoms that are potentially catastrophic, involve objective findings, or present as a classic constellation of symptoms. While the investigation is proceeding, the patient can be treated for panic disorder and the symptoms reassessed periodically. Effective pharmacological treatment reduces the cognitive and physical symptoms and lessens the patient's belief that the problem is caused by an undiscovered medical condition.

Panic disorder is a potentially debilitating disease with major complications. It leads to agoraphobia in one-third to one-half of cases, most often within 6 months of the first panic attack. Agoraphobia is a fear of being in a place or a situation where escape or rescue might be difficult if another attack occurs. This fear may cause many patients to avoid important activities of daily living. In Case Illustration 1, the patient avoided tasks that required her to leave home because she was afraid of the consequences of having another attack. Community-based studies have shown that suicide attempts are more common among patients with panic disorder than among patients with major depression. Because panic disorder is so frequently misdiagnosed by physicians, iatrogenesis can result from unnecessary procedures and treatments.

MANAGEMENT

In tailoring the treatment to the patient, several factors should be weighed, including the degree of avoidance present, the severity of physical manifestations of panic, and the presence or absence of overlapping psychiatric disorders. The clinician must balance patient education and supportive counseling with patients' beliefs about the cause of their symptoms. For example, if the physical symptoms are attributed to a cardiac problem, correcting this misinterpretation and emphasizing the biological basis of panic disorder may help the patient accept the diagnosis and thus improve adherence to treatment. The primary physician has a vital role to play in treatment, and many of the treatments, such as patient education and supportive counseling, can appropriately be incorporated into routine office visits.

Medications used to treat panic disorder include some antidepressants [selective serotonin reuptake inhibitors (SSRIs), tricyclics (TCAs), or monoamine oxidase inhibitors (MAOIs), in order of preference] and benzodiazepines (alprazolam, clonazepam). Benzodiazepines relieve symptoms rapidly, usually within the first week of treatment, and they have a relatively wide therapeutic index. Their main disadvantages are their potential for misuse and dependence, a high incidence of rebound panic attacks when the medication is discontinued, and interference with exposure-based cognitive-behavioral therapy. In contrast, SSRIs and TCAs are not associated with dependence and may have a synergistic effect with cognitive-behavioral therapy, but generally take 3–4 weeks or longer before reaching maximum effectiveness. In addition, some antidepressants may exacerbate symptoms of anxiety during the first 1–2 weeks of administration.

Antidepressants and benzodiazepines may be used in combination. A common practice is to initiate treatment with a low daily dose of an SSRI (eg, paroxetine, 10 mg orally each day), titrating the dose slowly upward to 20 mg daily over 1–2 weeks. If panic symptoms worsen in the initial week of therapy, alprazolam or clonazepam is started to control symptoms more quickly. After 3–4 weeks on therapeutic doses of antidepressant (eg, paroxetine, 20 mg daily, or sertraline, 50–200 mg daily), the benzodiazepine can be tapered and discontinued. Although MAOIs are effective, they are seldom used in primary care because of the extensive dietary restrictions needed to minimize the risk of tyramine-induced hypertensive crisis. It is recommended that antidepressants be continued for a minimum of 1 year. Because panic disorder tends to be chronic, longer treatment is often necessary; the length of treatment often depends on patient preference and ability to tolerate relapse.

Adjunctive cognitive-behavioral interventions (eg, relaxation training, challenging catastrophic thinking, and gradual exposures) can treat both the physical manifestations and avoidance behaviors and substantially decrease the likelihood of relapse when medications are discontinued. Patients should be helped to gradually face the situations and activities they feared and fully experience the physical sensations they once believed indicated a serious medical problem. For example, Gwen in Case Illustration 1 would be encouraged to drive, shop, and manage other tasks outside her home while experiencing and eventually managing her shortness of breath, racing heartbeat, and sensation of fainting. If patients are at first overwhelmed by the prospect of doing this, they can first initiate exposure mentally, using relaxation techniques and guided imagery. The patient should be instructed to imagine a frightening but tolerable aspect of the activity (in this case, driving) while doing a relaxation exercise and to repeatedly visualize successfully coping with the activity. In some cases, it may be necessary to enlist the assistance of a cognitive-behavioral therapist who can design and manage successive "exposure" exercises for overly frightened patients.

All patients benefit from a clear understanding of their problem. This eases anxiety, increases the strength of the therapeutic alliance, and increases the likelihood that the patient will follow the treatment plan. It is helpful to emphasize the biological nature of panic disorder, as most patients find it reassuring and destigmatizing to know that they have a recognized, treatable biological syndrome with a typically good prognosis. Patients should be referred to self-help books, support groups, and cognitive-behavioral resources, which are widely available (see Suggested Readings).

Phobias

DIAGNOSIS

Specific phobias and social anxiety disorder (formerly known as social phobia) are characterized by episodic anxiety in response to specific precipitants. Stimuli for specific phobias include places, things, or events, such as airplane flights, heights, insects, snakes, or rodents. Affected individuals are aware that their fears are exaggerated or unreasonable; nonetheless, when exposed to the precipitant, patients experience intense, excessive fear subsequently leading to avoidance behaviors. Social anxiety disorder involves excessive fear of embarrassment, failure, or humiliation before others. This sometimes becomes evident as a fear of speaking, performing, eating, or writing in public. Most often, social anxiety disorder involves a specific focus such as fear of public speaking; occasionally it presents as a generalized type that disables the patient in a wide range of social situations. Marked anticipatory anxiety can cause avoidance behaviors that significantly disrupt patients' functioning.

CASE ILLUSTRATION 2

Charlie, a man in his mid-thirties, presents to his primary care provider complaining of severe palpitations, sweating, and tremulousness. The symptoms occur when he is waiting in customs lines. As he approaches the front of the line, fear of talking with the customs official intensifies until the symptoms occur. The patient then flees to the end of the long line. Charlie realizes this cycle is silly and laughs anxiously as he describes it. This symptom is a major problem for him because his occupation is writing travel books. He has begun avoiding travel and is increasingly worried about his ability to meet writing deadlines and to continue working. A conservative medical work-up is unrevealing, and the primary care provider makes the diagnosis of specific social anxiety disorder, prescribing a trial of β-blockers to be used a short time before standing in the customs line. Charlie is also given a self-help book and a tape on relaxation techniques and the use of guided imagery as a way of visualizing success in the customs line. Charlie uses these treatment approaches successfully on his next trip and realizes that the problem is controllable. He incorporates them into his routine work schedule, and within 2 months has returned to full occupational functioning.

Specific phobias are perhaps the most common but least disabling anxiety disorder. Although many patients have them, most experience only minor related dysfunction, and therefore seldom seek medical care. When care is sought, the diagnosis is usually evident from the history and requires no further testing.

MANAGEMENT

Treatment of specific phobias and social anxiety disorder almost always involves some form of cognitive-behavioral therapy such as systematic desensitization in which the patient is gradually exposed to the feared object or situation. Generally accepted pharmacotherapy guidelines have not been established for specific phobias. As noted in Case Illustration 2, patients with phobia and specific social anxiety disorder are often prescribed β-blockers to be taken prior to an anticipated exposure to the phobic stimulus. Benzodiazepines are often given for exposures to infrequent events that have no complex performance requirements (eg, traveling by commercial airliner on an annual vacation trip). Patients should be informed of the risk of anterograde amnesia, or blackouts, associated with some of these drugs. Paroxetine is approved for the treatment of social anxiety disorder and it or other SSRIs may be helpful when given in standard antidepressant doses.

Obsessive-Compulsive Disorder

DIAGNOSIS

Patients with obsessive-compulsive disorder (OCD) experience regular, intrusive, anxiety-provoking thoughts—called obsessions—or are driven to repeatedly perform seemingly unnecessary or bizarre rituals—called compulsions. Aggression, sex, and religion are common obsessional themes. Compulsions may involve mental tasks, such as counting or praying, or they may involve physical rituals, such as repeated hand washing or checking the state of an object. In patients with both obsessions and compulsions, the ritualized compulsions are usually performed to control the anxiety generated by the obsessive thoughts (eg, obsessive fear about germs is eased by compulsive hand washing). Patients may become so preoccupied with their obsessions and compulsions that they become extremely anxious, slow, and disabled. In one instance, a patient wrung her hands so constantly she could not cook, work, or sleep. Another washed his hands every 10–15 minutes, which interfered significantly with his normal business and social activities. Although patients' level of insight is typically high—they generally experience obsessions and compulsions as intrusive, upsetting, and silly—such insight may diminish acutely when they are faced with the focus of an obsession.

Until the introduction of effective pharmacotherapies for OCD, the disorder was markedly underrecognized in both primary care and psychiatric practice. About 1–3% of the general population develops OCD during their lives. The disorder has been found to have a distinct biological component, a finding supported by the efficacy of biological therapies that selectively inhibit the reuptake of serotonin at CNS neurosynapses. Twin studies have shown a significantly higher percentage of monozygotic twins with diagnostic concordance than is the case for dizygotic twins. Additionally, there is a distinct and reciprocal association between OCD and Tourette's syndrome. Tourette's syndrome is a neurological disorder involving persistent motor and verbal tics. It is often treated with centrally acting dopamine antagonists, such as haloperidol and pimozide. Consequently it has been suggested that dopamine may also play a role in OCD.

MANAGEMENT

Pharmacological treatment of OCD includes four Food and Drug Administration (FDA)-approved medications: clomipramine, paroxetine (40–60 mg/day), sertraline (50–200 mg/day), and fluoxetine (40–80 mg/day). Clomipramine is a tricyclic antidepressant with relatively selective effects on serotonin reuptake. It is commonly prescribed for depression in Europe but in the United States is FDA approved only for OCD. Clomipramine shares the usual tricyclic antidepressant profile of anticholinergic, sedative, and orthostatic side effects.

Psychotherapy for OCD usually involves a form of cognitive-behavioral therapy called "exposure with response prevention" in which the patient is exposed to the anxiety-provoking obsessions or situation but does not engage in the subsequent compulsions or other maladaptive strategies to manage the anxiety. Patients are taught alternate ways of coping with the anxiety including diaphragmatic breathing and progressive muscle relaxation. The cognitive-behavioral therapist may also guide the patient in identifying faulty beliefs and assist the patient in testing those beliefs. The belief, "something terrible will happen if I don't check my lock a hundred times a day," is first rationally examined, then a behavioral test of that belief is collaboratively designed and executed—much as a scientist would design and run a test for any hypothesis.

Posttraumatic Stress Disorder & Acute Stress Disorder

DIAGNOSIS

Posttraumatic stress disorder (PTSD) and acute stress disorder (ASD) are the common mental sequelae of catastrophic trauma. ASD involves symptoms that occur within the first month after trauma. PTSD is essentially the same syndrome, but beginning or persisting beyond a month. Severe trauma of either ASD or PTSD entails an observed or experienced serious injury (actual or threatened). By definition, the trauma experience is accompanied by feelings of intense fear, helplessness, or horror. Patients subsequently develop a mix of flashbacks, nightmares, persistent avoidance of stimuli resembling (concretely or symbolically) the precipitating event, numbing of general responsiveness (restricted range of affect, feelings of interpersonal estrangement, anhedonia), and persistent signs and symptoms of physiological arousal. Secondary depression, panic attacks, substance abuse, unexplained physical symptoms, and aggressive behavior may also be present.

Overall, the lifetime prevalence for PTSD is 1–14% for the general population. Epidemiological studies suggest that about one-third of the population suffers some trauma, placing them at risk for PTSD, and one-fourth of those at risk develop PTSD, usually within a year, although occasionally PTSD may have a delayed onset of years after the trauma has occurred. Assault carries the highest risk for subsequent PTSD, but the most common precipitant is the sudden, unexpected death of a loved one. Although men experience more lifetime trauma, women are more likely to develop PTSD. Women who are sexually assaulted have the highest prevalance rate at 48%.

 CASE ILLUSTRATION 3

Jacques was a successful accountant with no psychiatric history until he had aortic valve surgery at the age of 42. Subsequently, he became totally dysfunctional, losing jobs and clients. He is always angry and suffers flashbacks about the postoperative period of pain and confusion. Jacques gradually became depressed, and his obnoxious, angry behavior alienated both friends and providers.

His primary care physician developed a trusting relationship with Jacques, and helped him disclose painful information about his personal fears and perceived failures triggered by the traumatic brush with serious illness. The doctor identified the association between the onset of symptoms and the surgery and helped Jacques recognize the role of the traumatic event in his life. The doctor explained the potential for improvement with psychotherapy and treatment for depression and encouraged Jacques to enter an established multidisciplinary treatment program.

MANAGEMENT

Treatment of PTSD is multifaceted and usually best accomplished with a multidisciplinary team. Typical team members include the primary care physician, a mental health professional, an addiction specialist, a social worker, and possibly community-based referral resources such as theme counseling groups (eg, veterans groups and abuse-survivor groups). It is helpful to label the problem as PTSD and thus legitimize the manifestations, as patients often blame themselves or others. The physician might say to the patient, "The kinds of feelings, thoughts, and problems you're having are not unusual—they're fairly common among people who have gone through a catastrophe." Aggressive treatment of substance abuse, using addiction specialists, is essential to maximize the patient's occupational and other functions. Support groups of persons who have suffered similar trauma help patients feel understood and normalize their symptoms as they share their experiences and solve problems together. Cognitive-behavioral therapy is the nondrug treatment of choice for PTSD. Patients are taught behavioral skills to manage their autonomic hyperarousal and then are guided through repeated and desensitizing retellings of their traumatic experience. Sertraline (50–200 mg/day) and paroxetine (20–50 mg/day) are approved for the treatment of PTSD.

There is little evidence of efficacy in using pharmacological agents for treating flashbacks and nightmares, although some practitioners advocate the use of clonidine or β-adrenergic antagonists for treating aggression and other psychophysiological arousal symptoms. Care should be taken to avoid use of benzodiazepines in patients with a substance-abuse history. The best pharmacological strategy is to initiate an SSRI and to diagnose and treat coexisting major depression, panic disorder, or substance abuse if indicated.

Generalized Anxiety Disorder

DIAGNOSIS

Generalized anxiety disorder (GAD) consists of almost constant, nonepisodic worry and anxiety that affect patients for more than 6 months and interfere with normal functioning. The worry and anxiety are difficult for the patient to control and are associated with edginess or restlessness, easy fatigability, difficulty concentrating, irritability, muscle tension, or sleep disturbance. Worries typically involve multiple domains and may include concern about routine life circumstances, with the magnitude of worry being out of proportion to the severity of the situation. Symptoms must not be due to the physiological effects of a medical problem such as hyperthyroidism or abuse of a medication or drug. Patients with GAD usually complain of feeling "up tight" or constantly nervous. Physical symptoms such as muscle aches, twitching, trembling, sweating, dry mouth, headaches, gastrointestinal symptoms, urinary frequency, and exaggerated startle often accompany the disorder (Table 22–3) and are often the patient's presenting complaint.

The 1-year prevalence of GAD in the community is approximately 3%; the lifetime prevalence is approximately 5%. About two-thirds of affected individuals are women.

Table 22–3. Specific symptoms associated with generalized anxiety disorder.

Symptom	Manifestation
Motor tension	Trembling, twitching, feeling shaky
	Muscle tension, aches, soreness
	Restlessness
	Easy fatigability
Autonomic hyperactivity	Shortness of breath, smothering sensations
	Palpitations, accelerated heart rate
	Sweating, cold clammy hands
	Dry mouth
	Dizziness, lightheadedness
	Nausea, diarrhea, other types of abdominal distress
	Flushes (hot flashes), chills
	Frequent urination
	Trouble swallowing, "lump in throat"
Vigilance and scanning	Feeling keyed up or on edge
	Exaggerated startle response
	Difficulty concentrating or "mind going blank" because of anxiety
	Trouble falling or staying asleep
	Irritability

Source: Reproduced, with permission, from McGlynn TJ, Metcalf HL (editors): *Diagnosis and Treatment of Anxiety Disorders: A Physician's Handbook,* 2nd ed. American Psychiatric Press, 1991.

The disorder tends to have a chronic, fluctuating course that worsens under stress. Secondary depression is common and predicts a better outcome.

MANAGEMENT

Paroxetine and venlafaxine are both approved by the FDA for treatment of GAD. Venlafaxine XR, an extended release serotonin and norepinephrine reuptake inhibitor, has been shown to effectively reduce the psychological and somatic symptoms associated with GAD and GAD with comorbid depression. Dosage should start at 37.5 mg/day for the first 4–7 days then increase to the usual dose of 75 mg/day (maximum dosage 225 mg daily). Venlafaxine is generally well tolerated and has few drug interactions.

Benzodiazepine therapy at doses lower than those required for panic disorder is usually rapidly effective with few adverse effects. Sedation is the most common side effect but diminishes over time. Tolerance to therapeutic effects is minimal. Minimum effective doses should be used, but care must be taken not to undertreat patients out of fear of making them drug dependent. As with benzodiazepine treatment for other anxiety disorders, rebound symptoms of anxiety are the rule as medication is discontinued. Often a lengthy (a month or more) taper is required. Buspirone is a nonsedating, nonbenzodiazepine anxiolytic specifically indicated for patients with GAD. It is not associated with tolerance, withdrawal, or dependence and has an onset of action of about 3–4 weeks. There is some evidence that buspirone is most effective for less chronic patients who have never tried benzodiazepines.

Short-term supportive psychotherapy can also be helpful. Many patients with GAD have focal life conflicts or stressors for which psychotherapy may be helpful. Basic primary care strategies include empathic listening; encouragement; and assisting patients to identify problems, discuss possible solutions, and solve the problem. Cognitive-behavioral techniques can be used to help patients examine the catastrophic beliefs that underlie their unrealistic worries. Biofeedback and relaxation techniques are useful for improving patient control over muscle tension and other physiological signs of anxiety.

Adjustment Disorder with Anxiety

DIAGNOSIS

Adjustment disorder with anxiety should be considered in patients who are responding with maladaptive anxiety to a recent situational stressor but who do not meet the criteria for another mental disorder. The stressor may be a medical event (eg, surgery, hospitalization, onset of an illness), but most often is a personal crisis such as a divorce, financial problems, or a job change. Symptoms usually begin within 2 months of the onset of the stressor and significantly impair social or occupational functioning. If symptoms persist for more than 6 months, then another diagnosis, such as GAD, is usually more appropriate. Sleeplessness and the physiological aspects of anxiety predominate, and the patient may seek care for somatic complaints. Eliciting the history of the stressful life event and ascertaining the relationship of symptoms to that event help to establish this diagnosis.

MANAGEMENT

The fundamental management of adjustment disorder with anxious mood is supportive counseling, in which the patient discusses the stressful event and the provider helps the patient actively identify and solve problems and/or find ways to more effectively manage the stress (eg, more effectively access social supports or engage in pleasant activities). Patients with adjustment disorder are generally well cared for by a primary care physician who has learned the details of the precipitating event and can incorporate brief supportive strategies into the office visit. Structured relaxation exercises and stress management or other support groups may also be helpful. Sometimes a brief trial of benzodiazepine (less than 3 weeks) can help improve patient coping by reducing the debilitating stress-related symptoms (eg, insomnia or overwhelming fear). Referral to mental health professionals may help if patients do not respond quickly, are severely incapacitated, show a repetitive pattern of maladaptive coping, or specifically request a therapist.

Many studies suggest that there is a substantial group of primary care patients who present with relatively minor complaints of anxiety and depression. Although they do not satisfy criteria for a mental disorder, they do experience associated poor functioning. Often psychosocial stressors or chronic medical problems exacerbate the emotional symptoms. Generally speaking, effective management should emphasize supportive psychosocial rather than pharmacological interventions.

MANAGEMENT OF ANXIETY: GENERAL PRINCIPLES

Most of the treatments for anxiety disorders were described previously along with the disorders for which they are characteristically used. Some general principles pertaining to the primary care treatment of anxiety disorders are, however, worthy of note.

Pharmacotherapy

Pharmacological treatment (Table 22–4) is appropriate when the patient's symptoms are severe enough to sig-

Table 22–4. Pharmacotherapy for anxiety disorders.

Disorder	Examples of Treatment Options	Comments
Panic	(1) Paroxetine, 20 mg a day (smaller doses may be effective, especially in the elderly) (2) Sertraline, 50–200 mg a day (3) Imipramine, 25 mg a day; increase up to 150–200 mg a day; maximum daily dose 300 mg Add alprazolam or clonazepam for 3–4 weeks while increasing antidepressant	Panic may increase in initial treatment
Simple phobias	(1) β-Blocker: propanolol 10–40 mg prior to anticipated exposure (2) Benzodiazepine as needed prior to anticipated, infrequent exposure	
Social anxiety disorder	(1) Benzodiazepine or β-blocker as needed (2) Paroxetine, 20 mg a day	Mild, nongeneralized cases
OCD	(1) Clomipramine, 25 mg a day; increase to 100 mg a day over 2 weeks; maximum daily dose 250 mg (2) Fluoxetine 40–80 mg a day (3) Paroxetine, 40–60 mg a day (4) Sertraline, 50–200 mg a day	Treatment often chronic
GAD	(1) Low-dose benzodiazepine (eg, lorazepam), 1–5 mg a day, divided (2) Buspirone, 5 mg three times a day; increase in 5-mg increments; maximum daily dose 60 mg (3) Venlafaxine XR, 75–225 mg a day	Tolerance develops to initial sedation Nonsedating, no dependence
Adjustment disorder	Brief benzodiazepine use as sedative or anxiolytic	Main treatment is support; medication treatment is time limited

nificantly interfere with functioning and the benefits of medication outweigh the risks for a given patient. The treatment must be carefully individualized, based on the patient's particular constellation of symptoms, complicating medical or substance-abuse problems, vulnerability to various side effects, and willingness to collaborate in a psychopharmacological approach to treatment.

When medications are prescribed, it is important to recognize, track, and document specific target symptoms. The dosage of medication should be titrated so as to minimize both the target symptoms and bothersome side effects. Lower than normal doses of psychoactive agents are recommended for the elderly; because these drugs have longer half-lives in this age group, accumulation can easily occur, and sensitivity to unwanted cognitive and other toxic effects is greater (see Chapter 11).

Although monotherapy is almost always preferable to medication combinations, a common exception is prescribing both ongoing antidepressants and 1–2 weeks of minor tranquilizers for patients with panic disorder. This strategy achieves rapid reduction of symptoms, avoids the intensification of anxiety sometimes seen in early antidepressant treatment of anxiety disorders, and allows discontinuation of benzodiazepines before dependence occurs. If patients are being referred to cognitive-behavioral therapy, a benzodiazepine taper and discontinuation are recommended. Benzodiazepines should seldom be used in patients with a history of substance abuse.

Psychosocial Therapies

Primary care providers should not underestimate the importance of basic supportive measures that can easily be performed in the general medical setting. The relationship between the doctor and patient usually plays a pivotal role for anxious patients in need of reassurance. Patient–provider trust is especially important for anxious patients, enhancing timely and accurate history taking, physical examination, diagnosis, and treatment adherence.

Symptoms of anxiety are extremely distressing to patients, who often fear that occult disease is causing their symptoms. Clinicians must try to view the symptoms through the eyes and perceptions of the affected patient—what seems trivial to a provider may be overwhelming for the patient. Listening to patients, expressing empathy for their feelings and concerns, and providing information about anxiety disorders are crucial ways to improve patient rapport (see Chapters 1 and 2) and should be routine in the course of care.

Equipping patients with basic information about anxiety disorders is essential (Table 22–5). Patients with anxiety are common enough that providers should be prepared with standard explanations such as the example described in the section on panic disorder. Most patients find such explanations and suggestions for appropriate lay publications reassuring.

INDICATIONS FOR REFERRAL

Multiple randomized, controlled trials have shown that pharmacotherapy and/or cognitive-behavioral therapy are effective treatments for most anxiety disorders. Patients should be considered for referral to a mental health professional under the following circumstances:

1. The treatment does not lead to improvement in the patient's symptoms within the expected timeframe.
2. The physician is confused about the primary diagnosis. It is particularly important to differentiate patients who have depression, alcohol abuse/dependence, or personality disorders from those with an anxiety disorder. Mental health consultation is appropriate if the primary care doctor is uncertain and the distinction has therapeutic implications.
3. Complicating substance abuse is suspected.
4. The patient has suicidal or homicidal thoughts or plans or exhibits intended suicidal or homicidal behavior.
5. The provider has questions about appropriate administration or tapering of benzodiazepines and questions regarding possible dependence.
6. The patient has an especially complicated set of ongoing psychosocial stressors whose resolution requires greater time and expertise than can be provided in primary care.

Table 22–5. Nonpharmacologic management of anxiety disorders.

Type of Treatment	Description	Indication
Education	Provides basic information and reassurance	Appropriate in all disorders Lay publications useful
Cognitive-behavioral therapy, eg, systematic desensitization	Gradually increases exposure to feared stimulus using relaxation techniques Helps patient reorganize way of thinking about symptoms	Useful in all disorders Particularly effective for panic disorder
Relaxation techniques	Uses muscle-relaxation therapy, including hypnosis, biofeedback, meditation	Particularly useful in panic disorders, GAD, adjustment disorder with anxious mood

In some circumstances, the primary care physician may be uncertain about whether a patient has another medical illness and believes a specialist is necessary to consider that possibility. It is helpful to select a specialist who understands anxiety disorders and will work with the referring physician to explain the nature of the specific anxiety disorder to the patient. It is imperative that the specialist bring a conservative approach to diagnostic studies, an understanding of the many physical manifestations of anxiety, and a respectful approach to treatment of the anxiety-disordered patient.

The primary care physician who is knowledgeable and skilled in the diagnosis and management of anxiety disorders can make an important contribution to the quality of patient care and to the appropriate use of health resources, particularly in the managed care environment. The accurate and prompt diagnosis of anxiety disorders can prevent unnecessary diagnostic testing.

SUGGESTED READINGS

Hales RE, Hilty DA, Wise MG: A treatment algorithm for the management of anxiety in primary care practice. J Clin Psychiatry 1997;58[Suppl 3]:76.

Lange JT, Lange CL, Cabaltica RBG: Primary care of post-traumatic stress disorder. Am Fam Physician 2000;62:1035.

McGlynn TJ, Metcalf HL (editors): *Diagnosis and Treatment of Anxiety Disorders: A Physician's Handbook,* 2nd ed. American Psychiatric Press, 1991.

Rakel RE: Anxiety and the primary care physician. Primary Psychiatry 2001;8:52.

REFERENCE BOOKS FOR PATIENTS

Bourne, EJ: *The Anxiety and Phobia Workbook,* 3rd ed. New Harbinger Press, 2000.

Davis M, McKay M, Eshelman ER: *The Relaxation and Stress Reduction Workbook,* 5th ed. New Harbinger Press, 2000.

Zuercher-White, E: *An End to Panic: Breakthrough Techniques for Overcoming Panic Disorder,* 2nd ed. New Harbinger Press, 1998.

WEB SITES

Anxiety Disorders Association
http://www.adaa.org
Cognitive-Behavioral Therapy
http://www.aabt.org/
Consumer Nonprofit
http://www.freedomfromfear.org

Somatization

John R. Chamberlain, MD, & Stuart J. Eisendrath, MD

INTRODUCTION

CASE ILLUSTRATION 1

Ms. A, a 57-year-old woman, makes an appointment with a new clinician. She presents with a 10-year history of multiple, unexplained symptoms. She has seen many physicians over the past decade, including several primary care physicians and numerous subspecialists. Her principal complaints today include abdominal pain, chest pain, headache, palpitations, fatigue, and intermittent dizziness. She brings a thick stack of records from some of her prior physicians. These records include multiple laboratory tests and diagnostic procedures, none of which has identified any cause for her symptoms.

Clinician: How can I help you today, Ms. A?

Patient (sighing): I don't know. A friend of mine saw you a few months ago and said you were very good. I hope you can help me. I've had these problems for years now, and no one seems to be able to figure them out. Maybe you can. I know there's something wrong. I've been so sick.

Clinician: Why don't you tell me about your symptoms?

Patient: Well, it all began about 10 years ago. . . .

Clinicians are taught that patients will present with symptoms (subjective complaints) and signs (objective findings) that suggest the presence of a pathophysiological process. They are trained to recognize these presentations and to diagnose the underlying disease so that they may institute the appropriate treatment. Satisfaction for the care provider arises from the ability to perform these tasks proficiently and to see the patient benefit. Patients typically come to the clinician's office seeking an explanation for and relief from their symptoms. Difficulties arise in the relationship when the patient presents with symptoms and the clinician can find no disease to explain them. Symptoms that lack discernible physical pathology have been referred to variously as medically unexplained, functional, or somatization symptoms.

The term *somatization* (as used in this chapter) refers to the experience and reporting of physical symptoms that cause distress but that lack a corresponding level of tissue damage or pathology and are linked to psychosocial stress. In contrast to this broad and inclusive view of the process, psychiatrists have developed strict diagnostic criteria that define several distinct disorders, which are collectively referred to as the *somatoform disorders*. In general, these conditions are chronic and reflect an enduring way for the affected individuals to cope with psychosocial stressors. However, it is much more common in the primary care setting to encounter patients who have somatization symptoms but do not meet the full criteria for a psychiatric diagnosis. In many individuals, the somatization might be a transient phenomenon during a particularly stressful period such as divorce consisting of an exaggeration of common physical symptoms such as headache. In other patients, the process may be more persistent and the symptoms may be disabling. The latter group of patients can be particularly difficult for clinicians. Although their symptoms are suggestive of an underlying medical or neurological condition, no such etiology is discovered upon appropriate diagnostic evaluation. Some patients do find reassurance in the provider's statements that no medical cause for their symptoms has been found. Other patients may become upset and accuse the clinician of not believing them or of being incompetent. Some patients demand continued diagnostic testing or referral to specialists. Further, the somatization symptoms do not respond to medical treatments that are prescribed for the disease suggested by the symptoms; this apparent therapeutic failure can lead to demands for more testing and requests for referral or different treatment regimens. The combination of increasing demands made by patients and their failure to respond to treatment can be very frustrating for the clinician.

HISTORICAL CONCEPTS

The existence of medically unexplained symptoms has been recognized throughout the history of medicine. Each historical period has described syndromes composed of such symptoms. The scientific knowledge and theories of the time have shaped the etiologies proposed for these disorders. The treatments advocated by medical practitioners were directed at attempting to correct the abnormality assumed to cause the illness. Each of these syndromes shared the recognition by medical authorities of the time that the illness lacked the demonstrable, pathologically defined tissue changes that characterize most medical conditions.

Prior to the Renaissance, medical theories were based on limited understanding of anatomy or physiology and, as a result, seem quite primitive to modern practitioners. Diseases lacking an apparent cause were believed to result from gross disturbances in the function and behavior of bodily organs. For example, hysteria was attributed to a "wandering uterus" as early as 1900 B.C. The treatments for hysteria flowed from this conceptual model and included the application of ointments to the labia or manipulation of the uterus to return it to its "natural" position. It was not until after the Renaissance that medical practitioners began to implicate disturbances of the nervous system in the genesis of medically unexplained symptoms. However, despite this change in the understanding of these disorders, the treatments utilized by clinicians did not become significantly more advanced. For instance, some practitioners in the latter half of the seventeenth century advocated hitting patients who had symptoms of hysteria with a stick.

By the end of the seventeenth century, and continuing into the eighteenth century, clinicians increasingly recognized the role psychological factors played in the origin and maintenance of somatization symptoms. More importantly, their treatments were beginning to reflect this appreciation. Medical authorities no longer focused exclusively on somatic therapies in the care of afflicted individuals. Instead, practitioners were encouraged to inquire about and demonstrate an active interest in their patients' mental state and welfare. Further, clinicians recognized the need to attempt to promote optimism about recovery in their patients.

In the nineteenth century there was awareness that despite many advances in the understanding of pathology, patients suffering from somatization syndromes lacked discernible anatomic abnormalities. As a result, the medically unexplained disorders were attributed to a subtle or "functional" pathological disturbance. This explanatory model of illness was associated with a return to predominantly somatic interventions for treating the symptoms. However, some practitioners maintained that psychological treatments were important for managing these patients. These clinicians also recognized that unless the therapy was delivered in a way that was consistent with the patients' belief that their illness had a physical etiology, the intervention would be rejected.

At the turn of the twentieth century, an exclusively psychological model for these disorders was developed. The idea of a functional pathological lesion of the nervous system was replaced with the concept of psychogenesis (ie, the somatization symptoms arose from the mind). Somatization was viewed as the means by which unconscious mental conflicts could be manifested in the

form of physical symptoms. As a result, mental health practitioners became responsible for the diagnosis and treatment of these disorders. However, the idea of physical complaints originating from the mind was also associated with implications that the symptoms were not "real." Further, many patients were not convinced of the value of this explanatory model.

Medically unexplained syndromes have persisted as clinical problems for practitioners. Patients often present with many symptoms that are not associated with abnormalities demonstrable by physical examination or laboratory or radiological studies. The symptoms are often clustered together as syndromes with a variety of proposed etiologies including environmental exposures, infections (eg, *Candida,* Epstein–Barr virus), or multiple chemical sensitivity. The broad range of advocacy and educational groups that try to promote various agendas with regard to the disorders makes the evaluation of these syndromes difficult.

 CASE ILLUSTRATION 2

Mr. B is a 32-year-old man who presents to his primary care physician with complaints about being tired, weak, and nauseated. He also complains about intermittent abdominal and chest pain as well as a feeling of "dizziness." He noted that he lived in an old building and was worried he had been exposed to lead or some other toxin. His physical examination and laboratory values were all normal. However, he was not relieved by these results and his complaints persisted. He began to phone frequently with questions about chronic Candida infections, postviral syndromes, and multiple chemical sensitivity syndromes. His physician would discuss each process with him and continued to perform appropriate medical evaluations of Mr. B's symptoms. The patient began to research his symptoms on the Internet. He was convinced that he suffered from sensitivity to multiple compounds in his home and became involved in a number of "on-line" support groups. He resisted other explanations for his symptoms and gradually became dissatisfied with his primary care physician and chose to seek care from "experts" on his disorder.

ETIOLOGY

Somatization can be understood from a number of different perspectives, each of which proposes a cause for the symptoms. However, because the precise cause of these symptoms is not known, none of the following models is fully explanatory. Rather, each model provides practitioners with insight into the genesis of these symptoms and suggests possible treatments as well. Unfortunately, each model is able to explain the symptoms of only a select group of patients. A more comprehensive understanding of patients comes from incorporating more than one perspective.

Neurobiological

According to the neurobiological perspective, the somatization symptoms result from dysfunction in the neuro-endocrine systems responsible for processing peripheral sensory and central emotional information. As a result, the affected individual misperceives normal bodily sensations or emotional signals as indicating a dangerous somatic process. The mechanism by which dysfunction in the nervous or endocrine systems results in the preoccupation with somatic symptoms is unknown. There is growing evidence of the role of such abnormalities in these disorders. For example, researchers have recently suggested that hypocortisolism plays a role in posttraumatic stress disorder, fibromyalgia, chronic fatigue syndrome, and some chronic pain disorders. Although hypocortisolism has been found in groups of individuals with the above diagnoses, the relationship between a deficiency of cortisol and the production of these symptoms is not understood. Additional research has examined the ability of individuals with somatization symptoms to habituate to novel stimuli. Individuals with somatization syndrome reported higher levels of tension in novel situations and were less likely to habituate to the situation over time. In addition, the affected individuals had a slower return to baseline heart rate upon leaving stressful situations. These studies suggest a relationship between physiological mechanisms involved in adapting to novel or stressful stimuli and the apparently psychological symptoms of individuals with somatoform disorders.

Psychodynamic

According to psychodynamic theory, the somatoform symptoms arise solely from the mind. They are believed to represent the outward expression of underlying, internal psychological conflicts. In support of this theory, studies have demonstrated that individuals with somatization symptoms have higher rates of prior emotional and physical abuse, depression, and anxiety than non-affected populations. It is hypothesized that abuse places individuals at risk for the types of internal conflicts that result in somatoform disorders. For example, women who have suffered sexual abuse in childhood have increased rates of chronic pelvic pain when compared with nonabused populations. Depression and anxiety may be both a product and a cause of these internal conflicts.

Cognitive-Behavioral

According to cognitive-behavioral theorists, somatoform symptoms arise from incorrect beliefs about bodily sensations, for example, believing that mild gastroesophageal reflux (or panic symptoms) represents myocardial ischemia. These misperceptions, in turn, result in certain maladaptive behaviors, such as going from emergency room to emergency room seeking evaluation of the symptom and reassurance that the heart is functioning normally. These symptoms are reinforced by factors in the individual's environment such as the responses of other people to the perceived illness. For instance, the affected individual may be excused from work or social obligations. As an example of this process, some researchers proposed that learning about a disease may lead certain individuals to attribute previously overlooked symptoms to the illness. The affected person seeks out confirmatory evidence of additional symptoms that both reinforce the belief in the illness and amplify the somatic symptoms. The person's self-validating review of symptoms may be augmented by contact with advocacy or educational groups that promote awareness of the disease. The processing of bodily information gradually becomes colored by the belief that the person has a disease and this can result in the affected individual embracing the sick role.

CASE ILLUSTRATION 3

Mr. C is a 53-year-old man who worked as a manual laborer. He had always been in good health. One day, while lifting a particularly heavy item, he experienced pain on the right side of his chest. A colleague said that his father had a similar experience and died of a heart attack shortly thereafter. Mr. C became focused on the idea he has heart disease and began to visit a number of emergency rooms, primary care physicians, and cardiologists. His evaluations were always completely negative. However, his concern has persisted and he now presents to a new clinician.

Clinician: How may I help you Mr. C?

Patient: Doc, I know that I have a problem with my heart.

Clinician: What are your symptoms?

Patient: Well, I sometimes feel like I am more out of breath and if I lift heavy things I can feel some pain in the muscle over my chest. Other times, I start to breath fast and my fingers get tingly. I've watched programs on TV and they say those are things that can mean I have angina. I've stopped working because I don't want to stress myself out and have a heart attack.

Sociocultural

According to the sociocultural perspective, individuals learn to express disease and distress in culturally sanctioned ways. In any culture the expression of certain bodily symptoms and illness behaviors are encouraged while others are discouraged. Although somatization is a universal process, an individual's culture can affect the manner in which somatic representations of emotional distress are utilized. Further, this theory maintains that because the patient and the clinician are often from different backgrounds, the cultural interaction between the clinician and the patient is important. This interaction often determines how the patient's symptoms are experienced and interpreted. The clinician's task in these meetings is to correctly recognize which of the patient's somatic complaints represent cultural idioms of emotional distress. Mistakes in this assessment can lead to misdiagnosis, unnecessary medical treatment or evaluation, frustration on the part of the provider when the patient does not respond as expected, and dissatisfaction on the part of the patient.

A DIFFERENT PARADIGM

Although the theoretical models discussed above have evidence to support them and have been used as the basis for treatment in cases of somatization, there is another way to conceptualize somatization and the associated disorders. This view begins with the clinician abandoning the either-or categories of "physical" and "psychological." That dichotomous framework leads to interactions in which the patient can feel that the clinician is rejecting them and the reality of their symptoms by concluding, "The doctor's saying its all in my head." Instead, the provider adopts a more comprehensive view of disease based on the biopsychosocial model of illness. In this paradigm, all illnesses are understood to have biological, psychological, and social dimensions.

Although the western medical model focuses on the biological aspects of disease, it often ignores the psychological and social facets of the patient's experience. In addition, this model, often very effective for understanding and treating acute disease processes, may fail to explain much of the complexity of chronic illness. For example, pain researchers have found that psychological factors are more important than physical factors in predicting future disability. Such research has led to the development of new treatment paradigms that recognize the interplay between the biological disease process and the psychosocial impact of symptoms. Treatment is focused on both relieving the biomedical symptoms and modifying the thoughts, feelings, and behavior associated with the pain and disability.

Using the more comprehensive biopsychosocial model, illness can be understood as occurring along a spectrum with disorders characterized by predominantly somatic problems at one end and disorders with predominantly psychological or social manifestations at the other end. Therefore, evaluation of patients should routinely include inquiries into both the physical and psychosocial dimensions of their illness. Using the biopsychosocial framework, the somatoform disorders can be viewed as arising when the patient neglects the psychosocial components of their illness and insists on viewing the problem solely from a somatic perspective. For example, an individual with a history of chronic pelvic pain who has undergone multiple thorough evaluations with no anatomic etiology identified but who insists on repeating the work-up rather than discussing psychosocial facets of the symptoms is likely to be experiencing somatization. Somatization itself is not a single entity. Like most illnesses it can be understood to have a continuum of expression. At one end is the transient, stress-related exaggeration of common physical symptoms and at the other end are the serious, persistent complaints that leave the patient disabled.

Patient: I don't know. Maybe I am crazy . . . that's what everyone else seems to think.

Clinician: Let me assure you that you're not crazy. I hear your concern. Why don't we talk about this a little bit?

Patient: Well, a friend of mine had a disease called Cushing's. Do you think I might have that?

Clinician: That's a good question. There are a great many diseases that can present with symptoms like yours. I want you to know that as I've listened to you and examined you, I've tried to think of rare diseases. I don't believe any of them are very likely, especially since you've had your symptoms for so long. I do want to be honest with you, though. There's no way to be absolutely certain. There are so many different diseases that it would be impossible to get tested for all of them. Let's get a few laboratory tests done, though. If they're normal, let's not do any more tests, but I'll keep an open mind as to these possibilities as we get to know each other during the course of the next few months. If you develop symptoms later that suggest one of these rare diseases to me, I'll certainly order more tests. How does that sound to you?

Patient: Okay, that sounds like it could work.

Clinician: Are there other things going on that add stress to your life?

Patient: Now that you mention it, there are some stressful things going on. . . .

In this brief dialogue the practitioner acknowledges uncertainty while communicating a sense of honesty and trustworthiness. By reinforcing the continuity of the relationship and the willingness to entertain different possibilities in the future, the provider helps the patient feel cared for without the need for multiple, and most likely unnecessary, diagnostic tests. Moreover, the clinician has helped the patient to entertain the idea of a connection between psychosocial and somatic factors in illness.

PREVALENCE

Somatization is frequently encountered in primary care clinics. Epidemiological studies have demonstrated that 25–35% of the patients in primary care settings will meet criteria for a recognized psychiatric disorder with the most common disorders being anxiety or depression. In addition, research has shown that 50–80% of patients who meet criteria for an anxiety or depressive disorder initially present to health care providers with physical symptoms. Other studies have found that somatoform disorders can be diagnosed in up to 22% of patients in primary care outpatient clinics. One study found that no organic cause was found in 80% of primary care visits scheduled for the evaluation of common symptoms such as dizziness, chest pain, and fatigue. Similarly, studies of medical inpatients have found that between 20 and 40% of these individuals meet the criteria for a coexisting mental disorder. A recent study actually found that somatoform disorders were the most common psychiatric diagnoses in a population of medical inpatients. These results indicate that the phenomenon of somatization, as well as more rigorously defined somatoform disorders, is very common among patients presenting for medical services.

IMPACT AND OUTCOMES

Somatization is not only a common, but also an expensive problem. One study estimated that patients with somatization disorder generate medical costs nine times those of the average medical patient. In addition, these patients often demand a great deal of time and attention and yet they frequently do not respond to the prescribed treatment. This can eventually lead to frustration for the practitioner and even feelings of incompetence or inadequacy. The patients' seemingly unending complaints can lead to feelings of anger at the individual or dread when their name appears on the appointment list. Thus, patients with somatization symptoms not only tax the health care system by disproportionately utilizing limited resources, but also burden health care providers who can feel overwhelmed by the needs of these individuals.

Research has consistently demonstrated that individuals who present with somatization symptoms have worse outcomes in regard to health status, physical functioning, and psychological well-being than those patients who do not manifest these symptoms. Patients with somatization symptoms have ongoing difficulties not only with their somatic complaints and concerns about physical illness, but also with emotional and social impairment. It is important to accurately diagnose these individuals so that appropriate management can be instituted.

DIFFERENTIAL DIAGNOSIS

Patients with somatization symptoms should be evaluated for a biomedical etiology that could explain the presenting complaints. The nature of the evaluation will depend on the patients' medical history, presenting symptoms, and age. In evaluating patients, it is important to remember that the onset of multiple physical symptoms late in life is almost always due to a general medical condition; somatoform disorders generally start decades earlier.

The American Psychiatric Association *Diagnostic and Statistical Manual of Mental Disorders,* 4th edition, *Text Revision* (*DSM-IV-TR*) classifies a number of syndromes together under the heading of "Somatoform Disorders." This classification is based on the common feature that the affected individuals report symptoms suggestive of a general medical condition but appropriate work-up either fails to reveal such a condition or, if the condition is present, does not explain the severity of the patient's complaints. In addition, the somatic complaints in these disorders are produced unconsciously and are not under the voluntary control of the patient (Table 23-1).

A number of other psychiatric disorders have been associated with somatization. These disorders should be considered when evaluating a patient who appears to have somatization symptoms. For example, panic attacks often involve symptoms in multiple organ systems such as palpitations, nausea, shortness of breath, and tingling in the extremities. Unlike symptoms of somatoform disorders, however, the symptoms of this disorder have an abrupt onset and are limited to the panic attack episodes. A careful history can often elicit this time course and prove helpful in making the diagnosis. Patients with generalized anxiety disorder may also present with multiple somatic complaints. Excessive worrying about multiple domains in life is the key feature of this disorder and helps to separate it from the somatoform disorders. Depressed patients often present to medical practitioners with unexplained physical symptoms, especially headache, pain, and gastrointestinal problems. In contrast to the somatic symptoms of the chronic somatoform disorders, the physical complaints in depression exist only in the presence of the mood symptoms. In such cases, the depression and the somatic complaints resolve contemporaneously. Studies have demonstrated a high level of comorbidity between depression and somatoform disorders, so clinically both disorders may be present. Patients with obsessive-compulsive disorder whose beliefs focus on bodily functions or organs can appear to be suffering from a somatoform disorder. The key to diagnosis is a careful history about the presence of the obsessions and compulsions. Patients with psychotic disorders, such as schizophrenia, may also present with multiple somatic complaints. In contrast to the concerns in the somatoform disorders, psychotic symptoms tend to be bizarre or completely irrational (eg,

Table 23–1. Somatoform disorders.

Somatization Disorder: Begins before age 30, endures for many years, and involves a combination of pain, gastrointestinal, sexual, and pseudoneurological symptoms. The defining feature of somatization disorder is the persistence of multiple system symptoms without the development of the structural abnormalities, laboratory abnormalities, or physical findings that are characteristic of the general medical condition suggested by the symptoms.

Undifferentiated Somatoform Disorder: Characterized by the presence of one or more physical complaints that persist for 6 months or longer and cannot be explained by any known substance or general medical condition or are grossly out of proportion to what would be expected by history, physical examination, or laboratory evaluation.

Conversion Disorder: Characterized by the presence of symptoms or deficits affecting voluntary motor or sensory function that suggest a neurological or other general medical condition. However, no underlying condition can be identified to explain the symptoms. It is important to emphasize that because many general medical etiologies for apparent conversion syndromes take years to become evident, the diagnosis should be viewed as provisional. In the past, studies have shown that up to 50% of patients with a presumed conversion disorder are later found to have a general medical condition. However, more recent studies suggest that this percentage is now less than 25%, perhaps because of improved diagnostic techniques and understanding of this disorder.

Pain Disorder with Psychological Factors: Characterized by pain in one or more anatomical sites as the focus of clinical attention. Psychological factors are judged to have an important role in the onset, severity, exacerbation, and maintenance of the pain.

Hypochondriasis: Characterized by the preoccupation with or fear of having a serious disease based on the individual's misinterpretation of bodily symptoms.

Body Dysmorphic Disorder: Characterized by preoccupation with an imagined or exaggerated defect in the individual's physical appearance.

Somatoform Disorder Not Otherwise Specified: Refers to any disorder with somatoform symptoms that does not meet the criteria for any of the other more specific somatoform disorders (eg, pseudocyesis—the false belief that one is pregnant often accompanied by signs of pregnancy such as missed menstrual periods and abdominal distention).

"My insides are rotting" or "I have pain from the dinosaur eggs in my stomach").

In contrast to the psychiatric disorders described above, there are conditions in which the individual's symptoms are consciously produced. Factitious disorders are diagnosed when the clinician determines that the symptoms are consciously or voluntarily fabricated or exaggerated. However, in these individuals there is no discernible external incentive to produce the symptoms such as financial compensation. The patient's only apparent goal is to assume the sick role. Malingering, on the other hand, is diagnosed when the clinician determines that the individual has consciously produced the symptoms for an apparent external gain such as obtaining a monetary award, acquiring drugs, or avoiding a noxious situation such as military duty or incarceration. Malingering is not considered a mental disorder.

EVALUATION

A stepwise evidence-based approach is invaluable to the evaluation of patients with suspected somatization symptoms. This framework can help the clinician avoid unnecessary and costly diagnostic procedures or referrals to specialists. In addition, it can spare the patient potential iatrogenic complications from any of the evaluation procedures. As with all of medicine, the first step in evaluating the patient with multiple somatic complaints is a detailed and thorough history of the presenting problem.

The clinician should, of course, include review of pertinent medical records in the history-gathering phase of the evaluation. The practitioner should then perform appropriate physical and neurological examinations. The provider may then consider what tests are indicated to confirm the diagnosis or rule out a predominantly biomedical disease based on the information obtained. The urge to order a wide variety of tests ("the shotgun approach") should be resisted and a rational determination of the patient's needs should be made. Obtaining an informal consultation from a colleague can be useful in appropriately evaluating these individuals.

Once the provider determines that the patient's physical symptoms are not explained by any underlying pathological abnormalities, the focus can turn to more predominantly psychological disorders. The assessment of psychiatric disorders can be accomplished through the use of a careful clinical interview or a semistructured interview tool or by referral to a mental health clinician. The clinical interview can be helpful in establishing the presence of psychiatric illness as well as in communicating to the patient that the clinician is taking an active interest in the individual's life. Instruments such as the PRIME-MD, which are designed for use in primary care settings, can help the provider diagnose somatoform disorders as well as depression, anxiety, eating disorders, and substance abuse. Such instruments have the advantages of rapid administration and established validity. Many patients refuse referral to a mental health specialist as an option because they fear that their complaints are being dismissed. Above all, when evaluating a patient the clinician should recognize and articulate the interplay between the physical and psychosocial realms.

> **Clinician:** Today I would like to talk about how you are doing.
>
> **Patient:** Well, my chest has been hurting again and I have been really worn down.
>
> **Clinician:** (after several pertinent questions about the symptoms) It sounds like this is the same pain you've had before, although I do understand that it's a little worse. I wonder if there is anything else that has changed in your life recently besides the intensity of the pain?
>
> **Patient:** Nothing . . . really. Well my wife and I are arguing about the mortgage again.
>
> **Clinician:** Oh, I remember that's been a problem before when you've been having pain.
>
> **Patient:** Yeah. I just get tired of her nagging and the stress of barely making ends meet.
>
> **Clinician:** I think its possible that the stress you've been under may be taking its toll on your body and your sense of well being.

TREATMENT

The treatment strategies to be described are not specific to a certain somatoform diagnosis. It is less important in most cases to make a specific psychiatric diagnosis of a somatoform disorder than it is to recognize that the patient's symptoms represent somatization. However, if a psychiatric disorder such as anxiety, depression, or psychosis is identified as driving the somatic symptoms, specific treatments for the identified disorder should be utilized.

Treatments Designed for Primary Care Providers

Nonsomatic therapies are the primary treatments for the somatoform disorders. Patients with somatization symptoms most often present to the primary care setting and are resistant to psychiatric referrals. Techniques are required that are effective, acceptable to primary care clinicians, and useful in busy primary care settings. Finally, the intervention must be congruent with patients' beliefs about the nature of their illness so that they are willing to engage in the treatment.

The most important aspect of managing patients with somatization symptoms is the development of an empathic, trusting relationship. Although it is not easy to form such a relationship with these individuals, establishing a therapeutic alliance is critical to both diagnosis and treatment. It can be helpful to remember that patients with somatization are reacting in the best and, without treatment, only way available to them. Before considering spe-

cific therapies for these individuals, it is useful to consider basic techniques for interacting with them.

The practitioner should never challenge the reality of the patient's physical symptoms. Somatization is an unconscious process and therefore the somatic complaints are very real to the patient. Further, because most of the symptoms are subjective in nature, there is no means to verify or dispute them. It can be helpful to explicitly acknowledge the patient's suffering to bolster the therapeutic relationship.

> **Clinician:** I can see how much you've suffered with all of these symptoms.
>
> **Patient:** You're the only one who seems to understand that.

Medical providers should avoid trying to convince the patient that the symptoms are psychological in origin. They should also avoid the use of psychological labels (eg, depression, anxiety). Instead, they should try to use easily understandable and mutually acceptable language to discuss symptoms. Each appointment should begin with a discussion of the somatic complaint. The provider can then use descriptive physiological explanations, which are more acceptable to these individuals, to describe the symptoms (eg, "abnormally tense muscles in your neck go into painful spasm"). It is important to note that although such descriptors imply a physiological component to the symptoms, they do not provide an etiology. Over time (often months or years), the patient and clinician may begin to explore possible explanations for the symptoms that integrate somatic and psychosocial aspects of the problem.

> **Patient:** I just don't get why my neck keeps getting spasms.
>
> **Clinician:** I have noticed that sometimes you mention this happening after your supervisor criticizes you. Sometimes our muscles react to emotions like anger or stress by tightening up. When this becomes extreme, they can spasm.
>
> **Patient:** You know that makes some sense. When he comes around I can feel myself grit my teeth and begin to feel stiff.

Another management suggestion is to have the provider evaluate the patients in an appropriate manner to rule out somatic causes of their symptoms. Once the somatization is identified, the clinician continues to schedule the individual for brief, regularly spaced intervals. These visits are time contingent; patients need not have new symptoms to be able to meet regularly with their medical practitioner. These visits allow for an initial brief check-in regarding the somatic symptoms followed by discussions of events in the patient's life and the patient's emotional well-being and relationships. The clinician can adopt a conservative approach toward new treatments or diagnostic work-ups when the patient presents with new or worsening symptoms. The goal is to focus the patient on behaviors promoting well-being and to help them discuss the psychosocial aspects of their life and illness. They are discouraged from pursuing new therapies or evaluations for their symptoms. At the same time, they are shown that the provider is taking an active interest in them. Moreover, they learn that they will receive this care and attention even without new symptoms or exacerbations of existing symptoms. The clinician may also ask the patient when they want to return for the next visit. This provides the patient with a sense of control and over time many patients will suggest lengthening the interval between appointments.

Establishing appropriate goals is also important when working with these patients. These disorders, like any chronic disease, are often not curable. However, clinicians often hope that another medication will relieve the symptoms or that one more diagnostic procedure will elucidate the cause of the patient's problem. However, these beliefs can lead to disappointment for both the patient and the clinician. Rather than aiming for complete resolution of the symptoms, it is better to set more realistic goals. For the primary care practitioner, these might include reducing the number of phone calls and visits with new symptoms, the number of requests for medications or referrals to specialists, and the number of emergency room visits. For patients, these goals might include an increased sense of control in their lives, improved social functioning, and better coping with day-to-day symptoms.

> **Clinician:** Today I would like to talk about what we should expect from each other in this relationship. From your perspective, I suspect that the best thing I could do would be to figure out what's causing these symptoms and make them go away completely. Given all of your years of suffering and the many doctors you've seen, however, I'm sad to say that I don't think that is very realistic. What do you think?
>
> **Patient:** Well, of course I was hoping that you could find a cure. So—does this mean that you can't help me?
>
> **Clinician:** No, I didn't mean to imply that. I do think I can help. First, I'd like to work on helping you learn to cope more effectively with your symptoms. We could also work to improve how you function from day to day. Whether you get better or not, I'm committed to helping you in the best way I can.

A novel treatment for somatoform disorders involves the use of a "written self-disclosure protocol." This therapy involves having the patient with somatoform symptoms periodically write in a journal format. The clinician convinces the patient to spend 20 minutes one time per week at home writing about distressing experiences in their lives. They are specifically encouraged to think about experiences involving relationships with others. The patients are also instructed to write about how these experiences have affected them in the past and how they may continue to affect them in the future. The journal

may be shared with others if the patient wishes, but it does not have to be shared to have a benefit. This technique has been found to be acceptable by both patients and providers. It has also been found to be helpful, time effective, and cost effective. The patients do the writing outside of the office and have demonstrated decreases in health care utilization.

Another recently developed technique for treating patients with somatization symptoms in the primary care setting is designed to help general practitioners teach these patients to reattribute and relate physical symptoms to psychosocial problems. The clinician is encouraged to take a history of the patient's illness including related physical, mood, and social factors. The clinician then broadens the view of the problem and the necessary treatment by reframing the complaint using the biopsychosocial information provided by the patient. The practitioner then links the patient's distress and the physical complaint using a coherent explanation of how psychosocial factors can give rise to physical symptoms. This intervention model has been found to be both cost effective and clinically effective.

Despite all of these interventions, it may be necessary to refer the patient to a mental health specialist. Many individuals with somatization will resist such a referral. Although this reluctance on the patient's part can be frustrating, the primary care provider should remember that many of these patients have experienced such referral as the first step in the termination of their relationship with a health care provider. The primary care clinician can address this concern by making a follow-up appointment with the patient prior to the referral. Once the continuity of the relationship is ensured, the referral can be discussed. Further, a consultation model in which the patient is asked to see the mental health provider for one or a few visits in order to "advise and help the primary care provider do a better job" is often more acceptable to patients than a referral for ongoing treatment. The consultation can be useful in confirming diagnosis or in providing advice on the use of psychotropic medications.

> **Clinician:** I'd like to see you in a month. In the meantime, I'd like you to consider seeing Dr. R, the psychiatrist we've talked about. I know that you don't think that your chest pain is caused by your depression. But we've both agreed to try to treat the depression. I still don't know if we've found the right antidepressant, and I'd really value Dr. R's opinion. What do you think?

Psychotherapy

Cognitive-behavioral Therapy (CBT) has been studied as a means of addressing the medically unexplained somatic symptoms. This technique is based on the theory that incorrect beliefs about bodily functioning and related dysfunctional behaviors underlie these symptoms. The first task in therapy is to identify these beliefs and behaviors. Next, the patient is encouraged to challenge the beliefs and is taught to adopt more accurate ideas about bodily functioning. This change is paired with adoption of more appropriate behaviors. A review of clinical trials utilizing CBT for the treatment of somatization symptoms found that in 71% of the studies treated subjects improved significantly more than controls. Further, there was a trend toward significance in another 11% of the studies. These benefits occurred independently of the effect of the therapy on psychological distress. This finding suggests that the improvement was not due only to improvement in depression or anxiety symptoms, but rather to some effect on the somatization itself.

Psychodynamic psychotherapy is based on the assumption that the individual is experiencing internal emotional conflicts and that the associated emotions cannot be expressed. As a result, the conflict is manifested through somatic symptoms. The therapy focuses on attempting to uncover these conflicts and having the patient express them openly in the therapy sessions. As the patient does this work, the somatic symptoms become unnecessary and resolve. Unfortunately, most somatizing patients are not enthusiastic about exploring unconscious conflicts. In general the psychodynamic perspective is a long-term, time-intensive approach that requires a referral to a specialist and a commitment by the patient.

In family-oriented approaches to therapy, therapists must integrate the biological and psychosocial aspects of the patient's illness. The care provider must collaborate with the patient and the patient's family in treating the illness. Further, the clinician must demonstrate true interest in and curiosity about the patient's symptoms, family, relationships, and life. These therapies attempt to help the patients and their families break down the distinction between physical and psychological and move their thinking from "either-or" (eg, it is either a physical problem or a mental problem) to "both-and" (eg, the problem has both physical and mental facets). Relational therapists argue that effective therapy involves validating the illness, involving the family, working closely with the healthcare team, and enhancing the patient's curiosity about symptoms. They also emphasize demonstrating interest in the patient's somatic symptoms, helping the patient to see the relationship between the somatic symptoms and psychosocial stressors, and using physical interventions (eg, biofeedback and relaxation techniques) to form an alliance with the patient to deal with the illness.

Medication

Data on the efficacy of using medications to treat somatoform disorders are limited to studies in certain disorders. Gabapentin, at a dose of 1200–1600 mg/day, was used to treat somatization disorder with pain as the main symptom in an open-label study protocol. Patients improved in ratings of pain, clinician-assessed global level of functioning, and clinician assessment of symptomatic improvement. Interestingly, there was no significant improvement in the subjects' anxiety and depression, suggesting that the improvement in other areas was independent of changes in these symptoms. Medications that increase the level of central nervous system serotonin have also been found to be effective in some somatoform disorders. For example, clomipramine (a tricyclic antidepressant with potent serotonin reuptake blocking action), at doses up to 250 mg/day, and fluvoxamine (a selective serotonin reuptake inhibitor), at doses up to 150 mg twice a day, have both been studied in patients with body dysmorphic disorder (BDD). The treated patients improved significantly, even if they were felt to have delusional beliefs about their bodies. Interestingly, clomipramine was demonstrated to be superior to desipramine (a tricyclic antidepressant with predominantly norepinephrine reuptake blockade properties). The conclusion is that the efficacy of these agents in treating BDD is related specifically to their serotonin reuptake blockade.

A summary of recommendations for managing patients with somatization symptoms is found in Table 23–2.

CLINICIAN–PATIENT RELATIONSHIP

Caring for individuals with somatoform disorders is difficult. The patients present with symptoms suggestive of a medical or neurological illness and require an appropriate evaluation. However, at the completion of the evaluation the clinician is faced with an individual who, by definition, does not have a physical condition or who has a condition that cannot account for the level of symptoms or disability that the patient experiences. However, the patients view the

Table 23–2. Management of somatization.

Interventions
1. Take a detailed history, perform a physical examination, and order appropriate diagnostic studies.
2. Screen individuals with multiple somatic complaints for psychiatric disorders.
3. Integrate the patient's physical and psychosocial concerns by inquiring not only about somatic symptoms but also about other events in the person's life.
4. Develop an empathic relationship.
5. Never challenge the validity of the patient's somatic symptoms.
6. Do not utilize psychological labels for the patient's symptoms.
7. Schedule the patient for appointments at regular intervals.
8. Establish realistic expectations.
9. Care for yourself.

symptoms as somatic and strenuously resist the idea that the symptoms have a psychological component. As a result, neither party is satisfied with the interaction.

Why is dealing with patients who experience somatoform disorders so difficult? One theory is that clinicians use terminology that was developed to promote communication with other health care providers. It is not meant to provide the patient with an explanation of or validation of their illness experience. Health providers focus on understanding the pathophysiology of disease in a scientific manner. Laypersons have different explanatory models of disease, and therefore, when they present to the clinician's office they may already have a theory about the origin of their symptoms. In the case of patients with somatization, this theory involves a physical cause. In contrast, the practitioner may feel that a physical cause for the symptoms is less likely than a psychological etiology. As a result, the patient and clinician possess models of illness that are not only competing but also conflicting. To work effectively with the patient, the provider must reconcile these theories.

> **Patient:** So you think I have "depression"? How is that causing me to be tired all the time? I don't understand how you can say that. I don't cry and I don't feel sad.
>
> **Clinician:** Depression is not just feeling sad. It is a medical illness, just like diabetes or epilepsy. It is caused by an imbalance in the chemicals in the brain that help the brain cells communicate with each other. When those chemicals, or transmitters, are out of balance the brain does not function correctly and people develop symptoms such as fatigue, sadness, changes in sleep and appetite, and changes in their ability to concentrate.
>
> **Patient:** Well what can be done?
>
> **Clinician:** The good news is there are a number of treatments. Medications can be very helpful by directly affecting the balance of the transmitters. Other treatments involve working with someone to help you train your brain to function better without medications.

It seems, then, that working with these patients is difficult because they do not share the clinician's explanatory models and they resist giving up their own model of illness. When providers are able to explain the patient's symptoms in a way that provides a holistic and empowering perspective, they are viewed as a positive and helpful influence. As a result, the patient is satisfied, an alliance is formed to address the symptoms in a collaborative manner, and the practitioner may feel more positive about the patient.

Research has also focused on the reasons clinicians experience certain patients as difficult. Patients who are rated as difficult by health providers have twice the prevalence of psychiatric disorders. Further, the presence of more physical symptoms, both those judged to result from medical causes and those judged to be somatoform in origin, contributes to the sense that the patient is difficult. In addition, clinicians expect physical symptoms to be associated with medical diagnoses and the lack of such an association leads to frustration over the "vagueness" of the symptoms and their own inability to make a diagnosis. Patients may have reasons for "holding onto" the symptoms. The assumption of the sick role may confer some benefits, through changes in social and family systems, that are difficult for the provider to discern or understand. The practitioner may feel that the patient is consciously faking symptoms. Clinicians should attempt to understand the role that the symptoms play in the patient's family and social systems to gain insight into why the symptoms persist despite the lack of a somatic etiology.

CARING FOR THE CLINICIAN

The care of patients with somatoform symptoms is a draining experience and the clinician must take care not to burn out. The patient's unending physical concerns, resistance to treatment, and complaints that the clinician is not doing enough can easily overwhelm the provider. The practitioner is well advised to remember that these are chronic disorders. As a consequence, it can be helpful to set reasonable goals for treatment such as "care and not cure." Clinicians must remember that they can provide support and effective treatment but that the patient will likely have some residual symptoms. The practitioner should feel comfortable setting limits with their somatizing patients. Once the clinician and patient have committed to regular follow-up appointments, it is appropriate to set limits on calls and drop-in visits. For example, the patient can be asked to reserve all but emergency complaints for the regular visits. If the patient calls between scheduled sessions, the discussion should be limited to ascertaining that there is no emergency. If there is none, then the patient can be gently urged to defer further discussion until the next visit.

Outside of work, practitioners should take time for exercise, family, friends, and other interests. They may also wish to discuss difficult cases with colleagues to manage the powerful feelings these patients can elicit. In this way, they can maintain a healthy life-style and balance in their life. Clinicians must remember that the illness belongs to the patient and not to them. They must not allow the patient's frustration or demands make them forget this. The combination of empathic listening, conservative (but appropriate) evaluation, and gentle limit setting can not only benefit these patients, but also improve the primary care provider's satisfaction with these relationships.

SUGGESTED READINGS

Barsky AJ, Borus JF: Functional somatic syndromes. Ann Intern Med 1999;130:910. PMID: 10375340.

Colegrave S, Holcombe C, Salmon P: Psychological characteristics of women presenting with breast pain. J Psychosom Res 2001;50:303. PMID: 11438111.

Garcia-Campayo J, Sanz-Carrillo C: Gabapentin for the treatment of patients with somatization disorder. J Clin Psychiatry 2001;62: 474. PMID: 11465526.

Hahn SR: Physical symptoms and physician-experienced difficulty in the physician-patient relationship. Ann Intern Med 2001; 134:897. PMID: 11346326.

Hansen MS et al: Mental disorders among internal medical inpatients: prevalence, detection, and treatment status. J Psychosom Res 2001;50:199. PMID: 11369025.

Heim C, Ehlert U, Hellhammer DH: The potential role of hypocortisolism in the pathophysiology of stress-related bodily disorders. Psychoneuroendocrinology 2000;25:1. PMID: 10633533.

Hollander E et al: Clomipramine vs desipramine crossover trial in body dysmorphic disorder. Arch Gen Psychiatry 1999;56:1033. PMID: 10565503.

Holloway KL, Zerbe KJ: Simplified approach to somatization disorder. Postgrad Med 2000;108:89. PMID: 11098261.

Katon W, Sullivan M, Walker E: Medical symptoms without identified pathology: relationship to psychiatric disorders, childhood and adult trauma, and personality traits. Ann Intern Med 2001; 134:917. PMID: 11346329.

Kirmayer LJ: Cultural variations in the clinical presentation of depression and anxiety: implications for diagnosis and treatment. J Clin Psychiatry 2001;62(Suppl 13):22. PMID: 11434415.

Klapow JC et al: Symptom management in older primary care patients: feasibility of an experimental, written self-disclosure protocol. Ann Intern Med 2001;134:905. PMID: 11346327.

Kroenke K, Swindle R: Cognitive-behavioral therapy for somatization and symptom syndromes: a critical review of controlled clinical trials. Psychother Psychosom 2000;69:205. PMID: 10867588.

Morriss RK et al: Clinical and patient satisfaction outcomes of a new treatment for somatized mental disorder taught to general-practitioners. Br J Gen Pract 1999;49:263. PMID: 10736901.

Phillips KA et al: Delusionality and response to open-label fluvoxamine in body dysmorphic disorder. J Clin Psychiatry 2001;62:87. PMID: 11247107.

Rief W, Auer C: Is somatization a habituation disorder? physiological reactivity in somatization syndrome. Psychiatry Res 2001;101:63. PMID: 11223121

Sharpe M, Carson A: "Unexplained" somatic symptoms, functional syndromes, and somatization: do we need a paradigm shift? Ann Intern Med 2001;134:926. PMID: 11346330.

Smith GR, Monson RA, Ray DC: Psychiatric consultation in somatization disorder. N Engl J Med 1986;314:1407.

Spitzer RL et al: Validity and utility of the PRIME-MD Patient Health Questionnaire in assessment of 3000 obstetric-gynecologic patients: The PRIME-MD Patient Health Questionnaire Obstetric-Gynecologic Study. Am J Obstet Gynecol 2000;183: 759. PMID: 10992206.

Watson WH, McDaniel SH: Relational therapy in medical settings: working with somatizing patients and their families. J Clin Psychol 2000;56:1065. PMID: 10946733.

Personality Disorders

Adriana Feder, MD, Seth Wigdor Robbins, MD, MPH, & Britta Ostermeyer, MD

INTRODUCTION

Establishing successful relationships with patients who are suffering from personality disorders can be quite challenging for health care providers, yet these patients are common in medical practice. Patients with personality disorders may over- or underuse medical care, and often have more difficulty complying with treatment. In addition, these patients are more likely to be hospitalized. An understanding of personality disorders allows physicians to anticipate the challenging interpersonal and behavioral problems that can arise in working with these patients and can help physicians work through the negative emotions that working with such patients may arouse. This facilitates the development and implementation of appropriate treatment plans.

The current edition of the American Psychiatric Association *Diagnostic and Statistical Manual of Mental Disorders,* 4th edition, *Text Revision (DSM-IV-TR)* defines personality disorder as:

> *an enduring pattern of inner experience and behavior that deviates markedly from the expectations of the individual's culture, is pervasive and inflexible, has an onset in adolescence or early adulthood, is stable over time, and leads to distress or impairment.*

People suffering from personality disorders are affected in their view of themselves, their ability to establish and maintain relationships with others, and their ability to function at work and to experience pleasure in life. These patients have difficulty negotiating complex situations and coping with stress and anxiety. The sick role and the demands of medical care can be particularly problematic for them. The stress of illness is often extreme and sets into motion defensive and inflexible emotional processes, cognitions, and behaviors—with negative consequences for their medical treatment. In addition, these patients' difficulties in relating to others manifest themselves in the doctor–patient relationship. They may be quite demanding or disrespectful of the needs of others, or they may experience such anxiety when they need to trust or confide in others that they avoid building relationships.

Personality theorists have long debated how best to understand and classify personality disorders. The debate has centered on two models. The **categorical model,** adopted by *DSM-IV,* views personality disorders as entities that are distinct from one another—that is, classified in separate categories—and also distinct from normalcy. This model blends more easily with traditional medical diagnosis than does the **dimensional model,** which views personality disorders as entities that overlap each other and that are not distinct from normalcy, so that the maladaptive traits of patients with personality disorders represent normal traits that are exaggerated.

In fact, both models hold some truth. Some personality disorders, such as schizotypal and paranoid, may belong to a spectrum of illness that includes psychotic Axis I disorders and are thus better explained by a categorical model. Other personality disorders, such as histrionic and obsessive-compulsive personality, may depict exaggerated normal traits, reinforcing the concept of a dimensional model.

Diagnostic Classification of Personality Disorders

DSM-IV classifies personality disorders on a separate axis, Axis II, and groups them into three clusters based on descriptive similarities. Cluster A includes paranoid, schizoid, and schizotypal personality disorders—individuals who often appear odd or eccentric; cluster B includes antisocial, borderline, histrionic, and narcissistic personality disorders—individuals who often appear dramatic, emotional, or erratic; and cluster C includes avoidant, dependent, and obsessive-compulsive personality disorders—individuals who often appear anxious or fearful. Given the unique nature of any individual personality, a patient can exhibit traits of two or more personality disorders, or meet the full diagnostic criteria for more than one disorder.

Diagnosing a personality disorder can be a difficult task. To make an accurate diagnosis, it is usually necessary for the physician to get to know the patient over time, to find out how the patient reacts in other situations, and to obtain collateral information from family and friends. Clinicians should attend to three key issues.

First, it is important to differentiate a true personality disorder from personality traits that become exaggerated under stress. The stress of illness on patients often causes them to behave in maladaptive ways; because of this, many patients, at one time or another, seem to have a personality disorder. Patients who do not suffer from a true personality disorder, however, are usually capable of more adaptive functioning. In these cases, the physician can successfully intervene by supporting and strengthening these patients' own natural coping skills.

Second, it is also important to differentiate personality disorders from such Axis I disorders as major depression or generalized anxiety disorder. For example, patients with panic disorder may—out of sheer terror—become extremely dependent on their physician. If their panic disorder is diagnosed and treated, they may reveal an underlying independent and self-sufficient personality. When patients who do have a personality disorder are evaluated, looking for Axis I disorders is particularly important as the latter are more frequent and difficult to treat if patients actually have a personality disorder. Treating an episode of major depression in a patient with borderline personality disorder, however, can alleviate suffering and lead to better coping with illness.

Third, the primary care provider must distinguish personality disorders from personality changes caused by general medical conditions, such as head trauma, stroke, epilepsy, or endocrine disorders. Patients with one of these problems may exhibit many of the characteristics of a personality disorder. These behaviors can be distinguished from a true personality disorder, however, in that they typically represent a change from baseline personality characteristics. Medical conditions such as these at times may also exacerbate preexisting personality traits (eg, obsessive mannerisms). Treatment of the underlying medical problem may bring about reversal of the personality changes.

Finally, personality disorder diagnoses, like other mental disorder diagnoses, are often misunderstood and may serve to stigmatize the patient. These diagnoses should therefore be made carefully, deferred in cases of uncertainty, and noted in medical records and correspondence only when their notation is likely to be helpful in enhancing patient care.

Doctor–Patient Relationship Issues

The primary care provider may find many challenges in working with patients with personality disorders. Personality disorders often significantly impair the quality of interpersonal relationships. Because the doctor–patient relationship requires effective communication about important health issues of a personal nature, tensions and at times overt conflict may develop between patients with personality disorders and their providers. These tensions may also affect other members of the health care team and may be especially pronounced in the context of acute illness or crisis situations. In fact, the first diagnostic clues suggesting personality dysfunction or disorder may appear as difficulties in the doctor–patient relationship.

For patients with personality disorders, physical illness can cause exaggerated degrees of emotional distress, not always expressed to the provider. Although some patients do tell their providers about their emotional distress, others may instead manifest distress as noncompliance with the agreed-upon plan of evaluation or treatment or as changed, unexpected, or undesirable behavior (as judged by the physician) toward the physician.

In response to patients' actions or statements, physicians may have a significant emotional reaction to the patients and may change their behavior toward them. Even when they experience no subjective distress from a medical condition or the doctor–patient relationship, patients with personality dysfunction may have such aberrant expectations of others that their statements or behavior are troubling or burdensome to the physician. Physicians must be aware of their own emotional responses to such patients so as to avoid reacting inappropriately. Physicians who deny their negative feelings toward the patients may fail to recognize a personality disorder or other psychiatric diagnosis, or fail to address the diagnostic and treatment needs of the patient with the necessary vigor and thoroughness. When clinicians recognize and deal with their negative feelings, they are better able to make thoughtful and appropriate responses to these patients' psychological symptoms and behavior, minimizing the emotional strain for both patient and doctor and optimizing the quality of the medical outcome.

A clear understanding by both patient and doctor of the role each expects the other to play can aid in identifying problematic behaviors and can help to maintain the necessary degree of cooperation and collaboration, even when the patient has significant personality dysfunction. In this regard, it is important to understand how patients with different personality disorders vary in their needs and expectations in this relationship. Table 24–1 outlines typical responses to illness by patients with each of the most common personality disorders, details troublesome reactions by physicians, and suggests strategies to avoid further problems with these challenging patients.

Management of Patients with Personality Disorders

In most cases, a stable therapeutic alliance with patients who have personality disorders can be maintained by implementing the behavioral strategies suggested in the following sections. Sometimes other factors must also be addressed. As mentioned earlier, comorbid Axis I diagnoses must be treated. The most common examples of this would be treatment of depression or anxiety disorders. Pharmacotherapy and psychotherapy (and their integration) are often more complex for patients with comorbid Axis I and II disorders. This difficulty is particularly evident (*text continues on page 237*)

Table 24-1. Common personality disorders and typical manifestations.

Personality Disorder	Paranoid	Schizoid	Schizotypal	Antisocial	Borderline
Prominent features of disorder	Distrust and suspiciousness of others, such that their motives are interpreted as malevolent	Pattern of detachment from social relationships and a restricted range of emotional expression	Odd beliefs, inappropriate affect, perceptual distortions and desire for social isolation	Disregard for and violation of the rights of others, beginning in adolescence	Pattern of instability in interpersonal relationships, self-image and affects, and marked impulsivity
Patient's experience of illness	Heightened sense of fear and vulnerability	Threat to personal integrity; increased anxiety because illness forces interaction with others	May have odd interpretations of illness, increased anxiety because of interactions with others, may become overtly psychotic	Sense of fear may be masked by increased hostility or entitled stance	Terrifying fantasies about illness; feels either completely well or deathly ill
Problematic behavior in the medical care setting	Fear that physician or others may harm them; Misinterpretation of innocuous or even helpful behaviors; Increased likelihood of argument or conflict with staff	May delay seeking care until symptoms become severe, out of fear of interacting with others; May appear detached and unappreciative of help	May delay care because of odd and magical beliefs about symptoms, may not recognize symptoms as a sign of illness; May appear odd and eccentric and paranoid toward others	Irresponsible, impulsive, or dangerous health behavior, without regard for consequences to self or others; Angry, deceitful, or manipulative behavior	Mistrust of physicians and delay in seeking treatment; Intense fear of rejection and abandonment; Abrupt shifts from idealizing to devaluing caregivers; splitting; Self-destructive threats and acts

(continued)

Table 24–1. Continued

Personality Disorder	Paranoid	Schizoid	Schizotypal	Antisocial	Borderline
Common problematic reactions to patient by caregiver	Defensive, argumentative or angry response that "confirms" patient's suspicions Ignoring the patient's suspicious or angry stance	Overzealous attempts to connect with patient Frustration at feeling unappreciated	Frustration about patient's misinterpretation of illness Not wanting to connect with an odd and eccentric patient	Succumbing to patient's manipulation Angry, punitive reaction when manipulation is discovered	Succumbing to patient's idealization and splitting Getting too close to patient, causing overstimulation Despair at patient's self-destructive behaviors Temptation to punish patient angrily
Helpful management strategies by caregiver	Attend to and be empathic toward patient fears, even when irrational in appearance Carefully detail care plan for patient with advance information about risks of procedures/treatments Maintain patient's independence when possible Professional, but not overly friendly stance	Appreciate need for privacy and maintain a low-key approach Focus on technical elements of treatment; these are better tolerated Encourage patient to maintain daily routines Do not become personally overly involved or too zealous in trying to provide social supports	Try not to be turned off by patient's odd appearance Try to educate patient about the illness and its treatment Do not become overly involved in trying to provide social support	Carefully, respectfully investigate patient's concerns and motives Communicate directly; avoid punitive reactions to patient Set clear limits in context of medically indicated interventions	Don't get too close to patient Schedule frequent periodic check-ups Provide clear, non-technical answers to questions to counter scary fantasies Tolerate periodic angry outbursts, but set limits Be aware of patient's potential for self-destructive behavior Discuss feelings with co-workers and schedule multidisciplinary

(continued)

Table 24–1. Continued.

Personality Disorder	Histrionic	Narcissistic	Avoidant	Dependent	Obsessive-Compulsive
Prominent features of disorder	Pattern of excessive attention seeking and emotionality	Pervasive pattern of grandiosity, need for admiration, and lack of empathy for others	Pattern of social inhibition because of fears of being rejected or humiliated by others	Pervasive and excessive need to be taken care of that leads to submissive and clinging behavior, and fears of separation	Pattern of preoccupation with orderliness, perfectionism, control
Patient's experience of illness	Threatened sense of attractiveness and self-esteem	Illness may increase anxiety related to doubts about personal adequacy	Illness may heighten sense of inadequacy and worsen low self-esteem	Fear that illness will lead to abandonment and helplessness	Fear of losing control over bodily functions and over emotions generated by illness; feelings of shame and vulnerability
Problematic behavior in the medical care setting	Overly dramatic, attention-seeking behavior, with tendency to draw caregiver into excessively familiar relationship Inadequate focus on symptoms and their management, with over emphasis on feeling states May provide answers they believe physician wants to hear Tendency to somatize	Demanding, entitled attitude Excessive praise toward caregiver may turn to devaluation, in effort to maintain sense of superiority Denial of illness or minimization of symptoms	May not be forthcoming about symptom severity, may easily agree with physician out of fear of not being liked	Dramatic and urgent demands for medical attention Angry outbursts at physician if not responded to Patient may contribute to prolong illness or encourage medical procedures in order to get attention May abuse substances and medications	Anger about disruption of routines Repetitive questions and excessive attention to detail Fear of relinquishing control to health care team

(continued)

Table 24–1. Continued.

Personality Disorder	Histrionic	Narcissistic	Avoidant	Dependent	Obsessive-Compulsive
Common problematic reactions to patient by caregiver	Performing excessive work-up (when patient is dramatic) or inadequate work-up (when patient is vague) Allowing too much emotional closeness, thereby losing objectivity Frustration with patient's dramatic or vague presentation	Outright rejection of patient's demands, resulting in patient distancing self from caregiver Excessive submission to patient's grandiose stance	Feeling overly concerned for the patient, taking on a paternalistic role that may increase patient's sense of inadequacy May feel angry and betrayed by patient if the patient's symptoms turn out to be more extensive than initially reported	Inability to set limits to availability, thus leading to burnout Hostile rejection of patient	Impatience and cutting answers short Attempts to control treatment planning
Helpful management strategies by caregiver	Show respectful and professional concern for feelings, with emphasis on objective issues Avoid excessive familiarity	Generous validation of patient's concerns, with attentive but factual response to questions Allow patients to maintain sense of competence by rechannelling their "skills" to deal with illness, obviating need for devaluation of caregivers	Provide reassurance, validate patient's concerns Encourage reporting of symptoms and concerns	Provide reassurance and schedule frequent periodic check-ups Be consistently available but provide firm realistic limits to availability Enlist other members of the health care team in providing support for patient Help patient obtain outside support systems Avoid hostile rejection of patient	Thorough history taking and careful diagnostic work-ups are reassuring Give clear and thorough explanation of diagnosis and treatment options Do not overemphasize uncertainties about treatments Avoid vague and impressionistic explanations Treat patient as an equal partner; encourage self-monitoring and allow patient participation in treatment

when patients with personality disorders have concurrent substance-abuse problems or psychotic symptoms (eg, hallucinations, delusions, paranoid ideation). In such cases, mental health consultation can be particularly helpful.

When a provider feels unable to continue productive work with a patient with a personality disorder, it may be appropriate to transfer the patient to another clinician. Although such transfers of care may be both necessary and helpful, they require consideration of the impact of the transfer on the well-being of the patient. Patients with certain personality disorders may experience such transfers as rejection or abandonment, perceptions that may exacerbate their emotional distress and potentially disrupt their medical treatment. Prior consultation with a mental health provider can be useful in determining whether such a transfer might be helpful and can aid in carrying it out smoothly.

The remainder of this chapter discusses the 10 personality disorders as they manifest in the primary care setting, and management recommendations.

PARANOID PERSONALITY DISORDER

Symptoms & Signs

Patients with paranoid personality disorder (Table 24–2) have a long-standing pattern of distrust and suspiciousness. They perceive the behavior and motives of others as malevolent in nature and expect others, in many situations, to disappoint or take advantage of them. They may perceive seemingly benign or innocuous statements or behavior by others as threatening, insulting, or hurtful. To defend against their perceived vulnerability, they usually adopt a rigid, distanced, or guarded position. In general, persons with this personality structure find intimate relationships undesirable and difficult, which often leaves them without any significant social supports.

Differential Diagnosis

Long-standing psychotic symptoms, such as delusions and hallucinations, suggest a diagnosis of paranoid delusional disorder or paranoid schizophrenia. Although persons with paranoid personality disorder usually do not have frank paranoid delusions, at times of extreme stress they may develop such symptoms. Brief paranoid ideation may be associated with medical causes or with alcohol or substance abuse or withdrawal.

Illness Experience & Illness Behavior

Illness is difficult for individuals with paranoid personality disorder because having to communicate personal information to the physician may challenge the self-protective, rigid way they approach social interactions. Patients may experience a heightened sense of vulnerability and fear of harm by the physician. In their fearful state, they may perceive innocuous or even overtly helpful behavior as threatening. They may then question or challenge the physician about the content of an intervention or the motives behind it. This can lead to possible conflict and argument between patient and doctor.

THE DOCTOR–PATIENT RELATIONSHIP

Physicians confronted with such a paranoid stance may react in ways that exacerbate the situation. If they feel that their intentions are inappropriately suspect they might argue with the patient or become defensive, perhaps using an angry tone. This kind of reaction may frighten the patient and may be perceived as confirmation of the patient's suspicion. Although such a response should be avoided, ignoring the patient's distrustful or angry behavior can also be problematic; the patient's concerns, however irrational, may increase if not addressed.

Table 24–2. Diagnostic criteria for paranoid personality disorder (301.0).

A. A pervasive distrust and suspiciousness of others such that their motives are interpreted as malevolent, beginning by early adulthood and present in a variety of contexts, as indicated by four (or more) of the following:
1. suspects, without sufficient basis, that others are exploiting, harming, or deceiving him or her
2. is preoccupied with unjustified doubts about the loyalty or trustworthiness of friends or associates
3. is reluctant to confide in others because of unwarranted fear that the information will be used maliciously against him or her
4. reads hidden demeaning or threatening meanings into benign remarks or events
5. persistently bears grudges, that is, is unforgiving of insults, injuries, or slights
6. perceives attacks on his or her character or reputation that are not apparent to others and is quick to react angrily or to counterattack
7. has recurrent suspicions, without justification, regarding fidelity of spouse or sexual partner
B. Does not occur exclusively during the course of schizophrenia, a mood disorder with psychotic features, or another psychotic disorder and is not due to the direct physiological effects of a general medical condition.

Source: Reprinted, with permission, from American Psychiatric Association: *Diagnostic and Statistical Manual of Mental Disorders,* 4th edition, *Text Revision* (*DSM-IV-TR*). American Psychiatric Association, 2000.

Specific Management Strategies

It is essential to address the patient's concerns and fears empathically, however irrational they seem. Although the physician may see the patient's concern as unrealistic, to the patient the fear is real. Dismissing these patients' concerns or calling them paranoid will not address their emotional needs and may instead create distance in the doctor–patient relationship. A professional stance is most reassuring to these patients. Excessive friendliness or reassurance may be misinterpreted and may intensify their paranoia. It is important to give these patients detailed information about their proposed treatment plan, allowing them to feel they are in control of the treatment and can make independent decisions. Provide factual information about risks associated with the treatment, whenever possible, before any major procedures or changes in treatment.

CASE ILLUSTRATION 1

Simon, a 42-year-old, single, male parking lot attendant, presents to his primary care provider, complaining of 3 months of tension headaches and fatigue in the context of what he calls "job stress." The only notable finding in the physical examination is a new, but mild, elevation of blood pressure. The physician also observes that Simon seems angry and anxious, in contrast to his previously distant and somewhat guarded demeanor. When asked about his job stress, Simon reveals anxieties about not being able to trust two new co-workers, along with fears that his supervisors are conspiring to dismiss him from his job. He also mentions, hesitantly, that he had not sought evaluation of his headaches sooner because he worried that the physician would dismiss his fears as unfounded or "crazy." Additional social history reveals difficulty with close relationships and recurrent problems adjusting to changes in the workplace.

The physician responds by listening in a nonjudgmental and empathic manner. An over-the-counter analgesic for the headaches and buspirone for anxiety and agitation are prescribed. The physician plans follow-up measurements of the blood pressure and suggests that Simon see a psychiatrist for further evaluation of his very stressful job situation.

Simon feels that his concerns have been taken seriously. He finds the referral to a psychiatrist acceptable because it has been proposed in a way that offers support and does not dismiss his fears as pathological. The physician's matter-of-fact responses to Simon's somatic complaints help increase the patient's trust in his physician.

SCHIZOID PERSONALITY DISORDER

Symptoms & Signs

Individuals with schizoid personality disorder (Table 24–3) remain detached from social relationships and exhibit a restricted range of emotional expression in their interactions with others, often appearing cold or indifferent. Because patients with this disorder find emotions, intimacy, and conflict threatening, they tend to isolate themselves and avoid close or sexual relationships. They prefer dealing with technical or abstract concepts to contact with people, and so they may devote their time to pursuits such as mathematical games. Work can be problematic if it involves

Table 24–3. Diagnostic criteria for schizoid personality disorder (301.20).

A. A pervasive pattern of detachment from social relationships and a restricted range of expression of emotions in interpersonal settings, beginning by early adulthood and present in a variety of contexts, as indicated by four (or more) of the following:
  1. neither desires nor enjoys close relationships, including being part of a family
  2. almost always chooses solitary activities
  3. has little, if any, interest in having sexual experiences with another person
  4. takes pleasure in few, if any, activities
  5. lacks close friends or confidants other than first-degree relatives
  6. appears indifferent to the praise or criticism of others
  7. shows emotional coldness, detachment, or flattened affectivity
B. Does not occur exclusively during the course of schizophrenia, a mood disorder with psychotic features, another psychotic disorder, or a pervasive developmental disorder and is not due to the direct physiological effects of a general medical condition.

interactions with others, but many individuals can perform quite well if they work with some degree of independence.

Differential Diagnosis

Patients with schizoid personality disorder do not exhibit prolonged psychotic symptoms. They may, however, suffer a brief psychotic decompensation during times of extreme stress. In addition, schizoid personality disorder may in some cases precede the development of psychotic Axis I conditions, such as schizophrenia or delusional disorder. It can also coexist with schizotypal, paranoid, or avoidant personality disorders.

Illness Experience & Illness Behavior

Illness can be especially stressful for these patients because it gives rise to strong emotions that they are not prepared to cope with. The necessity of interacting with caregivers when ill, often around quite personal issues, forces them to do the very thing they systematically avoid. They may therefore delay seeking care until their symptoms become more serious. When they finally present for medical attention, they may appear indifferent or detached as a way of protecting themselves from overwhelming emotion. They may show little facial expression and may not respond in kind to caregivers' empathic nods or comments—which may make establishing a therapeutic relationship difficult.

THE DOCTOR–PATIENT RELATIONSHIP

Because these patients often appear cold or indifferent, physicians may consider them as unappreciative of help. They may also be puzzled or frustrated by their patients' delay in seeking medical care and their apparent passivity in the face of illness. As a result, caregivers may make overzealous attempts to connect with patients by trying to be especially empathic, a tactic that may instead frighten them away. On the other hand, providers may themselves draw back and lose their enthusiasm for helping patients who seem so unappreciative or uninvolved in their own treatment.

Specific Management Strategies

Understanding that individuals with schizoid personality disorder have difficulty tolerating emotions and intimate interactions is important. Physicians should appreciate their patients' need for privacy and should maintain a low-key approach, avoiding attempts to reach out by becoming too close or by insisting on providing social support. It is helpful to focus on the more technical aspects of treatment, as these are better tolerated, and encourage patients to maintain daily routines. Caregivers should remain available and provide steady but nonthreatening help.

CASE ILLUSTRATION 2

Ben, a 44-year-old computer programmer, presents to a university outpatient clinic for evaluation of nausea, anorexia, and a 30-pound weight loss occurring over the previous several months. When asked why he hadn't sought treatment before, Ben states that he has always been healthy and thought he would probably regain the lost weight.

Throughout the interview, Ben makes poor eye contact and gives brief answers to questions. He appears to dislike being interviewed by both a medical student and a resident. He becomes more uncomfortable when asked questions about his personal life and how he likes spending his time. Ben states that he usually keeps to himself, with the exception of visiting his sister about once a month. He spends much of his time programming and playing with his computer.

Ben appears visibly anxious when the resident recommends a consultation with a gastroenterologist. He asks whether this is truly necessary, as it will be hard for him to take time off from work. The resident emphasizes the importance of this consultation, and Ben seems to calm down a bit when the conversation focuses more on the possible tests that might be done to evaluate his symptoms, thereby distracting his attention from his concerns about having to see yet another doctor.

The resident later explains to the medical student that it is important to minimize the number of doctors Ben sees over time and to avoid an overfriendly style, which might frighten him.

SCHIZOTYPAL PERSONALITY DISORDER

Symptoms & Signs

Patients with schizotypal personality disorder (Table 24–4) behave in an odd and eccentric manner, are socially inept and isolated, and experience cognitive or perceptual distortions. Their distortions include magical thinking, odd beliefs, ideas of reference, bodily illusions, or telepathic and clairvoyant experiences. These beliefs and distortions are inconsistent with subcultural norms, occur frequently, and are an important and pervasive core component of the patient's experience. The patient's enduring psychotic-like symptoms may worsen under stress. Patients often dress in an odd and peculiar fashion and their affect is often inappropriate, for example, they may laugh inappropriately during the visit while talking about their problems.

Table 24–4. Diagnostic criteria for schizotypal personality disorder (301.22).

A. A pervasive pattern of social and interpersonal defects marked by acute discomfort with, and reduced capacity for, close relationships as well as by cognitive or perceptual distortions and eccentricities of behavior, beginning by early adulthood and present in a variety of contexts, as indicated by five (or more) of the following:
   1. ideas of reference (excluding delusions of reference)
   2. odd beliefs or magical thinking that influences behavior and is inconsistent with subcultural norms (eg, superstitiousness, belief in clairvoyance, telepathy, or "sixth sense"; in children and adolescents, bizarre fantasies or preoccupations)
   3. unusual perceptual experiences, including bodily illusions
   4. odd thinking and speech (eg, vague, circumstantial, metaphorical, overelaborate, or stereotyped)
   5. suspiciousness or paranoid ideation
   6. inappropriate or constricted affect
   7. behavior or appearance that is odd, eccentric, or peculiar
   8. lack of close friends or confidants other than first-degree relatives
   9. excessive social anxiety that does not diminish with familiarity and tends to be associated with paranoid fears rather than negative judgments about self
B. Does not occur exclusively during the course of schizophrenia, a mood disorder with psychotic features, another psychotic disorder, or a pervasive developmental disorder.

Source: Reprinted, with permission, from American Psychiatric Association: *Diagnostic and Statistical Manual of Mental Disorders*, 4th edition, *Text Revision* (*DSM-IV-TR*). American Psychiatric Association, 2000.

These patients are socially isolated and usually have few or no close friends. Their social isolation stems from their odd behavior as well as from their persistent social anxiety due to suspiciousness or paranoia toward others.

Differential Diagnosis

Schizotypal personality disorder shares the symptom of suspiciousness and paranoia with paranoid personality disorder and that of social isolation with schizoid personality disorder. However, the latter two disorders do not present with odd and peculiar mannerisms and behaviors and also lack cognitive or perceptual distortions.

The differential diagnosis includes schizophrenia (Axis I disorder). Although patients with schizotypal personality disorder lack signs and symptoms of overt psychosis, the disorder is considered a schizophrenia-spectrum disorder. This means that it may be related to schizophrenia. Family studies show an increased risk of schizophrenia in relatives of patients with schizotypal personality disorder and an increased risk of schizotypal personality disorder in families of patients with schizophrenia.

Illness Experience & Illness Behavior

Patients with schizotypal personality disorder may present late in the course of their illness because they may have odd interpretations of their illness and may, therefore, not recognize the serious nature of their symptoms. Also, like patients with schizoid personality disorder, they do not like to interact with and seek the company of others. Illness forces them to interact with health care providers and their support staff, something they may not be prepared to do.

This may lead to increased paranoid ideation or overt psychotic symptoms.

THE DOCTOR–PATIENT RELATIONSHIP

These patients' eccentric appearance may cause the clinician to be hesitant in approaching them. Odd and weird interpretations of illness may lead to misunderstandings between patient and clinician. It may be challenging for the physician to improve these patients' understanding of their problems.

Specific Management Strategies

Clinicians should try to overcome their apprehension about treating these patients, often caused by their eccentric appearance. It is helpful to find out what these patients think about their symptoms and to help them obtain a better understanding of their illness. At the same time, the physician should not get overly involved in trying to increase their patients' social support or exposure to others. Knowing that patients with schizotypal personality disorder desire social isolation is important.

 CASE ILLUSTRATION 3

Donna, a 35-year-old single female, has developed a cough, high fever, and chills and her family noticed that she started to look ill. She was brought to the emergency room by her mother. She is oddly dressed in a long and colorful country style wrap-around shirt with military type boots. Her hair is unkempt

and pinned up with a number of different hairpins. During the interview, Donna laughs in a silly manner while discussing her problem with the physician and the nurse. She says that she does not like to see a doctor because she prefers to walk in the woods by herself and communicate with the birds and insects.

The physician focuses on the patient's presenting symptoms and explains to her that she may suffer from pneumonia. He explains to her in simple terms what pneumonia is and that she needs sputum cultures and a chest X-ray to confirm the diagnosis.

While Donna has her chest X-ray taken, the physician explains to the nurse that health care providers should help the patient understand her symptoms as well as the rationale for her medical work-up and treatment. The physician also recommends focusing on the patient's problems and respecting her need for distance from others.

ANTISOCIAL PERSONALITY DISORDER

Symptoms & Signs

Persons with antisocial personality disorder (Table 24–5) demonstrate a disregard for others and behavior that violates others' rights. The diagnosis can be made only in persons over age 18, and it requires a history of conduct disorder prior to that age. Characteristics include lack of conformity to social norms and laws, using lies or other deceitfulness for personal gain, and impulsiveness and irresponsibility in many settings. These individuals may be threatening, manipulative, or harmful to others, and they are generally not remorseful. Their tendencies toward ag-

gressive behavior may not be immediately evident, but contact with collateral sources frequently reveals a criminal record. These character traits affect relations with both strangers and family alike, as persons with antisocial personality disorder may engage in inconsiderate, angry, or harmful behaviors. These individuals may present themselves in a superficially grandiose manner, and they can also initially appear somewhat charismatic, until others recognize their charm as manipulative.

Differential Diagnosis

Antisocial personality disorder can overlap significantly with other personality disorder traits, most commonly narcissistic, histrionic, or borderline personality disorder. Because substance abuse is a frequent comorbid diagnosis, it is important to distinguish between the problems when making the diagnosis.

Illness Experience & Illness Behavior

To mask the fear that illness may cause, patients with antisocial personality disorder may unconsciously adopt an excessively self-assured, entitled, or hostile stance. Irresponsible, impulsive, or dangerous health behavior may help these patients deny their vulnerability to illness. This behavior can occur without regard for medical consequences, and many patients show blatant disregard for the health care personnel and resources from which they have benefited. Patients may assume a privileged, self-deserving stance and can become antagonistic if they fail to obtain the desired response. They may attempt to manipulate their physician, malingering to obtain things such as drugs or inappropriate disability benefits. This behavior can be an embellishment of a real illness, or it can occur when they are not ill.

Table 24–5. Diagnostic criteria for antisocial personality disorder (301.7).

A. There is a pervasive pattern of disregard for and violation of the rights of others occurring since age 15 years, as indicated by three (or more) of the following:
   1. failure to conform to social norms with respect to lawful behaviors as indicated by repeatedly performing acts that are grounds for arrest
   2. deceitfulness, as indicated by repeated lying, use of aliases, or conning others for personal profit or pleasure
   3. impulsivity or failure to plan ahead
   4. irritability and aggressiveness, as indicated by repeated physical fights or assaults
   5. reckless disregard for safety of self or others
   6. consistent irresponsibility, as indicated by repeated failure to sustain consistent work behavior or honor financial obligations
   7. lack of remorse, as indicated by being indifferent to or rationalizing having hurt, mistreated, or stolen from another
B. The individual is at least age 18 years.
C. There is evidence of conduct disorder with onset before age 15 years.
D. The occurrence of antisocial behavior is not exclusively during the course of schizophrenia or a manic episode.

Source: Reprinted, with permission, from American Psychiatric Association: *Diagnostic and Statistical Manual of Mental Disorders,* 4th edition, *Text Revision* (*DSM-IV-TR*). American Psychiatric Association, 2000.

THE DOCTOR–PATIENT RELATIONSHIP

Because these patients often behave in ways that are non-compliant, ungracious, or dishonest, they are frequently irritating to health care providers. Physicians may become angry with these individuals or reject them if they see that the treatments in which they have invested their knowledge and energy have not been followed, or if they discover they have been manipulated by these patients.

Specific Management Strategies

Managing manipulative patients can be particularly challenging. If the patient tricks the physician, the outcome is usually detrimental to the patient's overall health (broadly defined). On the other hand, although recognizing the manipulative behavior may avert a detrimental health outcome, the physician's confrontation can alienate the patient. The more authoritarian the physician's stance, the more likely it is that the patient will become oppositional, reducing the possibility for development of an effective therapeutic alliance.

The key here is to maintain an objective, thorough, nonauthoritarian, and respectful approach to investigating the patient's presenting complaints. If the patient's presentation or motives are suspicious, the provider should gather corroborating data from collateral sources (other providers or family members) when needed. It is important to avoid becoming angry, punitive, or rejecting toward the patient; these behaviors may recapitulate behavior the patient experienced earlier in life that contributed to the development of the antisocial personality disorder. Such behavior by the physician can cause the patient to become hostile, with additional deterioration in the doctor–patient relationship. If confrontation or disagreement is necessary, it is essential to avoid humiliating the patient while identifying the attempted manipulation. Communication should be direct and factual with these patients, based on what is medically indicated, and clear limits should be set on the diagnostic or treatment plan.

CASE ILLUSTRATION 4

On returning from vacation, the doctor's first patient is Randy, an angry 42-year-old man, well known to her for his problems with long-standing recurrent low back pain. Although his back pain is generally well controlled with back exercises and as-needed nonsteroidal analgesics, Randy frequently takes long motorcycle trips with friends, during which he does not exercise or take his analgesics. While the physician was away, Randy went on a motorcycle tour and had a recurrence of acute back pain. He then telephoned the clinic and became angry and abusive toward the on-call nurse practitioner, who would not submit to his demands for narcotics.

The physician, who has seen similar behavior from Randy in the past, listens carefully to his story, acknowledges his anger, and reflects empathically on how painful his back must be. She inquires, non-judgmentally, about the reasons for his failure to exercise. She then explains the benefits of a more preventive approach—using exercise and avoiding pain-inducing behaviors—compared with the long-term risks of relying on narcotics and failing to exercise. Finally, she offers him referral to a physical therapist for a review of the exercise plan, along with a refill of his nonsteroidal analgesic, emphasizing her view that this would offer the best long-term outcome. With some bitterness, Randy acknowledges the benefits of the physician's recommendations and agrees to try to follow through with them.

In dealing with Randy, the physician uses her past experience with him as a guide. Randy's self-destructive behavior, hostility, and disregard for others are met with clear limit setting by the physician, who responds in a calm and nonpunitive manner, emphasizing her concern for the patient's long-term well-being.

BORDERLINE PERSONALITY DISORDER

Symptoms & Signs

Patients with borderline personality disorder (Table 24–6) exhibit instability in their self-image, their affect, and their relationships with others. They can be quite impulsive and may engage in self-destructive behaviors, such as substance abuse, self-mutilation, and suicide attempts. These behaviors reflect a deep sense of emptiness and an intense fear of abandonment by others. On the other hand, patients with borderline personality disorder are often also fearful of closeness. They experience many contradictory emotions and feelings that are not integrated into a stable sense of who they are and that may be associated with rapid shifts in mood. This instability can cause frequent changes in goals and values. These patients usually have difficulty differentiating reality from fantasy and tend toward all-or-nothing thinking in their view of themselves and others, alternating between overidealization and devaluation.

Differential Diagnosis

Some patients with borderline personality disorder may suffer brief psychotic episodes when under stress. They may, for example, become very anxious or experience auditory hallucinations. Such episodes are distinguishable from Axis I psychotic disorders by psychotic symptoms of brief

Table 24–6. Diagnostic criteria for borderline personality disorder (301.83).

A pervasive pattern of instability of interpersonal relationships, self-image, and affects, and marked impulsivity beginning by early adulthood and present in a variety of contexts, as indicated by five (or more) of the following:

1. frantic efforts to avoid real or imagined abandonment; *Note:* Do not include suicidal or self-mutilating behavior covered in criterion 5
2. a pattern of unstable and intense interpersonal relationships characterized by alternating between extremes of idealization and devaluation
3. identity disturbance: markedly and persistently unstable self-image or sense of self
4. impulsivity in at least two areas that are potentially self-damaging (eg, spending, sex, substance abuse, reckless driving, binge eating); *Note:* Do not include suicidal or self-mutilating behavior covered in criterion 5
5. recurrent suicidal behavior, gestures, or threats, or self-mutilating behavior
6. affective instability due to a marked reactivity of mood (eg, intense episodic dysphoria, irritability, or anxiety usually lasting a few hours and only rarely more than a few days)
7. chronic feelings of emptiness
8. inappropriate, intense anger or difficulty controlling anger (eg, frequent displays of temper, constant anger, recurrent physical fights)
9. transient, stress-related paranoid ideation or severe dissociative symptoms

Source: Reprinted, with permission, from American Psychiatric Association: *Diagnostic and Statistical Manual of Mental Disorders,* 4th edition, *Text Revision* (*DSM-IV-TR*). American Psychiatric Association, 2000.

duration. In addition, patients with borderline personality disorder also often suffer from a concurrent Axis I mood disorder, such as major depression or bipolar disorder, which should, of course, be treated. Other personality disorders (eg, histrionic or narcissistic) may be confused with borderline personality disorder. Some patients, however, may have traits of more than one personality disorder.

Illness Experience & Illness Behavior

Patients with borderline personality disorder have difficulty distinguishing reality from fantasy, and they may have terrifying fantasies about illness. The complex and contradictory feelings engendered in response to illness can feel intolerable to these patients, so they may try to cope by pretending that they are completely well and denying the presence of illness. Alternatively, they may become convinced that they are deathly ill, even when suffering from a mild illness. Having felt wounded in earlier relationships, individuals with borderline personality disorder mistrust and fear caregivers. In an attempt to cope with their simultaneous intense wish for, and fear of, closeness, they tend to conceptualize caregivers as all good or all bad—a mechanism called "splitting." To complicate things further, these conceptualizations are not stable. Even an overidealized caregiver can abruptly be devalued if a borderline patient becomes angry and disappointed or feels abandoned. In addition, patients with borderline personality disorder may respond to feeling overwhelmed by engaging in impulsive and self-destructive acts, such as self-mutilation, substance abuse, and suicide gestures or attempts. They may also be noncompliant with treatment as a way to remain ill and thus maintain an ongoing relationship with the caregiver.

THE DOCTOR–PATIENT RELATIONSHIP

A common mistake clinicians make in treating patients with borderline personality disorder is getting too emotionally close. This occurs when clinicians feel intensely drawn to help patients through their suffering and spend a great deal of time with them. This usually causes overstimulation of the patient's emotions, leading to increased instability and acting out. It should be noted that the patient's emotional behavior can cloud the clinician's judgment, causing the clinician to succumb to the patient's idealization and splitting. The borderline patient's self-destructive or often provocative behaviors can cause despair and helplessness in caregivers. Caregivers may also feel tempted to punish the patient, for example, by becoming verbally hostile or withholding needed pain medication.

Specific Management Strategies

While providing basic support and reassurance, clinicians should be careful not to become emotionally overinvolved with the borderline patient. It is appropriate to counter the patient's frightening fantasies about illness by scheduling frequent periodic check-ups and providing clear, nontechnical answers to questions. Caregivers may have to tolerate periodic angry outbursts, but it is appropriate to set firm limits on both the patient's disruptive behavior and on the caregiver's response. When a multidisciplinary team of clinicians is involved, meetings of all providers should be arranged, to allow them to vent their feelings about the patient and to reach consensus on a treatment plan. It is helpful to select a small number of caregivers to interact with the patient directly and to present the same clear and consistent plan. This approach often prevents splitting. Finally, it is essential to remain aware of these patients' potential for self-destructive behavior and not to retaliate for their disruptions by displaying anger at them when setting limits.

CASE ILLUSTRATION 5

A primary care resident expresses concern about her patient Amanda to her clinic's attending physician. She is scheduled to leave the clinic in 3 months and believes that Amanda will find transferring to a new doctor difficult.

Amanda is a 35-year-old temporary clerical worker with a long-standing history of migraine headaches. She often delays taking medication until her migraine headaches become severe, and then calls the resident, complaining of unbearable pain, sometimes stating that the pain is so intolerable that she wishes to die. She sometimes comes to the clinic without a scheduled appointment, demanding to be seen right away. On the other hand, she often misses regularly scheduled appointments. During her visits, she expresses a fear of becoming homeless; she house-sits at other people's homes but doesn't have a stable place of her own.

The resident asks for a psychiatric consultation to help her work with Amanda. She is particularly concerned about Amanda's periodic statements that she wishes to die.

Following the psychiatrist's recommendations, the resident continues to schedule regular, brief follow-up appointments, and encourages Amanda to keep these appointments. She explains that this is not a walk-in clinic, and that Amanda will have to seek treatment for acute pain in the emergency room. She also reminds Amanda that taking medication early will likely keep the headache from becoming very intense.

Other helpful interventions include providing increased support to Amanda by referring her to a psychotherapist and asking the team social worker to assist her in finding a stable residence. It is also important to monitor Amanda for suicidal ideation. If she expresses a wish to die, the resident assesses her suicidal ideation and intent. One afternoon, Amanda drops in at the clinic expressing suicidal ideation, and a nurse practitioner calls for an urgent psychiatric consultation. After talking to the psychiatrist, Amanda gradually calms down and denies any suicidal intent; however, she refuses a referral for ongoing psychiatric treatment.

Over time, Amanda continues to miss some appointments, and occasionally becomes demanding or complains bitterly about the resident to the nurse practitioner. When both the resident and the nurse practitioner, however, firmly and supportively continue to reiterate their treatment plan—to meet with the doctor for regular appointments, to treat migraines early, and to go to the emergency room for acute pain—Amanda's unpredictable visits and noncompliance diminish. Periodic meetings between the resident and the nurse practitioner help them both present the same coherent plan to Amanda, thus minimizing splitting.

In planning ahead for her departure from the clinic, the resident and the attending physician discuss some helpful strategies to facilitate this transition, such as introducing the new resident to Amanda ahead of time and involving the nurse practitioner—who is staying at the clinic—in the process.

In this case, regular meetings of the resident, the attending physician, and the nurse practitioner allow them to present the same coherent plan to the patient, minimize the splitting, and reduce the patient's anxiety and unpredictable behavior. This approach successfully combines increased support and limit setting.

HISTRIONIC PERSONALITY DISORDER

Symptoms & Signs

Histrionic personality disorder (Table 24–7) is marked by excessive attention seeking and emotionalism. These patients may present with dramatic, theatrical shows of feeling, or they may dress or behave in a sexually provocative fashion in an unconscious effort to engage others and draw attention to themselves. The emotions they express may be shallow and inconsistent, but the patients may still believe that the sharing of those feelings creates a special closeness (which they often exaggerate) with the physician. These patients have a tendency to prefer subjective and intuitive impressions over objective, linear, logical thinking. They often have somatic complaints, with impressive—but inconsistent—presentations.

Differential Diagnosis

Histrionic personality disorder may be difficult to distinguish from narcissistic or borderline personality disorder, and patients in each of these categories may exhibit traits common to patients in the others. Patients with histrionic personality disorder are deeply affected by perceived frailties in relationship bonds, as are patients with borderline personality disorder. The latter, however, display less emotional stability and are more impulsive and self-destructive. Patients with histrionic personality disorder may crave attention—as patients with narcissistic personality dis-

Table 24–7. Diagnostic criteria for histrionic personality disorder (301.50).

A pervasive pattern of excessive emotionality and attention seeking, beginning by early adulthood and present in a variety of contexts, as indicated by five (or more) of the following:
1. is uncomfortable in situations in which he or she is not the center of attention
2. interaction with others is often characterized by inappropriate sexually seductive or provocative behavior
3. displays rapidly shifting and shallow expression of emotions
4. consistently uses physical appearance to draw attention to self
5. has a style of speech that is excessively impressionistic and lacking in detail
6. shows self-dramatization, theatricality, and exaggerated expression of emotion
7. is suggestible, ie, easily influenced by others or circumstances
8. considers relationships to be more intimate than they actually are

Source: Reprinted, with permission, from American Psychiatric Association: *Diagnostic and Statistical Manual of Mental Disorders*, 4th edition, *Text Revision* (*DSM-IV-TR*). American Psychiatric Association, 2000.

order crave admiration—but the former tend to be less grandiose, arrogant, and self-absorbed.

Illness Experience & Illness Behavior

Medical illness represents a particular threat to the emotional well-being of patients with histrionic personality disorder, who derive much of their sense of self-worth and personal desirability from their sense of physical attractiveness. To reduce the fear of being deemed less desirable by others, these patients may attempt to bolster their physical appearance or embellish their abilities.

As a result, patients of either gender may engage in flirtatious or seductive behavior. When they feel weak and vulnerable, they may express their emotions with more intensity, in an attempt to strengthen their bond with the physician. In addition, because these patients focus on feelings, rather than on carefully observed physical symptoms, they may present with a collection of loosely connected somatic complaints. Their descriptions of the symptoms may reflect their desire to capture the physician's interest.

THE DOCTOR–PATIENT RELATIONSHIP

In working with the histrionic patient, the physician may be drawn in by the patient's dramatic and somewhat dependent style, become overly involved, and perhaps embark on an excessive work-up. As the physician becomes increasingly engaged by the patient's style, the patient may then become anxious, distant, or noncompliant, puzzling and frustrating the physician. Alternatively, the physician may instead pursue too cursory an evaluation, because of a lack of objective information, or out of frustration with the patient's emotional and vague style.

Specific Management Strategies

Because the patient with histrionic personality disorder has an emotional (rather than a logical) style and may display contrasting behaviors—that range from excessive anxiety

about potentially minor symptoms to inappropriate indifference about significant medical problems—it is essential that the physician maintain an objective stance. The physician must offer a supportive and logical approach to the patient's problems. This requires being both sensitive to the patient's emotional concerns and sufficiently distanced to avoid any degree of closeness that the patient might misperceive as intimate or sexual.

 CASE ILLUSTRATION 6

Rita is 38-year-old, single, unemployed actress with lupus. She is excessively friendly and flirtatious with her 45-year-old male physician, calling him frequently with questions about her medical problems and dressing somewhat seductively for office visits. During these visits she asks for examinations of a variety of somatic complaints. Over time, the physician becomes increasingly uncomfortable. Finally, Rita complains that she would like more time to discuss her problems at each office visit, and asks the physician if he thinks her problems "deserve more time."

After reflecting on the chronicity of this pattern of behavior, the physician responds that Rita's medical problems are significant and deserving of attention. He states that he intends to evaluate each of them carefully, allocating time on the basis of his impression of their medical necessity. He also says that he understands that she would like more time to discuss her concerns, but that as a busy doctor he cannot make additional time available to her. He suggests, gently, that if he cannot provide adequate emotional support to her, he could refer her to a local clinic's health psychologist. Although she is rather disappointed, Rita is able to accept this limit setting and continues to work with this doctor.

This approach is successful because the physician shows positive regard for the patient and her problems—while clearly setting the limits of the doctor–patient relationship.

NARCISSISTIC PERSONALITY DISORDER

Symptoms & Signs

Narcissistic personality disorder (Table 24–8) is characterized by a long-standing pattern of grandiosity, with a need for praise and admiration that stands out in contrast to a lack of sensitivity to the feelings of others. These persons may have an exaggerated sense of self-importance and social status. They may be driven toward attaining an idealized position in terms of social, personal, romantic, or career accomplishment. In this regard, they may be envious and potentially devaluing of others whose accomplishments they perceive as exceeding their own.

Differential Diagnosis

Narcissistic personality disorder may be difficult to distinguish from borderline, antisocial, histrionic, or obsessive-compulsive personality disorders, and in many cases it may overlap with these disorders. When the differentiation is unclear, identifying a high degree of grandiosity and a need for admiration can help clarify the diagnosis. In contrast to persons with borderline personality disorder, persons with narcissistic personality disorder have a more stable self-image and display less impulsiveness and sensitivity to relationship losses. In addition, persons with narcissistic personality disorder are generally less aggressive and deceitful than are persons with antisocial personality disorder, who also display evidence of childhood conduct disorder. Persons with histrionic personality disorder, in contrast, may be relatively more dramatic and emotional than those with narcissistic personality disorder. Although persons with narcissistic personality disorder, like those with obsessive-compulsive personality disorder, may be perfectionists, the former often have a higher self-assessment of their accomplishments.

Clinicians must be careful not to misdiagnose a person with transient hypomanic or manic grandiosity as having narcissistic personality disorder. Similarly, it is important to distinguish between narcissistic personality disorder and transient substance-related personality changes (eg, from central nervous system stimulants) or personality changes caused by a general medical condition.

Illness Experience & Illness Behavior

Health problems are a particular blow to patients with narcissistic personality disorder. Illness threatens these patients' unconscious attempts to maintain an intrapsychic and external image of untarnished well-being and resiliency. Medical problems and physical limitations may disrupt this image, threaten their public personas, and leave them fearing disruption of their (unrealistically unchallengeable) sense of self. In an attempt to defend against this threat, patients may minimize the significance of symptoms or deny the presence of the illness. More commonly, as patients try to recapture their admired, idealized status, they may demand special treatment or ridicule the physician caring for them. These patients may devalue, criticize, or question the behavior or credentials of the treating physician, or they may fail to comply with treatment recommendations.

Table 24–8. Diagnostic criteria for narcissistic personality disorder (301.81).

A pervasive pattern of grandiosity (in fantasy or behavior), need for admiration, and lack of empathy, beginning by early adulthood and present in a variety of contexts, as indicated by five (or more) of the following:

1. has a grandiose sense of self-importance (eg, exaggerates achievements and talents, expects to be recognized as superior without commensurate achievements)
2. is preoccupied with fantasies of unlimited success, power, brilliance, beauty, or ideal love
3. believes that he or she is "special" and unique and can only be understood by, or should associate with, other special or high-status people (or institutions)
4. requires excessive admiration
5. has a sense of entitlement, ie, unreasonable expectations of especially favorable treatment or automatic compliance with his or her expectations
6. is interpersonally exploitative, ie, takes advantage of others to achieve his or her own ends
7. lacks empathy: is unwilling to recognize or identify with the feelings and needs of others
8. is often envious of others or believes that others are envious of him or her
9. shows arrogant, haughty behaviors or altitudes

Source: Reprinted, with permission, from American Psychiatric Association: *Diagnostic and Statistical Manual of Mental Disorders,* 4th edition, *Text Revision* (*DSM-IV-TR*). American Psychiatric Association, 2000.

THE DOCTOR–PATIENT RELATIONSHIP

Narcissistic patients' arrogant and grandiose behavior, combined with demands for special treatment, can be extremely irritating to physicians. Reactions to these patients can take many forms. Sometimes, in an attempt to avoid conflict, physicians submit to the demands. With particularly critical patients, providers may feel frustration, resentment, and even anger. Alternatively, they may feel devalued and question their own competence. Frustration may be especially great if the physician expends special energy on behalf of a charismatic or demanding patient, only to later become the butt of unfair criticism. Physicians may reject or avoid the patient, withhold treatment, or respond in an angry manner—responses that can harm both the patient and the doctor–patient relationship.

Specific Management Strategies

The most effective strategy for dealing with narcissistic patients is to be respectful and nonconfrontational about their sense of specialness and entitlement and to help them use their self-perceived talents in the service of their treatment. If narcissistic patients feel vulnerable and threatened by the illness, they are more likely to criticize and devalue the physician. Thus physicians should not take this devaluation personally, and instead understand it as the patients' attempt to cope with their own intense insecurity. Providers can appeal to the patients' narcissism by explaining that they chose a particular course of action because they believe it represents the best possible care—a course of action they feel the patients deserve. Physicians can further support the patients by validating their concerns about the illness and pointing to their patients' ability to respond competently to its challenges. This approach helps the patients feel more secure and able, allowing them to ally confidently with—rather than defensively attack—their physicians.

CASE ILLUSTRATION 7

Maggie, a 44-year-old married female lawyer who is quite prominent in the community, is an unusually demanding patient. She becomes very angry with her male physician, whom she accuses of not responding adequately to her complaints about menopausal symptoms. In fact, the physician has done all the necessary laboratory tests, has conferred extensively with the patient's gynecologist, and has answered numerous phone calls by the patient over a period of several months.

The physician, aware of Maggie's long-standing sense of entitlement and her extreme sensitivity to slights, responds by reviewing her concerns, discussing the treatment plan and rationale, and encouraging her to discuss some of her emotional reactions to this unexpectedly early menopause. He then emphasizes the special consideration he has put into her evaluation and treatment plan. He arranges more frequent office visits and tells Maggie that he predicts a relatively good response to treatment, given her active involvement in her own care.

This response is reassuring to the patient, because it validates her concerns and satisfies her narcissistic feelings of entitlement.

AVOIDANT PERSONALITY DISORDER

Symptoms & Signs

Patients with avoidant personality disorder (Table 24–9) have a long-standing pattern of excessive anxiety in social situations and in intimate relationships, and extreme hypersensitivity to what other people think about them. These

Table 24–9. Diagnostic criteria for avoidant personality disorder (301.82).

A pervasive pattern of social inhibition, feelings of inadequacy, and hypersensitivity to negative evaluation, beginning by early adulthood and present in a variety of contexts, as indicated by four (or more) of the following:
1. avoids occupational activities that involve significant interpersonal contact, because of fears of criticism, disapproval, or rejection
2. is unwilling to get involved with people unless certain of being liked
3. shows restraint within intimate relationships because of the fear of being shamed or ridiculed
4. is preoccupied with being criticized or rejected in social situations
5. is inhibited in new interpersonal situations because of feelings of inadequacy
6. views self as socially inept, personally unappealing, or inferior to others
7. is unusually reluctant to take personal risks or to engage in any new activities because they may prove embarrassing

Source: Reprinted, with permission, from American Psychiatric Association: *Diagnostic and Statistical Manual of Mental Disorders,* 4th edition, *Text Revision* (*DSM-IV-TR*). American Psychiatric Association, 2000.

patients desire relationships but avoid them because of fears of being rejected, humiliated, or embarrassed. If they do engage in social situations or relationships, they are constantly preoccupied with being rejected, criticized, and not being liked by others. As a result, these patients have low self-esteem, feel socially inept, have feelings of inferiority, and are shy and inhibited.

Differential Diagnosis

Patients with schizoid personality disorder also avoid social situations and relationships but they do desire social isolation. In contrast, patients with avoidant personality disorder strongly desire relationships but avoid them because of anxiety and fears of rejection and humiliation.

Avoidant personality disorder should be distinguished from social phobia (Axis I disorder). Whereas patients with avoidant personality disorder try to avoid social interactions in general, patients with social phobia usually have more specific concerns related to social performance, such as saying something inappropriate to unfamiliar people at a social gathering.

Illness Experience & Illness Behavior

Illness provokes anxiety and increases feelings of ineptness in patients with avoidant personality disorder. Patients may delay care out of fear of not being liked or being rejected by the caregiver. In their interactions with clinicians, they may be shy and not forthcoming about their problems out of fear of being rejected or humiliated by them. They may blame their physical discomfort on themselves and may actually not ask for appropriate pain relief. Because these patients feel that they may not deserve attention by their physician, they may be reluctant to undergo necessary medical procedures.

THE DOCTOR–PATIENT RELATIONSHIP

Physicians treating patients with avoidant personality disorder may initially not realize the full extent of their patients' symptoms. Because these patients are shy and easily agreeable to what their physicians propose, physicians may be prone to take a more paternalistic stance with them. If they discover later that the patient's symptoms are more severe than initially reported, clinicians may react with concern or feel betrayed by the patient for withholding information and for their passive attitude.

Specific Management Strategies

Patients with avoidant personality disorder need reassurance and permission to express their distress and concerns in a nonjudgmental environment. It is helpful for health care providers to explain that they are interested in knowing about the patient's problems.

CASE ILLUSTRATION 8

Michael, a 45-year-old single office clerk, presents 45 minutes early for his annual check-up with his primary care physician. While signing in at the reception desk, he asks whether he has arrived on time for his appointment.

The physician finds a marked rash over the patient's elbows upon physical examination. The patient has a known history of psoriasis. Michael's face turns red out of embarrassment. He starts to explain that he applied the cream that his physician prescribed for him last year but that he ran out of the prescription some time ago. When asked why he did not call the physician's office for a refill, Michael states that he felt that he should not bother his physician for just a rash.

The physician expresses concern about the patient's rash. He writes a new prescription and asks Michael to call his office for a refill once he finishes the prescription. The doctor explains to the patient that he does not feel bothered by the patient's phone calls and that communication between patient and doctor is necessary to ensure appropriate medical care. He again requests that Michael call him for any refills or problems in the future.

This reassuring and supportive approach encourages the patient to communicate with his physician and not hold back out of fear of being rejected.

DEPENDENT PERSONALITY DISORDER
Symptoms & Signs

Patients with dependent personality disorder (Table 24–10) have a pervasive and excessive need to be taken care of. They experience intense fear of separation and abandonment and feel great discomfort when they are alone. This leads to submissive and clinging behavior in their interpersonal relationships. These patients have difficulty making independent decisions without a great deal of advice and reassurance, and they are afraid of disagreeing with others.

Differential Diagnosis

It is important to distinguish dependent personality disorder from the dependency that arises from panic disorder, mood disorders, or agoraphobia. Patients suffering from medical illnesses may also become very dependent on others, without having this disorder. Dependent personality disorder can sometimes be confused with other person-

Table 24–10. Diagnostic criteria for dependent personality disorder (301.6).

A pervasive and excessive need to be taken care of that leads to submissive and clinging behavior and fears of separation, beginning by early adulthood and present in a variety of contexts, as indicated by five (or more) of the following:

1. has difficulty making everyday decisions without an excessive amount of advice and reassurance from others
2. needs others to assume responsibility for most major areas of his or her life
3. has difficulty expressing disagreement with others because of fear of loss of support or approval. *Note:* Do not include realistic fears of retribution
4. has difficulty initiating projects or doing things on his or her own (because of a lack of self-confidence in judgment or abilities rather than a lack of motivation or energy)
5. goes to excessive lengths to obtain nurturance and support from others, to the point of volunteering to do things that are unpleasant
6. feels uncomfortable or helpless when alone because of exaggerated fears of being unable to care for himself or herself
7. urgently seeks another relationship as a source of care and support when a close relationship ends
8. is unrealistically preoccupied with fears of being left to take care of himself or herself

Source: Reprinted, with permission, from American Psychiatric Association: *Diagnostic and Statistical Manual of Mental Disorders,* 4th edition, *Text Revision* (*DSM-IV-TR*). American Psychiatric Association, 2000.

ality disorders, and dependent personality traits may be the result of chronic substance abuse.

Illness Experience & Illness Behavior

Patients with dependent personality disorder fear that illness will lead to both helplessness and abandonment by others. In their interactions with caregivers, they may become very needy and make dramatic demands for urgent medical attention. If the response is not what they wish, they may display angry outbursts at the physician. They may also blame their physical discomfort on others, including their physician. In addition, they may use addictive substances or overuse medications in a desperate attempt to obtain immediate relief from their suffering. Because receiving medical care may fulfill their wishes for attention from others, some dependent patients may unconsciously contribute to prolonging their illness, or—in some extreme cases—they may encourage unnecessary medical procedures.

THE DOCTOR–PATIENT RELATIONSHIP

Clinicians treating patients with dependent personality disorder may initially react with aversion to their patients' clingy and demanding behavior. Alternatively, clinicians may find it difficult to set limits on their availability and may try to provide reassurance by attempting to meet every demand, which ultimately leads to burnout or feelings of inadequacy. Eventually, caregivers may react in a hostile fashion and openly reject these patients.

Specific Management Strategies

Effective ways to provide reassurance to dependent patients and allay their fear of being abandoned include scheduling frequent periodic check-ups and being consistently avail-

able. It is nonetheless important to provide firm, realistic limits to this availability early in treatment or as soon as the patient's dependent traits become apparent. To prevent burnout, enlist other members of the health care team in providing support for the patient. In addition, physicians should help these patients find outside support systems to lessen fears of abandonment. They must also be alert to the patients' potential contribution to prolonging their illness or to their possible abuse of substances or medications.

 CASE ILLUSTRATION 9

Terry, a 50-year-old divorced secretary, repeatedly presents to her primary care physician complaining of various somatic symptoms, including dizziness, headaches, blurred vision, and leg pains. Repeated work-ups of her symptoms are negative, and her evaluation for major depression is negative. Further inquiry into Terry's life reveals that after her divorce 6 years ago, her daughter became the focus of her life. Even though her history of occasional somatic symptoms goes back to her teenage years, there had been no appreciable change until 2 years ago, when her daughter got married and left her home.

Terry makes frequent phone calls to her doctor. She usually sounds nervous, expresses concern about some new symptom, and asks for medication. The doctor decides to schedule regular follow-up appointments to address Terry's concerns. Terry often complains during office visits that there is not enough time to evaluate all her symptoms and laments that her daughter no longer has much time for her. Her doctor listens in a supportive manner and acknowledges that the available appointment time is limited, explaining how he will ultimately address all the complaints. He also emphasizes the importance of continuing to meet for regular appointments. In addition, the doctor acknowledges Terry's increased sense of isolation after her daughter's marriage and evaluates her for possible major depression. He further suggests a referral to the clinic's social worker as a means of helping her pursue a volunteer activity and increase her social interactions.

This approach usually helps diminish the patient's anxiety and decreases the frequency of phone calls. If the patient's distress does not improve with such interventions, a referral for psychotherapy and evaluation for a possible underlying anxiety disorder are indicated.

OBSESSIVE-COMPULSIVE PERSONALITY DISORDER

Symptoms & Signs

Individuals with obsessive-compulsive personality disorder (Table 24–11) are preoccupied with orderliness, perfectionism, and control. They are excessively concerned with details and rules, tend to be overly moralistic, and are usually focused on work to the exclusion of leisure. They find it difficult to adapt themselves to others and instead insist that others follow their plans. Their general inflexibility and restricted emotional expression betray an underlying fear of losing control. Because they can be indecisive, they feel distressed when faced with the need to make decisions.

Differential Diagnosis

Obsessive-compulsive disorder (see Chapter 22) is distinguished from obsessive-compulsive personality disorder by the presence of actual obsessions (repetitive intrusive thoughts) and compulsions. Sometimes, however, both disorders coexist in one patient, and obsessive-compulsive personality disorder can also be confused with other personality disorders.

Illness Experience & Illness Behavior

Illness is threatening to persons with obsessive-compulsive personality disorder because it generates an intense fear of losing control over bodily functions and emotions. Patients may experience extremely unsettling feelings of shame and vulnerability. They may also feel anger at the disruption of their usual daily routines by medical appointments and treatments. They may fear having to relinquish control to health care providers. In the physician's office, their intense anxiety tends to drive them to ask repetitive questions and to pay excessive attention to detail.

THE DOCTOR–PATIENT RELATIONSHIP

Caregivers may react to patients with obsessive-compulsive personality disorder by becoming impatient at their repetitive questions, cutting their answers short. They may feel their competence challenged by their patients' insistence on knowing every single detail and reason for choosing a particular treatment. Clinicians may also inadvertently attempt to control treatment planning rather than making it a joint effort, without realizing how important it is for these patients to remain in control.

Table 24–11. Diagnostic criteria for obsessive-compulsive personality disorder (301.4).

A pervasive pattern of preoccupation with orderliness, perfectionism, and mental and interpersonal control, at the expense of flexibility, openness, and efficiency, beginning by early adulthood and present in a variety of contexts, as indicated by four (or more) of the following:

1. is preoccupied with details, rules, lists, order, organization, or schedules to the extent that the major point of the activity is lost
2. shows perfectionism that interferes with task completion (eg, is unable to complete a project because his or her own overly strict standards are not met)
3. is excessively devoted to work and productivity to the exclusion of leisure activities and friendships (not accounted for by obvious economic necessity)
4. is overly conscientious, scrupulous, and inflexible about matters of morality, ethics, or values (not accounted for by cultural or religious identification)
5. is unable to discard worn-out or worthless objects even when they have no sentimental value
6. is reluctant to delegate tasks or to work with others unless they submit to exactly his or her way of doing things
7. adopts a miserly spending style toward both self and others; money is viewed as something to be hoarded for future catastrophes
8. shows rigidity and stubbornness

Source: Reprinted, with permission, from American Psychiatric Association: *Diagnostic and Statistical Manual of Mental Disorders*, 4th edition, *Text Revision* (*DSM-IV-TR*). American Psychiatric Association, 2000.

Specific Management Strategies

Helpful strategies in working with patients with obsessive-compulsive personality disorder include taking a thorough history, performing a careful diagnostic work-up, giving patients a clear and thorough explanation of their diagnosis and treatment options, and providing and explaining laboratory test results. It is important not to overemphasize uncertainties about treatments or the patient's possible response to treatment. Patients find it reassuring when clinicians cite literature reports and avoid vague and inexact impressionistic explanations. It is helpful to treat these patients as equal partners, encourage self-monitoring, allow their participation in treatment, and give them recognition for their clear reasoning and high standards.

CASE ILLUSTRATION 10

Sam, a 42-year-old biochemist, requests an appointment with his primary care physician for evaluation of an uncomfortable lump in his left groin. The physician is familiar with Sam's mild nervousness during routine medical check-ups and his tendency to ask detailed questions about his health. After a physical examination, the doctor diagnoses an inguinal hernia and recommends a surgical consultation for further evaluation and possible surgery. Sam, in his usual formal and somewhat restricted manner—but this time appearing visibly more anxious—repeatedly asks several questions about surgical repair, whether the literature discusses any alternative treatments, and what guidelines physicians follow to recommend one treatment over another. He then asks questions about the risks of general anesthesia and whether this procedure can be performed under local anesthesia.

When the physician tries to reassure him that this is a routine procedure, Sam asks him whether he is sure of his diagnosis; he also asks him to list the criteria he used in diagnosing the inguinal hernia. Sam also talks at length about his responsibilities at work and expresses concern that surgery might disrupt ongoing projects at his laboratory, as several people depend on him for regular supervision. He also wants to know how long his doctor has known the recommended surgeon, and whether they have worked together in the past.

Reassurance is essential here. The doctor explains that the surgeon is both trustworthy and well known to him. He praises Sam for his thoroughness and initiative in finding out about treatment alternatives before making a decision. He answers basic questions in a precise manner and defers some questions to the surgeon, explaining that these will be better answered by a specialist. He reassures Sam that he will not wait for a written report but will personally contact the surgeon after the consultation to discuss treatment options. The physician also suggests a follow-up appointment to help Sam with his decision.

Although Sam continues to express concern that the surgery will disrupt his work, his anxiety decreases somewhat after the physician takes his concerns seriously. His questions are answered precisely, and the physician further suggests an article in the literature that he can read to learn more about the treatment of inguinal hernias.

PSYCHOPHARMACOLOGICAL TREATMENT OF PATIENTS WITH PERSONALITY DISORDERS

There is no consistent effective psychopharmacological treatment for patients with personality disorders. Nevertheless, medication can be beneficial in targeting symptom clusters within the disorder and in treating comorbid Axis I disorders, for example, depression.

Symptoms such as paranoid ideation and suspiciousness in patients with cluster A disorders (paranoid, schizoid, and schizotypal personality disorder) may improve by low-dose treatment with an antipsychotic (eg, haloperidol, risperidone, or olanzapine). In case of overt psychotic symptoms, a psychiatric consultation and treatment with an antipsychotic medication should be considered.

Patients with cluster B disorders (antisocial, borderline, histrionic, and narcissistic personality disorder), who often appear dramatic and emotional, should be evaluated for prominent mood symptoms and the coexistence of an Axis I disorder.

Patients with prominent depressive symptoms should be treated with an antidepressant. The newer and better tolerated selective serotonin reuptake inhibitors (SSRIs) such as fluoxetine, sertraline, paroxetine, or citalopram should be considered the first-line choice antidepressants. Patients with prominent mood swings, irritability, or impulsive behaviors may be candidates for treatment with a mood stabilizer (eg, valproate or lithium). However, a psychiatric consultation is recommended for this type of treatment. Medications have been most extensively used in patients with borderline personality disorder. Borderline patients with more affective dysregulation can be considered for treatment with an antidepressant and/or a mood stabilizer. Antipsychotics can be considered in borderline patients with dissociative or psychotic symptoms.

Anxiety and fear are the most dominant symptoms of patients with cluster C disorders (avoidant, dependent, and obsessive-compulsive personality disorder). Symptoms in these patients may improve by treatment with an SSRI. Time-limited symptomatic treatment with a benzodiazepine might be considered.

SUGGESTED READINGS

Cohen-Cole SA: Difficult interviews: Personality disorders, psychosis, delirium, and dementia. In: Cole SA, Bird J (editors): *The Medical Interview: The Three-Function Approach.* Mosby-Year Book, 2000.

Fogel BS: Personality disorders in the medical setting. In: Stoudemire A, Fogel BS (editors): *Psychiatric Care of the Medical Patient.* Oxford University Press, 2000.

Geringer ES, Stern TA: Coping with medical illness: the impact of personality types. Psychosomatics 1986;27(4):251.

Gabbard GO: Psychotherapy of personality disorders. J Psychother Pract Res 2000;9:1.

Gross R et al: Borderline personality disorder in primary care. Arch Intern Med 2002;162:53.

Groves JE: Taking care of the hateful patient. N Engl J Med 1978; 298:883.

Gunderson JD: *Borderline Personality Disorder. A Clinical Guide.* American Psychiatric Publishing, 2001.

Hori A: Pharmacotherapy for personality disorders. Psychiatry Clin Neurosci 1998;52:13.

Kahana R, Bibring G: Personality types in medical management. In: Zinberg N (editor): *Psychiatry and Medical Practice in the General Hospital.* International Universities Press, 1964.

Markovitz P: Pharmacotherapy. In: Livesley WJ (editor): *Handbook of Personality Disorders: Theory, Research, and Treatment.* Guilford Press, 2001.

Marmar C: Personality disorders. In: Goldman H (editor): *Review of General Psychiatry.* McGraw-Hill, 2000.

Oldham JM: Personality disorders: current perspectives. JAMA 1994;272:1770.

Putnam SM et al: Personality styles. In: Lipkin M, Putnam S, Lazare A (editors): *The Medical Interview: Clinical Care, Education, and Research.* Springer-Verlag, 1995.

Dementia[1]

William L. Lyons, MD, & Kristine Yaffe, MD

INTRODUCTION

Dementia is an increasingly common disorder, affecting about 1% of individuals aged 60 years; its prevalence doubles every 5 years after this mark. Despite this, the diagnosis is often missed by primary care providers, perhaps because patients in the early stages frequently retain their social graces. Dementia is defined as an acquired, persistent, and usually progressive impairment in intellectual function, with compromise in multiple cognitive domains, at least one of which is memory. The deficits must represent a significant decline in function, and must be severe enough to interfere with work or social life for the diagnosis to be formally applied. As the disorder progresses, individuals with dementia fail to recognize family members, are unable to express themselves clearly and meaningfully, and often undergo dramatic personality changes. Table 25–1 lists some of the more common causes of dementia. Important tasks for the primary care provider working with individuals with dementia are to recognize and correctly diagnose the condition, to rule out any reversible or treatable disorders, to treat any associated complications such as difficult behaviors, to ensure that the patient is as comfortable and safe as possible, to recognize when referral for specialist care is needed, and to work with family and other caregivers to help them understand and care for the patient. Furthermore, with several pharmacological treatments available for Alzheimer's disease (AD) and more in development, it has become important for the primary care physician to know how to diagnose this etiology of dementia, and to be familiar with available drug therapies.

TYPES OF DEMENTIA

Alzheimer's Disease

Alzheimer's disease is the most common form of dementia, accounting for about 60–70% of cases. The age of onset varies considerably; many cases occur between ages 50 and 60, but it is more common for symptoms to arise after age 70. Incidence of the disease increases with age. Clinicians who encounter patients with AD in their 40s and 50s

should take a careful family history, as early-onset disease may show an autosomal dominant pattern of inheritance. Women are at a slightly higher risk of developing the disorder than men.

AD usually follows a slow, but progressive and insidious, course (Table 25–2). Life expectancy following the appearance of the disorder ranges from 3 to 15 years, but considerable variation may occur, and survival of up to 20 years has been reported. Memory deficits are prominent in all dementias, but especially so in AD, and are typically the first and most obvious manifestation of the disorder. AD affects both the encoding and retrieval of new information to a profound degree such that these patients do not appear to benefit from cueing and prompting of memory. For example, a patient asked to remember the words "piano," "carrot," and "green" may not be helped by hints such as "musical instrument," "vegetable," or "color." AD is a "cortical dementia" in which the areas of the brain associated with specific cognitive functions and the integration of these functions are directly affected. Although diagnostic certainty is less than 100% without pathological examination of the cerebral cortex, careful clinical and neuropsychological evaluation often allow reliable diagnosis of the disease. A computed tomography (CT) or magnetic resonance imaging (MRI) scan often shows cerebral atrophy and hippocampal volume loss; the electroencephalogram (EEG) may show diffuse slowing. These are nonspecific findings.

CASE ILLUSTRATION

Gertrude is 74 years old. She is brought by her family to a medical clinic for evaluation. Since the death of her husband 2 years ago, Gertrude has become increasingly absentminded, withdrawn, and sedentary. Her family assumed at first that she was grieving and would eventually readjust. Gertrude's condition has continued to deteriorate, however, until she is now confused and disoriented and has difficulty recognizing family members. Physical examination and routine laboratory tests are essentially normal, but Gertrude shows clear signs of cognitive deficits on the mental status examination. For example, given three

---

[1] David M. Pope, PhD, and Alicia Boccellari, PhD, were authors of the first edition version of this chapter.

Table 25–1. Common causes of dementia.

Alzheimer's disease
Multiple infarcts and other cerebrovascular disease
Lewy body dementia
Frontotemporal dementia
Parkinson's disease
Metabolic and potentially reversible disease (eg, chronic vitamin B_{12} deficiency, hypothyroidism)
AIDS
Neurodegenerative disorders (eg, Huntington's chorea, progressive supranuclear palsy)

---

words to remember she is unable to recall any of them after several minutes. She cannot give the correct month and year and thinks she is in the city where she had lived many years ago. Asked to repeat several sentences, she makes a number of verbal slips. When she is given a geometric design to copy, her drawing is dis-

torted and unrecognizable. Other causes of the patient's deficits are ruled out, and a diagnosis of AD is eventually made.

In retrospect, her family recalls that Gertrude had been having some mild difficulties in memory and functioning prior to her husband's death and had been dependent on him for helping her to manage things. Recognition of Gertrude's emerging dementia had been made more difficult by her grief and possible depression after her husband's death.

The physician spends some time with family members discussing the nature of Gertrude's condition and options for future care. She inquires about immediate concerns such as agitation and other behavioral disturbances, none of which is currently present. The physician then refers the family to a social worker specializing in geriatric issues and indicates the availability of groups such as the Family Caregiver Alliance for education and support. She also advises Gertrude not to drive, and, in accordance with the law in her state, notifies the government of the new diagnosis

Table 25–2. Stages of Alzheimer's disease.

Stage	General Changes	Specific Changes
Early	Patients show relatively subtle changes in memory, along with declining clarity of thought and ability to perform everyday tasks. These changes may go largely unnoticed by the patient and significant others. Patients typically retain some ability to compensate for the cognitive changes.	• Mild memory problems such as missed appointments, failure to pay bills. • Occasional mild and transitory confusion and disorientation. • A "slowed-down" quality to thinking, personality, and life-style. • An increase in personal rigidity and intolerance of changes. • Social isolation, loss of interest in usual activities. • Possible increase in restlessness and impulsivity.
Middle	Cognitive deficits become more prominent during this stage and the loss of functioning becomes obvious to others.	• Severe memory impairment. • Frank and persistent confusion and disorientation. • Aphasia, apraxia, and visuospatial disturbances. • Serious difficulties in the ability to manage everyday activities. • Agitation, simple paranoia, other delusions.
Late	In the third, and terminal, stage of the disorder, the patient becomes very inactive, is extremely withdrawn, and loses nearly all ability to engage in purposeful activities.	• Profound loss of short- and long-term memory. • Severe confusion and disorientation. • Bladder and bowel incontinence. • Patient eventually is bedridden and nonresponsive. • Primitive reflexes such as grasping, rooting, and sucking. • Seizures. • Signs of gross neurologic impairment, such as hemiplegia, tremor, pronounced rigidity. • Bodily wasting in the face of adequate nourishment just prior to death.

Note: The signs and symptoms of dementia include the progressive loss of cognitive abilities, especially memory, and a decline in everyday functioning. Dementia is generally a deteriorating condition, and its progression is best described in terms of several stages. The stages outlined above are based on the most common form of dementia, Alzheimer's disease.

of dementia. Finally, the physician initiates a trial of donepezil, which, by family report, appears to have slowed Gertrude's cognitive and functional decline.

Dementia with Lewy Bodies (DLB)

Although not often seen in the primary care setting, DLB is the second most common cause of dementia in autopsy studies, accounting for 15–30% of cases. It is defined by the presence of cognitive impairment, parkinsonism, delusions, prominent (often bizarre) hallucinations, and fluctuations in alertness. Patients with DLB are often intolerant of traditional antipsychotics, and use of such neuroleptic agents has caused fatalities. Preliminary data suggest that anticholinergic agents such as donepezil may be useful in treating the disorder.

Vascular Dementia

Previously known as multiinfarct dementia, the condition is characterized by the development of multiple areas of infarction in both cortical and subcortical areas. Patients with a history of hypertension and noncerebral atherosclerotic cerebrovascular disease are at increased risk for the disorder, and many patients who go on to develop vascular dementia have a previous history of stroke. A patchy and inconsistent pattern of deficits may be seen initially, with relative preservation of some cognitive areas. As strokes accumulate, impairment becomes more widespread and generalized in nature. A so-called stepwise course is typical, with fairly stable periods of functioning interrupted by sudden deteriorations and the establishment of a more impaired level of functioning.

Focal neurological signs are more common in vascular dementia than in AD, and lateralized motor and sensory findings may be seen. CT and MRI scans frequently reveal multiple areas of infarction in the brain, often with diffuse white matter changes. Later in the course of the disorder atrophy from loss of brain tissue may be seen.

The diagnostic criteria for vascular dementia need additional research. Many elders show diffuse white matter changes on brain imaging, and yet are cognitively intact. Other demented elders, who were thought by their clinicians to have vascular dementia because of cognitive decline following cerebral infarcts, are subsequently found to have Alzheimer's pathology at autopsy, in addition to the known infarcts. Such individuals, with elements of both AD and vascular dementia, are considered to have mixed dementia. In short, current diagnostic instruments and criteria are often inadequate for clinicians to confidently employ or reject the "vascular dementia" label.

Other Causes

Frontotemporal dementias (FTD) are a group of disorders characterized by personality change (eg, apathy, or socially inappropriate behavior), hyperorality, and cognitive decline. Some studies have demonstrated reduced visualspatial deficits compared with AD patients. FTD tends to affect individuals at a younger age than AD, with many persons receiving the diagnosis in their 50s or 60s. Imaging studies may show marked atrophy in frontal and temporal lobes.

Advanced Parkinson's disease commonly results in dementia. These patients frequently display mental sluggishness and a general lack of spontaneity. Language functions (compared with those of AD patients) are relatively preserved.

Chronic alcohol abuse can result in serious cognitive deficits if drinking is severe and prolonged, although it is not clear whether the dementing process occurs in the absence of coexisting thiamine deficiency. Severe head trauma can also result in permanent cognitive impairment, which might be viewed as static dementia.

Human immunodeficiency virus (HIV)-1-associated dementia (HAD) is caused by the direct infection of the brain by the HIV-1 virus. It is associated with late-stage AIDS and is generally seen in individuals whose T cell count has fallen below 200. Features of this form of dementia are summarized in Table 25–3. HAD is discussed further in Chapter 31.

Reversible Conditions

A number of medical conditions can result in cognitive impairment. These may be treatable and partially or completely reversible. Assessing the patient for these conditions is one of the most important parts of the dementia workup. Reversible brain syndromes are usually the result of depression or a toxic or metabolic disorder. The most common types of primary and secondary syndromes are listed in Table 25–4.

Table 25–3. Signs and symptoms of advanced HIV-1-associated dementia.

- Impaired attention and difficulty learning new information.
- Slow, soft, and impoverished speech.
- Ataxia, decreased manual dexterity, and motor slowness.
- Poor judgment.
- Flat and unspontaneous facial expression with fixed gaze.
- Personality changes that may include apathy or increased impulsivity.

Table 25–4. Possibly reversible syndromes that impair cognition.

Hydrocephalus	Chronic hematoma
Metabolic disease	Toxic states
Thyroid	Medication toxicity
Adrenal	CNS infections
Renal failure	Meningitis
Hepatic failure	Encephalitis
Deficiencies	Neurosyphilis
Vitamin B_{12}	Cerebral abscess
Folate	Mild head trauma
Niacin	Dementia syndrome of depression
Thiamine	

Differential Diagnosis

Persons suspected of having dementia are encountered in a number of medical settings. For example, a patient who presents to the emergency department with confusion, disorientation, and hallucinations should be evaluated for delirium (eg, from infection, metabolic derangement, or use of or withdrawal from medications or recreational substances) and psychotic disorders. An older adult with a history of recent bereavement, withdrawal, and increased forgetfulness may indeed be demented, or may be suffering from cognitive deficits related to major depression. Other problems that initially may be confused with dementia include sensory deficits (severe visual or hearing impairment), aphasia, developmental disability, and low levels of literacy or education.

Normal Aging

As people age, some degree of decline in cognitive functioning is common. The presence of mild memory impairment among older adults has been reported to occur among a very wide range (11–96%) of participants in various research studies. Normal aging often brings minor word-finding difficulties, slowed memory retrieval, and some changes in the speed and efficiency of thought. These changes, however, typically do not cause significant problems in everyday functioning or produce confusion or disorientation, which are signs of impaired cognition (see Chapter 11).

Some individuals demonstrate greater-than-expected cognitive decline for their age, yet they do not meet the criteria for a formal diagnosis of dementia. The labels mild cognitive impairment (MCI) or cognitive impairment not demented (CIND) have been applied to this group. These patients tend to have subjective complaints of forgetfulness and objective evidence of memory impairment or deficits in other cognitive domains. Nevertheless, they have normal overall cognitive function and capabilities for performing activities of daily living. Importantly, such individuals are at substantially increased risk of subsequently becoming demented. The American Academy of Neurology recommends that these patients be identified and monitored by their providers.

Dementia versus Delirium

Delirium is a rapidly evolving state of cognitive impairment associated with fluctuations in mental status and behavior, inattention, disorganized thinking, and an altered level of consciousness. Because dementia is a significant risk factor for delirium, the two syndromes are closely linked. A significant number of demented individuals become delirious when admitted to a hospital with an acute illness. Similarly, a substantial number of delirious, hospitalized elders are found (after the delirium has cleared, or by chart review) to be demented as well. Table 25–5 distinguishes delirium from dementia.

Acute confusional states are usually caused by toxic and metabolic derangements or infections. In determining the cause, a clinician should consider reviewing the medication record (looking for recent changes); checking blood cell counts, electrolytes, renal function, glucose, calcium, and urinalysis; and reviewing a chest film and electrocardiogram.

Table 25–5. Delirium versus dementia: Signs and symptoms.

Delirium	Dementia
Rapid onset; short duration	Insidious onset; progressive deterioration
May show heightened autonomic arousal	No impairment in autonomic arousal
Clouded consciousness or gross confusion	Alertness retained in early stages
Prominent waxing and waning	Consistently impaired mentation except in late stage dementia
Often restless, agitated, hypervigilant, or lethargic	Agitation less prominent; varies with stress
Gross perceptual distortions and hallucinations common	If psychotic, usually vague paranoid ideas

Table 25–6. Differentiating between dementia and dementia syndrome of depression (DSD).

Dementia	DSD
History	
• Slow, insidious onset • Precipitating event not necessarily present • Family complains of problem	• Rapid onset • Recent stress, loss • Previous depression • Patient complains of problem • Multiple somatic complaints
Evaluation	
• Often indifferent or anxious • Willing to put forth good effort on mental status examination • Excuses or denies deficits • Psychotic symptoms usually not with depressive content	• Sad, withdrawn, hopeless • Little motivation, poor effort on mental status examination • Complains of deficits • If psychotic, has depressive quality

Dementia versus Depression

Especially among older adults, symptoms of depression may masquerade as dementia (Table 25–6) making it difficult to distinguish between dementia and the dementia syndrome of depression (DSD), once referred to as pseudodementia. One of the reasons for the change in terminology is that there is nothing "pseudo" about the cognitive problems seen in these individuals. They may be quite profoundly impaired, even confused and disoriented, and at times it can be very difficult to tell them apart from patients with genuine dementia. Cognitive deficits of this magnitude are generally seen only among the severely depressed. Individuals with milder depression—even when they are elderly—usually have mild, if any, cognitive deficits. It is important to note that individuals with depression and recent losses do become demented, just as individuals with early-stage dementia can be depressed. It may be difficult to distinguish between the withdrawal and apathy that can accompany depression and that seen with dementia. Both depressed and demented patients may appear quite impaired cognitively. Formal neuropsychological testing and/or an empiric trial of antidepressant medication may provide the best means of distinguishing between dementia and DSD.

Persons with DSD whose cognition improves following treatment of their mood disorder are nevertheless at increased risk of developing "true" dementia later in life.

Dementia versus Psychotic Disorders

The symptoms of psychotic disorders such as schizophrenia or bipolar disorder may resemble the disorganization, confusion, delusions, and agitation that sometimes accompany dementia. The typical presence of more consistent and systematized delusions and the increased likelihood of previous psychosis and a family psychiatric history among individuals with non-dementia-related psychotic disorders are important in making this differentiation.

DIAGNOSTIC WORK-UP

A dementia work-up should include a careful history (Table 25–7) and physical, neurological, and mental status examinations. In many cases additional tests and procedures may be helpful; these are discussed later.

History

A complete history should be elicited from both patients and their families. In many cases it is helpful to ask both about the same topics. Although many demented individuals are unreliable historians, they may be able to provide much useful information, including symptoms of which family members are not aware. In addition, patients' abilities to provide a coherent and organized account of their complaints and recent history can often tell you much about their conditions.

A complete social and family history that includes native language; family history of dementia; and educational, marital, and employment background can also be useful. An educational and occupational history, for example, may provide information about a patient's previous level of functioning. A quality of vagueness in patients' reports or inconsistency in the information supplied may suggest less blatant memory deficits. Particular attention should be paid to patients' accounts of more recent events. Individuals with mild or moderate dementia often show intact recall for older, overlearned information (eg, family, education, work) but cannot provide accurate information about the immediate past.

Table 25–7. Dementia work-up: history.

- Time course and nature of symptoms and functional decline.
- Slow and insidious versus more sudden/dramatic changes.
- Current ability to function.
- Accompanying mood or personality changes.
- Presence or absence of confusion, agitation, and disorientation.
- Psychotic symptoms.
- Complicating factors, such as alcohol or substance abuse.

Ask patients about their regular activities, appetite, and sleep habits, as well as any physical or cognitive complaints. Information about their mood can be gained by inquiring directly, but also by asking about things that they enjoy and look forward to, any worries or concerns they may have, and their plans for the future.

Family members may be able to supply a more complete and balanced impression of the patient's symptoms, behavioral changes, and level of functioning. Individuals with dementia typically lack insight into their cognitive problems and minimize or deny any difficulties. In fact, it is the family that most frequently raises concerns about the patient. Because family members may feel more comfortable discussing their observations away from the presence of the patient, they should be interviewed separately. It is especially important to inquire about both current and potential safety issues, such as driving (Table 25–8).

Physical & Neurological Examinations

In addition to a routine physical examination, a complete neurological examination should be done, although the results of the latter are generally unremarkable in cases of early AD. Parkinsonian signs may be apparent during the later course of many dementing illnesses. Individuals with a developing vascular dementia may show focal signs on the neurological examination.

The Mental Status Examination

Because cognitive impairment is the hallmark of dementia, it is necessary to add additional screening items to the traditional mental status examination. Several brief dementia screening instruments offer the advantages of both a structured format and a scoring system. These instruments must be used with caution, however, for the reasons discussed here.

The Mini-Mental State Examination (MMSE) is the most commonly used dementia-screening instrument and is recommended for use by the primary care provider. It takes about 5 minutes to administer and samples a

Table 25–8. Dementia work-up: potential safety issues.

- Ambulation and balance
- Dizziness
- Ability to live independently
  Leaving stove or running water unattended
  Wandering behavior
  Confusion/agitation
  Ability to manage finances
- Ability to drive
- Level of supervision available

wide range of functions, including orientation, immediate and delayed memory, concentration, basic language and reading functions, and visual construction abilities (Table 25–9). Patients are asked to count backward by 7, write a sentence, follow concrete directions, and copy geometric figures. A maximum score of 30 is possible; a score lower than 24 (some clinicians recommend 27) is suspicious for dementia. Because the MMSE is not sensitive for early dementia, a significant number of false-negative results occur among individuals with mild disease. Conversely, low scores may be obtained from individuals who are not demented but are uncooperative, psychiatrically impaired, not formally educated, or lacking in English proficiency. Consequently, results should be interpreted cautiously. Other brief dementia-screening instruments include the Blessed Dementia Scale and the Neurobehavioral Cognitive Status Examination.

Other Tests

Multiple infectious and metabolic insults can cause or exacerbate cognitive deficits, and laboratory tests (Table 25–10) may help to uncover these. Unfortunately, it is extremely unusual for an individual with longstanding dementia to show complete recovery after treatment of a potentially reversible cause.

Whether to routinely order brain imaging when evaluating a demented patient is controversial. Some clinicians restrict imaging to those patients with acute or subacute cognitive changes, focal neurological findings, or onset at a relatively young age. Recently, the American Academy of Neurology recommended that structural neuroimaging (with noncontrast CT or MRI) be employed in the initial evaluation of most patients with dementia, as some 5% of such patients have been found to have important but clinically unexpected structural lesions. An EEG is helpful if the differential diagnosis includes status epilepticus or postictal confusion. On the other hand, the major dementing disorders, especially early in their course, do not generate characteristic EEG patterns, and a normal EEG cannot be taken as definitive evidence of the absence of brain pathology.

Lumbar punctures are indicated when there is a question of an infectious process or when a rapidly progressing condition is present. In rare instances brain biopsy may be employed to help with diagnosis.

Neuropsychological Testing

Neuropsychological testing involves the use of psychometric tests designed to detect and characterize a wide variety of cognitive problems. The testing requires the patient to be able to attend for a minimum of 20–30 minutes; some patients may be too agitated, withdrawn, or resistant to comply. Consider referring a patient for neuropsychological testing in the following circumstances:

Table 25–9. Dementia work-up: Mini-Mental State Examination.

Function	Question or Task	Maximum Score
Orientation	What is the year, season, date, day, month? (5 points) Where are we: state, county, town, hospital, floor? (5 points)	10
Registration	Name three objects and ask the patient to repeat the names of the objects (correct response = 1 point). Repeat the names of the three objects until the patient learns them.	3
Attention and calculation	Ask the patient to recite serial 7s backward from 100. Stop the patient after five responses (correct response = 1 point).	5
Recall	Ask the patient to repeat the names of the three objects learned above (correct response = 1 point).	3
Language	Show the patient two common objects, eg, a pencil and watch, and ask the patient to identify them (2 points). Ask the patient to repeat "no ifs, ands, or buts" (1 point). Instruct the patient to follow the three-stage command: "take a paper in your right hand, fold it in half, and put it on the floor" (3 points). Ask the patient to read and obey the following: "close your eyes" (1 point). Instruct the patient to write a sentence (1 point). Ask the patient to copy a design (1 point).	9

Source: Reprinted, with permission, from Folstein MF, Folstein SE, McHugh PR: "Mini-Mental State": A practical method for grading the cognitive state of patients for the clinician. J Psychiatr Res 1975;12:189.

- When the reported deficits are subtle or equivocal and the impairment is mild.
- When the differential diagnosis is difficult to resolve (eg, distinguishing between dementia and depression).
- When a baseline is needed to measure the degree of cognitive deterioration over time.
- When a greater understanding of the patient's everyday level of functioning, limitations, potential safety issues, and the appropriate level of supervision is needed.
- When deficits or competency issues must be documented, such as in conservatorship proceedings.
- To monitor effects of treatment.

Table 25–10. Dementia work-up: recommended laboratory tests.

Complete blood count	Calcium
Thyroid studies	Albumin
Blood urea nitrogen	Vitamin B$_{12}$
Creatinine	Electrolytes

Consider: liver function, rapid plasma reagin, HIV serology, glucose, medication serum levels, toxicology screens, folate, urinalysis, lumbar puncture.

TREATMENT & MANAGEMENT ISSUES

Treatment of dementia consists of identifying and addressing a treatable basis for the underlying condition (if one exists), treating secondary disorders such as anxiety or depression, educating patients and their families as to the nature of the condition, and assisting caregivers with safety and management issues. In addition, clinical trials have demonstrated benefits of pharmacological agents that may directly improve cognition and functional capacity of AD patients, or at least slow their decline. Table 25–11 summarizes overall principles of dementia management.

Behavioral Issues

Management of patients with dementia involves matters of self-care, safety, and communication. Individuals with dementia are disorganized, forgetful, and inefficient in many of their activities. They have difficulty following directions, in managing everyday activities, and in expressing themselves clearly. They are frequently impulsive, may have limited insight into their abilities, and generally do not learn well from experience. Emotionally, they may be labile and unstable, irritable, or anxious; they may be fearful, easily frustrated, or apathetic and withdrawn. Because of circadian rhythm disturbances, patients with AD may tend to be awake and wandering during the night, leading to sleep deprivation in caregivers.

Table 25–11. Overall principles of dementia management.

- Periodically assess safety and self-care function.
- Assess caregiver each visit.
- Address advance directives early.
- Educate patient and caregivers about dementing condition.
- Refer to Alzheimer's Association and supportive community organizations.
- Treat secondary disorders (anxiety, depression).
- "Fine-tune" comorbid illnesses (eg, congestive heart failure).
- Trial of cholinesterase inhibitors for mild-to-moderate Alzheimer's disease.

These traits create special problems in managing and caring for patients with dementia, and many interactions with family and caregivers therefore focus on day-to-day management issues and behavioral problems. The following sections provide some general guidelines for addressing these issues. It is useful in many situations to refer patients and their families to groups that can provide counseling, home evaluations, and case management. (In some instances there may be no more important knowledge for the primary doctor than familiarity with the capabilities of local support agencies.)

SELF-CARE

This area includes dressing, grooming, and hygiene. The best approach is to provide sufficient structure and guidance so that the patient can manage, while allowing some preservation of independence and choice. Individuals with mild cognitive impairment often get by with prompts and reminders. For individuals with more severe impairment, caregivers should offer a limited choice of clothing, food, or activities; use signs or pictures to identify important objects and locations; and emphasize routine and predictability. The caregiver may need to modify clothing, eg, by incorporating sweatshirts to avoid buttons, and using shoes with Velcro closures rather than laces.

SAFETY ISSUES

Individuals with dementia are at increased risk for accidents because of their problems with attention, perception, and judgment. The following guidelines are designed to minimize the risk of household accidents:

- Carefully supervise use of medications.
- Keep things simple: reduce clutter; keep passageways clear.
- Install railings and other safety equipment, such as shower chairs and tub rails.
- Use a night light where necessary.
- Remove stove and oven controls if necessary.

- Use safety gates or install keyless locks on exterior doors if wandering is a problem.
- Make sure patients wear medical and personal identification bracelets.

Another important safety issue concerns driving and dementia. Deficits in attention, reaction time, visual spatial abilities, and judgment typically impair the ability of individuals with marked cognitive deficits to operate a motor vehicle safely. Individuals with advanced dementia who continue to operate a car seriously endanger others as well as themselves. Unfortunately, patients with dementia may insist on driving because of their lack of insight into their problems, and caregivers may be reluctant to press the issue. Because driving is symbolic of independence, this often becomes an emotional issue for everyone involved.

Confidentiality must be weighed against issues of competency, safety of the public, and the duty to warn. Legal responsibilities may also be involved. For example, in California, physicians are required by law to report patients who are unable to operate a motor vehicle because of "Alzheimer's or other related dementias." In the case of accident or injury, physicians who have failed to make such a report may be legally liable. Primary care providers should inform themselves of the legal requirements in their own state regarding this issue.

COMMUNICATION

Individuals with brain impairment may have specific deficits in language comprehension and expression similar to the various forms of aphasia that occur in stroke patients. More common may be a generalized difficulty in communication secondary to a short attention span, memory problems, or confusion. Some guidelines for communicating with the cognitively impaired are presented in Table 25–12.

SEVERE BEHAVIORAL AND PSYCHIATRIC PROBLEMS

When serious psychiatric symptoms occur, such as severe depression, agitation, or psychosis, psychotropic medications may be indicated. Some general guidelines should be followed:

- Because these medications have the potential to further disrupt cognitive processes and worsen the problem, use considerably lower doses than those used for younger or nondemented individuals. Older adults in particular are particularly susceptible to side effects from these medications, especially when there are concurrent medical problems.
- Avoid benzodiazepines, especially for more than brief periods, as they have significant potential for causing sedation, confusion, and ataxia.
- Haloperidol (Haldol) may be a good choice for addressing symptoms of psychosis, as it does not promote anticholinergic effects and is a high-potency

Table 25–12. Tips for communicating with the cognitively impaired.

- Make sure you have patients' attention when you speak with them. Keep distractions, such as television, radio, or other conversations, to a minimum by meeting with patients in a quiet place.
- Keep communications brief, simple, and concrete. Break more complex information down into smaller pieces.
- Give patients several options to choose among, or phrase questions in multiple-choice format.
- Have patients paraphrase back the information to make sure they have understood what was said.

medication. An initial dosage of 0.5 mg is often used, with gradual and slow increases if symptoms persist. Newer antipsychotics such as risperidone (starting 0.5 mg orally every night) and olanzapine (starting 2.5 mg orally every night) are probably preferable when treating the elderly, as they are less frequently associated with rigidity and other extrapyramidal side effects. If the problem continues, consider another agent or obtain consultation with a psychiatrist, preferably one specializing in geriatric psychiatry.

- Nonpsychotic agitation deserves careful evaluation before a drug is prescribed. New agitation may represent delirium, undertreated pain, a distended bladder, or fecal impaction. If these disorders are not contributing and if nonpharmacological approaches are inadequate, an empiric trial of trazodone or carbamazepine (or another antiepileptic drug) may be worthwhile. Again, recalcitrant cases may benefit from consultation with a geriatric psychiatrist.

Drugs for Improving Cognition

Cholinesterase inhibitors have been the class of drugs most extensively studied for use with AD patients. Currently,

there are four Food and Drug Administration (FDA)-approved medications: tacrine, donepezil, rivastigmine, and galantamine. Most studies have tested these agents in patients with mild to moderate dementia, which may roughly correspond to MMSE scores of 10 to 24. On the whole, statistically significant benefits have been demonstrated, but clinical effects tend to be modest. Patients, families, and caregivers should not expect dramatic results. Table 25–13 gives dosing recommendations for the four medications. The drugs have not yet been studied in head-to-head comparisons, so drug choice may best be made based on half-life and side effects. If a patient is started on one of these drugs and shows no benefit (as gauged by clinicians' and caregivers' impression of behavior and function, and confirmed by some form of neuropsychological testing, such as the MMSE) after a few months, the drug should be discontinued. For this purpose, "benefit" might practically be defined as a slowing in the rate of decline, if not frank improvement.

Caregivers

Caring for cognitively impaired individuals is often exhausting and stressful. Primary care providers should ensure that caregivers also attend to their own needs and guard against fatigue and burnout. A number of support services, such as the Family Caregiver Alliance (website http://www.caregiver.org), offer education, support groups, and information about resources. Specialized case management and home consultation services can also be very helpful in assessing patient and family needs and locating additional services. Respite-care and day-activity programs may be invaluable in allowing stressed families and caregivers time off and providing needed stimulation and increased structure for the patient. Many experienced clinicians often assess stressed caregivers at each clinic visit.

Nursing Home Placement

In the management of demented patients, the issue often arises as to whether the patient can continue to be man-

Table 25–13. Cholinesterase inhibitors for Alzheimer's disease.

Drug	Initial Regimen	Dose Escalation
Donepezil	5 mg orally every day	10 mg orally every day after 4–6 weeks
Rivastigmine	1.5 mg orally twice a day	Adjust every 2 weeks to 3 mg orally twice a day, then 4.5 mg orally twice a day, maximum 6 mg orally twice a day
Galantamine	4 mg orally twice a day	Adjust every 4 weeks to 8 mg orally twice a day, maximum 12 mg orally twice a day
Tacrine[1]	10 mg orally four times a day	Adjust upward to 20 mg orally four times a day or higher at 4 week intervals

[1] Tacrine use has been associated with episodes of serious hepatotoxicity. If employed, liver function tests should be monitored every 2 weeks.

aged at home. This is an area fraught with strong feelings on the part of patient and caregiver alike, and it is often difficult to make objective decisions. Major predictors of nursing home placement include the presence of behavioral problems, dementia severity, and extent of caregiver burden. Some important considerations related to nursing home admission are as follows:

- Can the necessary level of supervision and care required by the patient be realistically and dependably supplied at home? Such issues as wandering and the potential for neglect and abuse should be considered here.
- Is sufficient assistance available to caregivers for them to continue to care for the patient without becoming overstressed and burned out?
- What financial resources are available for the patient's care?

All things being equal, allowing patients to remain in their own homes is desirable. In many cases, however, doing so creates other significant problems, and however desirable this goal, it must be carefully weighed against issues of safety and practical limitations. In the advanced stage of dementia, when the patient becomes mute, bedbound, and incontinent, very often the services of a skilled nursing facility are required to ensure that the patient receives proper care. Nursing facilities should be chosen carefully; obviously, cost must be considered, but the quality of care must also be investigated. Information about both complaints and compliance with state regulations can be found through government agencies, advocacy groups, published reviews, and organizations (eg, geriatric-care programs) that frequently place patients in such facilities. Although definitive data are lacking, some studies suggest that Alzheimer's special care units reduce behavioral disturbances and use of restraints.

SUMMARY

Dementia is an increasingly common syndrome characterized by a progressive loss of cognition and functioning. Given the aging of the population, it is essential that primary care providers become comfortable with diagnosis, counseling, community and specialist referral, and treatment. Early diagnosis may allow for identification of (unfortunately rare) reversible causes, improved symptom management, and planning for the future.

When patients present with cognitive complaints, the primary care provider must consider differential diagnoses including dementia, delirium, depression, and psychosis. Diagnostic workup includes a careful history from patient and family, physical examination, mental status examination, labwork, and, on occasion, referral for brain imaging or neuropsychological testing

Treatment and management consist of ruling out treatable conditions, treating secondary disorders such as anxiety or depression, providing information to patients and families, and assisting caregivers with safety and management issues. Use of medications may modestly slow the rate of cognitive decline or help with management of severe psychiatric symptoms, but interventions also consist of adjusting the environment to make the patient as comfortable and safe as possible, and providing support for the stressed caregiver.

Taking care of demented patients and their caregivers can be extremely rewarding. Further, with abundant research efforts under way, there is reason to be optimistic that improved methods of preventing and treating dementing disorders are just over the horizon.

SUGGESTED READINGS

Carlson DL et al: Management of dementia-related behavioral disturbances: a nonpharmacologic approach. Mayo Clin Proc 1995;70:1108.

Crum RM et al: Population-based norms for the Mini-Mental State Examination by age and educational level. JAMA 1993;269:2386.

Doody RS et al: Practice parameter: management of dementia (an evidence-based review). Neurology 2001;56:1154.

Gomez-Tortosa E et al: Dementia with Lewy bodies. J Am Geriatr Soc 1998;46:1449.

Knopman DS et al: Practice parameter: diagnosis of dementia (an evidence-based review). Neurology 2001;56:1143.

Mintzer JE, Hoernig KS, Mirski DF: Treatment of agitation in patients with dementia. Clin Geriatr Med 1998;14(1):147.

Nyenhuis DL, Gorelick PB: Vascular dementia: a contemporary review of epidemiology, diagnosis, prevention, and treatment. J Am Geriatr Soc 1998;46:1437.

Petersen RC et al: Mild cognitive impairment: clinical characterization and outcome. Arch Neurol 1999;56:303.

Petersen RC et al: Practice parameter: early detection of dementia: mild cognitive impairment (an evidence-based review). Neurology 2001;56:1133.

Raskind MA, Peskind ER: Alzheimer's disease and related disorders. Med Clin North Am 2001;85(3):803.

Teri L et al: Treatment of agitation in Alzheimer's disease: a randomized, placebo-controlled trial. Neurology 2000;55:1271.

WEB SITES

Alzheimer's Association
http://www.alz.org

Alzheimer's Disease Education and Referral Center
http://www.alzheimers.org

American Geriatrics Society
http://www.americangeriatrics.org

Brain Injury Association of America
http://www.biausa.org

Eldercare Locator (nationwide toll-free service helps older adults and caregivers to fine local services for seniors)
http://www.eldercare.gov

Family Caregiver Alliance
http://www.caregiver.org

Gerontological Society of America
http://www.geron.org

Sleep Disorders

26

Clifford Milo Singer, MD, & Robert Sack, MD

INTRODUCTION

Thirty-five percent of adults in the United States experience sleep-related symptoms over the course of a year, making insomnia and daytime sleepiness among the most common symptoms seen in primary care practice. Sleep disorders are more than just a large part of clinical practice, however, they also pose a major public health threat. Sleepiness impairs work performance and is the underlying cause of many industrial and motor-vehicle accidents. Sleep-related breathing problems lead to hypertension, cardiovascular disease, and sudden death. Sleep medications themselves carry morbidity risks of falls, daytime anxiety, and worsened sleep apnea. The diagnosis of insomnia is based on the duration and nature of the symptoms. Treatment depends on the underlying disorder contributing to the sleep disturbance: depression, pain, restless legs syndrome, periodic leg movements, alcohol abuse, circadian rhythm disorders, and poor sleep hygiene are all part of the differential diagnosis. Clinicians clearly need to be knowledgeable about sleep to treat patients effectively and advocate sound public policy.

Normal Sleep Physiology

ADULTHOOD

The sleep–wake cycle is a complex electrophysiological process consisting of alternating periods of wakefulness, rapid eye movement (REM) sleep and non-REM sleep. Each of these periods has a characteristic electroencephalogram (EEG), peripheral muscle, and autonomic nervous system pattern. These sleep stages can be documented by polysomnographic recording (PSG), which usually occurs in hospital-based sleep laboratories, although newer technology allows in-home recordings. PSG allows clinicians to make specific diagnoses based on electrophysiological monitoring of EEG, electrooculogram, and electromyogram of submentalis and anterior tibialis muscles, respiratory muscles, nasal airflow, ear oximetry, and electrocardiogram.

Sleep has a structure, or architecture, that consists of four stages of non-REM and REM sleep cycles. The wake EEG consists of low-voltage, high-frequency waveforms that become dominated by alpha waveforms (8–12 cps) as a person becomes drowsy. Stage 1 sleep is defined by the disappearance of the alpha pattern and the establish-

ment of theta waveforms (2–7 cps) and slow, rolling eye movements. Stage 2 is defined by the appearance of low-frequency, high-amplitude discharges (K complexes) and brief high-frequency (12–14 cps), variable-amplitude discharges (sleep spindles) on a background of theta waveforms similar to stage 1. The emergence of slow waves [high-amplitude, low-frequency (0.5–2 cps)delta waveforms] heralds stage 3 sleep, when they make up at least 20% of sleep time, and stage 4 sleep when they comprise more than 50% of sleep time. These two stages are known as the "deep stages" of sleep, because they are associated with high-arousal thresholds. REM sleep is a distinct state of sleep characterized by wake-pattern EEG, skeletal muscle paralysis, and rapid, conjugate eye movements.

With the initiation of sleep, the healthy adult will descend through the non-REM stages within 45–60 minutes before beginning the first REM cycle, which tends to be brief. As the night progresses, less time is spent in slow-wave sleep and REM cycle duration increases, eventually comprising 20–25% of total sleep time. The non-REM/REM cycle typically lasts 90–110 minutes, with about four complete cycles per night.

The timing and duration of sleep are controlled by many factors. Although most adults have some control over when to go to sleep and when to wake up, they have less control over how much sleep they need and when they become sleepy. Although stimulants such as caffeine and habituation to a state of chronic fatigue can help people cope with inadequate sleep, they must ultimately pay the price of diminished energy and mental efficiency. People's sleep requirements vary and the human range is thought to be from 3 to 12 hours, but most people need 6 to 9 hours of sleep per night. Children generally need more sleep than adults, but after adolescence, daily sleep requirement remains fairly stable until late life. In old age, sleep need may increase or decrease, but the most dramatic changes are in sleep quality and duration. There is a gradual reduction in the amount of time spent in deep sleep as we age, plus a tendency to have more awakenings at night and more naps during the day.

The body clock, located in the suprachiasmatic nucleus of the hypothalamus, functions as the circadian pacemaker. It superimposes a rhythm of sleepiness and alertness to days and nights and determines whether a person is a night owl, morning lark, or somewhere in between. The

263

light–dark cycle and nightly rhythm of melatonin secretion by the pineal gland act synergistically to keep the body clock synchronized with the day–night cycle, allowing alertness during the day and sleepiness at night.

CHILDHOOD

Newborns typically spend about 70% of each day asleep, with more time in REM than older children and adults. A circadian pattern does not develop for several weeks—sometimes months—after birth. Sleeping through the night is one of the first maturational milestones. Sleep continues to be polyphasic, with daytime naps, until the child is 5 or 6. From ages 5 to 10, children are usually consummate sleepers with few arousals. Total sleep time gradually decreases throughout childhood, but for hormonal and psychosocial reasons the amount and quality of sleep drop sharply with puberty. Sleep can be erratic—brief on some nights with long "recovery" sleep periods on others.

There has been some renewed interest in household arrangements for children's sleep. Anthropologists point out that isolating a newborn in a separate bedroom is almost unique to western cultures and that cosleeping with infants is more natural and may be beneficial. Sleeping alone is a desirable mark of independence, but at what age this should occur varies considerable, depending on the child and the family.

OLD AGE

As people age, sleep tends to be lighter, with more frequent awakenings and the near disappearance of deep or slow-wave sleep. Sleep onset and awakening come earlier. Many people experience this change in early midlife; it may progress as they grow older, and waking at 4 AM is normal for many older adults. Sleep disorders also increase with age, including insomnia and disorders causing excessive daytime sleepiness, especially obstructive sleep apnea.

CLASSIFICATION OF SLEEP DISORDERS

Sleep disorders are generally grouped into three categories: disorders of initiating and maintaining sleep (insomnias), disorders of excessive daytime sleepiness (hypersomnias), and abnormal sleep behaviors (parasomnias) (Table 26–1).

Every clinician's review of systems should include screening patients for daytime sleepiness and nighttime sleep problems. Three basic questions give clinicians a head start in diagnosing sleep disorders and determining whether they are severe enough to warrant treatment:

- How are you sleeping?
- How much sleep do you get in a typical night?
- Do you feel alert during the day?

Follow-up questions should sharpen the differential diagnosis of specific disorders.

Table 26–1. The sleepless patient: disorders of initiating and maintaining sleep.

Category	Disorders
Insomnia	Transient and persistent insomnia, chronobiological insomnia, restless legs syndrome, periodic leg movements, mood and anxiety disorders, alcohol and drugs, and medical disorders affecting sleep
Hypersomnia	Sleep apnea syndrome, narcolepsy, idiopathic CNS hypersomnolence, delirium, advanced dementia, and traumatic brain injury
Parasomnia	Pavor nocturnus (sleep terrors), nightmares, somnambulism (sleepwalking), and REM behavior disorder

The Sleepless Patient: The Insomnias

TRANSIENT AND PERSISTENT INSOMNIA

Insomnia is one of the most common complaints in primary care practice. It is best to think of insomnia as a symptom rather than a diagnosis. Many factors combine to produce insomnia, which often occurs when a delicate balance is tipped; for example, a constitutionally light sleeper may be fine until he or she enters a period of stress or uses a medication that has alerting effects. It may be necessary to deal with several causative factors concurrently to restore a natural sleep cycle.

Temporary insomnia caused by stress, environment (cold, noise, new baby), acute illness, or pain is easy to identify and usually needs no special intervention. A brief course of sedative-hypnotic medication is occasionally warranted and may reduce the risk of developing long-term insomnia. Travel across time zones brings about a mismatch between the body clock and the time clock and induces transient insomnia known as "jet lag," which can ruin the first few days of a trip. Shift workers may experience the same phenomenon and can suffer severe health and social consequences because of it.

In a large multicenter study, the diagnosis of chronic insomnia accounted for 40–88% of patients in medical, psychiatric, and sleep clinics who presented with a primary complaint of insomnia. Chronic insomnia is a diagnosis of exclusion, and must be differentiated from the many other causes of long-term sleep disruption (see later discussion). Chronic insomnia goes by many names: psychophysiological insomnia, conditioned insomnia, learned insomnia, and primary insomnia. These terms all imply what is known about this condition: it is a chronic ailment that develops over time in what is conceived as operant conditioning to an arousal state incompatible with deep, sustained, restful sleep. It may develop after a period of sleep disruption from stress, infant care, medical illness, pain, or psychological stress.

Long-term dependence on sedative-hypnotics is often one result of chronic insomnia, as is cumulative sleep deprivation and daytime fatigue and dysphoria. Psychophysiological insomnia requires a holistic approach that can include use of medication as well as cognitive-behavioral treatment. The latter, which is successful with motivated patients, including the elderly, involves cognitive techniques to reduce anxiety and behavioral changes to improve sleep hygiene (see Table 26–2). Short-term use of sedative-hypnotic medications is appropriate to break the cycle of anxiety, arousal, and insomnia (see the section on "Medical Treatment"). In some patients, the symptoms suggest another disorder that can be targeted separately (depression, restless leg syndrome).

CHRONOBIOLOGICAL DISORDERS OF THE SLEEP–WAKE CYCLE

The timing of sleep is influenced by the hypothalamic circadian pacemaker or "body clock." Disturbances in the circadian timing of sleep may only be transient, as in jet lag and shift work syndromes, or chronic, as in delayed-sleep phase syndrome, advanced-sleep phase syndrome, and free-running sleep syndrome. The last is most common in blind persons, who lack the critical input of the light–dark cycle in regulating circadian rhythms. Diagnosis of chronobiological disorders is based on the understanding that except for its timing, sleep is normal in these conditions. Given the freedom to choose sleep times based only on internal cues of sleepiness, persons with chronobiological insomnias usually sleep well on weekends or while on vacation. A mismatch between the body clock and the hours that a person attempts to sleep may cause insomnia. Successful treatment can require strategically timed exposure to bright light. Morning shifts the pacemaker ahead (advances), whereas bright light in the evening delays the clock. Commercial light boxes are recommended for this purpose (see the section on "Chronobiological Treatment"). The pineal hormone melatonin, sold in the United States in health food stores as a "food supplement,"

may achieve this same goal with greater convenience, although probably with less robustness and with opposite timing. For example, people with delayed sleep-phase syndrome who want to advance the timing of their sleep might take synthetic melatonin (0.5–3 mg) in the evening at 8:00 or 9:00 PM—hours before their own phase-delayed melatonin secretion begins and more synchronous with the timing of melatonin onset in people with earlier sleep—to reset their body clock to the desired phase position.

CASE ILLUSTRATION 1

Greg is a 27-year-old man who presents with a complaint of insomnia. He describes having great trouble getting up in the morning. He is chronically late for work and his job is in jeopardy. No matter what time he goes to bed, Greg cannot fall asleep until about 2:00 AM and then sleeps through the alarm set for 7:00 AM. His wife has given up trying to wake him, and although he has arranged for an answering service to call him, the ringing telephone does not awaken him either. He is often tired and sleepy during the day, but in the evening gets his second wind just as his wife goes to bed. He craves weekends and vacations when he sleeps until noon and feels alert the rest of the day.

Greg has delayed-sleep-phase syndrome (DSPS). Persons with this disorder are extreme night owls and lack the chronobiological flexibility to adjust their sleep times according to school, work, and social demands. Origins of DSPS are probably multifactorial. Sleep timing is delayed, there is a surge of energy in the evening, sleep onset is late, and there is severe morning hypersomnia.

This syndrome is extremely common in teenagers and young adults, in whom the insomnia complaint is usually prolonged sleep onset, with an inability to fall asleep until several hours past midnight. Parents or spouses may de-

Table 26–2. Cognitive-behavioral treatment for insomnia.

Essential Cognitive Techniques	Essential Behavioral Changes
1. Talk about the frustration of not falling asleep and put this into perspective, ie, decatastrophize being awake	1. Bed restriction (out of bed if awake more than 30 minutes, no TV, reading, or eating in bed)
2. Education about sleep requirements (not everyone needs 8 hours) and day napping (OK if very sleepy)	2. No caffeine, alcohol, or nicotine late in the day
3. Confront patient's belief that they are "defective" in sleep and will always be a poor sleeper	3. Mild to moderate exercise in the afternoon

scribe their frustration with getting the patient out of bed in the morning. Treatment involves bright light exposure in the morning (to phase-advance the body clock) and short-term use of a sedative-hypnotic medication to facilitate earlier sleep onset and make getting up for bright light exposure manageable. Properly timed melatonin intake may also be helpful. Successful management calls for fairly strict adherence to a life-style that avoids late-night activity, because deviation from the early-to-bed schedule will result in relapse to a phase-delayed sleep cycle. This last requirement is, of course, especially difficult for teenagers and young adults.

RESTLESS LEGS SYNDROME (RLS)

This condition comes on with rest and produces an irresistible need to move, stretch, or rub the lower extremities. Severe dysesthesia may occur, sometimes described as "creepy-crawling sensations," aching, tension, tingling, or prickling. Most people with RLS also have periodic limb movements during sleep, leading to further sleep disruption. RLS can interfere with plane travel, deskwork, reading, and especially sleep onset. The syndrome is common, affecting at least 5% of the population, and may be even more common in periodic or subclinical form. In females it sometimes first appears during pregnancy, but in both genders it can run in families and tends to worsen with age. It is especially common in patients with Parkinson's disease. Many physicians do not think to ask about this symptom and hence fail to recognize it as a source of discomfort and insomnia for their patients.

The first-line treatment of RLS involves the use of the newer nonergotamine dopamine agonist agents [eg, pramipexole (Mirapex), ropinirole (Requip)]. Dopamine precursor treatment [levadopa/carbidopa (Sinemet)] is effective as well, but may be associated with "rebound" or "augmentation" effects, with a tendency for the symptoms to develop earlier in the day. Anticonvulsant and sedative-hypnotic drugs may be helpful. Opiates may be indicated in severe or refractory cases. The syndrome is so distressful for some of its sufferers that there is a national support group and newsletter (see "Resources" at the end of the chapter for reference to the RLS Foundation on web-link to the National Sleep Foundation).

PERIODIC LEG MOVEMENTS DURING SLEEP (PLMS)

These are repetitive myoclonic movements of the lower extremities that come in bursts lasting from a few seconds to many minutes; they are more common in, but not limited to, the first half of the night. The movements are usually associated with brief arousals and can lead to nonrestorative sleep and daytime somnolence. The prevalence of PLMS increases with age—5% in people 30–50 years of age, 29% in those 50–65, and 44% in those over 65—and is often seen in metabolic and neurodegenerative dis-

eases. PLMS should be distinguished from nocturnal leg cramps, which are painful, prolonged involuntary contractions of the muscles of the lower legs often treated with quinine sulfate. Tricyclic antidepressants, lithium carbonate, and withdrawal from benzodiazepines and alcohol can induce or worsen PLMS. It is often asymptomatic, but in severe form patients may have sleep-onset insomnia, nonrestorative sleep, or frequent arousals during the night from more robust myoclonic movements. Not infrequently, the bed partner is the one complaining about the jerking leg movements at night.

Whereas RLS is primarily a symptomatic diagnosis, PLMS is best documented by polysomnography in the home or sleep laboratory. PLMS responds to some of the same treatments as RLS. Sedative-hypnotics can improve sleep continuity in PLMS patients, but not reduce the number of leg movements. Dopaminergic agents may be the treatment of choice, but rebound of symptoms in the second half of the night or during the following day may make dosing a challenge. Opiates, such as a bedtime dose of codeine, work well in PLMS (as in RLS), but should be reserved for patients with severe symptoms.

MENTAL ILLNESS AND INSOMNIA

Sleep disturbances are among the most common symptoms of mental illnesses, particularly mood disorders. Major depression must always be considered in patients complaining of frequent nighttime awakenings and early morning arousal, particularly when those arousals are accompanied by anxiety and worry. On the other hand, many depressed patients complain of hypersomnia with fatigue and difficulty getting going in the morning. This symptom is especially characteristic of seasonal affective disorder and so-called atypical depression. Both are common in young and middle-aged adults.

Mania is frequently accompanied by a reduced need for sleep, making change in sleep a cardinal diagnostic symptom of the disorder, although patients will not usually complain about this change. Depressed patients, however, find their sleep changes very distressing. Sedating antidepressant medications may help with the insomnia symptom, but can also lead to daytime sedation. Mirtazepine and nefazodone are reasonable choices of antidepressants in depressed patients with insomnia. When cost is an overriding consideration, the older tricyclic antidepressants (eg, doxepin, amitriptyline, and nortriptyline) may be considered. They combine moderate to severe sedation with effective antidepressant activity but must be used with caution due to overdose toxicity and anticholinergic effects. Serotonin reuptake inhibitors (eg, fluoxetine, sertraline, paroxetine, citalopram, escitalopram, and venlafaxine) are much less likely to improve nighttime sleep initially, but are also less likely to cause daytime drowsiness. A brief course of a sedative-hypnotic agent for help with sleep is a comforting strategy for some patients.

The sleep medication can be tapered and discontinued as the depression and secondary insomnia improve.

Anxiety disorders can also present with insomnia. Nightmares, particularly in posttraumatic stress disorders, frequently complicate the picture. Treatment is often challenging and may require intensive psychotherapy as well as psychotropic medications. Antidepressant medication, and prazosin or clonidine, may be helpful with the sleep-related symptoms.

Bereavement is usually accompanied by anxiety and insomnia. Short-term use of sedative-hypnotic medications may help patients who struggle to get through long nights.

CASE ILLUSTRATION 2

Francine is a 47-year-old patient complaining of anxiety. She feels restless and fidgety during the day, but she is also tired. She cries easily and has trouble concentrating, making decisions, and getting things done, all of which are out of character for her. Although quite fatigued, it can take her an hour to fall asleep. When sleep finally comes, it is restless and interrupted by many awakenings, filled with worried thoughts.

Francine's diagnosis is likely to be major depression, presenting with prominent symptoms of anxiety and insomnia. All patients with these symptoms need to be screened for depression, with a few questions regarding their mood, sense of the future, appetite, and libido. A primary medical or neurological disease presenting with comorbid depression also needs to be considered. If the diagnosis does turn out to be depression, disease education, emotional support, and antidepressant medication are indicated. Short-term use (several days to weeks) of a sedative-hypnotic medication [eg, zolpidem (Ambien) or zaleplon (Sonata)] should be offered if a less-sedating antidepressant is chosen as the primary agent. The antidepressant medication trazodone, although considered to be less effective for depression, is commonly prescribed at bedtime to augment other antidepressants and help patients sleep. This is a widespread clinical practice, but its safety and efficacy have not been studied in randomized, placebo-controlled trials.

ALCOHOL AND DRUGS

Alcohol has variable affects on sleep patterns, but it generally impairs both alertness and sleep. Like other sedatives, alcohol suppresses slow-wave sleep, making sleep lighter. With its short half-life, alcohol also tends to pro-

duce a rebound arousal in the second half of the night and can reduce total sleep time.

Other drugs can affect sleep. Amphetamines and cocaine cause marked reduction in sleep during acute intoxication and profound hypersomnia during the withdrawal phase. Opiates have acute tranquilizing effects and improve sleep when nighttime pain contributes to insomnia. Caffeine causes longer sleep latency (time needed to fall asleep) and increased wakefulness during the night. Some persons may not perceive the effects of caffeine on sleep even when they are documented on sleep EEG; others are very aware of these effects. Caffeine can even affect sleep when ingested several hours before bedtime.

Both prescription and over-the-counter (OTC) sedative-hypnotic medications can contribute to rebound insomnia when doses are missed. Drugs with short half-lives can lead to rebound insomnia in the second half of the night, whereas drugs with long half-lives can cause daytime sedation. Although they are common geriatric problems, memory impairment and unexplained falls should cue the physician to consider alcohol or sedative-hypnotic abuse in elderly patients. For example, the antihistamine diphenhydramine, a component of many OTC sleep-promoting products, has potent anticholinergic effects and can induce delirium in old people.

Education about the effects of these substances on sleep may motivate patients to reduce their intake. Patients with more severe dependency and abuse problems need referral to specific treatment programs for chemical dependency (see Chapter 20).

MEDICAL DISORDERS

Pain, rheumatological disorders, neuromuscular diseases, cardiac disease, pulmonary diseases, dyspepsia, inflammatory bowel diseases, and nocturia are all common medical causes of insomnia. One of the classic medical syndromes affecting sleep is fibromyalgia, a condition in which sleep is characterized by alpha-wave intrusion into non-REM sleep. This syndrome produces nonrestorative sleep, in which patients complain of feeling tired despite sleep duration in the normal range. Acquired immunodeficiency syndrome (AIDS) has been associated with daytime sleepiness, decreased total slow-wave sleep with alpha-wave intrusions, increasing arousals, and frequent nightmares. Patients with chronic disease are often desperate for good sleep, making adequate nighttime analgesia and sedating antidepressants very welcome.

Acute illnesses often cause diffuse cerebral dysfunction in the frail elderly. The resulting delirium is almost always accompanied by disruption of the sleep–wake cycle and alertness. In many patients, the confusion and sleepiness of delirium are the first clues of illness.

Medications can also cause insomnia and daytime drowsiness. Bronchodilators, activating antidepressants, and steroids, for example, often interfere with sleep, whereas many psychotropics, opiates, and clonidine can cause daytime drowsiness.

NEURODEGENERATIVE DISEASE AND SLEEP

There is no localized sleep center in the brain; rather, there are several neuronal circuits that function in maintaining sleep or alertness. Diseases that affect diffuse brain functions invariably affect sleep and alertness; Alzheimer's disease (AD) and Parkinson's disease (PD) have been studied more than most others. AD causes the same kinds of changes in sleep as normal aging does, but they are more severe: less clear day–night difference with more daytime and less nighttime sleep. Complete day–night reversal is rare, but sleeping nearly as much during the day as at night is common. This is very stressful for caregivers, who must continue to supervise their charges for safety during these nocturnal wanderings. Sleep disruption is among the most stressful aspects of caring for a person with dementia at home.

PD patients also have severe sleep problems. Akinesia causes physical discomfort over pressure points that normally would be relieved by tossing and turning in sleep. Medications used to treat PD can also impair sleep. Furthermore, the neurodegenerative and neurotransmitter changes caused by the disease adversely affect sleep quality.

The Sleepy Patient: Disorders of Excessive Somnolence

Patients are more likely to complain about insomnia than about excessive daytime sleepiness. They may complain of fatigue or feeling tired, but sleepiness per se may not be acknowledged without specific inquiry by the clinician. Two questions that should be included in every sleep-related "review of systems" are:

- Do you struggle to stay awake while driving, reading, watching television and movies, or listening to lectures during daytime hours?
- Do you feel tired, fatigued, and lacking in energy during the day, especially in the morning?

If the answer is "yes" to either question, follow-up questions should be directed at determining if the problem is inadequate nighttime sleep from insomnia, drowsiness from medications, narcolepsy, or sleep-related breathing problems.

Sleep-Related Breathing Problems

SNORING

Apart from being a nuisance to bed partners, snoring may herald the development of serious respiratory obstruction during sleep along a continuum of partial to complete airway closure. Males snore more than young females, but after menopause females snore almost as much as

men. Aside from male gender, other factors associated with snoring include anatomic narrowing of the airways, body habitus (obese) and sleep position (supine), the use of alcohol and sedative-hypnotics, endocrinopathy (hypothyroidism, acromegaly), smoking, and, possibly, genetic factors. The view of snoring as a mild form of obstructive sleep apnea (OSA) is supported by the transient drop in SaO_2 and rise in pulmonary and systemic pressure that can occur. Weight loss, the avoidance of sedating medications or alcohol, and appliances to prevent back sleeping (tennis ball sewn at the back of nightshirt) are warranted in severe cases. A number of different dental appliances that thrust the tongue or mandible forward during sleep may be helpful. Laser surgery to enlarge the oropharynx is increasingly popular, but the long-term effects are unknown. Because surgery can eliminate the noise of snoring without affecting an associated obstruction, PSG evaluation prior to an operation should be performed to rule out OSA.

OBSTRUCTIVE SLEEP APNEA SYNDROME

OSA is a significant cause of cardiovascular morbidity and daytime somnolence in adults. Originally thought of as a relatively rare disturbance in severely obese patients with the classic "Pickwickian Syndrome" of somnolence, hypoventilation, and polycythemia, OSA is now known to represent a wide range of severity in upper airway narrowing in sleep that begins earlier in life and is more prevalent than previously thought. In midlife, 2% of women and 4% of men have OSA with serious daytime sequelae. Nighttime symptoms of OSA include loud snoring (often beginning early in adulthood and progressively worsening with age and increased weight), snorting and gagging sounds, tossing and turning, night sweats, abrupt awakenings with a feeling of choking, and profound sleep disruption. The arousals triggered by the apneic episodes cause daytime fatigue and sleepiness. In mild cases, subjective insomnia may be the chief complaint. Patients are often unaware of the severity of the sleep disruption and may attribute their sleepiness to some other cause, such as working too hard. The degree of sleepiness is variable, but is a key symptom. People may be so accustomed to living with fatigue that they are not fully aware how sleepy they are. Questions about dozing while reading or watching television, nodding off at the wheel, or poor concentration need to be posed directly to patients. Untreated OSA leads to hypertension and maybe a significant risk factor for lethal cardiovascular events including myocardial infarction and stroke. Clinical assessment by PSG, either at home or in a sleep laboratory, confirms the diagnosis and helps determine the proper setting for positive airway pressure devices, which are the major form of treatment. Surgical uvuloplasty, tracheostomy, and dental devices designed to keep the tongue from falling back and occluding the airway are other forms of treatment available for those who cannot tolerate continuous or bilevel positive airway pressure (CPAP or BIPAP). The correct diagnosis of OSA can help improve quality of life and may prevent serious accidents and cardiovascular disease.

Obstructive apneas also occur in children. Enlarged tonsils and adenoids are usually responsible, but craniofacial abnormalities and obesity can be the underlying causes. As in adults, loud snoring, restless sleep, and witnessed pauses in breathing are symptomatic. Children with OSA may not complain of sleepiness; instead they may manifest daytime irritability, decreased attention, or declining school performance. Some children have even been misidentified as intellectually impaired. Nocturnal enuresis may be another symptom of OSA in children. Parents should be asked about snoring and breath-holding during sleep. Consultation with an ear, nose, and throat specialist is advised whenever OSA is suspected. Tonsillectomy (if the underlying cause) is usually completely curative. Other causes of OSA can be treated with CPAP. Surgical approaches such as tracheostomy or craniofacial reconstruction may be necessary in rare cases.

CENTRAL APNEA

Central apnea is defined as the cessation of airflow for at least 10 seconds with no ventilatory effort. Patients with predominantly central apnea tend to complain more of insomnia than of the hypersomnolence that is so typical of patients with obstructive apnea. Arterial oxygen desaturation usually occurs with central apnea, but serious cardiovascular sequelae are less common than in obstructive apnea. Predisposing factors to central apnea are congestive heart failure (mechanism unknown) and neurodegenerative diseases that affect the central nervous system's respiratory control or induce profound hypoventilation from respiratory muscle weakness.

Central apneas are often seen in sleeping neonates, especially premature infants, and can be fatal [eg, sudden infant death syndrome (SIDS)]. The cause of SIDS remains a tragic mystery; obstructed breathing has long been suspected as an important etiology in at least some cases, but it is far from proven. There is currently an ongoing public information campaign to encourage mothers to avoid placing infants face down (prone), especially in soft bedding. Epidemiological assessments will determine whether this intervention is effective.

CASE ILLUSTRATION 3

Jim, who is 64 years old, visits his primary care physician for a follow-up of his hypertension treatment. His wife has accompanied him to the office to ask whether there is any medical explanation for her husband's fatigue. Close questioning reveals that the fatigue predates the antihypertensive medication and is not clearly attributable to the drug. The tiredness is accompanied by true sleepiness; Jim can fall asleep anytime during the day while reading or driving. He minimizes the problem, yet acknowledges having trouble with memory and concentration. He falls asleep easily after getting into bed at night, but his wife describes him as a restless sleeper who snores loudly.

Jim probably has OSA. The clues are his snoring, daytime sleepiness, and hypertension. Referral to a sleep disorders specialist should help confirm the diagnosis and provide a review of the best treatment options.

NARCOLEPSY

Narcolepsy is a syndrome consisting of four primary symptoms: excessive daytime sleepiness, cataplexy, and, less frequently, sleep paralysis and hypnagogic hallucinations. It occurs in approximately 1 in 2000 people. Narcolepsy usually begins in the teens or early twenties but later onset has been reported. It is more common in males than females. A formal diagnosis is frequently not made until 5 or 10 years after the onset of symptoms. If the syndrome is not diagnosed and treated, people with the disorder may be perceived as lazy and unmotivated. Additional sequelae of a missed diagnosis include poor school and work performance, social stigma, and accidents. Genetic factors play an important role in the development of narcolepsy, with at least two genes involved, one of them HLA related. The cardinal symptom is sleepiness that comes on suddenly and irresistibly in what are called "sleep attacks." Low-grade, persistent sleepiness affecting concentration, thinking, and memory may also occur. Sleep episodes may be brief (several minutes to an hour), but the person usually awakens feeling more alert and the next sleep episode usually does not come on for at least an hour. Narcolepsy can impair nighttime sleep with frequent awakenings, vivid nightmares, and intense, realistic hallucinations prior to sleep onset (hypnagogic). The hallucinations are usually visual, but may involve any sensory modality.

Cataplexy, the brief, sudden loss of muscle tone leading to buckling of the knees or complete collapse, is triggered by strong emotional reactions such as laughter or anger. **Sleep paralysis** is transient immobility on awakening, often accompanied by the vivid hallucinations of REM dreaming, all while the patient is lying in bed perfectly alert. The spells are brief, lasting several minutes at most.

Although there is no universal agreement on diagnostic "threshold," many sleep doctors will make the diagnosis on clinical grounds: excessive daytime sleepiness and symptoms of cataplexy. The finding of sleep-onset REM periods during daytime sleep polysomnography in a patient with excessive daytime sleepiness and cataplexy confirms the diagnosis. Without the symptoms of cataplexy, the diagnosis becomes less certain. In ambiguous cases, it is advisable to refer to a sleep disorders specialist, since diagnosis often means a commitment to long-term medication treatment.

Patients should have a formal evaluation by a sleep disorders specialist before treatment of narcolepsy is initiated. The diagnosis usually requires documentation of sleep-onset REM by PSG. Excessive daytime somnolence is treated with modafinil (Provigil) at doses of 100–200 mg each morning and mid-day and clearly improves daytime function. The older central nervous system (CNS) stimulants, dextroamphetamine (5–60 mg/day), methamphetamine (20–25 mg/day), and methylphenidate (10–90 mg/day), are still widely used as well. Cataplexy and sleep paralysis are treated with REM suppressant drugs such as tricyclic antidepressants. Joining a narcolepsy support group will help patients cope with the psychological sequelae, which result from the social and occupational stigma of having little control over sleep onset.

Patients with Abnormal Nighttime Behavior: The Parasomnias

An accurate diagnosis of the underlying causes of bizarre nighttime behavior can be challenging. Possible considerations include seizure disorders, psychosis, delirium, and intoxication, but parasomnias, the least common class of sleep disorders, but perhaps the most dramatic in their presentation, need to be included in the differential.

PAVOR NOCTURNUS

Sleep terrors (pavor nocturnus) are very disconcerting to parents but are usually quite benign. The child (usually aged 3–6) awakens with a scream and appears terrified, with signs of autonomic arousal: eyes bulging, heart racing, sweating. Although episodes usually last a few minutes, they can go on for half an hour. Attempts at comfort are to no avail. Finally, the child falls asleep. In the morning, the child is amnestic for the episode or may have a fragmentary memory of a bad dream. Sleep terrors involve partial arousals from stage 4 (deep) sleep. Reassurance of the parents is the usual treatment; in persistent night terrors, however, benzodiazepines may be justified.

NIGHTMARES

True nightmares occur in REM sleep and involve a narrative story people can often relate once awake. Nightmares are usually a transient problem, presumably triggered by stressful personal events. Persistent nightmares are a serious concern, however, and may require referral to a mental health specialist.

SOMNAMBULISM

Like sleep terrors, sleepwalking is a partial arousal from stage 4 sleep. Occasional sleepwalking is very common in childhood and may follow a period of stress or sleep deprivation. The main concern is accidental injury, and protective measures, such as placing gates in front of a stairwell, may be needed.

REM-BEHAVIOR DISORDER (RBD)

In this syndrome, loss of normal REM sleep muscle atonia leads to dream-enactment behavior. The diagnosis is made in patients with sudden bursts of excited, intense, sometimes violent, activity during sleep. The syndrome may be subtle, in the form of leg movements and talking, or dramatic, with punching, kicking, grabbing, strangling, running, and moving about the bedroom. Dreams of an intense, violent nature are typical. RBD is seen frequently in toxic or metabolic delirium, but most persistent forms of the syndrome occur in old age, and are presumed to be idiopathic, ischemic, or neurodegenerative in etiology. The syndrome is especially common in patients with Parkinson's disease and Lewy body dementia.

DIAGNOSTIC EVALUATION AND REFERRAL

Most types of insomnia are diagnosed on the basis of history, and polysomnographic evaluation of insomnia is rarely necessary or reimbursed. Primary care clinicians should be able to accurately diagnose and treat transient and psychophysiological insomnia without referral or consultation. Sleep difficulties secondary to medical and psychiatric disorders can also be successfully managed by the primary practitioner. Referral to a sleep specialist should be considered for patients with persistent symptoms who do not respond well to initial treatment attempts. Patients with severe restless legs syndrome and chronobiological sleep disorders should usually be referred. Sleep-related breathing problems, periodic leg movements, narcolepsy, and the adult parasomnias all require polysomnographic validation and expert management and will require a sleep specialist to validate the diagnosis and initial treatment plans.

TREATMENT OF INSOMNIA

Medical Treatment

Treating insomnia should involve the clarification of specific target goals, such as shorter sleep latency, delayed wake-up, or fewer nocturnal awakenings. Insomnia of recent onset should be treated with the expectation that short-term therapy will be effective. Sedative-hypnotic drugs should be used in conjunction with a sleep-hygiene program to maximize efficacy and reduce the dosage and duration of treatment (see Table 26–1). These medications should not be used in pregnancy. Patients with insomnia secondary to depression, pain, substance abuse, medication, or circadian rhythm disorders should also receive treatment for the primary cause of the insomnia.

BENZODIAZEPINES

All benzodiazepines have sleep-promoting effects, although only five are currently marketed as sedative-hypnotics. These drugs work well for short-term treatment of insomnia; tolerance to their sleep-promoting effects can develop quickly and some authorities recommend avoiding long-term use. However, some patients—especially those with an anxiety component to their insomnia—may benefit from long-term use. Benzodiazepines alter sleep structure, reducing both REM and slow-wave sleep, but the clinical significance of this is uncertain. They are generally safe for younger adults, even in overdose, although combining them with alcohol and other depressants can produce potentially catastrophic synergistic effects. In older individuals, the safety profile is less benign; amnesia, ataxia, confusion, and worsening sleep apnea may develop.

Choosing one benzodiazepine over another for a specific patient is partly based on drug half-life, and this will require prioritizing goals. Short-acting drugs such as triazolam are useful for the treatment of sleep-onset insomnia, but many individuals will have rebound insomnia in the second half of the night or anxiety the following day. Longer acting drugs such as flurazepam may work better for middle of the night insomnia, but some persons will have morning "hangover" effects. Longer acting drugs can be particularly troublesome in the elderly, as drug accumulation will lead to ataxia, confusion, and daytime sedation. Temazepam and estazolam are intermediate in half-life and represent reasonable compromises for patients with sleep maintenance insomnia who get hangover effects from the longer acting drugs.

These drugs should not be prescribed for patients with sleep apnea, severe respiratory disease, gait and balance problems, or alcohol abuse. Doses should be kept low in elderly patients and those with hepatic insufficiency. Rebound insomnia can complicate withdrawal from these drugs, causing patients to return to their use.

ZOLPIDEM AND ZALEPLON

These drugs are structurally unrelated to benzodiazepines, but share some characteristics with them due to the fact that they have some activity at benzodiazepine receptors. They have short half-lives (zolpidem, 1.4–3.8 hours; zaleplon, 1.0 hours), so they are most suitable for patients with sleep-onset or initial sleep maintenance problems. These medications preserve natural sleep architecture, which provides at least a theoretical advantage over benzodiazepines. The dose is 5–10 mg at bedtime, and patients should be cautioned to get into bed shortly after taking these drugs because of their fast onset. Precautions similar to benzodiazepines apply to the long-term use of these medications.

SEDATING ANTIDEPRESSANTS

Many clinicians use sedating antidepressants such as trazodone, nefazodone, mirtazapine, doxepin, and amitriptyline for long-term treatment of severe insomnia, although this has not been well studied. Theoretical advantages over benzodiazepines include less cognitive impairment and more slow-wave sleep. Treatment of underlying depression in many insomnia patients provides another advantage. Tolerance to the sedating effects of these drugs develops in many patients, but some clinicians believe this develops more slowly than with benzodiazepines. Side effects of these drugs are numerous, and special care must be taken in elderly patients, especially with amitriptyline, because of its potent anticholinergic effects.

BARBITURATES

Similar to benzodiazepines in mechanism and efficacy, these drugs are extremely dangerous in overdose and tolerance develops quickly. They should generally be avoided.

ANTIHISTAMINES

Diphenhydramine is sedating and is found in many over-the-counter preparations. It is generally safe and effective for short-term use, although tolerance develops very quickly after nightly ingestion. Diphenhydramine has some anticholinergic properties and can cause confusion and urinary retention in elderly persons.

ALTERNATIVE SUBSTANCES

L-Tryptophan was taken off the market some years ago because some preparations were found to cause eosinophilic-myalgia syndrome; however it is starting to become available again. Various other homeopathic and folk remedies have become popular treatments for insomnia. Teas and capsules containing volarian root extracts may be the most effective of these alternate substances. The pineal hormone melatonin, whose secretion declines as people age, has sleep-promoting effects in some people. Melatonin is the best studied of the food supplements and other remedies for insomnia and is commonly available at health food stores and pharmacies. Patients should be cautioned that melatonin remains an experimental drug and a naturally occurring hormone with potential neuroendocrine, immunological, and reproductive effects, although it appears to be quite safe with short-term administration. Results from placebo-controlled trials of melatonin for insomnia in various populations suggest it has only modest efficacy. Certain individuals respond quite well, however. Moreover, when taken at the correct point in the circadian cycle, melatonin can be an effective remedy for jet lag and can help people adapt to shift work (see next section). Commercial preparations may contain 1–5 mg of melatonin per capsule (sometimes in combination with vitamins). The most effective dose is unknown, and may vary from person to person. Doses in the 1–10 mg range are reasonable. Preparations containing "pineal extracts" should be avoided in favor of synthetic melatonin.

Chronobiological Treatments

Sleep–wake cycle disorders can be treated with scheduled exposure to bright natural or artificial light. Patients with advanced sleep-phase syndrome need to have a corrective phase delay with exposure to bright light in the evening. Bright light exposure must be carefully timed so that the circadian pacemaker is phase shifted to move sleep propensity to later hours, allowing these patients to be more alert in the evening. For the more common delayed sleep-phase syndrome, patients need to force themselves awake by receiving appropriately timed light exposure, which should begin around the time they want to wake up. The first few days are very difficult, but after several mornings of 30–60 minute light exposure, patients can begin falling asleep before midnight and wake up for morning classes or work. Light fixtures for treating these syndromes are available from numerous commercial vendors. The Society for Bright Light and Biological Rhythms (see "Resources" at the end of the chapter) can provide a list of vendors and more details about using bright light exposure in treating sleep disorders and winter depression.

Psychosocial Treatment

Sleep problems in children and adolescents usually affect the rest of the family, causing sleep loss in parents and siblings who may in some respects suffer as much as the patient. Because misinformation and inappropriate blaming may confound the problem, the disturbed sleep of such patients needs to be addressed as a problem for the whole family.

Modifying family routines may be helpful. Good sleep hygiene, including well-maintained bedtime rituals such as bathing, story-telling, and rocking a small child can facilitate the winding-down process that is an important prelude to sleep. Occasionally a child becomes overly dependent on a particular routine (eg, repeated drinks of water every time he or she wakes up) and the parents must set limits. After an expected period of protest, most children relinquish the need for unnecessary attention. These benign disruptions must be differentiated from the more serious panic that some children experience with separation. For this latter kind of anxiety, parental access through the night may be necessary, at least for a time.

In adolescence, sleep is often shortened at both ends. In the evening, there are the demands of homework, telephone socializing, school athletic events, and family life. In the morning, high school schedules often begin quite early, sometimes preceded by an even earlier bus ride. For many teenagers, the morning includes a formidable grooming ritual. Add to this the increasing tendency for teenagers to take part-time jobs after school, and the result is an epidemic of chronic sleep deprivation that is an increasing societal concern. Weekend sleeping-in may recover some of the lost sleep, but it tends to produce a phase delay that reinforces the tendency to stay up late during the week. In one experiment, high school students increased their IQ scores by 20 points after a week in which they systematically extended their sleep time.

In counseling teenagers, some flexibility and compromise are usually most effective. Adding naps during the day may improve alertness. A warning about the dangers of driving while sleepy, intoxicated, or both is important. Chronobiological interventions, such as light therapy, may be needed to counteract extremely delayed sleep. Outside the office, informed and politically active physicians may be able to influence public policy to help alleviate the problem, such as adopting sensible work rules for teens and scheduling school activities at reasonable hours.

Adults with sleep complaints need to feel that their health care practitioners take the problem seriously and understand the effect the disorder has on their lives. At the same time, clinicians can reassure the insomnia patient without severe daytime sleepiness that the problem of nighttime awakenings is more a nuisance than a serious health problem. Educating patients about appropriate sleep hygiene and cognitive measures helps them regain some sense of control over their symptoms (see Table 26–2). Persons with more persistent insomnia or those who appear to have severe emotional distress as a result—or cause—of the sleep disturbance may warrant evaluation by a mental health specialist.

As they do in children, sleep disorders in adults can affect family members. Partners and caregivers of patients with severe sleep disorders may need both emotional support and education about the nature of the sleep disturbance. Understanding the problem can help them to support the patient in following treatment recommendations.

RESOURCES

The National Sleep Foundation publishes a newsletter for physicians and health professionals, and has an outstanding website (www.sleepfoundation.org). The website offers information on many sleep-related topics, access to educational resources, and direct linkages to other relevant websites, including those of the American Sleep Apnea Association, Narcolepsy Network, RLS Foundation, and American Academy of Sleep Medicine.

The Society for Light Treatment and Biological Rhythms offers information on treating chronobiological sleep disorders and seasonal affective disorder. Contact information of vendors of bright light fixtures for clinical use is also available. The society has a Web site (www.sltbr.org).

The official website of the National Institutes of Health (www.nih.gov) provides many opportunities to learn about the ongoing research and resources of the National Center for Sleep Disorders Research (NCSDR), a part of the National Heart, Blood and Lung Institute (NHBLI).

SUGGESTED READINGS

Carskadon MA, Dement WC: Normal human sleep: an overview. In: Kryger M, Roth T, Dement W (editors): *Principals and Practice of Sleep Medicine,* 3rd ed. W.B. Saunders, 2000.

Czeisler CA, Richardson GS, Martin JB: Disorders of sleep and circadian rhythms. In: Isselbacher KJ et al (editors): *Harrison's Principals of Internal Medicine,* 13th ed. McGraw-Hill, 1992.

Morin CM et al: Cognitive-behavior therapy for late-life insomnia. J Consult Clin Psychol 1993;61:137.

Young T et al: The occurrence of sleep disordered breathing among middle-aged adults. N Engl J Med 1993;328:1230.

Sexual Problems

27

David G. Bullard, PhD, & Harvey Caplan, MD[1]

Sex is a problem for everyone. . . . Indeed, for a couple of weeks or a couple of months, or maybe even for a couple of years, if we are lucky, we may feel that we have solved the problem of sex. But then, of course, we change or our partners change, or the whole ballgame changes, and once again we are left trying to scramble over that obstacle with this built-in feeling that we can get over it, when actually we never can. However, in the process of trying to get over it, we learn a great deal about vulnerability and intimacy and love. . . . (Peck, 1993, Further Along the Road Less Traveled*)*

INTRODUCTION

Primary care providers are in an optimal position to evaluate sexual problems, as they often have the most comprehensive and long-lasting relationship with the patient. In contrast to most other medical diagnoses, however, it is the patient who usually defines when a sexual problem exists. Although referral to medical or mental health specialists (or both) may be indicated in certain situations, many problems can be diagnosed and treated by the primary care practitioner. When questions about sexuality are approached in an open, matter-of-fact manner, most patients are relieved and respond positively. They appreciate the affirmation that these issues are valid and important, whether or not they have current sexual concerns or are sexually active (Table 27–1).

■ CHALLENGE FOR PRIMARY CARE PROVIDERS

To provide patients with helpful responses to their sexual health concerns health professionals need to have the following:

[1]The authors would like to thank Linda Perlin Alperstein, LCSW, Jean M. Bullard, RN, MS, Lisa Capaldini, MD, Deborah Grady, MD, MPH, and William B. Shore, MD, for reviewing earlier drafts of this chapter. Our appreciation especially goes to the coeditors of this book for their valuable comments and suggestions. Finally, the contributions to the study of sexuality by Raymond C. Rosen, PhD, have been inspiring to us.

- A willingness and ability to discuss sexual topics comfortably.
- Awareness of the range and diversity of human sexual practices and concerns, as well as the importance of the circumstances or conditions under which individuals function best.
- The ability to separate their own personal beliefs and values from those of patients. Unless the practitioner encounters information indicating objective harm to someone involved, it is important to maintain a nonjudgmental demeanor.
- Skill at taking a sex problem history in appropriate detail.
- Knowledge of simple interventions, such as permission-giving, and the ability to transmit accurate information, make specific suggestions (eg, for making sex less pressured and more pleasurable), and make referrals to other resources, when appropriate.

Health professionals may have limited sexual experience, as well as questions and problems of their own, and consequently may be uncomfortable in discussing particular sexual material. Time, thought, and experience, however, can build confidence and expertise in talking about sexual problems. Health care providers can increase their comfort level by examining their own attitudes, beliefs, assumptions, and experiences; reading in the literature; discussing these issues with friends and colleagues; and routinely incorporating sexual health questions into the general health assessment of patients.

Of course, no one—patients *or* caregivers—should be forced to talk about sexuality. It is important for everyone to recognize the limits of their own interest, comfort, and competency. Sexual health is an integral part of health care, however, and all who deal with patients should be alert to the possibility of sexual concerns and, at a minimum, be able to respond with nonjudgmental listening and reassurance or by referring patients to a colleague who is comfortable and competent in discussing sexual issues.

■ PERSPECTIVES ON HUMAN SEXUALITY

Although a knowledge base of human sexual response is developing, even the most scholarly sexual research is rarely

Table 27–1. Sexual concerns of patients.

- **Common sexual worries about normalcy,** such as: *Am I O.K.? What is a "healthy" sex life? How do I compare? Is my sex life satisfactory?*
- **Sexual identity questions** relevant to life-style, orientation, and preference.
- **Developmental issues of sexuality** for children, adolescents, parents, and the elderly, including the development of gender identity, masturbation, genital exploration, child sex play, sexuality and the single life, marriage, divorce, and death of a partner.
- **Reproductive concerns** covering infertility, family planning, contraception, pregnancy, and abortion.
- **Sexual desire, satisfaction and dysfunctions,** such as a couple's differing levels of desire, and problems with vaginal lubrication, erections, orgasm, and pain.
- **Sexual changes** due to physical disability, medical illness, and treatment.
- **Sexual trauma** resulting from molestation, incest, and rape.
- **Safe sex practices:** AIDS and sexually transmitted diseases.
- **Paraphilias and sexual compulsions.**

value free. Sexuality encompasses an enormous range of behaviors, beliefs, desires, experiences, and fantasies that patients may discuss with their health care providers. Sexuality can also have legal, medical, moral, political, and religious aspects. It is difficult to find a more controversial area of human experience!

Motivations for human sexual expression are complex and numerous, existing throughout the life cycle in times of illness as well as health and varying from culture to culture and from individual to individual. Included are the need to express love; the need for physical release, reproduction, and recreation; and the need to increase self-esteem. Conversely, sexuality can also be used to coerce, control, or degrade others, or in the service of addiction or compulsion.

Sexual worries or difficulties are probably experienced by most people at some periods of their lives and may result from developmental growth and changes in life circumstances rather than from pathology alone. Sexual problems are sometimes a blessing, such as when they compel a person to get help for symptoms that indicate underlying medical problems, problems with self-esteem, or problems with a relationship. For some people, seeking help for problems involving erection or orgasm may be more acceptable than seeking help for issues involving self-esteem such as not liking themselves.

Because the language of sex is broad and varied, it is helpful to become familiar and comfortable with the vernacular and to be able to discuss calmly and in detail matters such as masturbation, sexual positions, oral sex, anal sex, penis size, and breast size. The following section discusses a few of the areas in which misconceptions about these subjects can be resolved.

COMMON SEXUAL ISSUES

From a medical viewpoint, **masturbation** is "normal," universal, and physically harmless at all ages. It is highly correlated with self-acceptance and sexual adjustment, and is often used to further sexual self-awareness in sex therapy. Some people freely choose not to masturbate, perhaps following personal or religious tenets. Guilt about masturbation, however, continues to affect many patients. Some may use masturbation compulsively to avoid personal or relationship issues. Sex offenders may reinforce their antisocial fantasies via masturbation. Those who are truly addicted to some sexual behaviors may suffer from a variety of life difficulties common to other addictions.

There is no standard for what constitutes acceptable **sexual frequency.** Individuals who are celibate may still consider themselves sexual beings, whereas others may have sex rarely but find it satisfying and enjoyable when they do. Compulsively frequent sex can become unrewarding for some, whereas others thrive on a frequent and active sex life. What is "right" for a particular individual or couple must be determined based on the various meanings and expectations they associate with sex.

Sexual fantasies are limited only by human imagination and may be enjoyed for their own sake. They may be exciting to a person who would never want to experience them in real life, or they may be yearned for. Obsessive and intrusive images that cause discomfort may need to be addressed with psychotherapy.

The majority of women enjoy and need direct **clitoral stimulation** manually or orally to reach orgasm. Unfortunately, many men assume that their female partners enjoy only intercourse. A result of this overemphasis on intercourse is that many women and men are uncomfortable with genital caressing alone. Couples can benefit from encouragement and permission to learn about and enjoy non-coital sex.

Most gay, lesbian, or bisexual patients do not wish to have their **sexual orientation** changed or challenged and often present the same concerns as heterosexuals about normalcy, dysfunction, and intimacy.

Normal changes in sexual response with **aging** include the following:

1. More direct genital stimulation and more time are needed for arousal (lubrication or erection).
2. Women may experience irritation and pain with intercourse, especially after menopause or periods of abstinence.
3. Erections may become less rigid.
4. Orgasm may not occur with each sexual encounter and the urge to ejaculate may become less intense.

5. The refractory period (the time interval between a man's ejaculation and his next erection) increases.

Many adults in their 70s, 80s, and even later years are willing to experiment in response to changes in their interest, sexual physiology, and partner status. Some older men and women become less focused on intercourse, finding increased enjoyment in petting, oral sex, and masturbation. Currently sildenafil (Viagra) and other oral medications in late-stage development such as tadalafil (Cialis) and vardenafil enhance erectile functioning in many men and may, in the future, be found to benefit select groups of women. Others may be happy to have retired from an active sexual life, or may be comfortable with relatively fixed beliefs as to what is sexually appropriate.

■ DISCUSSING SEXUALITY IN THE GENERAL MEDICAL EXAMINATION

Some patients may be more reluctant to discuss their diet or exercise patterns than the details of their sexual life, whereas others feel they risk disapproval or judgment when talking with a medical authority about sexuality.

It is often helpful to introduce the topic of sexuality and acknowledge that the patient might feel some embarrassment. By routinely asking questions about sexual health in an initial history-taking a caregiver shows acceptance of sexual health as an integral part of a person's well-being and removes much of the "charge" around sexuality.

The following is a potential way to initiate a discussion about sexuality:

Doctor: One area of health care that is often neglected is sexual health, yet it can be important to people. Do you have any questions about your sex life that you would like to discuss?

A "no" response can be accepted, without ruling out possible future discussion.

Doctor: If you have any questions later on, I'd be glad to talk with you or help you find someone with whom you would be comfortable talking.

When providers are uncomfortable about a sexual topic, they can make comments such as "I feel somewhat awkward bringing this up," or "I haven't had that experience, but let me find out," or "Can you educate me about that?" These phrases are acceptable to most patients and can extricate the clinician from some difficult situations, as well as foster patient rapport.

As part of the psychosocial component of the general medical examination, a brief sex history should cover the following:

• "Are you sexually active now?" "How many current partners do you have?" If none, "When was the last time you had sex?" "Is that O.K. for you at this point in your life?"

• "Are you sexually active with men, women, both, or neither?" To encourage the confidence of lesbian, gay, or bisexual patients, ask about the patient's "partner" rather than using the gender-specific terms "wife," "husband," "boyfriend," or "girlfriend." And ask about "sexual encounters" rather than "intercourse."

• "How satisfied are you with your sexual experiences and functioning?" (Frequency, variety, who initiates, etc.)

• "Do you experience any problems with lubrication, orgasm, erection, or ejaculation?"

• Before assessing type of contraception and consistency of use, ask "Do you have a need for contraception?" rather than assuming contraception is necessary.

• History of sexually transmitted diseases (STDs) and their treatment.

• "Have you ever been tested for human immunodeficiency virus (HIV), and if so do you know if you are positive?" "Are you aware of safer sex precautions?"

• "Have you ever had a difficult, disturbing, or abusive sexual experience?"

Use questions that show openness to other than the modal heterosexual preferences. Making assumptions about a person's sexuality based on age, gender, race, marital status, or sexual orientation may be diagnostically misleading and send damaging messages to the individual [eg, an elderly patient assumed to be sexually inactive may in fact have multiple sexual partners, and important risk factors for STDs and acquired immunodeficiency syndrome (AIDS) may be missed; a monogamous gay male may feel stereotyped or misunderstood if it is assumed that he has multiple partners]. Make sure that the terminology is *mutually understood.* Overly general or euphemistic terms such as "having sex," "getting it on," "making out," "making love," or "losing one's nature" may obscure important details. Terms that are too technical ("coitus," "copulation," "cunnilingus") or too colloquial ("cunt," "cock," "fucking") may be inappropriate for use in the professional relationship.

Avoid words that convey *moral judgments or indicate little* about what an individual is actually experiencing (eg, "adultery," "frigid," "impotent," "nymphomaniac," "perversion"). Clinicians can help patients discard demeaning labels by substituting behavioral descriptions such as "having sex outside of your primary relationship," "difficulty getting erections or getting aroused," or "trouble learning to have orgasms." Again, time and experience with a variety of patients provide a sense of what terms are most useful in conveying information to a given patient.

Patients may bring up vague or psychosomatic-like complaints (eg, insomnia, fatigue, musculoskeletal aches, indigestion, headaches, or any specific symptoms of depression or anxiety) as a veiled request to talk about sexual concerns. Others mention a sexual concern at the end of a visit in an offhand manner, when there is little time for the problem to be adequately evaluated. The provider may then choose to assess the problem briefly and validate the importance of investigating this as soon as a new appointment can be scheduled.

Because sexual problems are often the result of a distressing gap between the patient's expectations and experiences, the effective sexual interview aims to elucidate both sides of the equation: if expectations are unrealistic, the treatment is education; if the experience fails to meet realistic expectations, intervention or referral is indicated. Often education and other clinical interventions are combined.

CASE ILLUSTRATION 1

One couple sought help from a sex therapist because, after 30 years of enjoyable and satisfying sex (involving intercourse that would last less than 5 minutes), they had read an article extolling the virtues of extended intercourse and began to feel inadequate. When encouraged to value their own unique sexual patterns, versus what might be right for someone else, they were relieved and decided they didn't have a problem after all. They then felt freer to build upon what was already satisfying to them in a spirit of exploration, rather than of attempting to be more "normal."

SEX PROBLEM INTERVIEW

As with any other medical problem, five basic areas need to be addressed for the patient presenting with a sex problem (Table 27–2):

1. Explicit symptom or question
2. Onset and course of the symptoms
3. Patient's perception of the cause and maintenance of the problem
4. Medical evaluation, including medical history, past treatment, and outcome
5. Current expectations and goals for treatment

Answers to the preceding inquiries can help guide the clinician to specific interventions.

PHYSICAL EXAMINATION

The detailed examination of the genitourinary system should include checking for signs of androgen or estrogen deficiency or excess, neurological dysfunction, genital abnormalities, and vascular disease.

For men, the examination should include the penis (to exclude conditions such as Peyronie's disease, penile discharge, and hypospadias); testes and scrotum (for masses, atrophy, hernia, or varicoceles); and skin, prostate, and rectum. Testing should be conducted for evidence of gynecomastia, peripheral vascular disease, and neuropathy. Testicular self-examination should also be taught.

For women, the examination should look for evidence of atrophic vaginitis; vaginal atresia; defective vaginal repair; pelvic inflammatory disease; endometriosis; and signs of cystitis, vaginitis, urethritis, and vulvitis. For dyspareunia, the patient can use a mirror to help identify painful areas. Breast self-examination should also be taught.

When pathology can be excluded, patients can be reassured that their genitals look "quite healthy" and are in the normal range. This can help counter the shame that many people feel about these vulnerable areas of the body. Naming specific genital parts, such as the foreskin and glans of the penis and the clitoris and labia, may give increased permission for the patient to ask any questions or express any concerns they may have about them. Men concerned about the size of their penis or women with worries that their genitals are somehow abnormal are more likely to voice these concerns after the clinician has comfortably used these words.

LABORATORY TESTS

In general, few laboratory tests are necessary for patients presenting with the most common sexual problems. For complaints of low sexual desire, patients should be screened for depression and tested for anemia, endocrine, liver, and renal disease, or any other debilitating medical problems suggested by the history and physical examinations.

Tests for women with sexual problems might include measurement of serum estradiol (<35 ng/mL is predictive of low sexual frequency), follicle-stimulating hormone (FSH), prolactin, luteinizing hormone (LH) levels, and androgen.

Some authorities recommend evaluation of serum testosterone and prolactin levels in all male patients with erectile failure or low libido. Elevated prolactin levels can be the result of many medical conditions, including pituitary tumors; renal dysfunction; sarcoidosis; thyroid disease; trauma; pelvic surgery; or use of medications such as cimetidine, haloperidol, and phenothiazines. If any of these tests are abnormal or other endocrine problems are

Table 27–2. Sex problem interview.

Description of Current Symptom in Detail

- Signal that you are glad the patient brought up the problem (to give approval, counteract shame, and encourage the patient).
- Help the patient specify exactly what the problem is, being careful to use understandable language—low desire, not getting wet or lubricating, difficulty getting or losing a "hard-on" or erection, difficulty "coming" or having orgasm, "coming too quickly" or rapid ejaculation, etc.
- *I'd like to ask a few questions to help us sort it out.*
- *Tell me what happens.*
- *How is that a problem for you?*
- *Anything else that has changed?*

Onset and Course

- *Does it happen alone with self-pleasuring or masturbation, with a specific partner, or with any partner?*
- *How does your partner respond when the problem occurs?*
- *Was there a time it was more enjoyable and then changed?*
- *Any situations when it's not a problem?*

Patient's Perception of Cause and Maintenance of Problem

- *Anything you **think** might be causing it or that you worry might be causing the problem or keeping it going?*

Medical Evaluation, Past Treatment, and Outcome

- *Do you smoke or use prescription or over-the-counter medications, drugs, or alcohol?*
- *Do you have any medical illnesses or treatments, depression, anxiety, or relationship problems?*
- *For women: Are your menses normal, regular? Have you had any children? Were any problems associated with pregnancy, delivery, breast-feeding?*
- *For men: Do you notice morning or nocturnal erections? Are they firm enough for penetration?*
- *Do you have a need for birth control; if so, what methods do you use?*
- *Are you concerned you might have gotten a sexually transmitted disease?*
- *Any history of physical, emotional, or sexual abuse?*
- *What have you already tried to help to change the problem?*
- *Have you ever had psychotherapy, couple or sex therapy? If yes, was this sexual problem addressed in the treatment?*
- *Have you discussed this problem openly with your partner?*

Current Expectations and Goals for Treatment

- *How important is it to you to get help with this problem and are you interested in trying to change it now?*
- *What would be the minimum improvement you would need in order to feel it was worth your time and effort in dealing with this problem?*
- *Most everyone has sexual concerns at one time or another. Talking about them is the most important first step. I'm glad you've felt comfortable talking with me and I suggest . . . (or will suggest some things after I've had a chance to review the best resources for you). Many people have been helped with these issues.*

suggested by the history or physical examination, the additional relevant tests should be performed.

Depending on the problem, additional diagnostic studies for men with erectile dysfunction may be conducted by a urologist and include monitoring of nocturnal penile erections (NPT) in a sleep laboratory or, more commonly and less expensively, with a home monitoring unit or simple snap-gauge. Increasingly, a trial with a phosphodiesterase inhibitor such as sildenafil (Viagra) is recommended for diagnostic information as well as treatment.

ORGANIC & PSYCHOGENIC FACTORS

Rather than describing sexual problems with a simple differential diagnosis of either organic *or* psychogenic etiology, it is useful to identify *both* categories of causal factors. These can be assessed with the psychosocial history, sex problem interview, physical examination, and laboratory testing. A symptom that is generalized (occurring in all circumstances) may indicate major organic or psychogenic involvement, whereas situational symptoms tend to be psychogenic (Table 27–3).

ORGANIC FACTORS

Organic factors may be suspected when a man reports an absence of nocturnal or morning erections or is unable to get erect with masturbation. For painful intercourse, important situational variables to identify include whether the woman has been adequately stimulated and aroused prior to penetration, whether she feels pain with masturbation or when having sex with another partner, and whether she is able to direct the extent and timing of thrusting or is passive. Also, organic factors should be considered when a patient has not responded to an adequate course of sex therapy.

Medical Conditions & Treatments

Medical conditions and treatments affecting sexuality are listed in Table 27–4.

Medications

Medications of many kinds have been implicated in sexual dysfunction (Table 27–5). Older antidepressants such as amitriptyline (Elavil) and doxepin (Sinequan) have anticholinergic properties that undermine sexual arousal. The widely used selective serotonin-reuptake inhibitors (SSRI)—antidepressants such as fluoxetine (Prozac), ser-

traline (Zoloft), and paroxetine (Paxil)—may inhibit orgasm for women and ejaculation and orgasm for men, while decreasing sexual desire for both. Strategies to alleviate such dysfunction include (1) reducing the dosage, (2) taking a weekend "holiday" in which the last dose for the week is taken on Thursday morning and the medication is resumed at noon on Sunday, (3) switching to another medication, or (4) *co*administering other medications, such as bupropion-S.R. (Wellbutrin-S.R.), neostigmine (Prostig-

Table 27–4. Medical conditions commonly associated with sexual disorders.

- Arthritis/joint disease
- Diabetes mellitus
- Endocrine problems
- Injury to autonomic nervous system by surgery or radiation
- Liver or renal failure
- Mood disorders, including depression, anxiety, and panic
- Multiple sclerosis
- Peripheral neuropathy
- Radical pelvic surgery
- Respiratory disorders (eg, COPD[1])
- Spinal cord injury
- Vascular disease

[1] COPD, chronic obstructive pulmonary disease.

Table 27–3. Symptom patterns and etiology.

Symptom Patterns Suggestive of Principally Organic Etiology

- Generalized (especially for absent desire, erectile disorder, secondary premature ejaculation, and painful intercourse. Even when generalized, however, primary rapid ejaculation and primary female orgasmic disorder in otherwise healthy individuals are rarely organic)
- Gradual onset
- Rapid onset when associated with certain medications

Symptom Patterns Suggestive of Principally Psychological Etiology

- Situational
- Rapid onset (unless medications are suspected)
- Sexual phobia and aversion

Table 27–5. Medication and drug categories commonly associated with sexual disorders.

- Alcohol
- Anticancer drugs and hormones
- Anticonvulsants
- Antihypertensives, including beta blockers (at high dosage), excluding ACE[1] inhibitors
- Carbonic anhydrase inhibitors
- Cytotoxic drugs
- Digitalis family
- Diuretics
- H$_2$ receptor antagonists
- Nonsteroidal antiinflammatory agents
- Opiates
- Pain medications
- Psychedelic and hallucinogenic drugs
- Psychiatric medications (benzodiazepines, tricyclic antidepressants, monoamine oxidase inhibitors, selective serotonin reuptake inhibitors, antipsychotics, lithium carbonate)
- Recreational drugs (tobacco, alcohol, and opiates)
- Sleep medications
- Tranquilizers

[1] ACE, angiotensin-converting enzyme inhibitors.

min), cyproheptadine (Periactin), bethanechol (Duvoid), and yohimbine (Yohimex) 1–2 hours prior to sexual activity. Newer antidepressants being developed will hopefully have fewer negative sexual side effects.

PSYCHOLOGICAL FACTORS

Psychological factors often play a causal role in maintaining sexual dysfunction even when there has been identification of a medical condition or medication commonly known to cause problems (Table 27–6). For example, a female patient experiencing difficulty reaching orgasm since being treated with an SSRI antidepressant may continue to have this problem even after switching to a lower dosage or different medication, because of a conditioned performance anxiety.

Following hysterectomy, some women report increased sexual enjoyment because of the relief from uncomfortable physical symptoms and bleeding, whereas others find the surgery difficult and have a psychological response to the loss of these organs and to their reproductive capacity. These women may then experience a decrease in sexual desire, arousal, or orgasmic responsiveness. The research is mixed as to the effects of hysterectomy on orgasm in women; it has been proposed that women differ in the extent to which they perceive uterine and cervical contrac-

Table 27–6. Psychological conditions commonly associated with sexual disorders.

I. Immediate causes (of most concern for the general medical practitioner)
   A. Performance anxiety—fear of inadequate performance
   B. Spectatoring—critically monitoring one's own sexual performance
   C. Inadequate communication with partner regarding sex
   D. Fantasy—absence of fantasy, antifantasy incompatible with sexual arousal, or distracting thoughts
II. Deeper causes (for referral)
   A. Intrapsychic issues—early conditioning, sexual trauma, depression, anxiety, guilt, fear of intimacy, or separation
   B. Relationship issues—lack of trust, power and control issues, anger at partner
   C. Sociocultural factors—attitudes and values, religious beliefs
   D. Educational and cognitive factors—Sexual myths or expectations (gender roles, age and appearance, proper sexual activity, performance expectations), sexual ignorance

---

Source: Adapted, with permission, from Plaut SM, Lehne GK: Sexual dysfunction, gender identity disorders, and paraphilias. In: Goldman HH (editor): *Review of General Psychiatry*, 5th ed. McGraw-Hill, 2000.

tions during orgasm, with differing sense of loss after the surgery. There is similar variability in men after prostatectomy. For many, orgasm may feel satisfactory even with a "dry" or retrograde ejaculation, with semen going into the bladder, but others may complain of a loss of orgasmic sensation.

 CASE ILLUSTRATION 2

Juan, a 38-year-old male patient complaining of erectile dysfunction with a possible organic component (type II diabetes) and performance anxiety, declined treatment with sildenafil (Viagra), saying that he wanted help without more medication. By quitting smoking cigarettes and engaging in noncoital caressing with his partner to decrease his pressure to perform, he was able to experience satisfying erections firm enough for intercourse. In this case, the diabetes by itself was not the determining factor in maintaining the problem.

Some medical illnesses and treatments are believed to decrease sexual desire or to cause sexual dysfunction *directly*. Psychosocial adaptations to virtually any medical condition, however, can *indirectly* affect sexual desire or functioning. For example, fears of rejection by a sexual partner because of a stoma or mastectomy or concerns about sexual functioning may lead to a suppression of sexual feelings and avoidance of sexual opportunities. Of course, many medically healthy men and women either choose to be sexually inactive or refrain out of a sense of inadequacy. The capacity to enjoy one's sexuality cannot therefore be predicted on the basis of medical diagnosis alone.

Psychological problems such as depression or anxiety can either be the *cause* or the *effect* of diminished sexual desire or functioning. Both may be true to some degree. In other instances, depression and sexual problems may both be the result of a third underlying factor, such as an endocrine disorder.

Sexual problems might have remote psychological causes, such as childhood trauma or prohibitions about sexual pleasure, but almost all such problems can be seen as having current maintaining variables of anxiety or depression. In general, psychological etiology is primarily suggested when the problem is situational; seems related to performance anxiety, depression, or guilt; or is associated with significant relationship and communication problems.

PSYCHOLOGICAL MANAGEMENT & BRIEF SEX COUNSELING

A paradigm shift occurred in the treatment of sexual dysfunctions with the publication in 1970 of Masters and Johnson's signal work on sex therapy. The previous emphasis on the diagnosis and treatment of individual psychopathology, with somewhat poor treatment results for the sexual dysfunctions, gave way to an understanding of the importance of the **conditions** (internal variables such as attitudes, expectations, and lack of knowledge, as well as external factors related to the partner or the situation) under which people attempt to function sexually. Education and suggestions for focusing on pleasure rather than on performance were found to lower anxiety and to promote improved sexual functioning and enjoyment.

Anxiety is considered one of the major psychological causes of the sexual dysfunctions, whether stemming from individual or relationship issues. Are patients comfortable, at ease, and feeling close to their partners or are they anxious due to lack of information, strained relationships, unrealistic attitudes about and focus on sexual performance goals, or other conditions? In these cases, modern sex therapy commonly provides anxiety-reduction interventions, many of which can be adapted for use by primary care providers. These include validating that most people at some time experience sexual problems and that such problems are often an understandable response to stress, worry, and concerns about performance; encouraging open communication between partners; dispelling maladaptive beliefs about sex; suggesting ways that patients can increase their level of comfort and safety and their ability to relax during sex; and encouraging the view that noncoital sex can be very satisfying and does not have to be considered "second best."

THE P-LI-SS-IT MODEL

Annon's P-LI-SS-IT model is a useful hierarchical guide to anxiety-reduction approaches to sexual problems and can be used by primary care practitioners. The letters in the acronym stand for different levels of intervention:

P = Permission

The fundamental intervention is to give patients permission to discuss their sexual concerns. Empathic listening, including verbal and nonverbal reassurance, helps give patients permission to talk openly about sexual issues and may encourage and enable them to discuss the problem more directly with a partner. Reassurance and permission can help validate that having a sexual problem is normal rather than pathological. Inquire into positive exceptions: patients can describe those areas of sex about which they do

feel good; for example, a woman can appreciate her ability to become aroused despite difficulty reaching orgasm, and a man can be a skillful lover despite his erectile disorder. Permission to choose not to be sexually active may be very helpful for patients who feel pressured to have sex or who feel inadequate if they don't care to be sexually active.

LI = Limited Information

Facts can add to the effectiveness of reassurance and can be at the disposal of any clinician who has done basic reading about sexuality and keeps up through the literature or review courses. Keeping responses focused and limited to the expressed concern saves time and does not overwhelm the patient with extraneous information (Table 27–7). Such information gives the patient the choice of maintaining or changing sexual practices or attitudes. A simple explanation of the psychophysiology of sexual arousal and the importance of conditions for relaxation helps "normalize" the symptoms and refocuses attention on conditions that can be changed to alleviate the problem rather than on trying to determine what is wrong with the patient. This can be conveyed by the following "rhinoceros" story about sexuality:

> Imagine you are lying on a blanket in a secluded meadow with a loving partner after having had a wonderful picnic lunch on a beautiful sunny day. You start kissing and feel arousal in your genitals, when, all of a sudden, a rhinoceros charges out of the jungle straight for you. What happens to your arousal (lubrication or erection)? The fight-or-flight response causes a rapid redirection of blood to the brain and large-muscle groups, with a corresponding loss of erection or genital arousal. The rhinoceros represents worrisome thoughts and anxieties about having erections, arousal, or orgasm, or fears that you won't please your partner or be seen as a good lover. Some simple suggestions can help you keep the rhinoceros out of your bedroom!

SS = Specific Suggestions

Where permission and limited information do not suffice, the patient may benefit from specific suggestions to help overcome a sexual problem. Most sex counseling interventions are designed to help the patient (and partner, if available) communicate better about sex and enjoy increased sexual pleasure by reducing performance anxiety about attaining the goals of arousal, lubrication, erection, and orgasm. Helpful interventions taken from sex therapy include (1) temporary agreement not to have intercourse; (2) suggestions for focusing on pleasurable touch, genital caressing, Kegel exercises (tensing and relaxing the pubococcygeal muscles), and progressive muscle relaxation methods; (3) correction of cognitive distortions

Table 27–7. Maladaptive ideas and therapeutic responses to them.

Maladaptive Idea	Therapeutic Response
My sexual problems are because I'm too old.	For those who are interested and willing to be creative, sex can be an enjoyable part of life in their seventies, eighties, and beyond!
I should be interested only in survival, not sex (for someone with terminal or chronic illness).	If sex was important to you before your illness it can remain so or become so again.
I am *asexual* because I don't have an active sex life.	We are *all* sexual beings. You can be aware of and enjoy your sexual feelings without being sexually active.
Sex equals love.	Many people have very loving relationships without being sexually active, and, of course, some people have sex without having loving feelings.
Sex equals intercourse.	There is no one *right* way to be sexual, and many people enjoy touching and caressing more than intercourse.
Having sex is the same as *enjoying sex.*	Many people have to learn to enjoy their sexuality.
It is not proper to talk about sex, either with your partner or a health care provider.	It is often a great relief when people can talk confidentially about their sexual feelings and concerns.
You shouldn't talk about sex because it will destroy the mystery.	Most people find that talking about their important feelings deepens intimacy, and trust develops when you know you can be vulnerable with another. You can create more mystery from deeper sharing.
You should be interested in having sex with any willing partner.	It is most important to be able to respect yourself. Your sexuality is a gift that you share only with those you truly want to share it with.
You should be able to enjoy sex with a partner even when you are tired, angry, or feel hurt.	We all have our own conditions for what makes a sexual encounter enjoyable, and feeling close to and loved by your partner is important to most of us.
I try not to masturbate and feel guilty when I give in because I have a partner and shouldn't need to do that.	Most married people continue to masturbate and find it does not interfere with the pleasure they have with their partner.
Sex is a performance, and it would be grim and catastrophic to "fail."	Sexual sharing can be playful, with the goals of giving and receiving feelings of pleasure and caring. If things don't go as planned, there is always next time!
A new partner will not like the size of my (breasts/penis).	Most men and women enjoy having sex with a person, not a body part. Most men compare themselves to other men when their penises are soft . . . size differences are usually not as great when erections are compared. Vaginas accommodate different penis sizes, with the outer third and the clitoris the most responsive areas for many women.
Sex should result in orgasm every time.	Does *not* having dessert ruin a fine meal? Orgasm is only one of the pleasurable aspects of a sexual encounter. Many people find it a relief to not have "should's" in their sex life.
Sex should never be a problem. Experiencing a problem is not normal.	Sex is perfectly natural, but not naturally perfect. Probably everyone has "problems" with sex at some time or another.

("self-talk"); and (4) suggestions to improve emotional and sexual communication.

Even for couples who previously enjoyed certain patterns of lovemaking, predictable repetition over time can lead to sexual boredom. Suggesting that a couple agree, for example, to temporarily forego intercourse or otherwise change their usual sexual pattern often helps them focus on moment-to-moment pleasure. Rather than making assumptions about what the other wants, the couple can communicate their likes and dislikes. Many people remember how arousing and exciting it was when they were younger and were "making out" (sexual petting) without intercourse. If agreeable to both, they can take turns exploring other ways of caressing and pleasuring each other. The **sensate focus** exercise, from Masters and Johnson, is done for the interest of the person doing the touching, rather than for the pleasure of the receiver. To minimize performance anxiety, each is encouraged to take turns "savoring" the experience of touching and exploring the other's body, in contrast to worrying about "turning on" or performing for the partner. For many people, permission for **genital caressing** in this way increases sexual pleasure and satisfaction.

Arranging for follow-up after giving specific suggestions keeps the health care provider informed as to their effectiveness, helps the patient stay focused on problem solving, and informs the clinician about the necessity for further intervention.

IT = Intensive Therapy

This is the last step in the hierarchy and involves referral to an appropriate specialist when the previous three levels of intervention have not been effective (see later section).

ADDITIONAL PATIENT EDUCATION

Pamphlets detailing approaches for safe sex for the prevention of AIDS can supplement discussions and should be made readily available for patients. Many good self-help books dealing with common sexual disorders enable patients to move at their own pace. Often people who are reluctant to enter counseling or who are hesitant about discussing their problems in depth are willing to read about the problems in the privacy of their home where they can be relaxed and comfortable. Several books are recommended at the end of this chapter (see Patient Bibliography).

INDICATIONS FOR REFERRAL

Refer patients to an appropriate medical specialist if the brief treatment suggestions in this chapter fail to help or if the history and physical examination suggest primarily an organic component. Refer patients to a mental health specialist trained in sex therapy if the problem is situational, occurring only with a certain partner; if functioning is adequate under certain conditions; or if significant emotional distress is present.

Primary care clinicians can develop a resource list of providers for sex-related problems. Colleagues, teachers, friends, and clinical societies can be asked for recommendations. Identify medical and mental health specialists with expertise in treating sexual issues. Practitioners can be licensed in psychiatry, psychology, social work, psychiatric nursing, or marriage and family counseling. Most states do not license "sex therapists" or "sex counselors."

■ COMMON SEXUAL DISORDERS

LOW OR ABSENT SEXUAL DESIRE & SEXUAL AVERSION

The range of issues concerning sexual desire is wide (Table 27–8). Some people simply put a low priority on sex, some are inhibited or find sex aversive, and some are clinically phobic. These problems can be of recent origin or reflect a long-standing pattern. Lack of desire may pertain only to certain sexual partners or practices (such as oral sex). Couples with different levels of desire may disagree as to which partner's level is "abnormal." In this situation, each side has valid feelings, and it is important not to stigmatize the patient with the lower level of desire. Most couples occasionally deal with periods of discrepancy in desire or mutually low desire and feel they should have sex more often than they do. Demands of family, career, and friends often take precedence over sex.

Problems with desire or sexual aversion can derive from deeper relational power struggles or reflect childhood sexual, physical, or emotional abuse that requires couple counseling or individual psychotherapy for resolution. The following case example, however, demonstrates how permission and encouragement to talk about sex directly, together with specific suggestions, can have a powerful positive influence.

CASE ILLUSTRATION 3[2]

Alice, a healthy 33-year-old primary school teacher, reported having lost her desire for sex. Her sex problem history established that although she had enjoyed sexual activity with her husband for the first 2 years of their marriage, in the past year it had become a chore that she never put on her extensive "to do" list. Because sex was seen as a bedtime activity, when she was usually tired, their sexual frequency dropped from weekly to once every several months. They did not address the problem directly, and Alice and her husband's feelings of estrangement from each other continued to grow.

When asked what steps they had taken to address these problems, Alice disclosed that she and

[2] Cases 3–10 described in this chapter were of actual patients seen in primary care settings as reported in consultation with the first author. Although some identifying characteristics of the patients have been changed to ensure confidentiality, the essential clinical issues presented are accurately portrayed. We thank all the patients and their health providers who helped us gather these examples.

Table 27–8. DSM-IV-TR sexual disorders and treatment approaches.

Disorder	Diagnostic Criteria	Treatment Approaches
Hypoactive Sexual Desire Disorder (302.71)	Persistently or recurrently deficient (or absent) sexual fantasies and desire for sexual activity. The judgment of deficiency or abscence is made by the clinician, taking into account factors that affect sexual functioning, such as age and the *context of the person's life.*	After organic causes ruled out or if situational: **Permission and Limited Information:** (a) Restate problem in behavioral terms, (b) Explore patient conditions for good sex (rhinoceros story), including whether patient receives adequate direct stimulation, (c) Validate patient's right to say "no" to sex, (d) May be secondary to depression, anxiety, panic, or phobic disorder (occasionally related to childhood sexual abuse), or (e) May be symptomatic of hidden arousal or orgasmic disorder (if so, treat appropriately). **Specific Suggestions:** (f) Listening exercises to increase *communication* with partner, (g) Suggested *readings* (Barbach, 2000, 2001; Gottman, 1999; Schnarch, 1998; Zilbergeld, 1999). **Intensive Therapy:** Refer to mental health professional trained in sexual therapy.
Sexual Aversion Disorder (302.79)	Persistent or recurrent extreme aversion to, and avoidance of, all (or almost all) genital sexual contact with a sexual partner.	
Female Sexual Arousal Disorder (302.72) Male Erectile Disorder (302.72)	Persistent or recurrent inability to attain, or to maintain until completion of the sexual activity, an adequate lubrication-swelling response of sexual excitement (female) or erection (male).	**Permission and Limited Information:** (a–d) Above, (h) Give brief explanation of the physiology of arousal and the need for relaxation. (i) Is sexual desire present? (if not, treat as desire disorder). **Specific Suggestions:** (f–h) Above, (j) Enough and desired kind of direct stimulation by partner? (k) Use of lubricants (Astroglide, K-Y, etc) or vaginal moisturizers (Replens), (l) Suggest temporary intercourse ban, (m) Sensate focus, (n) Genital caressing, (o) Progressive relaxation and Kegel exercises, (p) Explore ways other than intercourse of pleasuring partner, (q) Hormonal therapy, (r) Low-dose beta blocker (10 mg Inderal) if high performance anxiety, (s) Vacuum device, especially if organic and older male, (t) Intracorporeal penile injection or intraurethral application of PGE_1, (u) Penile implant, (v) Sildenafil (50 mg Viagra) for males.
Premature Ejaculation Disorder (302.75)	Persistent or recurrent ejaculation with minimal sexual stimulation before, on, or shortly after penetration and before the person wishes it. The clinician must take into account factors that affect duration of the excitement phase, such as age, novelty of the sexual partner or situation, and recent frequency of sexual activity.	**Permission and Limited Information:** As above, and explore masturbation patterns—may have conditioned himself to ejaculate rapidly. Explain connection between rapid ejaculation and anxiety versus relaxation and longer lasting erections. **Specific Suggestions:** (l–p) Above, (w) Increase frequency of ejaculation, (x) Stop-start exercises (Zilbergeld, 1999), (y) Clomipramine (Anafranil 25 mg as needed) or SSRI antidepressant medication, (z) Prilocaine-lidocaine cream with condom.

(continued)

Table 27–8. *Continued*.

Disorder	Diagnostic Criteria	Treatment Approaches
Female and Male Orgasmic Disorder (302.73)	Persistent or recurrent delay in, or absence of, orgasm following a normal sexual excitement phase. Women exhibit wide variability in the type or intensity of stimulation that triggers orgasm. The diagnosis of female orgasmic disorder should be based on the clinician's judgment that the woman's orgasmic capacity is less than would be reasonable for her age, sexual experience, and the adequacy of sexual stimulation she receives. For the male, the clinician should take into account the person's age, and judge the stimulation to be adequate in focus, intensity, and duration.	**Permission and Limited Information:** (a–e) Above. **Specific Suggestions:** For primary preorgasmic woman, recommend Barbach (2001); for male, Zilbergeld (1999). If orgasmic disorder is secondary (at one time patient was orgasmic), then evaluate and treat for desire or arousal disorder or relationship problems. (f) (j), (l–p) Above.
Dyspareunia (302.76) Vaginismus (306.51)	Recurrent or persistent genital pain associated with sexual intercourse in either a male or a female (dyspareunia). Recurrent or persistent involuntary spasm of the musculature of the outer third of the vagina that interferes with sexual intercourse (vaginismus).	**Permission and Limited Information:** (a–e) Above. **Specific Suggestions:** (f–k), (m–p) Above, (aa) Encourage explicit communication with patient's partner about her need to have enough stimulation prior to penetration, give control to the woman to choose when penetration occurs and timing of thrusting. **Intensive Therapy:** Sex therapy may be necessary for long-standing dyspareunia and vaginismus, due to conditioned expectation of pain.

her husband had never had an open discussion about sex. Her primary care physician validated that this was common among for couples and that most people have to learn to talk more comfortably about their sexual needs (*Permission and Limited Information*). The physician also explained that everyone has certain conditions that need to be met to be interested in sexual activity (*P and LI*) and encouraged Alice to think about her conditions and then, with her husband, to "set some private time aside outside of the bedroom and let yourselves have a discussion about this, even if it is awkward" (*Specific Suggestions*).

Doctor: It can be good for relationships when people risk being a little uneasy. You don't have to have the same perspective. You are each entitled to your own separate feelings about the situation, but together you can talk it out, try to understand each other, and see what other choices you have (**P, LI,** and **SS**).

The physician also recommended a self-help book (**SS**) and offered to refer them to a therapist who treats

couples, should their attempts to communicate falter (**Intensive Therapy**).

 CASE ILLUSTRATION 3 (CONT.)

At her 1-month follow-up appointment, Alice reported significant progress. When the couple set time aside to discuss their sex life, they had a very meaningful and tender talk. The husband was relieved to learn about the major sources of Alice's lack of desire and she acknowledged feeling resentful that he seemed unresponsive to her needs. He admitted that he had taken her lack of desire very personally, secretly and painfully interpreting the problem as her lack of desire for him. With these hidden resentments expressed, they could set aside their power struggles and cooperate in addressing these issues. Recognizing how they had both felt lonely and uncared for allowed them to take specific actions, such as planning a regular evening each week just for the two of them to talk and nurture their intimacy.

Management

PERMISSION AND LIMITED INFORMATION

Some couples can learn to accept that low desire may be understandable given their immediate circumstances (eg, the months prior to and after childbirth) and that their previous levels of desire can be expected to return over time. Validate the patient's right to say "no" to sex.

SPECIFIC SUGGESTIONS

A "prescription" to go away on a weekend or to arrange a sleepover for children with relatives may help couples "break the ice" and reexperience intimacy. Suggest that patient and partner set time aside to talk about each other's feelings and discuss conditions for more enjoyable sex, with each taking an uninterrupted amount of time for self-expression. Self-help books may also be recommended.

OTHER MEDICAL INTERVENTIONS

Hormonal replacement therapy, especially testosterone, may be helpful for those with low levels. For example, vaginal application of testosterone cream may be useful to some women who experience a loss of desire following chemotherapy for breast cancer, unless otherwise contraindicated.

FEMALE SEXUAL AROUSAL DISORDER

Symptoms & Signs

Problems with female arousal are primarily manifested as vaginal dryness and may be reported separately from or together with lack of desire, difficulty reaching orgasm, or pain experienced during intercourse. The most common medical cause in older women is estrogen deficiency with resulting signs of vulvar irritation and atrophic vaginitis. Side effects of medication may also inhibit arousal and this should be explored (see Table 27–5).

CASE ILLUSTRATION 4

Betty, a 78-year-old woman patient, had an appointment with her female physician. She brought along her 82-year-old husband because she wanted to discuss what she called her "sexual problems." Betty said she did not care about sex, that her husband was often angry with her lack of enthusiasm, and that this pattern had existed throughout the 50 years of their marriage. She believed she was not "a sexual person" because she had never been very excited by intercourse. She did enjoy kissing and caressing and mentioned that on several occasions she had been able to have orgasm when he stroked her labia and clitoris, but that she had never had orgasm from the "real sex" (intercourse) that he preferred. The physician

responded that there really is no one way to be a "sexual person," that many people cherish the sensual and emotional aspects of sex, and that Betty did not need to consider herself asexual just because she preferred different aspects of sexual intimacy than her husband (P and LI). The physician further explained that the majority of women reach orgasm more often from manual caressing than from coitus, and that many couples enjoy bringing each other to orgasm without intercourse (P and LI). The couple was relieved and admitted to having curiosity about trying this petting more. They were given brief instructions to take turns at home touching and stroking each other without the goal of orgasm (sensate focus), to get reacquainted with each other's body, and to refrain from any attempts at intercourse for two weeks (SS).

A follow-up telephone call confirmed that they were enjoying taking turns caressing each other, that orgasm often happened for each, and that they occasionally progressed to intercourse. A 1½-year follow-up was especially poignant—the husband reported that Betty had recently died from a stroke, and, although grieving her loss, he expressed profound appreciation for having gotten help for their sexual conflicts from the physician.

Husband: Settling those old battles over sex made our last year together more loving and caring than ever before in our marriage.

Management

PERMISSION AND LIMITED INFORMATION

Is the patient getting stimulation in the way that works best for her? Feeling distant from or angry with a partner can inhibit sexual arousal, and such relationship concerns need to be addressed.

SPECIFIC SUGGESTIONS

Homework may be suggested for her to identify what stimulation works best. The goal is to experience the pleasure of arousal in that mode—not to reach orgasm. Inquiry should be made into the quality of the patient's relationship. Commercial lubrication (Astroglide, KY Jelly, etc) and vaginal moisturizers such as Replens can be suggested and self-help books can be recommended.

INTENSIVE THERAPY

Recommend couple or individual therapy.

MALE ERECTILE DISORDER

Symptoms & Signs

Generally, a man with a significant psychological component is aware of nocturnal or morning erections, is able to maintain his erection for a reasonable time and then ejaculate with masturbation, or has good erections in some situations but not in others. He may be able to get a firm erection but lose it after penetration or may not get an erection with a partner at any time. The original cause of the problem is often distinct from the maintaining variable, which is generally anxiety. Consider possibilities such as performance anxiety, lack of direct physical stimulation of the penis, conscious or unconscious guilt (eg, "widower's syndrome"), anger at his partner or other relationship issues, or childhood issues such as sexual abuse.

 CASE ILLUSTRATION 5

*Carl, a 58-year-old HIV-negative gay male, confided to his physician that he had been "impotent" since the death of his partner of 17 years, with whom he had had an active and monogamous sexual life. Attributing this problem to aging and worries about HIV infection, Carl nonetheless asked for any help the primary care physician could provide. A full session was scheduled for talking only. His partner had died suddenly from cardiac arrest a year before. In the past month Carl had attempted sex on four occasions with two different men and was unable to get an erection. After a thorough sociosexual history, Carl was seen to fit the "widowers' syndrome." Clearly, he was still grieving the loss of his partner but attempted to control his tears with statements such as "I should be over this by now" and "Life has to go on; he wanted me to go on." Carl then revealed that he was very afraid of feeling such loss, fearing that he would never be able to come out of the sadness. His grieving was acknowledged and validated (**P**), and it was explained to him that temporary sexual problems were common after such loss because of a number of factors: performance pressure of being with a new partner, continuing feelings of loyalty to a deceased partner, subsequent guilt at having sex with new people, and concerns about HIV infection with a new partner (**LI**). The physician encouraged Carl to join a grief support group or to contact a psychotherapist comfortable with gay sexuality (**SS**). In addition, the doctor referred Carl to a book on male sexuality, with suggestions on how to talk to a potential partner about both safer sex practices and ways they could reduce the pressure to have erections (**LI and SS**). At a follow-up visit 4 months later, Carl reported he had been able to cry more about his loss and was enjoying sex and intimacy with a new friend who had also lost a partner.*

Management

PERMISSION AND LIMITED INFORMATION

Many patients over 40 years old report previous successful sexual encounters when they were younger in which they became erect without direct physical stimulation of the penis. If their pattern for sexual interaction has rarely or never included direct touching by a partner, it might help them to learn that such touching becomes more necessary as men age, and that it can be an enjoyable part of sex.

SPECIFIC SUGGESTIONS

Institute a temporary ban on penetration and suggest sensate focus, progressive relaxation, and Kegel exercises. The couple should agree *not* to attempt penetration or intercourse even if the patient gets an improved erection.

> **Doctor:** For every minute you are relaxing with your partner and have an erection, your body is remembering just what it needs to do to get and maintain an erection. Your mind can be free to enjoy the pleasurable feelings and sensations of being caressed and kissing your partner. You might even *allow* your erection to go away. If you stay relaxed, it will likely return again with resumed stimulation.

OTHER MEDICAL INTERVENTIONS

Phosphodiesterase (PDE5) inhibitors. Sildenafil (Viagra) and other oral medications under development such as tadalafil (Cialis) and vardenafil are popularly known to have revolutionized the medical treatment of male erectile dysfunction. Although contraindicated in men taking organic nitrate medication for angina, these medications have been found to have broad spectrum effectiveness across men of all ages and medical conditions, including diabetes, hypertension, neuropathy, postprostatectomy, and depression.

Testosterone replacement therapy. For men with demonstrated low levels of serum testosterone, hormone replacement therapy may be helpful. This does not benefit men whose serum testosterone is within normal limits. Side effects can be serious, including increase of any existing prostatic cancer, enlargement of the prostate, retention of fluids, and liver damage. Careful monitoring and follow-up prostate-specific antigen (PSA) screening and prostate examinations are necessary.

Antidepressant medication. Antidepressants, especially bupropion-S.R. (Wellbutrin-S.R.), can be effective treatment for some, but other patients may find that SSRI antidepressants hinder erection and ejaculation.

Low-dose beta blocker therapy. For some men whose performance anxiety is very high, 10 to 20 mg of propranolol (Inderal) as needed has been effective.

External penile vacuum device. With the aid of a vacuum cylinder a tension ring is placed around the base of the penis after it has become erect. This device may work better for men who clearly have a major organic component to their erectile problem, such as severe diabetes, multiple sclerosis, or spinal cord injury. Although this device can create erections functional for intercourse, men with a more psychogenic etiology may be disappointed when the erections are not as firm as they had been expecting. Side effects may include bruising of the penis.

Intracorporeal penile injections or intraurethral delivery of prostaglandin E_1 (PGE$_1$). These methods were originally used diagnostically by urologists. However, patients can now be taught to inject themselves prior to sexual encounters, resulting in firmer erections that often do not disappear at orgasm or ejaculation and last about an hour. Side effects are priapism in less than 3% of patients and pain. In addition, scarring may be a concern with repeated injections over time.

Penile implant surgery. Since the advent of effective oral medications, implants with semirigid silicone rods or inflatable cylinders are less commonly utilized. Total costs are high, ranging from $6,000 to $15,000. Complications include device failure (requiring additional surgery) and infection.

RAPID EJACULATION (PREMATURE EJACULATION)

Symptoms & Signs

Terms such as *rapid,* or *early ejaculation* are clinically preferable to the established *premature ejaculation,* as they highlight the subjective nature of the problem and are less pejorative. No absolute measure—either in number of minutes or thrusts—is applicable to the diverse numbers of men presenting with this problem. Factors to be assessed include a patient's subjective evaluation, degree of sexual satisfaction, and sense of control.

CASE ILLUSTRATION 6

*Donald, a 45-year-old divorced male, reported ejaculating after 1 minute or less of intercourse. This had been his pattern since becoming sexually active in his late teens. He reported proudly that he never masturbated but had a high sex drive, which led him to multiple sexual partners including prostitutes. His primary care physician gave Donald a supportive talk about how he could teach himself to last longer with certain physical exercises (**P, LI,** and **SS**). The patient was willing to do "self-stimulation" or "self-pleasuring" exercises for this "medical reason" and was comforted that as with the physical fitness regimen that he valued, he could tone up his pubococcygeal (p.c.) muscles and learn to relax the pelvic muscles during sexual stimulation. Donald was advised to increase his frequency of ejaculation, was told about the importance of relaxation for maintaining erection, and was encouraged to read Zilbergeld's self-help section on "stop-start" exercises for lasting longer (**P, LI,** and **SS**). As his confidence grew through the solo exercises, and as he increased the frequency of ejaculation, Donald was able to try the stop-start exercises with a partner with increasing success. He said that it also helped him to read about the experiences of other men (getting validation from the universality of sexual concerns) and about how many women enjoy a variety of forms of sexual stimulation in addition to intercourse.*

Management

PERMISSION AND LIMITED INFORMATION

Point out that early ejaculation is a very common problem—one study found 35% of married males reported that they ejaculated too quickly. Tell the patient that men with this problem have a high success rate when they try one or more specific suggestions that will be given to him for this problem. Give a *brief explanation of the psychophysiological mechanism.*

> **Doctor:** Men aren't supposed to be able to have long-lasting erections if they are too nervous or distracted. The fight-or-flight response generally makes men more likely to ejaculate. Most men have trained themselves through rapid masturbation to get erect and ejaculate quickly; so it makes sense that they would continue to ejaculate quickly when they are with a partner.

Assure the patient that men often report more intense orgasms after they have learned to last longer and that it is highly likely that he will gain greater ejaculatory control by following these suggestions.

SPECIFIC SUGGESTIONS

The patient may need to *increase his frequency of ejaculations,* alone or with a partner, perhaps masturbating to orgasm earlier on a day that a sexual encounter with a partner is anticipated. Discuss *other ways he can please his partner,* so he doesn't feel pressure to do it all with an erect penis. Discuss the importance of muscle relaxation in achieving a prolonged erection. Suggest *breathing exercises and progressive muscle relaxation exercises,* targeting the p.c. muscles or those in the buttocks.

In contrast to common attempts by men to diminish sensations in hope of lasting longer, they actually need to *increase their tolerance for the good sensations and feelings* and can best do this by concentrating on their feelings and getting more "turned on." Focusing on these feelings in a relaxed "practice" atmosphere can increase the threshold of enjoyment before ejaculation and orgasm.

He and his partner can read about and practice the *"stop-start technique."* Encourage the patient to change positions and to go from intercourse to oral or manual stimulation of his partner, and then back to intercourse (following the desires of his partner); changing positions and pleasuring a partner to orgasm without intercourse helps many men last longer.

OTHER MEDICAL INTERVENTIONS

Clomipramine (Anafranil, 25 mg as needed) or SSRI antidepressants help men prolong their erections prior to ejaculation.

Prilocaine-lidocaine cream applied to the penis and then used with a condom has been recommended by some clinicians (although "numbing" of the genitals may detract from enjoyment for both partners).

FEMALE & MALE ORGASMIC DISORDER
Symptoms & Signs

Many women do not learn to have orgasms until they are in their 20s, 30s, or even later. A **primary anorgasmic** or **preorgasmic** woman is not yet able to reach orgasm reliably either with a partner or by herself. A woman with **secondary orgasmic disorder** was previously able to reach orgasm but is no longer able to do so. **Situational orgasmic disorder** refers to a condition in which a woman can have orgasm with masturbation but not with a partner, or with one partner but not with another. She may reach moderate to high levels of arousal without experiencing the pleasure and release of climax. If no arousal or interest is present, she should be evaluated for a desire or arousal disorder.

CASE ILLUSTRATION 7

Ethyl's complaint of low sexual desire and difficulty feeling aroused led the physician to do a brief sex problem interview. With this more open discussion, Ethyl revealed that she had never been able to climax, but had been highly aroused in the first year of her 5-year marriage. Their lovemaking style was focused on intercourse, and Ethyl's husband didn't seem to understand why she didn't enjoy it as much as he did. She had not faked orgasm but had never told him about her feelings of frustration about not reaching orgasm. Ethyl had never masturbated and remembered vague attitudes conveyed by her parents and her church that masturbation was not a correct thing to do. The physician then validated that many women first learn about self-pleasuring as adults and that the information she could get about how her own body worked would then be useful in her sexual relationship with her husband. It was suggested that Ethyl read a self-help book for women who want to learn to have

*orgasms (**P, LI,** and **SS**). At a visit 3 months later Ethyl reported that she had proudly experienced her first orgasm by herself and felt so encouraged by this that she was able to talk more openly with her partner, who then agreed to go with her to see a marital/sex therapist to discuss ways they could bring more pleasure into their own lovemaking.*

For males, this *American Psychiatric Association Diagnostic and Statistical Manual of Mental Disorder,* 4th edition, *Text Revision* (*DSM-IV-TR*), category primarily refers to delayed or absent ejaculation despite prolonged intercourse or other stimulation. Some report ejaculation without the sensation of orgasm (see Table 27–8).

CASE ILLUSTRATION 8

*Frank, a 24-year-old man, confided that he had never reached orgasm with a partner. A sex problem history revealed that he had never ejaculated during intercourse and that his partners had never tried to bring him to orgasm manually or orally. Frank was able to ejaculate with masturbation, describing a vivid sexual fantasy (which he did not allow himself to have when with a partner) and a lifelong pattern of stimulation in which he rubbed his penis back and forth against a pillow without using his hands. He was congratulated for bringing this problem to his physician's attention (**P**) and was told that anxiety was often a cause of this problem, together with a masturbation pattern that did not simulate the type of sensations he would have during intercourse (**LI**). The physician encouraged Frank to take a stepwise approach to the problem by enlisting the help of a willing partner and starting with those elements that had been successful for him. He was also encouraged to expand on the kind of physical stimulation he received during masturbation by gripping his penis with his hand and stroking it. With his partner, Frank was to focus on the goal of having high arousal while his partner stimulated his penis manually and he was imagining his "tried-and-true" fantasy. The next step was to reach higher levels of arousal in this manner and to stimulate an orgasmic response (**SS**). Frank was also referred to a self-help book (**P, LI, SS**). Follow-up indicated that Frank had successfully reached orgasm with manual stimulation with a partner in 3 weeks and was following suggestions in the book on his goal toward ejaculation during intercourse.*

Management

PERMISSION, LIMITED INFORMATION, AND SPECIFIC SUGGESTIONS

Both men and women may present with difficulties in achieving orgasm because of a repeated pattern of masturbation that does not approximate the stimulation they receive from a partner. Although physical arousal may be apparent (erection or lubrication), these patients may not be feeling excited if they have to forego the fantasies or kinds of stimulation that had worked for them while masturbating. Encouraging them to incorporate the conditions under which they can reach orgasm when alone into their sexual play with a partner is the first step in their expanding their sexual enjoyment. In some instances, use of a vibrator may be recommended to provide the more intense stimulation needed for some people.

OTHER MEDICAL INTERVENTIONS

Currently, *sildenafil (Viagra)*, *tadalafil (Cialis)*, and vardenafil are undergoing clinical trials for the treatment of arousal and orgasm difficulties in women. Whereas these medications are broadly effective with men, research efforts are being made to identify selective subgroups of women who might also benefit from them.

SEXUAL PAIN: DYSPAREUNIA, VAGINISMUS, & MASTURBATORY PAIN

Symptoms & Signs

Female dyspareunia—pain associated with penile–vaginal intercourse or other forms of vaginal penetration—may be one of the most common and perhaps most underreported of the female sexual dysfunctions. **Vaginismus,** the involuntary spasm of muscles around the vagina, may cause dyspareunia and is highly curable with psychological and physical interventions. Little if any systematic, controlled research has been conducted on the etiology of dyspareunia. Manual–visual examination is of course important, but Meana and Binik warn against assuming that observed pathology causes the pain. Also factors that originally caused the pain may not be the maintaining variables. Psychological causes of vaginismus vary and may include fears of penetration because of confusion about genital anatomy and physiology, or fears resulting from other trauma or irrational fears, causing a conditioned response of involuntary spasm of the vaginal muscles.

 CASE ILLUSTRATION 9

*Nineteen-year-old Gina complained to her primary care provider that she had dyspareunia, was losing interest in sex, and was worried that her boyfriend was becoming impatient with her avoidance of sex. The physician then encouraged her to describe this problem behaviorally and in detail (**P**). Gina said that she had enjoyed intercourse since age 17 and always used latex condoms, but on one occasion 6 months ago she suddenly felt as if her vagina "was being rubbed with sandpaper" when her partner penetrated her. Although the physical pain had not actually returned in subsequent lovemaking sessions, Gina's fear of the pain recurring diminished both her interest in and her enjoyment of sex. When asked what she would do if the pain happened again during intercourse, Gina replied that she "would have to ask him to hurry up, but sometimes he lasts longer then." The physician asked how she would feel about telling him to stop all movement immediately and to withdraw when she felt discomfort or pain. Gina expressed concern that an abrupt withdrawal from intercourse might result in her boyfriend having testicular pain. She was reassured that this would create no lasting discomfort for him, and that there were alternatives for reaching ejaculation and orgasm, either with her or alone (**P, LI, and SS**). She was also offered some suggestions for reading about how couples learn to increase their enjoyment of sex (**SS**). The physician also praised Gina for having shown the courage to discuss this personal issue and encouraged her to bring up any future concerns (**P, LI**).*

Management

SPECIFIC SUGGESTIONS

These issues can be approached gradually, by encouraging the woman to speak with her partner about her needs and to be a full participant in the sexual encounter. She and her partner should be educated about the need for sufficient stimulation and arousal prior to attempted penetration, and about the importance of her being in control of the sexual movement, so that she can stop it instantly if pain is felt. Instruction in Kegel's pubococcygeal muscle exercises increases the woman's awareness and control of her vaginal muscles. Vaginal self-dilatation can be accomplished with graduated cylinders or with fingers, from the little finger to multiple fingers, while practicing muscle relaxation and calming mental imagery. The patient should be encouraged to be the one in control by bearing down on the finger(s) or penis as if pushing something out of the vagina, then relaxing. It helps for some women to imagine "capturing" the penis or other object in this manner, instead of being "penetrated."

OTHER MEDICAL INTERVENTIONS

Other medical suggestions include the use of artificial lubricants, such as Astroglide, Gyne-Moistrin, or KY Jelly (not good with latex); vaginal moisturizers, such as Replens; vaginal and vulvar application of estrogen creams; surgical repair of the vulvar region; and excision of abnormal growths in the genital area. Diseases thought to cause the pain, such as vaginitis, condylomata, endometriosis, pelvic inflammatory disease, and other gynecological or pelvic diseases, all may be treated directly. When painful intercourse has been a long-standing problem, however, medical intervention alone is seldom adequate and should be followed by sex therapy directed at the probable fear and expectation of pain that have been conditioned.

SEXUAL DISORDERS DUE TO A GENERAL MEDICAL CONDITION

 CASE ILLUSTRATION 10

When Hannah was 22, she was diagnosed with clear cell adenocarcinoma of the vagina and had surgery that removed one ovary, her uterus, tubes, the upper two-thirds of her vagina, and her bilateral pelvic lymph nodes. None of her health care team was able to comfortably discuss sexuality with her. She was completely unprepared for the first attempts at intercourse several months following the surgery and was shocked and distraught to discover how little genital sensation she had left. She sought help from a male psychiatrist who listened as she expressed her grief and fears that she would never find a man because of her sense of diminished sexual self-worth. After rapport was established, he acknowledged her fears by saying that she might never have a "clitoral" orgasm again, but that there were other routes to orgasm and sexual pleasure. He discussed with her ideas that have been helpful to others who have sustained the loss of genital sensation: that her brain knew how to feel pleasure and have orgasms, that men and women can learn to focus on sensations from other, nongenital parts of the body, such as breasts, neck, ears, and lips, and that with or without accompanying fantasy, one can thus relearn to enjoy a sense of orgasmic release and pleasure. Twelve years after her surgery, Hannah wrote, "The growth in my ideas and experiments with sexuality have increased many fold since my surgery. What was most helpful was being able to share my experiences with people who could understand and be accepting, and finding people who were trained and had accurate information on how I could help myself. Health professionals don't have to have all the answers, but they should know their own limitations and be able to refer when necessary."

OTHER SEXUAL PROBLEMS NOT OTHERWISE SPECIFIED

Other more serious sex-related human problems may be best dealt with by a psychotherapist trained in sexual issues. A patient with truly **compulsive sexual behavior**—sometimes described as **sexual addiction**—may be suffering from a form of obsessive-compulsive disorder and may require intensive psychotherapy, use of support groups, and medications such as the SSRI antidepressants. Patients with **gender identity disorders,** patients who have experienced **spousal abuse, incest,** and **rape,** and patients troubled by **paraphilias** require referral for specialized treatment.

■ CONCLUSION

For every human being, sexuality—like health—is a challenge at some point. Feelings of personal vulnerability are inherent in sexual interactions and help to make sexuality a powerful and unique part of life. Problems of sexual desire, arousal, or functioning can lead us to confront and overcome our fears of not being lovable and to seek better communication and increased intimacy with others. The deepest expressions of love often result from just such a sharing of our vulnerabilities or problems.

SUGGESTED READINGS

Annon J: *Behavioral Treatment of Sexual Problems.* Harper & Row, 1976.

Bokhour BG et al: Sexuality after treatment for early prostate cancer: exploring the meanings of "erectile dysfunction." J Gen Intern Med 2001;16:649.

DeBusk R et al: Management of sexual dysfunction in patients with cardiovascular disease: recommendations of The Princeton Consensus Panel. Am J Cardiol 2000;86:175.

Finger WW, Lund M, Slagle MA: Medications that may contribute to sexual disorders. A guide to assessment and treatment in family practice. J Fam Pract 1997;44:33.

Heiman J (Ed): Medical advances and human sexuality. J Sex Res, Special Issue 2000;37:193.

Kloner RA et al: Effect of sildenafil in patients with erectile dysfunction taking antihypertensive therapy. Sildenafil Study Group. Am J Hypertens 2001;14:70.

Leiblum SR: What every urologist should know about female sexual dysfunction. Int J Impot Res 1999;11(Suppl 1):S39.

Leiblum SR, Rosen RC: *Principles and Practice of Sex Therapy,* 3rd ed. Guilford Press, 2000.

Masters WH, Johnson VE: *Human Sexual Inadequacy.* Little, Brown, 1970.

Maurice WL: *Sexual Medicine in Primary Care.* Mosby, 1999.

Meana M, Binik YM: Painful coitus: a review of female dyspareunia. J Nerv Ment Dis 1994;182:264.

Peck MS: *Further Along the Road Less Traveled.* Touchstone, 1993.

Phillips NA: Female sexual dysfunction: evaluation and treatment. Am Fam Physician 2000;62:127.

Rosen RC: Prevalence and risk factors of sexual dysfunction in men and women. Curr Psychiatry Rep 2000;2:189.

Rosen RC: Sexual pharmacology in the 21st century. J Gend Specif Med 2000;3:45.

Seidman SN et al: Treatment of erectile dysfunction in men with depressive symptoms: results of a placebo-controlled trial with sildenafil citrate. Am J Psychiatry 2001;158:1623.

Shifren et al: Transdermal testosterone treatment in women with impaired sexual function after oophorectomy. N Engl J Med 2000;343:682.

Sipski ML et al: Sildenafil effects on sexual and cardiovascular responses in women with spinal cord injury. Urology 2000;55:812.

PATIENT BIBLIOGRAPHY

Barbach L: *For Yourself—Revised.* Signet, 2000.

(A revised classic that empowers women to enjoy their own sexuality, with suggestions for women who want to learn to become orgasmic.)

Barbach L: *For Each Other.* Signet, 2001.

(Encouragement and suggestions for couples wanting to enhance their sexuality and intimacy.)

Butler RN, Lewis MI: *Love and Sex After 60* (revised). Ballantine, 1996

Carnes P: *Out of the Shadows: Understanding Sexual Addiction.* Hazelden, 2001.

Carnes P et al: *In the Shadows of the Net: Breaking Free of Compulsive Online Sexual Behavior.* Hazelden, 2001.

Ellison CR: *Women's Sexualities.* New Harbinger, 2000.

(Respectful and helpful exploration of female sexuality from women of all ages.)

Gottman J, Silver, N: *The Seven Principles for Making Marriage Work.* Three Rivers, 1999.

(Results of over 20 years of research pointing out the danger signals for troubled marriages, with helpful suggestions.)

Holstein, L: *How to Have Magnificent Sex, The 7 Dimensions of a Vital Sexual Connection.* Harmony Books, 2001.

Leiblum SR, Sachs J: *Getting the Sex You Want: Becoming the Sexual Woman You Want to Be.* Crown, 2002.

(Great insights and suggestions from some of the most experienced sex therapist/educators.)

Mellody P et al: *Facing Love Addiction: Giving Yourself the Power to Change the Way You Love.* HarperCollins, 1992.

Person E: *Dreams of Love and Fateful Encounters.* Penguin USA, 1989.

(Literate and wise exploration of romantic love.)

Schnarch DM: *Passionate Marriage: Sex, Love, and Intimacy in Emotionally Committed Relationships.* Holt, 1998.

Schover LR: *Sexuality and Fertility After Cancer.* Wiley & Sons, 1997.

(Compassionate and hopeful resource for women and men who have had cancer.)

Schover LR: *Overcoming Male Infertility: Understanding Its Causes and Treatments.* Wiley & Sons, 2000.

Weinberg M, Williams C, Pryor D: *Dual Attraction: Understanding Bisexuality.* Oxford University Press, 1995.

Zilbergeld B: *The New Male Sexuality—Revised.* Bantam, 1999.

(A common-sense, practical, and sane antidote to media pressures on males to be sexual superstars. Excellent discussion of the fantasy model of sex and myths of male sexuality, the importance of an individual's conditions for good sex, and specific self-help chapters dealing with common male sexual problems.)

WEB SITES

Sexuality Organizations

American Association of Sex Educators, Counselors and Therapists
www.aasect.org
Kinsey Institute
www.indiana.edu/~kinsey/
Sex Information and Education Council of the United States
www.siecus.org
Society for the Scientific Study of Sexuality
www.sexscience.org

Sexuality Education

CDC (Centers for Disease Control) National Prevention Information Network
www.cdcnpin.org
Sexual Health Network
www.sexualhealth.com

Electronic Journals

Electronic Journal of Human Sexuality
www.ejhs.org
International Journal of Transgenderism
www.symposium.com/ijt

Section V
Special Topics

Complementary & Alternative Medicine

28

Ellen Hughes, MD, PhD, & Susan Folkman, PhD[1]

DEFINITIONS

Various terms have been used to describe a broad range of healing approaches that are not widely taught in medical schools, not generally available in hospitals, and not routinely reimbursed by medical insurance. Many of these approaches have their roots in nonwestern cultures. Others have developed within the west, but outside what is considered conventional medical practice. Complementary and alternative medicine (CAM) is the name chosen by the National Institutes of Health for these healing approaches.

Classification of CAM Modalities

The National Institutes of Health National Center for Complementary and Alternative Medicine (NCCAM) classifies CAM modalities under five domains (see Table 28–1).

EPIDEMIOLOGY OF CAM
Who Seeks CAM & Why?

Nearly half the U.S. population turns to complementary and alternative practices to maintain or improve their health. The total number of visits to CAM practitioners actually exceeds the total number of visits to primary care physicians each year. CAM is attractive to many people be-

cause it treats the "whole person" (body, mind, and spirit), emphasizes health promotion/prevention, and values the uniqueness of each individual. Independent predictors of CAM use in one survey included higher level of education, poorer health status, and a "holistic" interest in health, personal growth, and spirituality. People with conditions such as anxiety and chronic pain were also more likely to have used CAM in the previous year. Dissatisfaction with conventional medicine is not an independent predictor of greater use, so it appears that patients are more "pulled toward" CAM rather than "pushed away" from conventional medicine.

Epidemiology of Herbal Medicine Use

More than 39 million Americans take dietary supplements on a weekly basis. Many are drawn to herbal products because they appear "safe and natural." Regular users hold strong beliefs about what they take. In one survey, more than 70% reported that they would continue to take their favorite supplement, even if there were government research data that indicated it was not effective!

REGULATION OF HERBAL MEDICINE

In 1994, Congress passed the Dietary Supplement Health and Education Act (DSHEA), which limited regulatory control over botanicals. DSHEA classifies herbs, vitamins, minerals, and amino acids as nutritional or dietary supplements. It allows these products to be marketed without proof of efficacy, safety, or quality, as long as no claims to

[1] The authors gratefully acknowledge Dr. Bernard Lo for his valuable input in the preparation of this manuscript.

Table 28–1. NCCAM classification of complementary and alternative medicine.

Domain	Examples
Alternative medicine systems	Traditional Oriental medicine, acupuncture, ayurveda, naturopathy, homeopathy
Mind–body interventions	Meditation, dance, art and music therapy, spiritual healing
Biological-based therapies	Herbal medicines and dietary supplements, special diets
Manipulative and body-based methods	Chiropractic, massage, other "body-work" systems
Energy therapies	Reiki, therapeutic touch, magnets, methods that affect the body's "bioelectric" field

diagnose, treat, cure, or prevent disease are made. As a result, consumers taking herbal medicines have no guarantee that the plant was accurately identified, another plant part/species was not substituted, the herb is pure (ie, no microbial, pesticide, or heavy metal contamination), safe, and effective, or that the next bottle will contain the same ingredients at the same dose. In addition, in contrast to prescription drugs, the Federal Food and Drug Administration must first prove that an herbal preparation is unsafe before it can be taken off the market. Examples of some of the potential risks associated with botanical products are summarized in Table 28–2.

COMMUNICATING WITH PATIENTS ABOUT CAM

Despite the growing numbers of patients seeking CAM, less than 40% of alternative therapies used are disclosed to physicians, even though the majority of people who use CAM do so along with conventional medicine because they perceive the combination to be superior to either alone. The absence of disclosure is alarming, at the very

least, because some CAM therapies can interact adversely with conventional treatments. Discussions about CAM also offer valuable opportunities for the practitioner to explore a patient's health care beliefs and concerns.

This chapter will focus primarily on communicating with patients about their use of herbal medicines, because these are among the most popular CAM modalities and because of the potential for interaction of botanicals with conventional drug therapies.

Barriers to Disclosure

Patients are reluctant to disclose CAM practices to their primary care physicians for a number of reasons. In a study of CAM use among breast cancer patients the most frequently cited reason was the belief that the physician was not interested in the patient's use of CAM. Even when patients attempted to disclose CAM use, the physician was unresponsive, which prevented further discussion. Patients say, "I did tell the doctor . . . and he didn't say 'Good,' or 'Not good,' or 'Okay,' or anything." It's like, "We're looking at the platelets here, and the white count—let's not get

Table 28–2. Potential risks of botanical products.

Lack of quality assurance	Variable quality and quantity of herb in the product Lack of batch-to-batch consistency
Misidentification of herb	Renal failure when *Aristolochia*, a renal toxic herb, is misidentified as *Stefania* in a diet preparation
Adverse effect of herb itself	Hepatitis/liver failure with germander, comfrey, kava Stroke, myocardial infarct, death with *ephedra*
Contamination of herb Adulteration of product	Twenty-five percent of Asian patent medicines contain heavy metals Seven percent of Asian patent medicines contain undeclared prescription medicines (benzodiazepines, nonsteroidal antiinflammatory drugs, steroids)
Herb–drug interactions: herb decreases level of prescription drug	St John's wort with indinavir, cyclosporin, digoxin, warfarin, ethinyl estradiol
Herb increases potential for bleeding	Ginkgo, ginger, garlic, feverfew
Herb may interact with anesthetics	Some anesthesiologists recommend discontinuation of herbs 2–3 weeks before surgery
Herb has additive effect with prescription medications	St John's wort and selective serotonin reuptake inhibitors, kava and benzodiazepines, ginkgo and warfarin

too far afield!" Many patients believe that disclosure will not yield any benefit because their physician has inadequate training in or knowledge of CAM or may be biased against alternative health systems. Physicians may also communicate a reluctance or unwillingness to work with an alternative practitioner. Without such consultation, patients may feel that disclosing their interest in CAM will not be fruitful. Some patients believe that their physicians will actively disapprove of their use of CAM. Disapproval can be interpreted as disrespect for the CAM practice, and even worse, as disrespect for patients because they sought out nonconventional care.

Not all barriers to disclosure have to do with negative expectations about how physicians will respond. Some patients believe that their CAM use is not relevant to medical decision making. They may be using an herb, for example, to help regulate anxiety, which is not the problem for which they are seeing their physicians. This is borne out in a recent survey of patients who sought care from both a conventional and a CAM practitioner. Sixty percent of these patients did not reveal their use of CAM to their physician, giving the following reasons for their nondisclosure: "It wasn't important for the doctor to know" (61%), "The doctor never asked" (60%), "It was none of the doctor's business" (31%), "The doctor wouldn't understand" (20%), "The doctor would disapprove" (14%), and "The doctor wouldn't continue to take care of me" (2%).

Facilitating Disclosure

It is important for physicians to recognize that CAM practices are not limited to specific demographic groups. CAM practices are widespread, and all patients have the potential to be interested in or use a wide variety of treatments.

Patients are more likely to disclose their CAM practices if they anticipate that their physicians will be respectful, open-minded, and willing to listen. Behavior that conveys respect and open-mindedness includes asking questions nonjudgmentally or initiating a dialogue with patients' alternative practitioners. Lack of respect and closed-mindedness can be conveyed subtly through nonverbal behavior such as frowning or cutting off a response. If patients perceive that physicians disapprove of CAM, they may be reluctant to discuss other issues, such as noncompliance or substance use, of which the physician may disapprove. It is also easier for patients to disclose CAM use if they perceive that their physicians expect such use to be common and routine. This expectation can be conveyed by physicians through the use of questions about CAM practices. For example, "People use a variety of different methods to maintain or improve their health. What kinds of things are you doing to take care of [your health/this problem]?" Preoperative evaluations provide another opportunity to ask about CAM. Up to 50% of patients may not reveal that they are taking herbal medicines during presurgical evaluations, so it may be helpful to prompt

them with examples of specific CAM therapies. "Many patients take herbal medicines like gingko or use acupuncture for their health. Have you found any of these useful?" Finally, patients' comfort with disclosure is also facilitated by honest acknowledgment by physicians of the limitations of their own knowledge. "I'm not familiar with this specific therapy, but will try to find out more about it before our next visit." "Even though there may not be a lot of data available, I want to work together with you to come up with a good plan." Patients can be encouraged to contribute knowledge to the discussion and thereby strengthen the therapeutic relationship. "Why don't you bring in the information you've gathered about this therapy, so we can go over it together?" Ways in which physicians can facilitate disclosure are summarized in Table 28–3.

Communicating with Patients Interested in Herbal Medicines

In the following case, a patient asks her physician about an herbal remedy she is interested in trying. It presents a typical conversation that might occur when there is uncertainty on the part of the physician regarding the effectiveness and safety of an herbal medicine. Although the physician is acting in the patient's best interests, her responses have the effect of constraining rather than facilitating communication that could lead to more satisfactory outcomes.

 CASE ILLUSTRATION 1

Near the end of her annual check-up visit, a 57- year-old teacher with well-controlled type 2 diabetes mentions that she's considering taking an herbal supplement she found at the health food store.

Patient: A friend of mine told me about this new supplement that gives her more energy and boosts her immune system. I'm thinking about trying it.

Doctor: Oh. What is it?

Patient: Here, I brought the bottle in for you to see.

Doctor: Hmm. Unfortunately, I don't recognize the ingredients that are listed here, so I can't tell if they're safe or if they might affect your diabetes. As you may be aware, many claims made about these kinds of products are not backed up with scientific data, so I'm not sure that it's a good idea for you to take this.

Patient: I've actually been feeling a little bit better since starting it and my blood sugars have been fine.

Doctor: So. You're already taking the supplement. It's important for me to know everything you're taking, because of possible interactions with your prescription medications. I am happy to hear that your sugars haven't been affected by this medicine, but given that I don't know if it's safe or even what it does, I still don't feel comfortable with you taking it.

Table 28–3. Suggestions for talking with patients about CAM.

1. Ask if the patient is considering or using CAM.
   "Many patients use a variety of alternative medicines for their health. Are you taking any herbs such as ginkgo, or seeing a practitioner such as an acupuncturist?"
2. Explore patients' concerns and wishes that led them to be interested in CAM.
   "Tell me more about this therapy."
   "Can you share with me how you hope this therapy will help?"
   "You mentioned that this medicine helps people feel more energy. Have you been feeling less energetic lately?"
3. Establish a connection with the patient. Help identify, validate, and reflect back underlying emotions/concerns to the patient.
   "It's clear that you're interested in improving your health."
   "I sense that using something 'natural' is important to you. Is that right?"
   "It sounds like you're experiencing some difficulty with this prescription and might prefer something with fewer side effects. Is that true?"
4. Acknowledge that there is often inadequate information about safety and efficacy to guide clinical decision making.
   "Why don't you bring in the information you have gathered about this therapy, so we can go over it together?"
   "Even though there isn't a lot of data available, we can work to make a plan together."
5. Identify good resources (see Suggested Reading).
6. Explore potential risks and benefits of CAM with the patient (to the extent that they are known) as well as how CAM will interface with their ongoing care.
   "From what we found out about this supplement, it looks like it will be safe for you to add into your program of a low fat diet and exercise."
7. Encourage the patient to keep a diary of symptoms and schedule follow-up for ongoing assessment of safety and efficacy.
   "If you're willing to keep track of your blood pressures at home as you start this new supplement, we can see if it has any effect. If your pressure starts to go up before our next appointment, I'd recommend you stop the supplement and give me a call."
8. Be clear when you are concerned that a CAM intervention may be harmful.
   "I care about your well-being and understand your desire to stop your prescription medication and start this herbal therapy. This is a difficult situation, though, because I feel there are some dangers associated with this."
   "I want to support you in your desire to lose weight, but I'm worried that this medicine could be harmful to your health. How do you think we could best work together on this?"

Patient: When I checked out the manufacturer's website, I saw that many people who take it find it to be very safe. They feel better, have more energy, and catch fewer colds. My friend feels great after taking it for just two weeks.

Doctor: Commercial websites often contain testimonials, but rarely mention potential side effects. I don't think you can trust these kinds of sites on the Internet. It's certainly your choice, but I don't feel comfortable with your continuing to take this product.

Patient: OK. I guess I'll stop it then, even though I think it's safe and would like to have given it a chance.

In this interaction, the physician does most of the talking. At no time does she ask any exploratory questions to determine her patient's needs and concerns. She sees herself as an expert whose responsibility it is to communicate information and give clear recommendations. The doctor is legitimately concerned about the lack of reliable product information and the potential risks of taking the supplement for her diabetic patient. She responds to this uncertainty by deciding that it's not a good idea for her patient to take the herbal medicine, although she admits to not being familiar with its ingredients. By focusing exclusively on issues of safety, the doctor misses several opportunities to explore and validate her patient's underlying concerns. No doors are left open for further discussion, so this patient may be less likely to ask questions about CAM or other potentially sensitive issues in the future. Further, the patient may continue to use the product "in secret," and not tell the physician.

 CASE ILLUSTRATION 2

This case presents the same patient interacting with a physician whose style of communication is very different.

Patient: A friend of mine told me about this new herbal supplement that gives her more energy and boosts her immune system. I'm thinking about trying it.

Doctor: Many of my patients take herbal supplements for their health. How do you think this one might help you?

Patient: Well, for the past two months I don't seem to have any energy, so I was hoping this could make me feel better.

Doctor: Can you tell me more about what it means when you say you don't have any energy?

Patient: I'm sleeping OK, but get up each morning feeling tired. I keep catching colds. I can't afford to feel run down like this all the time.

Doctor: Do you have any idea what might be causing you to feel run down?

Patient: My sugars have been fine, so I know it's not my diabetes. I'm worried that with all the stress I've been under at work, my immune system isn't working. I'm not feeling depressed, just run down. That's why I started taking the herbal medicine. Do you think it will help?

Doctor: I understand better now why you're interested in taking something to boost your energy and immunity. Truthfully, I'm not familiar with the ingredients in this supplement, but I'm happy to try to find out more about this remedy before our next visit. More importantly, I'd like to understand better what's been going on for you. Is there anything else that's concerning you?

Patient: Well, I guess I'm worried that my being run down may be a sign that something more serious is wrong. My mother's cancer was first diagnosed when she went to the doctor with low energy.

Doctor: I can imagine how this might be scary for you. The good news is that your exam today and all your recent tests have been normal. And there are things you can do to help manage your stress. I'd like us to be able to talk more about this, but we don't have time now. Let's schedule another appointment as soon as possible. How does that sound?

By focusing on the patient and not on the herbal supplement, this physician was able to uncover important concerns that were completely missed by the first physician. She listened more than she talked, asked open-ended questions, validated her patient's concerns, and responded with empathy. From the onset, this doctor helped create a "safe" and respectful environment for her patient. She normalized the patient's interest in supplements by mentioning that many of her patients used herbal therapies. She was genuinely interested and attentive each time the patient spoke. Her goal was to help identify and explore her patient's concerns and needs, rather than to serve as an expert conveyer of information and advice.

Like the first physician, she was unfamiliar with the ingredients in the supplement. She dealt with her lack of knowledge in a different way, however. Instead of immediately concluding that the supplement wasn't a good idea, she kept the door open by offering to learn more about it. She also reacted empathetically, rather than defensively, when the patient admitted she had already started taking the supplement ("I understand better now why you'd want to take something that boosts your energy and your immunity" rather than "So, you've already started taking it.")

Lack of time in a busy clinical practice can be a significant barrier to discussing CAM. Some physicians fear that asking patients about "one more thing" will result in a conversation that cannot be completed in the limited time available to them. This is a legitimate concern, but using a

patient-centered communication style may not always take more time. The second doctor–patient interaction takes approximately 15 seconds longer than the first. Discussions of CAM with patients who are less insightful and articulate certainly might take more time. As well, an additional follow-up appointment was generated in the second case. Some would argue, though, that an additional visit to deal with a patient's concerns and fears would be worth the investment, particularly when the patient will be working with the physician on a long-term basis.

Communicating with Patients When CAM May Be Potentially Harmful

Physicians regularly help their patients assess the risks and benefits of different therapies. Their responsibility to "first, do no harm" applies to CAM as well as to conventional medical interventions. In the previous case, the physician and patient were discussing a supplement for which there was no clear information about its safety and efficacy. The conversation would be more challenging if the supplement had known toxicity and the patient wanted to continue using it. The same strategies that allowed the second physician to identify and address the patient's concerns would hopefully forge an alliance with the patient strong enough to allow them to negotiate a mutually acceptable plan. Openly acknowledging that the situation is difficult or challenging may be helpful.

Doctor: I care about your well-being and understand your desire to stop taking your prescription medication and start this herbal therapy. This is a difficult situation, though, because I feel there are some dangers associated with this.

Doctor: I want to support you in your desire to lose weight, but I'm worried that this medicine could be dangerous for your health. How do you think we could best work together on this?

Helping Patients Inform Themselves about Herbal Medicines

One of the principles of integrative medicine is the concept of self-care. Patients are encouraged to become knowledgeable participants in their treatment programs. Table 28–4 provides some practical advice for patients with respect to herbal medicines.

Communication Regarding Other CAM Modalities

Exploratory questions about CAM use may reveal that the patient is using other CAM practices, such as acupuncture, massage, or energy therapy. As with the use of botanicals, asking why the patient is turning to these practices can elicit additional information about the patient's total situation that can be helpful in treatment. The physician may be concerned about the safety of the alternative treatment,

Table 28–4. Practical advice for patients taking herbal medicines.

Communication
  Discuss use of all therapies with your medical and CAM providers, especially if you are pregnant or taking any prescription medications.
  Talk with your physician to reevaluate efficacy and safety on a regular basis.
  Report any adverse reactions to the FDA MedWatch.
Product selection
  Choose products that have the following information on the label:
    Common and scientific names of the herb(s)
    Part(s) of the plant used
    Indication
    Dose and frequency
    Potential side effects and interactions
    Name and address of the manufacturer
    Lot number
    Date of expiration
  Use products that are standardized to specific marker compound(s).
  Select formulations that have been studied in clinical trials, when available.
  Select products made by larger companies that have been in business for at least several years, as they have a reputation to protect.

---

in which case the physician can offer to contact the CAM practitioner to learn more about the treatment and its potential risks and benefits. This response shows a respect for the patient's concerns, which should strengthen the relationship between the patient and the physician. The physician can offer to discuss what is learned in a subsequent appointment.

CONCLUSION

Approximately half of the U.S. population is using some form of CAM, most often in combination with the conventional medical care they receive from their primary care provider. It is important for physicians to facilitate rather than constrain discussions about CAM so they can understand how it impacts care that they are providing. By taking the time to discuss a patient's interest in CAM, the physician may uncover important concerns and needs that impact ongoing care and medical decision making. Exploring and responding to these concerns can also significantly strengthen the provider–patient relationship.

SUGGESTED READINGS

General Reference Books

Blumenthal M et al: *Herbal Medicine: Expanded Commission E Monographs*. American Botanical Council, 2000.

Ernst E et al (editors): *The Desktop Guide to Complementary and Alternative Medicine: An Evidence-Based Approach*. Mosby, 2001.

Rotblatt M, Ziment I: *Evidence-Based Herbal Medicine*. Hanley & Belfus, 2001.

Schulz V, Hansel R, Tyler V: *Rational Phytotherapy: A Physicians' Guide to Herbal Medicine*, 4th ed. Springer, 2001.

General Reference Articles

Adler SR, Fosket JR: Disclosing complementary and alternative medicine use in the medical encounter: a qualitative study in women with breast cancer. J Fam Pract 1999;48:453. PMID: 10386489.

Eisenberg DM: Advising patients who seek alternative therapies. Ann Intern Med 1997;127:61. PMID: 9214254.

Eisenberg DM et al: Trends in alternative medicine use in the United States, 1990–1997: results of a follow-up national survey. JAMA 1998;280:1569. PMID: 9820257.

Eisenberg DM et al: Perceptions about complementary therapies relative to conventional therapies among adults who use both: results from a national survey. Ann Intern Med 2001;135:344. PMID: 11529698.

Fugh-Berman A: Herb-drug interactions. Lancet 2000;355:134. PMID: 10675182.

Lazar JS, O'Connor BB: Talking with patients about their use of alternative therapies. Prim Care 1997;24:699. PMID: 9386251.

WEB SITES

FDA Center for Food Safety & Applied Nutrition
  http://www.cfsan.fda.gov
FDA MedWatch
  http://www.fda.gov/medwatch
HerbMed
  http://www.herbmed.org
NIH National Center for Complementary and Alternative Medicine
  http://nccam.nih.gov
NIH Office of Dietary Supplements
  http://dietary-supplements.info.nih.gov
The Longwood Herbal Task Force
  http://www.mcp.edu/herbal
U.S. Pharmacopoeia
  http://www.usp.org

DATABASES

CAM on PubMed: Developed jointly by the National Library of Medicine and the National Center for Complementary and Alternative Medicine. Contains 220,000 citations with links to text.
  http://www.ncbi.nlm.nih.gov/entrez/query.fcgi?
    CMD=Limits&DB=PubMed
Cochrane Library (fee for access): Cochrane Collaboration is published quarterly on CD-ROM, the Internet, and on a subscription basis; contains reports of over 5000 randomized controlled trials and more than 60 systematic reviews of CAM.
  http://www.cochranelibrary.com
Cochrane Registry of Randomized Controlled Trials in CAM:
Cochrane Complementary Medicine Field.
  http://www.compmed.ummc.umaryland.edu/Compmed/
    Cochrane/Cochrane.htm

Stress & Disease

John F. Christensen, PhD, & Jeffrey L. Boone, MD, MS

INTRODUCTION

Human history is replete with stories of the connection between stress and disease. In the biblical Book of Acts (5:1–11) Ananias and his wife Sapphira both succumbed to stress-related sudden death. Confronted by the apostle Peter, Ananias "fell down and died" on hearing the words, "You have not lied to men, but to God." Sapphira died instantly 3 hours later when judged by Peter to be a willing accomplice in "testing the Spirit of the Lord."

More recently, a review of coroner's records in Los Angeles in 1994 revealed a marked increase in deaths, including sudden death, related to atherosclerotic cardiovascular disease on the day of the 1994 Northridge earthquake. In 1999 during a 7.3 earthquake in Taiwan, patients on Holter monitors showed heart rate variability derangement due to withdrawal of parasympathetic activity and increase in sympathetic arousal.

The psychological sequelae of exposure to life-threatening stressors are also problematic and disruptive to people's lives. The terrorist attacks on the World Trade Center and the Pentagon on September 11, 2001, were witnessed directly by an estimated 100,000 people and vicariously by millions of Americans and others worldwide. In the period of time bewteen October 16 and November 15, 2001, it is estimated that 7.5% of Manhattan residents south of 110th street were suffering from posttraumatic stress disorder (PTSD) and 9.7% were suffering from depression. In a representative sample of the American population surveyed 3–5 days following the attacks, 44% reported one or more substantial symptoms consistent with acute stress disorder (ASD), and 90% had one or more symptoms to some degree. Refugees and prisoners of war who have been exposed to torture are also likely to develop symptoms of PTSD, anxiety, and depression.

Less dramatically, research since the late 1960s has demonstrated correlations between significant changes in individuals' lives and the subsequent onset of various types of physical and psychological illness. A consistent relationship has even been found between daily hassles and the onset of illness.

The interrelationship between mental stress and physical disease is complex and multifactorial. As a result, the study of stress and disease embraces a wide range of behavioral, emotional, cognitive, physiological, hormonal, biochemical, cellular, environmental, and even spiritual interconnections not easily understood or encapsulated in the controlled clinical trial.

It has been estimated that up to 70% of visits to primary care physicians are for problems related to stress and life-style. Most clinicians, however, have not been trained to extend their diagnostic work-up and treatment interventions into the psychosocial context of these illnesses. Yet adequate treatment and prevention require that primary care providers regard their patients' illnesses and suffering in the context of their life struggles. This perspective allows the clinician to intervene at multiple points along the continuum from mind to molecule.

This chapter offers a framework for clinicians to think broadly and clinically about the stress–illness connection and suggests some approaches to assessing and treating stress-related illness. It offers a brief background of the research base for this new perspective; provides a conceptual framework to guide diagnosis and treatment; suggests methods for communicating with patients about stress; and offers some options for stress assessment, prevention, and intervention.

DEFINITIONS

The concept of stress was borrowed by physiology and psychology from physics, where it generally refers to a force acting against some resistance. Hooke's law of elasticity states that "stress-$K \times$ strain," where K is a constant (the modulus of elasticity) that depends on the nature and type of stress used to produce the strain. This constant K (ie, the stress–strain ratio) is called Young's modulus. In materials science, stress is what is imposed on a material by the outer world; strain is the reaction of the material to the stress.

Hans Selye is generally credited with introducing the concept of stress into physiology. He defined stress loosely as "the rate of wear and tear in the body" and more rigorously as "the state manifested by a specific syndrome which consists of all the nonspecifically induced changes within a biologic system." In this specific syndrome, termed by Selye the **general adaptation syndrome** (GAS), glucocorticoids are secreted by the adrenal cortex in response to adaptational demands placed on the organism by such disparate stressors as heat, cold, starvation, and other environmental insults—hence the expression "nonspecifically induced changes."

Various other definitions of stress have been offered by researchers. Some, like Selye's, refer to a state of the organism; others refer to the stressful stimuli; and still others refer to a combination that includes stimuli, organismic responses, and intervening variables. Currently, a distinction is usually made between stress and stressors. Although **stress** is sometimes loosely used to refer to the environmental sources of threat to the organism, the term **stressor** is more appropriate in reference to these agents.

More recent definitions of stress in humans emanate from a transactional model that takes into account the interactions between persons and their environment. In this view stress occurs when a situational demand presents a call for action that the individual perceives as exceeding available resources. One of the authors (JFC) has proposed the following working definition: "Stress is a process of interchange between an organism and its environment that involves self-generated or environmentally induced changes that, once they are perceived by the organism as exceeding available resources (internal or external), disrupt homeostatic processes in the organism–environment system." This definition includes the traditional notion of stress as originating with an external demand (environmentally induced change) that exceeds the coping resources of the organism. It also includes, however, those expectations of events that arise from within, that are seen as essential to one's life project, and that cannot be accommodated by the environment (exceeding external resources). The disruption of homeostasis in the organism–environment system can have its primary manifestation as a pathological end-state in the organism (illness or tissue damage) or as a destructive alteration of the environment (domestic violence as a stress response).

RESEARCH BACKGROUND

Stressful Life Events

In the 1930s Adolf Meyer advocated the use of a life chart in medical diagnosis. Data were entered on date of birth, periods of disorders of various organs, and various life situations and the patient's reactions to them. In 1954, a program of studies in life changes and illness patterns was initiated at Cornell University. These studies found that illnesses appeared to be associated with definite periods of life change, although illness patterns varied among those who had been through major life changes. In 1967, Holmes and Rahe published a scale of 43 life events, along with a method of quantifying life changes according to the amount of readjustment they require for the average person. This scale allowed greater quantitative precision in life change and illness studies and provided a pivotal methodological leap that broke through the circularity in which

the stressful life changes had been measured in terms of illness outcome, rather than in terms of the inherent magnitude of the stressor. Questionnaires based on this and similar scales have gathered data on several populations globally. Retrospective studies have shown a relationship between recent life change and a host of pathological outcomes, such as sudden cardiac death, onset of myocardial infarction, occurrence of fractures, pregnancy and birth complications, aggravation of chronic illness, tuberculosis, multiple sclerosis, diabetes, onset of leukemia in children, and onset of mental disorders such as depression and schizophrenia. Prospective studies, particularly those conducted on U.S. Navy populations while deployed at sea, predicted future illness based on life change scores prior to deployment and subsequently verified the accuracy of those predictions by inspection of medical records.

Although a consistent relationship has been found between stressful life events and illness patterns, this does not account for why some individuals who undergo significant change develop illnesses but others undergoing equally intense changes remain healthy. A typical correlation between life change and illness reported in these early studies was 0.30, which leaves 91% of the variance unexplained. Recent attention has focused on individual and situational variables that may mediate the relationship between life change and illness. Among the psychological variables that seem to mediate the stress response are locus of control (including the extent to which individuals prefer control in their lives and how much control they perceive they have over specific life events), need for stimulation, openness to change, stimulus screening, self-actualization, the use of denial, the presence of social supports, and emotional self-disclosure. In one study of Illinois Bell executives during the divestiture of AT&T, those executives who experienced high stress while remaining healthy differed from those with high stress and high illness on a dimension of "hardiness." This personal characteristic consists of "the 3 Cs": a strong *commitment* to self, work, family, and other important values; a sense of *control* over one's life; and the ability to see change as a *challenge* rather than a threat. More recently researchers suggest a "fourth C": *coherence,* a belief that one's internal and external environments are predictable and that things will work out as well as can be expected.

Timing of Cardiac Events

Data from the Framingham study, the Massachusetts Death Certificate Study, and other large epidemiological studies provide information regarding the timing of cardiovascular events such as angina and sudden cardiac death. Such events tend to occur with a greater frequency during the morning hours before noon with a second peak in the early evening hours. From the perspective of stress medicine, this circadian frequency data may be an objective description of the stress response as it affects the presentation of serious cardiovascular events.

A closer look at the data reveals that the death rate during the daytime work hours plummets over the noon hour to less than half the rate seen at 9:00 AM. The stress model suggests this may be more than coincidence. The peak death rates occur in the early hours of the work day and in the early evening hours when workers return home. These peaks are substantially blunted during the corresponding hours of the weekend days when people are moving toward recreation. Furthermore, circadian peaks in cardiac events are steeper and more deadly on Monday than on other days of the week. Employed workers die more frequently on Monday, whereas age-matched unemployed workers die on random days of the week.

Cardiac death also tends to occur on days that are more psychologically stressful than others. One study that examined death certificates in the United States found that among Chinese and Japanese, who are more likely to consider the number "4" unlucky, a peak of cardiac-related mortality occurred on the fourth day of the month, in contrast with white controls who showed no such peak. This was consistent with the hypothesis that cardiac-related mortality tends to increase on psychologically stressful occasions.

Coronary-Prone Behavior Pattern

In the 1950s Friedman and Rosenman began studying the relationship between coronary heart disease and a personality style they labeled "Type A"—hard driving, time urgent, and hostile. This was contrasted to a personality style they labeled "Type B," which was defined as the absence of Type A characteristics, ie, easy-going, patient, and soft-spoken. Their initial findings were that Type As were more than twice as likely as Type Bs to develop heart disease in the form of angina, silent heart attacks, overt heart attacks, and coronary death. Although subsequent large-scale studies failed to show this relationship, more recent research has isolated a "toxic core" of Type A that includes hostility, anger, cynicism, suspiciousness, and excessive self-involvement. This personality constellation predicts blockages in the coronary arteries as well as death from heart disease. It may be that this style, in the face of uncontrollable stressors, generates an excessive rise and fall of catecholamines that influence the development of arterial plaque.

Psychoneuroimmunology

Psychoneuroimmunology (PNI) involves the study of the interactions of consciousness, the central nervous system (CNS), and the immune system (involving the body's defense against infection and aberrant cell division). The compelling evidence of these studies is that the CNS influences immune function and that, conversely, the immune system can influence the CNS. It is likely that the brain is normally part of the immunoregulatory network. Specifically, stimulation of the hypothalamic–pituitary–adrenal (HPA) axis leads to down-regulation of immune system function in response to stress. Stressful thoughts and emotions may reach the hypothalamus by axons projecting from the limbic system or from the forebrain. Corticotropin-releasing factor (CRF), produced in the hypothalamus under conditions of stress, acts on the anterior pituitary to form adrenocorticotropin hormone (ACTH), which in turn stimulates the production of corticosteroids in the adrenal cortex. Corticosteroids have immunosuppressive effects on the lymphoreticular system and marked antiallergic and antiinflammatory effects.

In addition, CRF leads to release of catecholamines, which themselves may produce changes in lymphocyte, monocyte, and leukocyte functions. Opiates are also elevated with stress, and they are generally reported to be immunosuppressive. Finally, growth hormone and prolactin, which are immunoenhancing factors, are initially elevated at the onset of stress, but under conditions of prolonged stress their secretion is inhibited. Thus the combined effect of elevated corticosteroids, catecholamines, and opiates, along with inhibition of growth hormone and prolactin, is to down-regulate the immune system.

Effect of Psychological Interventions on the Immune System

A recent meta-analytic review showed that three classes of interventions could reliably alter immune function. *Hypnosis with immune suggestions* showed a positive influence on total salivary immunoglobulin A (IgA) concentration and neutrophil adherence, along with a modest suppression of intermediate-type hypersensitivity erythema. These effects were mediated through relaxation. *Conditioning interventions,* in which a neutral stimulus is initially paired with an immune-modulating stimulus and later elicits the immune changes on its own, were able to enhance natural killer cell cytotoxicity. *Disclosure interventions,* which encourage patients to write essays about previously inhibited stressful experiences, have shown some success in reducing antibody titers to Epstein–Barr virus and enhancing the body's control over latent herpes simplex virus production.

Expressive Writing about Stressful Experiences

Recent research has demonstrated the effectiveness of expressive writing about stressful events in improving the health status of patients with asthma (improved lung function) or rheumatoid arthritis (reduction in desease severity). These improvements were assessed 4 months after the intervention and were beyond those attributable to standard medical care.

Gender Differences

Females have been noted to respond to stress with a "tend-and-befriend" way of coping, in contrast with the "fight-or-flight" model that may be more characteristic of males. When confronted with stress females tend to engage in nurturing activities that protect themselves and their offspring and that enhance social support, which has been identified as a powerful stress buffer. In particular there may be links between estrogen and a blunting of oxytocin, which is implicated in the fight-or-flight response. The "tend-and-befriend" response may also lower blood pressure.

Positive Cognitive Styles

Evidence is accumulating from a variety of studies that optimism, perceptions of personal control, and a sense of meaning are protective of physical health. These cognitive resources assume special significance in helping people cope with intensely stressful events. Even unrealistically optimistic expectations appear to slow down the progression of disease in men infected with human immunodeficiency virus.

A STRESS MODEL FOR PRIMARY CARE

The etiology of illness and its waxing and waning course are multifactorial. Any given illness episode is determined by many circumstances. The complex pathway by which stress influences the outcome of illness is subject to the ongoing accumulation of data and elaboration of heuristic and clinical models. A model of stress that can aid diagnosis, prevention, and intervention is shown in Figure 29–1. Adapted from an optical model first proposed by Rahe and Arthur (1978), it depicts stressors as light rays filtered through successive lenses representing the individual's perception (threat appraisal), coping, physiological processes, and arousal reduction activities, and then projected onto illness outcome screens. Each lens either augments or diminishes the intensity of light (heavy bold lines or dotted lines, respectively) on its pathway to illness outcome, and represents a potential focal point for the clinician's diagnosis of a stress influence or risk factor for patient illness. Each lens also represents a potential focus of preventive health care or intervention.

Perception refers to the person's appraisal of the threat involved in various stressors. Several personal variables that may affect the degree of perceived threat are shown in Figure 29–1. For example, the degree of a person's openness to change or the extent to which he or she values change influences whether a particular life change, such as a child leaving home, is perceived as a threat to the self or an opportunity for growth. The degree of control individuals prefer to have in their lives, as well as the amount of control they perceive they have over specific stressors, also in-

fluence their perception of threat. Thus a parent with a high need to control an adolescent child's outside activities experiences more stress when the child struggles toward emancipation than does a parent who has less of a need for control and who trusts the child's judgment.

Coping refers to methods an individual uses to mitigate the influence of stressors perceived as threatening. One approach to coping is "exposure management," or attempts to increase or decrease the amount and intensity of stressors encountered. Thus an overworked, overcommitted manager might attempt to mitigate stress by withdrawing from some commitments and by reducing work hours by delegating more responsibility to subordinates. Social supports are an important stress buffer, and successful coping with stressors may involve both developing confiding relationships and increasing the amount of one's self-disclosure about the effect of stressors in one's life. There is some research evidence that emotional self-disclosure about stressors enhances immune functioning. In the aftermath of the September 11, 2001, attacks, it is estimated that 98% of Americans coped by talking with others, 90% by turning to religious or spiritual practices, 60% by participating in group activities to memorialize the events, and 36% by making donations. "Stimulus screening" involves techniques to focus attention on relevant stimuli and to regulate the overall flow of stimulation to one's optimal level of functioning.

Two major classes of **physiological response** to stressors that lead to target organ pathology are autonomic hyperreactivity and immunosuppression. Both are cortically mediated through the individual's perceptions and methods of coping. **Hyperreactivity** in the presence of stress, sometimes called the **defense reaction,** has been shown to be a factor in disease processes specific to vulnerable organ systems in persons with established disease. Thus exaggerated pressor responses in hypertensives, increased electromyelogram readings in those suffering from tension headaches and chronic back pain, disturbances in glucose metabolism in insulin-dependent diabetics, and bronchoconstrictive responses in asthmatics are all examples of hyperreactivity in the presence of a definable stressor. In the case of hypertension, hyperreactivity is present in normotensives at risk for the disorder and in some studies has predicted future blood pressure levels. Other examples are increased levels of serum cholesterol seen in studies of tax accountants in the 2 weeks prior to April 15 and of fighter pilots landing on aircraft carriers compared with pilots on long commercial airline flights.

One of the adaptive functions of sympathetic activation is to prepare the organism for large-muscle movement to either attack or flee a threat. In twenty-first century human society, these somatomotor responses are often voluntarily suppressed or sublimated, leading to delayed elimination of released glucose and fatty acids and often bringing more powerful and prolonged increases in blood pressure. In

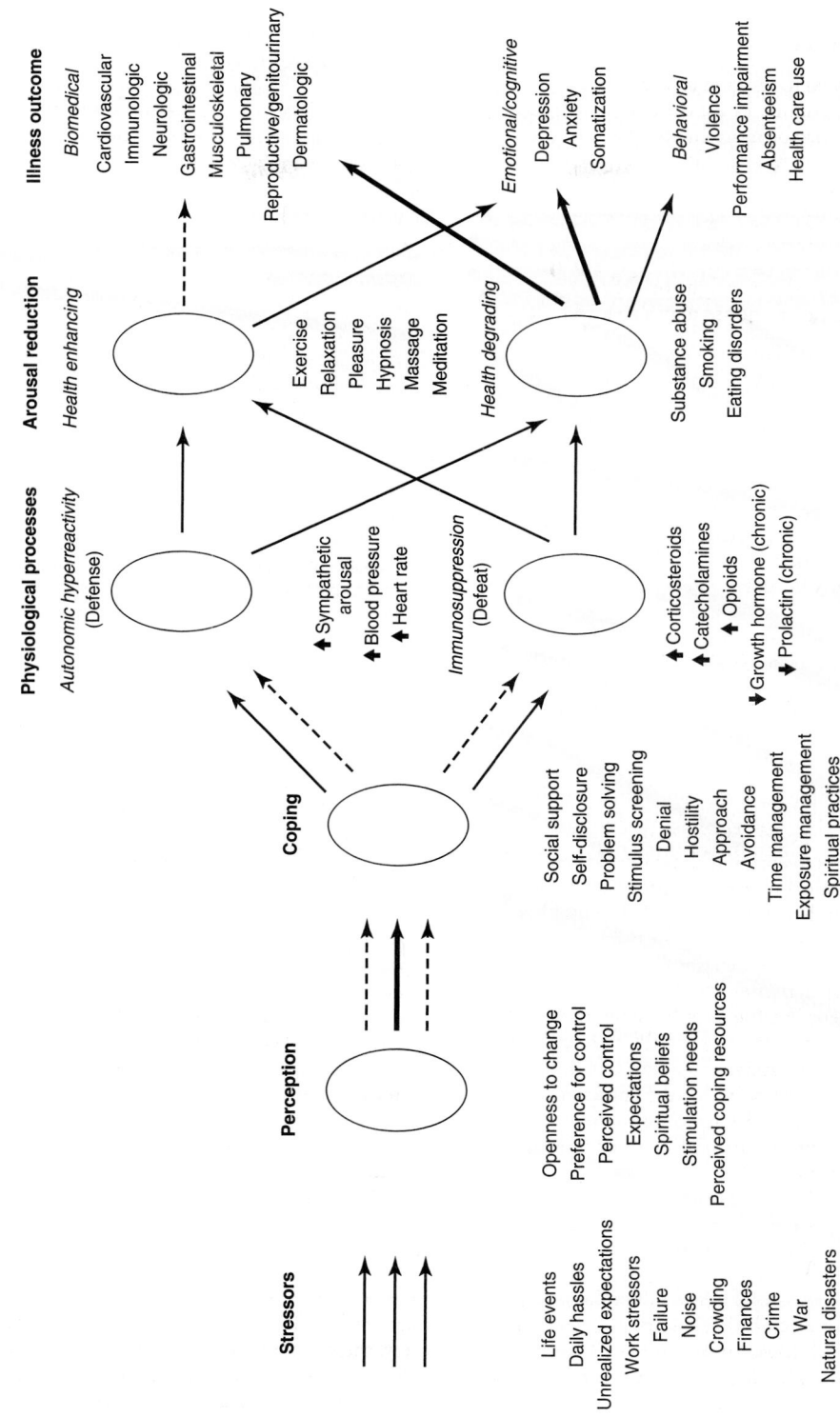

Figure 29–1. An optical model of stress pathways.

The following labels appear within the figure:

Stressors

Life events
Daily hassles
Unrealized expectations
Work stressors
Failure
Noise
Crowding
Finances
Crime
War
Natural disasters

Perception

Openness to change
Preference for control
Perceived control
Expectations
Spiritual beliefs
Stimulation needs
Perceived coping resources

Coping

Social support
Self-disclosure
Problem solving
Stimulus screening
Denial
Hostility
Approach
Avoidance
Time management
Exposure management
Spiritual practices

Physiological processes

Autonomic hyperreactivity (Defense)

↑ Sympathetic arousal
↑ Blood pressure
↑ Heart rate

Immunosuppression (Defeat)

↑ Corticosteroids
↑ Catecholamines
↑ Opioids
↑ Growth hormone (chronic)
↓ Prolactin (chronic)

Arousal reduction

Health enhancing

Exercise
Relaxation
Pleasure
Hypnosis
Massage
Meditation

Health degrading

Substance abuse
Smoking
Eating disorders

Illness outcome

Biomedical

Cardiovascular
Immunologic
Neurologic
Gastrointestinal
Musculoskeletal
Pulmonary
Reproductive/genitourinary
Dermatologic

Emotional/cognitive

Depression
Anxiety
Somatization

Behavioral

Violence
Performance impairment
Absenteeism
Health care use

addition, the relative absence of skeletal muscle exertion in affluent societies (without compensatory aerobic exercise) prevents the activation of endorphins that normally accompanies muscle exertion. Because these endorphins dampen mental arousal and sympathetic activity, in the absence of skeletal muscle exertion these arousal and activation states are prolonged.

Immunosuppression, as discussed previously, occurs through the mechanisms of increased levels of circulating corticosteriods, catecholamines, and opioids and decreased levels of growth hormone and prolactin under conditions of prolonged stress. Sometimes referred to as the **defeat reaction,** this response pattern occurs when patients are exposed to long-term stressful situations that tend to overwhelm ordinary coping mechanisms, thus leading to despair or deep sorrow in situations that appear to be beyond all hope and rescue. Rather than working directly on target organ systems as in the case of hyperreactivity, downregulation of the immune system in the defeat reaction increases vulnerability to external invasive organisms and endogenous neoplasms.

Several **arousal reduction** strategies are available to individuals to mitigate physiological activation and disruption of homeostatic processes in conditions of stress. These include both **health-enhancing** and **health-degrading** activities. Among the health-enhancing arousal-reduction strategies are exercise, which expends accumulated corticosteriods and dampens sympathetic activation through the release of endorphins, and various approaches to stimulating the parasympathetic nervous system. This latter category includes relaxation exercises, abdominal breathing, self-hypnosis, meditation, soothing music, massage, and contact with nature.

Health-degrading activities, which may be attempts at physiological arousal reduction but that actually magnify the stress response and lead to target organ disease, include substance abuse, tobacco use, and eating disorders. Intensification of all of these behaviors may coincide with stressful life episodes. An example is the mediating role of increased alcohol intake in the relationship between occupational stress and hypertension seen in studies of air traffic controllers.

Various **illness outcomes** of stress include **biomedical disease** manifested in specific organ systems, such as cardiovascular, immune, and neurological disorders; **emotional and cognitive disorders,** such as depression, anxiety, and somatization; and **behavioral disorders,** such as violence, performance impairment, absenteeism, and overuse of health care resources. These stress outcomes are the usual focus of medical and mental health intervention, but the larger model of the stress pathway provides primary care clinicians with potent opportunities for comprehensive preventive health care.

STRESS OUTCOMES IN ORGAN SYSTEMS

Each organ system has a unique susceptibility to stress. The following is a brief overview of some of the stress implications in specific systems.

Cardiovascular

Cardiovascular disease is the leading cause of mortality in the United States. Stress contributes to all expressions of heart disease, including coronary artery disease, congestive heart failure, and sudden cardiac death. Because fully a third of sudden cardiac deaths and myocardial infarctions cannot be explained by the severity of the standard cardiac risk factors—family history, hypertension, dyslipidemia, diabetes, or tobacco use—stress may explain some of this variance. Table 29–1 outlines the pathways that may mediate between stress and cardiovascular disease. For example, one of the hemodynamic risk factors, hypertension, is partially the result of mental stress. Changes in vessel caliber contributing to vascular constriction, coupled with surges in cardiac output under conditions of stress, often lead to circadian variation in blood pressure levels. The assessment of these peak levels of blood pressure may be helpful in identifying patients at risk for stress-related cardiovascular disease.

Table 29–1. The cardiovascular consequences of mental stress and intensity.

1. **Hemodynamic**—blood pressure elevations caused by deleterious change in vascular constriction or cardiac output increasing susceptibility to endothelial damage and plaque fracture
2. **Hypertrophic**—the dangerous thickening of the walls of the left ventricle accelerated by catecholamine excesses and hemodynamic overload
3. **Lusitropic**—the stiffening of the left ventricle, reducing cardiac compliance and ease of filling
4. **Arrhythmogenic**—catecholamine-driven increases in heart rate and cardiac electrical instability
5. **Metabolic**—deleterious derangements of cholesterol, insulin, glucose, electrolyte, and hormonal profiles
6. **Coagulative**—accelerated clotting due to enhanced platelet activation and decreased fibrinolytic activity during stress
7. **Cardiotoxic**—catecholamine myocarditis resulting in coagulative myocytolysis with direct nonischemic damage to cardiac muscle cells
8. **Ischemic**—dynamic coronary vascular constriction during stress, leading to ischemic perfusion defects and often chest pain

Immune

Clinical expressions of immune deficiencies are in part the result of stress. They range from the common cold to some forms of cancer. Although research on the relationship between stress and cancer is still inconclusive, there is a suggestion that stress may interact with personality traits, such as a helpless, hopeless way of responding to stressors and a rational, nonemotional response to stressful events, in the etiology of cancer. Other immune-mediated diseases such as rheumatoid arthritis and systemic lupus erythematosus may show a pattern of exacerbation brought on by stress. Another manifestation of immune dysfunction is the effect of psychological stress on the slowing of wound healing.

Neurological

All forms of stroke show a circadian expression in their presentation, with peaks during the early morning hours when catecholamines are highest. Dizziness, vertigo, and other balance disorders often have stress as a causative or contributing factor. One of the most common neurological expressions of stress in clinical practice is headache. Both tension headache and migraine headache are substantially influenced by patient stressors.

Gastrointestinal

Peptic ulcer disease may have an association with stress. Gastric hyperacidity and excess pepsin production are hallmarks of the sympathetic arousal that occurs during stress. Irritable bowel syndrome (IBS), which is characterized by abdominal pain with altered bowel habits (constipation or diarrhea) in the absence of a definable lesion or structural abnormality, frequently correlates with periods of emotional stress. The human "defense reaction" (fight-or-flight response) promotes activation of the cardiovascular system along with inhibition of gastric motility.

Musculoskeletal

Some forms of arthritis show stress-related exacerbations. Complex syndromes such as fibromyalgia seem to have a psychosocial trigger. Temporomandibular joint (TMJ) dysfunction and its related pain syndrome are frequently associated with mental stress. Chronic pain tends to correlate with stress in a person's life.

Pulmonary

Asthma and chronic obstructive pulmonary disease appear to be worsened by stress. Conversely, one of the more powerful self-regulatory stress-control techniques is relaxed abdominal breathing. Asthmatics who participate in stress reduction programs have shown improved physical activity and decreased medical visits. Hypnosis has helped some asthmatics decrease their use of bronchodilators (see Chapter 6).

Reproductive & Genitourinary

The neurohormonal, vascular, and immunological effects of stress significantly impact the reproductive and genitourinary systems. Changes in estrogen and testosterone levels can show marked association with environmental and psychological stressors. Amenorrhea frequently occurs during stressful times in the lives of women. Fertility also can be affected by stress. Dysmenorrhea, dyspareunia, endometriosis, and impotence all have substantial stress and strain connections.

Dermatological

A variety of skin lesions and rashes have been associated with the stress response. Stress-induced vasomotor changes may aggravate inflammatory dermatoses. Vasodilation is considered to be responsible for the thermal aggravation often expressed as pruritus. This lowering of the itch threshold by vasodilation may account for the pruritus seen with many dermatological syndromes. Emotional stress, fear, and pain are all accompanied by substantial drops in skin temperature of the fingers.

DIAGNOSIS

Given the multivariate, multiple-pathway nature of the stress response, clinical diagnosis of stress assumes a multifactorial approach. Traditional medical diagnosis and treatment occur at the point of illness manifestation in target organ systems. From the broader perspective of stress medicine, however, each of the lenses in the optical model (see Figure 29–1) is a potential focus of diagnosis.

The Medical Interview

The richest source of data concerning stressors, perception, coping, and arousal reduction strategies is the medical interview (see Chapter 1). Having the stress model in mind allows the primary care clinician to inquire about current and recent life stressors and to make note of significant clusterings of stressors that precede illness onset. A careful history should uncover whether life stressors are temporally related to the onset of chronic disease and to periods of disease exacerbation.

During the interview, the clinician can ask patients about their beliefs, expectations, self-perceptions, and needs that influence how stressors are perceived. For example, asking patients how much control they prefer in their lives and how much control they perceive that they have over specific life events can determine whether there is congruence or incongruence between preferred control and perceived control. Incongruence tends to amplify the effect of stressors. It is also helpful to ask patients how they view their own resources (internal and external) for coping with stressors, since the more the perceived threats exceed the perceived personal resources, the greater the stress involved.

Patients' approaches to coping with stressors should also be probed in the interview. The presence or absence of social supports as well as the ability of patients to access these supports through self-disclosure are critical data for facilitating stress management. The perceptual and coping styles uncovered in the interview have implications for primary care management of the patient's health, both in prevention and intervention.

It is also important to assess patients' approaches to arousal reduction and to ascertain the balance of health-enhancing and health-degrading strategies. The following questions can be helpful in this regard: "What are the signs indicating that you are experiencing stress?" "What are the physical symptoms?" "What happens in your emotional life?" "How do you act differently when you are stressed?" Methods used to mitigate this arousal can then be ascertained: "When you notice these signs of stress, what do you do to reduce the intensity of the physical symptoms?" It is also important to elicit the short- and long-term outcomes of these strategies: "How does this strategy work for you?" "How does it affect the way you feel immediately? Several hours later? The next day?" Sometimes it is helpful to ask about specific arousal reduction techniques: "Do you practice a form of meditation or relaxation exercise?" "Do you get regular physical exercise?" When questioning patients about substance use or tobacco use, it is helpful to ask whether their use is associated with periods of stress.

Self-Report Questionnaire

A multitude of self-report questionnaires and inventories have been developed for research purposes that measure stressors and many of the variables listed in Figure 29–1 related to perception and coping. Given the limitations of patient and support staff time in primary care settings, it is recommended that any questionnaire be simple, brief, and provide data that can be used by the provider in counseling patients in the area of stress management. An example of such an instrument is the Life Stress Inventory developed by one of the authors (JFC) and shown in Appendix 29–A. Borrowing from the life event scaling studies and the critical role that perceived control plays in mediating stress, this inventory asks patients in an open-ended way to list the major events (and expected nonevents), changes, and stressors that have occurred during the previous year. They are asked to check those stressors that are current, ongoing problems. In addition, patients are asked to rate each stressor on a scale of 1 to 10, indicating the extent of perceived control they had over these events. The provider can take the mean of the control ratings and place that number (1 to 10) in the "control score" blank. This instrument provides both qualitative and quantitative data on the nature of patients' stressors, those that are a current source of struggle, and their perceived control over these events. The higher the external control score, the more at risk the patient is for adverse consequences of stress. Examining with patients those stressors that seem under their control can allow the clinician to suggest life-style changes in those areas. In some instances, patients can be counseled to adjust their perceptions of no control in the direction of greater control. For example, a patient who perceives that she has no control over her work hours can be helped to see areas in which limits can actually be set. In other cases patients can be led to consider changing their expectations and accepting areas that are truly beyond their control.

Assessing Blood Pressure Responses to Stress

In addition to patient self-reporting in the medical interview and on questionnaires, stress can be assessed in the office setting by direct measurement of physiological responses. Of all the physiological consequences of mental stress, blood pressure and heart rate may be the most clinically accessible. Blood pressure—both systolic and diastolic— tends to elevate during times of mental stress and fall during periods of calm and relaxation. Heart rate varies in a similar fashion. Both the absolute values of the peak pressures and pulses during stress and the variation from the resting state may have clinical diagnostic and prognostic significance in the analysis of stress and disease in primary care medicine. The "defense reaction," a common response to challenges in everyday life, occurs whenever interesting, irritating, or otherwise challenging mental stimuli are at hand. In the laboratory setting the peak ambulatory blood pressure levels associated with defense reactions have been approximated by standardized stress tests. One of the authors (JLB) has developed the MOST protocol (Mental Office-based Stress Testing), which consists of measuring blood pressure at rest, during mental arithmetic and time-reaction tests (β-adrenergic challenge that increases cardiac output), and during a cold pressor test (α-adrenergic or vasoconstrictive challenge). These blood pressure readings have been found to correlate with ambulatory blood pressure variations obtained in the same subjects during the work day. Blood pressure reactions to the challenge tests have been demonstrated to be predictive of future cardiovascular events.

The mathematics challenge has been shown to induce cardiac ischemia in susceptible patients and cause blood pressure elevations equivalent to those that occur with exposure to environmental stress. The cold pressor test, which has been used in research settings for several decades, has been shown to reliably predict coronary heart disease (CHD). A diastolic blood pressure rise of more than 20 mm Hg was associated in one study with hyperreactors 2.4 times more prone to CHD than their normal-reactor counterparts.

MANAGEMENT: PREVENTION & INTERVENTION

The model of stress shown in Figure 29–1 offers the clinician various foci for illness prevention and intervention, just as it does for diagnosis. The clinician familiar with this model should be able to tailor specific psychological, social, behavioral, and pharmacological strategies to the unique needs of individual patients. This is preferable to referring the patient for "stress management," since this generic term does not address the multiplicity of stress-related variables and pathways discussed earlier.

Communicating with Patients about Stress

A primary component of stress prevention and treatment involves the way stress is discussed with patients. Avoiding the implication that "it's all in your head" is of great importance. Equally important is avoiding the message that "you are responsible for your illness," which implies greater personal control over somatic processes than is realistic. Here the risk is inducing guilt in patients who become ill and who feel they have failed at being a "better person." Avoiding negative emphases, for example, "Your hectic pace is going to kill you," in favor of a positive framing of the health benefits of stress management is more likely to have a positive influence (see Chapter 6). For example, the clinician can express optimism about the patient's ability to influence health as follows: "Fortunately there are many avenues available for examining and changing your habits of thought and ways of responding to life challenges. I'd like to give you an overview of some strategies that we can discuss now and in future appointments." Showing the patient a model such as that in Figure 29–1 can be helpful as part of this discussion.

It is also important to frame beneficial life-style changes as the patient's choice. Rather than using the stress model to assume more responsibility for patients' lives, the primary care provider can act as a consultant and coach, clearly giving feedback to patients about the patterns of stress revealed by the diagnostic work-up and offering concrete strategies for health promotion along with likely consequences for adherence and nonadherence (see Chapters 15 and 16).

Counseling about Perception & Coping

The perception and coping variables listed in Figure 29–1 represent potential topics for primary care counseling with patients. Depending on the clinician's expertise, inclination, and time, this could be done during a portion of several primary care visits. For example, a parent who is feeling stressed because of a teenager's oppositional behavior could be invited to reflect on how much parental control is needed and coached on ways of setting realistic limits. With an accountant feeling overwhelmed about a recent promotion to senior management, the clinician could elicit his recollections of previous adaptations to challenging life changes in order to help him become cognizant of his own resources.

Referring a parent of a child with recently diagnosed leukemia to a support group of other parents is an example of a coping strategy. Encouraging a widower to confide feelings of sadness to close friends is an example of helping a patient improve his use of social supports. Referring a teacher with a chronically explosive temper for short-term anger management therapy would potentially reduce a cardiac risk factor.

Counseling patients about time management offers a rich opportunity for clinicians to raise questions concerning the patients' values and missed opportunities for personal renewal. For example, the clinician can ask the patient to reflect on those important but nonurgent activities that can contribute to personal well-being (eg, time spent playing with a child), but which are consistently postponed in favor of more urgent but less important tasks (eg, keeping track of the performance of stocks). A list of potential nonpharmacological strategies related to perception and coping that can be suggested to patients is shown in Table 29–2.

Nonpharmacological Strategies for Improving Physiological Processes

Once identified in clinical practice, sympathetic hyperreactors may benefit from both nonpharmacological and pharmacological treatment interventions. The nonpharmacological treatment of elevations in blood pressure related to stress is outlined in Table 29–3. Included are strategies for exercise, diet, and weight control.

Table 29–2. Nonpharmacological interventions related to perception and coping.

1. Improve time management.
2. Improve sense of humor.
3. Pursue personal and vocational activities consistent with life values.
4. Explore the meaning and purpose of life.
5. Cultivate spiritual and transcendent activities:
   a. Prayer
   b. Communal religious observances
   c. Spiritual retreat
   d. Seasonal ritual celebrations.
6. Increase emotional self-disclosure.
7. Pursue short-term psychotherapy.
8. Clarify values.
9. Cultivate social support network.
10. Increase assertiveness.
11. Reduce exposure to unnecessary stressors.
12. Monitor sensory input.
13. Help others.

Arousal Reduction Strategies

For patients showing a high degree of autonomic hyper-reactivity, the clinician can provide or suggest several arousal reduction strategies that can work synergistically with perception and coping skills, as well as with pharmacological interventions. These strategies are listed in Table 29–4. Mindfulness meditation in particular is an effective method of stress reduction that not only activates the parasympathetic response, but builds a mental habit of staying present to the task at hand while assuming a non-judgmental stance toward the progression of one's thoughts and emotions. Referring patients to introductory books on mindfulness meditation, such as those listed at the end of this chapter, or encouraging them to take a meditation class, can provide them with a powerful stress management resource.

Referral for Psychotherapy

The clinician may choose to refer patients for psychotherapy or to educational groups to achieve some of the desired outcomes in the areas of perception, coping, and arousal reduction techniques. These referrals are more effectively targeted to the unique needs of patients if the clinician uses the multifactorial model in Figure 29–1. This model can also aid the primary care clinician in communicating with the psychotherapist about possible foci for treatment. Psychotherapy may be more effective than primary care counseling for altering dysfunctional belief systems (eg, no control of one's life) or coping habits (eg, excessive need for achievement) that amplify stress. In addition it may offer focused training in the acquisition of arousal reduction skills such as meditation and self-hypnosis.

Table 29–4. Health-enhancing arousal reduction techniques.

1. Meditation
2. Self-hypnosis
3. Relaxation exercises
4. Time in nature
5. Massage
6. Abdominal breathing
7. Singing
8. Tai-chi
9. Listening to soothing music

CASE ILLUSTRATIONS

 CASE ILLUSTRATION 1

History: A 46-year-old manager of a computer store presented with concern over palpitations that occurred the previous week at work. He noted "skipped" heart beats intermittently during the previous 2 months, but they intensified during the previous week as the work pace accelerated. The patient played racquetball once a week and noticed no chest pains or palpitations during the game. He had no history of hypertension or lipid abnormalities, and denied nausea, shortness of breath, or diaphoresis.

Related History: As the holiday season approached, the patient also noted sleep disturbance, eczema of the hands, heartburn, and unusually loose stools. He also gained 8 lb and noted increased irritability with his children. Screens for depression and anxiety disorder were negative.

Medical Assessment: Physical examination revealed a normal male 20 lb overweight with a resting pulse of 92. No other abnormalities were noted except for an occasional "skipped" beat during manual heart rate monitoring. The resting blood pressure in the sitting position was 141/92 but rose to 166/102 with a mathematics challenge (Serial 7's).

Recommendations: The patient was encouraged to hire extra help for his retail business during the holiday season. He agreed to ask a trusted employee to remind him to leave the store each day by noon for an hour of walking, reflection, and relaxation. The nursing staff provided brief instructions in diaphragmatic breathing techniques. A sleeping medication was given to be used as needed.

Disposition: Over the next 2 months the daily hour program of walking and relaxation resulted in a 6-lb weight loss. Heartburn, loose stool, and sleep disturbance improved. The patient's palpitations resolved. The sleeping medication was discontinued. At

Table 29–3. The nonpharmacological treatment of blood pressure elevations related to stress.

Exercise

1. Pursue daily aerobic exercise.
2. Improve physical fitness and stamina.

Diet and Weight Control

1. Reduce excess body weight and fat.
2. Reduce alcohol intake to less than one ounce per day.
3. Reduce dietary sodium.
4. Increase dietary potassium.
5. Increase dietary calcium.
6. Increase dietary omega-3-rich fish.

follow-up his resting blood pressure was 126/84, and after mathematics challenge was 143/90.

 CASE ILLUSTRATION 2[1]

History: A 54-year-old female with a history of chronic migraine headaches, hypertension, hypercholesterolemia, mild obesity, and smoking presented to a new primary care physician. She was treated by her previous physician with Tylenol #3, 1 tablet twice a day, for the migraines, and she routinely called in halfway through the month for extra refills. Other medications included propranolol 10 mg twice a day for blood pressure elevation and migraine prophylaxis, as well as over-the-counter antacids for occasional heartburn.

Patient Interview: The patient appeared angry and complained that the medication was not helping her pain. The new physician listened to her complaints and agreed at the end of the visit to refill her medications, but told her he would not prescribe more than the previous doctor. He asked her to return for her annual Pap smear, at which time he would take a history and do a physical examination.

Social History: At the follow-up appointment the physician took a social history, which revealed that the patient had been smoking a pack of cigarettes every day for the last 35 years but did not use alcohol or street drugs. Although never married, she had been involved in a 10-year relationship with her current boyfriend, who suffered from severe emphysema and was dependent on oxygen. Three years previously this man had assumed responsibility for raising his two granddaughters (ages 8 and 11) because his daughter, the girls' mother, was a drug addict serving time in prison. The patient was not consulted about this custody decision. She accepted the stressor out of love for her partner, who was also dependent on her. The oldest granddaughter was now 14 and had become unruly, rebellious, sexually active, and aggressive. She had asked the patient for help obtaining birth control. Although the patient wanted to leave this demanding social situation, she saw it as her responsibility to care for her partner and the two children. The history correlated these recent life events with increased frequency of migraines and initiation of daily use of Tylenol #3.

Physician Facilitation of Emotional Self-Disclosure: The physician actively listened to the patient's self-disclosure, which was accompanied by crying. At the end of the interview the patient thanked the physician, who noted that she had not complained of migraines during that visit.

Brief Counseling and Referral for Family Therapy: In the follow-up visit the physician counseled the patient to realize that she was not isolated. He validated her efforts to work with the situation, even though she had the real option of leaving. He recommended family therapy, to which the patient agreed. Further medical treatment was deferred until after the family had engaged in therapy. The patient made no mention of pain medication during this visit.

Change of Medication and of Life-Style: Prior to the next visit, which was several months later, there were no further calls for pain medication refills. At that visit the patient stated that the migraines, although still present, were not as disabling. The focus of the visit was on improving management of hypertension, high cholesterol, and migraines. They discussed starting an exercise program, initiating a low-fat diet and weight loss, and quitting smoking. The physician discontinued the propranolol and Tylenol #3 and started the patient on a low-dose calcium channel blocker. They discussed starting hormone replacement therapy to treat her menopausal symptoms. The physician remarked that the patient appeared to be gaining control over the life events involving her family.

Disposition: After several months of family therapy the patient had established a primary care relationship with a pediatrician to help her with the medical and hormonal issues of the grandchildren. Her boyfriend had increased his level of help. She had lost 8 lb over 4 months, started walking 4 days a week for 30 minutes, and began a low-fat diet. She began hormone replacement therapy, and her headaches and blood pressure were well controlled without pain medication. She agreed to start a smoking cessation program within the year. The patient demonstrated a marked change in attitude and treatment of office staff, and the primary care provider developed a changed perception of her and an appreciation of the healing potential in "drug-seeking patients."

CONCLUSION

The relationship between stress and disease is well established, although the specific pathways are complex and multifactorial. Primary care clinicians increasingly are asked to examine the cost-effectiveness of the time spent with their patients with a view to improving outcomes within the constraints of available financial and human resources. Attention to the function of stress in patients' illnesses creates the potential for improving treatment outcomes and

[1] The authors are grateful to Kerry Kuehl, MD, for sharing this case.

preventing or delaying the onset of costly target organ disease or the exacerbation of chronic illness. Applying a multidimensional stress model that includes patients' perceptions, coping strategies, physiological arousal mechanisms, and arousal reduction strategies offers the primary care provider multiple opportunities for influencing the ecology of disease.

SUGGESTED READINGS

Beaton R, Murphy S: Psychosocial responses to biological and chemical terrorist threats and events. AAOHN J 2002;50:182.

Black PH: Central nervous system-immune system interactions: psychoneuroendocrinology of stress and its immune consequences. Antimicrob Agents Chemother 1994;38(1):1.

Boone JL: Stress and hypertension. In: Boone JL (editor): *Primary Care: Clinics in Office Practice: Hypertension.* Saunders, 1991.

Boone JL: Mental intensity and your heart. In: Barko WF, Vaitkus MA (editors): *U.S. Army War College Guide to Executive Health and Fitness.* Army Physical Fitness Research Institute, 2000.

Christensen JF: The assessment of stress: environmental, intrapersonal, and outcome issues. In: McReynolds P (editor): *Advances in Psychological Assessment,* Vol 5. Jossey-Bass, 1981.

Friedman M, Rosenman R: *Type A Behavior and Your Heart.* Knopf, 1974.

Galea S et al: Psychological sequelae of the September 11 terrorist attacks in New York City. N Engl J Med 2002;346:982.

Hafen BQ et al: *Mind/Body Health: the Effects of Attitudes, Emotions, and Relationships.* Allyn & Bacon, 1996.

Hanh TN: *The Miracle of Mindfulness: A Manual on Meditation.* Beacon Press, 1987.

Holmes TH, Rahe RH: The Social Readjustment Rating Scale. J Psychosom Res 1967;11:213.

Kabat-Zinn J: *Wherever You Go There You Are: Mindfulness Meditation in Everyday Life.* Hyperion, 1994.

Kiecolt-Glaser JK et al: Emotions, morbidity, and mortality: new perspectives from psychoneuroimmunology. Annu Rev Psychol 2002;53:83.

Kobasa SC: Stressful life events, personality and health: an inquiry into hardiness. J Pers Soc Psychol 1979;37:1.

Leor J, Poole WK, Kloner RA: Sudden cardiac death triggered by an earthquake. N Engl J Med 1996;334:413.

Lin LY et al: Derangement of heart rate variability during a catastrophic earthquake: a possible mechanism for increased heart attacks. Pacing Clin Electrophysiol 2001;24:1596.

Miller GE, Cohen S: Psychological interventions and the immune system: a meta-analytic review and critique. Health Psychol 2001;20:47.

Nice DS et al: Long-term health outcomes and medical effects of torture among US Navy prisoners of war in Vietnam. JAMA 1996; 276:375.

Phillips DP et al: The *Hound of the Baskervilles* effect: natural experiment on the influence of psychological stress on timing of death. BMJ 2001;323:1443.

Pickering TG: Terror strikes the heart—September 11, 2001. J Clin Hypertension 2002;4:58.

Rahe RH, Arthur RJ: Life change and illness studies: past history and future directions. J Hum Stress 1978;4:3.

Ringel Y, Drossman DA: Psychosocial aspects of Crohn's disease. Surg Clin N Am 2001;81:231.

Schuster MA et al: A national survey of stress reactions after the September 11, 2001, terrorist attacks. N Engl J Med 2001;345:1507.

Seyle H: *Stress in Health and Disease.* Butterworth, 1976.

Shrestha NM et al: Impact of torture on refugees displaced within the developing world: symptomatology among Bhutanese refugees in Nepal. JAMA 1998;280:443.

Smyth JM et al: Effects of writing about stressful experiences on symptom reduction in patients with asthma or rheumatoid arthritis. JAMA 1999;281:1304.

Sobel D: Mind matters, money matters: the cost-effectiveness of clinical behavioral medicine. Ment Med Update 1993;1.

Taylor SE et al: Biobehavioral responses to stress in females: tend-and-befriend, not fight-or-flight. Psychol Rev 2000;107:411.

Taylor SE et al: Psychological resources, positive illusions, and health. Am Psychol 2000;55:99.

Yehuda R: Post-trumatic stress disorder. N Engl J Med 2002;346:108.

WEB SITES

Summary of a lecture on psychoneuroimmunology by Steven Maier at the American Psychological Association 2001 convention. http://www.apa.org/monitor/dec01/anewtake.html

Article for lay public from NIH on stress and disease. http://www.nih.gov/news/WordonHealth/oct2000/story01.htm

Website of the PsychoNeuroImmunology Research Society. http://www.pnirs.org/

Summary of a 1999 lecture by Robert Ader, one of the founders of PNI research, on the growth of the field since 1970. http://www.apa.org/monitor/jun99/pni.html

Webpage on psychoneuroimmunology with helpful links to other sites. http://web.indstate.edu/nurs/mary/pnipage.htm

Institute of Science, Technology, and Public Policy http://www.istp.org/coalition/stressprevention.html

Center for Mindfulness in Medicine, Health Care, and Society http://www.umassmed.edu/cfm/

Appendix 29–A. Life Stress Inventory

In the blanks below list the major events, changes, or stressors that have happened to you within the last year. Also list those events that you expected but that failed to occur. In the next column place a check next to those stressors that are current, ongoing problems. In the last column opposite each stressor, indicate the degree to which this event has been under your control by writing a number corresponding to the scale at the top.

Life Event or Stressor	Current Problem	Within Your Control	Outside Your Control
		1 2 3 4 5 6 7 8 9 10	
1. _____	_____		_____
2. _____	_____		_____
3. _____	_____		_____
4. _____	_____		_____
5. _____	_____		_____
6. _____	_____		_____
7. _____	_____		_____
8. _____	_____		_____
9. _____	_____		_____
10. _____	_____		_____
		Control Score _____ (mean of ratings)	

John F. Christensen, PhD

Pain

Gregory T. Smith, PhD, & Douglas Beers, MD

> *There are among us those who haply please to think
> our business is to treat disease. And all unknowingly
> lack this lesson still 'tis not the body, but the man is
> ill. S. Weir Mitchell (cited in Turk, Meichenbaum, and
> Genest, 1983).*

INTRODUCTION

Pain is commonly a symptom of an underlying disease process or injury. It usually and initially derives from nociceptive input and is always modulated by (1) central nervous system activity (arousal), (2) physical movement, (3) psychological status (depression, anxiety), (4) environmental consequences (stressors, reinforcers), and (5) conditioning history. Pain is not directly measurable, and its significance for treatment is therefore not fully understood.

Pain is often the central complaint in somatization disorder and psychophysiological reactions (Chapter 23). Pain is often accompanied by a sleeping disorder (Chapter 26) and depression, anxiety and fear (Chapters 21 and 22) are common reactions to pain. Pain associated with a somatization disorder or psychophysiological reaction may not derive initially from injury or illness (nociceptive input) but rather may be an expression of the psychological conflicts that define the disorder.

Pain perception, that is, the patient's verbal description of the pain (or use of a 0–10 pain rating scale) will likely be a consistent report of changes in pain and suffering as a result of treatment only with that patient. Treatments will however influence pain perception variably between different patients based primarily on the modulation effects on the pain. In other words, patients will experience pain and respond to treatment differently depending on their unique conditioning histories, current psychological states, central nervous system (CNS) arousal patterns, activity levels, and environmental consequences related to pain behavior. Pain behavior is the best measure of the modulation effects on the pain, which often guide medical decision making concerning pain treatment.

Pain behavior is the verbal and nonverbal expression of pain that describes both the nociceptive input and the modulation and suffering that together comprise the problem of pain (Table 30–1). Chapter 29 on stress and disease and Chapter 34 on chronic illness further describe the influence of stress and coping with stress on disease states as well as pain behavior.

This chapter addresses treatment concepts of several different pain problems:

Acute pain
Chronic periodic pain, such as migraine headaches
Chronic intractable benign pain, such as chronic low back pain
Chronic progressive pain such as cancer pain.

Special attention is given to issues of evaluation and treatment related to cross-cultural differences, worker's compensation, and appropriate use of interventions including multidisciplinary pain rehabilitation center treatment. Guidelines, tools, and techniques are highlighted to better assist the primary care physician in the treatment of various pain problems.

This chapter assumes that the primary care physician has the primary responsibility for treatment and use of appropriate referrals and consultations. Behavioral management of patient care and use of appropriate referral sources in a timely way is cost-effective as well as good patient care.

A patient dealing with pain comes to medical attention with a number of possible feelings and goals:

1. The patient may simply want to discover the cause of the pain to allay his or her fears about serious disease.
2. The patient may be interested only in relief from nociceptive stimulis.
3. The patient may want to regain impaired function in order to return to normal work or recreational activities.
4. The patient may want medical and social acknowledgment that the pain is preventing or interfering with normal activities.

Establishing a good doctor–patient relationship is key to treating problems with pain. The effectiveness of the doctor–patient relationship is defined largely by the physician's ability to acknowledge the patient's problem, address the patient's goals, and establish a collaborative approach on which both the doctor and patient can agree. Because the primary concerns of the doctor and patient are often different, the potential for miscommunication can occur with patients suffering from acute as well as chronic pain. Pain is a symptom not perceivable to the observer. Pain behaviors are the functional medium for observing pain.

Table 30–1. Pain behaviors.

Pain behaviors can be separated into four categories:

1. **Pain complaints:** Verbalizing the presence of pain, complaining, moaning, grimacing.
2. **Posturing:** The nonverbal expression of pain; limping, leaning, use of a cane.
3. **Impaired functioning:** Reduction of activities, avoidance of certain activities, impaired personal and sexual relationships.
4. **Somatic interventions:** Taking medications or seeking treatment.

Moreover, pain behaviors are often embedded in family interactions and dynamics that can lead unintentionally to reinforcing a sick role or to family dysfunction, which can promote increases in pain behaviors (see Chapter 8). It is therefore important to modify the "three-function model of the medical interview" as an ongoing format for the evaluation and treatment of patients presenting with pain (Table 30–2) (see Chapter 1). In this model, all functions are openly and simultaneously pursued throughout treatment.

The three-function model allows for a streamlined diagnostic evaluation, ongoing relationship building, and early return to function. Patient anxieties about pain and use of medical resources often stem from unrealistic expectations of the doctor–patient relationship. Establishing a diagnosis and a mutually agreed upon expectation for return to function can help control excess use of both pain medications and diagnostic and consultative services.

Table 30–2. Three-function model of the medical interview.

1. **Data gathering:** Elucidate the etiology (physical and psychological) of the pain. Arrive at a tentative working diagnosis even while considering alternative hypotheses.
2. **Relationship building:** Collaborate on the meaning the pain has in the patient's life and on the understanding of "pain behaviors" and pain dysfunction (both physical and social).
3. **Management:** Explain the role of pain medications, including the duration of their use, the importance of time contingency, and an expectation of the degree of relief.
   a. Plan the use of physical and other therapies designed to improve function.
   b. Acknowledge the roles and limitations of rest.
   c. Establish the value of return to normal work and recreational activity to overcome pain behavior and dysfunction.

Medications that are commonly used to treat pain include short-acting opiates, long-acting opiates, anticonvulsants such as gabapentin, and other central nervous system drugs such as valproic acid and sumatriptan (for treatment of migraine headaches), muscle relaxants, nonsteroidal anti-inflammatory drugs (NSAIDs), and antidepressant medications both tricyclic and selective serotonin reuptake inhibitors (SSRI) (Table 30–3). Use of epidural and trigger point injections as well as sensory and somatic nerve blocks can facilitate making an appropriate diagnosis with complicated pain problems and can influence the patient's perception of pain on a short-term basis (hours to a few weeks). The use of implantable morphine pumps and implanted nerve stimulators is controversial. Although patients often report some reduced pain with use (pain perception), the continued use of oral pain medications with ongoing reduced function (pain behavior) is common.

Throughout the course of treatment of the pain the agreed upon expectations should always include an increase of function and return to as normal a life-style as possible. Rehabilitative treatments (Table 30–4) are designed to improve function and increase functional independence as much as possible. Although rehabilitation can and should occur at any point during the course of treatment, a logical continuum of integrating both treatments designed to reduce pain complaint (pain perception) while improving function (pain behaviors) should always be the systematic approach to treatment (Table 30–5). In summary, integrating medical, behavioral, and social influences in the assessment and management of chronic pain can help avoid a lengthy, expensive, and seemingly endless "rule-out" process. The next section discusses four cases representing common pain types (Table 30–6). In each case the approach to evaluation and treatment uses the three-function model. We suggest specific questions representative of the three functions that can be asked initially and at any time during treatment (Table 30–7).

ACUTE PAIN: CARPAL TUNNEL SYNDROME

 CASE ILLUSTRATION 1

Ann is a 28-year-old woman with insulin-dependent diabetes mellitus who presented with bilateral hand and wrist pain with radiation to the elbows and shoulders. The pain began 2 months earlier and increased with work (data entry) and in the morning. Pain and tingling in the median nerve distribution were increased with Tinel's and Phelan's maneuvers, consistent with carpal tunnel syndrome. There was no discernible weakness or wasting in the hands.

Table 30-3. Some common oral medications used to treat pain.

Medication	Primary Effect	Comment
Short-acting opiates (eg, acetaminophen/hydrocodone, codeine, morphine)	For acute and periodic pain	Has CNS effects, abuse potential, tolerance is an issue
Long-acting opiates (eg, oxycodone, morphine SR, methadone)	Used with chronic pain conditions	Has CNS effects, less abuse potential in lower doses, tolerance is an issue
CNS medications (eg, gabapentin, sumatriptan, valproic acid)	For diseases of the nervous system, migraine headaches, and pain arising from nerve damage	Has CNS effects, need to closely monitor to evaluate for toxic effects
Muscle relaxants (eg, carisoprodol, diazepam, cyclobenzaprine)	For acute musculoskeletal conditions and periodic flare-ups	Has CNS effects, can potentiate effects of opiates, tolerance is an issue
NSAIDs (eg, acetaminophen, ibuprofen)	For acute and chronic musculoskeletal conditions and pain arising from rheumatic disease	In high doses can cause GI complaints
Antidepressant medications SSRI (eg, paroxetine, fluoxetine) Tricyclic medications (eg, amitriptyline, doxepin) Trazodone	For treatment of depression/anxiety that accompanies the pain; can also be helpful to reduce pain and improve sleep	Has CNS effects and can be combined with opiates, muscle relaxants, or NSAIDs for effect

Wrist splints afforded no relief. Nerve conduction studies confirmed slowing in the median nerve at the carpal tunnel. She had stopped work at the time of the first visit and filed a worker's compensation claim for carpal tunnel syndrome. She was advised by her doctor to rest her wrists.

She does not want to return to her previous job and would like to use the time to identify an alternative employer. She is not eager to consider surgery at this time.

Several common pain management traps are evident in this case:

1. The overprescription of rest as a treatment modality.
2. Failure to build restoration of activity level into the treatment regimen.
3. Positive reinforcement of pain behaviors.

To engage this patient in collaborative management of the pain problem, a number of behavioral techniques can be used. Although there is a very close link between nociceptive input and pain behavior in the acute phase of the

Table 30-4. Commonly used rehabilitative treatments for pain.

Rehabilitative Treatment	Most Effective Use
Physical therapy Passive (eg, hot packs, ultrasound, massage) Active (eg, stretching, strengthening, and endurance exercises)	Passive techniques useful to treat acute pain or flare-ups Active treatment useful to improve physical function
Occupational therapy: primarily *active* treatment	To improve physical function specific to activities of daily living (ADL) and return to work (RTW)
Multidisciplinary pain rehabilitation treatment	Combines coordinated team active and passive rehabilitative approaches with medical, behavioral, and psychosocial treatments to maximize improvement in function
Single-modality treatments Massage therapy	Passive treatment for muscle soreness to treat acute musculoskeletal pain and periodic pain flare-ups
Acupuncture	Passive treatment to reduce report of pain
Chiropractic treatment	Passive treatment to improve function and reduce report of pain

Table 30–5. The logical continuum of care in the treatment of pain.

Acute onset

1. Diagnosis and treatment of acute injury or illness as soon as possible after the injury or illness onset.
2. Use of analgesics and other appropriate medications (see Table 30–3) to reduce pain perception.
3. Active exercise-based rehabilitation (from 2 to 12 weeks after onset).
4. Single modality (chiropractic or acupuncture) and implantable treatment may be considered here to assist with rehabilitation and to improve function.
5. Multidisciplinary pain rehabilitation evaluation. A biopsychosocial assessment to further guide treatment planning.
6. Multidisciplinary pain rehabilitation treatment.

Chronic pain

injury, the doctor should discuss with the patient how pain behaviors can, in the chronic phase, become a more prominent problem. In the acute phase, this patient has been conditioned to believe that the persistence of pain means a continuation of the precipitating factor. As a behavior, pain is readily conditioned. For example, pain behaviors in the subacute condition can become linked to anticipating positive consequences (worker's compensation), avoiding aversive consequences (unpleasant work environment), and excessive guarding (significantly reduced activity level). It is important to note that persistence of the pain does not imply an emotional problem.

CASE ILLUSTRATION 1 (CONT.)

Further evaluation reveals that during the weekends or time away from work Ann holds her hands in a somewhat immobilized position that greatly reduces her pain. She reports that after this period of "rest" she can resume many of her activities around the home. Her husband expresses concern about her pain but is uninvolved in her daily activities. Ann does report maintaining her exercise and diet program throughout, even with the reduced mobility of her hands. She also indicates that she hopes to better control the pain and to locate alternative employment that would not exacerbate her pain. Further inquiry reveals that she feels too much pressure from her boss, sees little chance for advancement, and dislikes her co-workers.

The significance of the pain complaint in the patient's life has become clearer. Although she reports an acute onset

Table 30–6. Pain types.

1. **Acute pain:** usually self-limiting and of less than 6 months' duration (eg, postsurgical pain, dental pain, pain accompanying childbirth).
2. **Chronic periodic pain:** acute but intermittent (eg, migraine headaches, trigeminal neuralgia).
3. **Chronic, intractable, benign pain:** present most of the time, with intensity varying (eg, low back pain).
4. **Chronic, progressive pain:** often associated with malignancies.
5. **Experimentally induced pain:** nociceptive stimulation produced in a laboratory setting (eg, electric shock, radiant heat, muscle ischemia).

of carpal tunnel symptoms, she also reports a method of managing the symptoms that was initially effective. The influence of her injury was largely felt in the work setting rather than at home. Although it may be appropriate for her to consider changing employment, the consequences of doing so while filing for worker's compensation may have the effect of increasing and prolonging the pain behavior.

During the patient's first appointment and evaluation a realistic projection of the probable duration of the pain should be agreed on (4–8 weeks) as well as a plan for active physical therapy and a resumption of normal activity. An early elucidation of the expectations of treatment allows the patient to focus on work dissatisfaction independent of the pain behavior. Appropriate referral for behavior therapy and vocational rehabilitation may be considered. Addressing all of these issues during the first session also decreases the patient's uncertainty and therefore the need to use further diagnostic and consultative resources.

Table 30–7. Five questions to ask patients.

1. What does pain keep you from doing that you would otherwise do (work, sex, etc—all can mean something about the effect or etiology of pain behaviors)? Conversely, what do you do in spite of the pain?
2. How has pain affected those around you? When you're hurting what does your spouse (partner) do?
3. What is your goal in seeking help for this pain? What do you hope will be the benefit of coming here today? (Diagnosis, fear reduction, pain relief, return to work, remain out of work, etc.)
4. How has this pain affected other health issues? Do you have other physical problems that are now worse since the pain has started? (Exercise program; obesity; unrelated aches and pains; worry; eg, cancer; heart disease; etc.)
5. What told you that this pain was one that warranted medical attention? What's different about this pain from other pain problems you've had in the past?

CHRONIC PERIODIC PAIN: MIGRAINE HEADACHE

CASE ILLUSTRATION 2

Lisa is a 39-year-old woman who sought care for her long-standing migraine headaches. These headaches first appeared at age 18, at which time they were characterized by severe left orbital and temporal pain associated with nausea, nasal stuffiness, and photophobia. They were often preceded by a scintillating scotoma in the right temporal visual field. Her work-up included a normal lumbar puncture, several normal electroencephalograms (EEGs), computed tomography (CT) scans, and blood chemistries. She was virtually headache-free for 1 year following a pregnancy in her early twenties. Headaches gradually recurred but remitted again for a year after a hysterectomy for endometriosis in her early thirties. She now reports that the headaches have increased in frequency, duration, and severity over the past 2 years, with more photophobia, nausea, and vomiting.

Treatment modalities have included analgesia (aspirin, acetaminophen, NSAIDs, narcotics), abortive agents [DHE injections, ergotamines (Cafergot), sumatriptan], prophylactic medication (amitriptyline, cyproheptadine, phenytoin, valproic acid, propranolol), and vitamins that have had only transient benefit. Dietary and activity prescriptions have also been of minimal success. Her main source of relief over the past year has been repeated after-hours visits for intermuscular narcotics. She has seen multiple internists, neurologists, allergists, and emergency room physicians.

Long-standing, recurrent, incapacitating, nonmalignant pain provides a number of management traps:

1. Doctor "shopping" or seeking assistance from a series of caregivers without resolution.
2. A clear fluctuation in the frequency and intensity of the headache seemingly due to physiological changes, but without an exploration of possible behavioral or social changes associated with these fluctuations.
3. Failure to explore the significance the headache has had in the patient's life.

CASE ILLUSTRATION 2 (CONT.)

Further history revealed that Lisa's headaches in late adolescence were infrequent (several per year) and were managed conservatively. Her single severe at-

tack resulted in a hospitalization that was a source of embarrassment to her and her husband. During the early years of her marriage, she continued to have infrequent, but more severe headaches. During a period of 6 months of treatment with oral contraceptives, she suffered a transient exacerbation. As her daughter grew older and her job responsibilities increased, the frequency and severity of headaches grew. She further reported that she was best able to control her pain by being alone in a quiet room, reading, or listening to quiet music.

The patient is now identifying what may be a clear relationship between marital or social stress and her headache complaint. Whereas the headache can provide "time-out" from the conflicts at hand, it does not interfere with other activities such as listening to music or reading. She further indicates that the headaches did not have a significant effect in her early life.

The headache pattern remained unchanged until 1½ years ago. At that time Lisa and her husband relocated as a result of her husband's work and they moved into a home that required major remodeling, the responsibility of which was largely the patient's. She had difficulty replacing her former employment and considered a new career. Although she reported enthusiasm for the remodeling and the relocation, Lisa also reported a marked increase in the frequency of the headaches. She was unable to work around the house remodeling or participate in stressful family discussions when she had the headache but was otherwise able to prepare meals, do housework, and drive as far as 30 miles one way for social or medical visits. She reported that when she retreats to her room with a headache her husband and children attend to her until she starts to improve. She also indicated that her husband returned home early from work during times of severe headache. She has seen a cascade of physicians in various specialties with a variety of diagnostic tests and specialty work-ups. Her average length of adherence with any one physician was five visits; new referrals were made after several visits. She reported with embarrassment that she had been unable to keep up with her diet and exercise program and was increasingly overweight. Otherwise she was in good health, with no other medical problems.

Although the headache event is likely to have both muscle contraction and vascular components, there appear to be a number of clear situations or conditions that accompany its onset. Moreover, it is clear that in early adulthood the headache was manageable without medications and with minimal medical attention. The primary behavioral reinforcing events for the headache complaint therefore appear to be (1) avoidance of stressful marital or environmental situations and (2) increased attention from others. A possible secondary reinforcer may be the conditioned use of opiates in a failed effort to control the headache.

The following treatment course of action was undertaken:

1. It was agreed that the best course of treatment was to use as little opiate medication as possible. Even though opiates were found to be useful by the patient, she recognized their addictive potential and agreed to use them only with the direction of the primary care physician. Patient and physician medication management responsibilities were also outlined, which specified the number and frequency of use of the opiate.

2. It was agreed that the patient would not seek additional medical evaluation or treatment without discussing it with her primary care physician first.

3. The primary care physician agreed to be available within a 12-hour period of being contacted about a headache to discuss the headache and the possible situation surrounding it. It was agreed that these conversations were to last no longer than 5–10 minutes.

4. An effort was made to encourage active patient participation. A course of biofeedback training and instruction in neck exercises was arranged to place a share of control with the patient.

5. A family conference affirmed to all that the headaches were to be treated as both symptoms of stress and as problems in themselves. A referral for specialized behavior therapy was provided to the patient.

6. If this plan did not show significant reduction in headaches in a month, referral to a multidisciplinary pain rehabilitation center would be made.

7. Finally, the physician would be available for treatment of other medical complaints.

In this way, the primary care physician redefined the headache complaint: It does not need immediate or intensive medical care, it does not need further diagnostic evaluation, and it does not need different medication trials. By establishing a meaningful relationship with the patient, acknowledging the severity of her complaint, setting clear expectations for how to respond to symptoms, and securing the patient's commitment to work within these limitations, a patient and physician agreed upon framework for pain management. Appropriate referral for pain management to a pain rehabilitation program should be the next contingency plan.

CHRONIC INTRACTABLE PAIN: CHRONIC LOW BACK PAIN

 CASE ILLUSTRATION 3

Michael is a 45-year-old man with known controlled hypertension who presented with low back pain. He reported that while working on a farm a year ago he experienced a motor vehicle accident that resulted in a herniated disc in his lumbar spine. A lumbar laminectomy and discectomy followed with some recovery for approximately 3 months. Since that time he had been seen twice a week for 6 weeks for passive physical therapy (hot packs, ultrasound massage, gentle stretching) and he was provided with additional pain medication, including oral narcotics and anti-inflammatories by his surgeon. He had not returned to work since the day of injury and was currently involved in vocational rehabilitation.

On physical examination the patient was tender to palpation across his low back bilaterally. Passive straight leg raising was normal. Sharp, dull, and light touch sensations were intact throughout, with symmetric reflexes in both lower extremities.

Imaging studies revealed old surgical repair of a herniated disc without other abnormalities. Recent nerve conduction studies were unremarkable for nerve slowing. The patient's surgeon, who had "nothing more to offer," referred him back to his primary care physician for continued treatment.

Chronic low back pain commonly displays the following characteristics:

1. Subjective complaint of pain without substantial objective findings.

2. Prominent pain behaviors (eg, avoidance of work).

3. Use of "passive" instead of "active" physical therapy.

4. Continued use of narcotic medication to manage the pain.

 CASE ILLUSTRATION 3 (CONT.)

The patient went on to report that he spends much of the day sitting in his reclining chair either watching television or reading. He moves from the chair two or three times each day, primarily for meals. He frequently naps during the day and reports disrupted sleep at night, averaging 5–6 hours. He feels depressed and hopeless about his recovery, and believes that

unless his pain is relieved he will be unable to return to work. He acknowledges that his spouse and children are angry with him and his inability to return to work.

On further questioning it is discovered that the social "cost" of the pain is high. Michael's daily activities are greatly impaired, his self-esteem and affect have plummeted, and he is further emotionally isolated from his family by his pain. In a circumstance in which a patient's pain behaviors are well entrenched the doctor must accurately establish the expectations for recovery and the outcome of treatment. Because the patient is probably still focused on the pain as a continuation of the original precipitating injury, it becomes necessary to identify and deal more with the patient's pain behaviors.

Although Michael reported feelings of depression, it is inaccurate to say that the pain is caused by the depression. It has been shown, however, that the intensity of pain often diminishes with a trial of an antidepressant medication.

The treatment for chronic low back pain is primarily focused on improving patients' activity level, diminishing their reliance on medications, and reducing pain behaviors (eg, changing the focus of treatment from decreasing pain-enhancing activities to increasing activity level for meaningful tasks). In this way the doctor assists in "managing" the pain behavior.

After a careful explanation by the doctor of the anatomy, physiology, and probable cause of Michael's low back pain, a collaborative discussion followed, leading to an agreement on the following treatment plan:

1. A course of physical therapy using primarily active exercises (eg, aerobic exercise, walking, strengthening, and stretching) would be started. In addition, the patient agreed to take progressively longer walks each day. It was expected that with increased activity there would be an initial increase in pain. For that reason, it was agreed that the patient could continue to use his opiate medication for a short time.

2. Opiate oral medication was placed on a time-contingent basis, extending the number of hours between pills without increasing the dose. This regimen avoided linking the patient's pain perception with the timing and amount of dosing. This was managed through weekly dispensing of the medications through the pharmacy. It was agreed that any request for change in his medication regimen would be directed only to the doctor, not to emergency rooms or other physicians.

3. The patient would be seen once monthly by the doctor. It was agreed that after the first 4 weeks of physical therapy, a reducing medication taper would begin. A primary focus of future visits would be discussion about daily activities or return to work goals rather than the pain.

4. If, by the end of the second month, functional activity levels were not substantially greater, progress toward return to work was not made, or the patient was not yet off opiate medication, then referral to a multidisciplinary pain rehabilitation facility would be made.

The doctor has now, in collaboration with the patient, established the parameters of treatment, clarified the expected outcomes in terms of function, reduced or discontinued the use of opiate medications, and progressed toward meaningful employment goals. These steps define the treatment effort to reducing pain perception and pain behaviors. In this way the doctor becomes a "change agent." Patients who respond favorably to treatment of pain behavior usually report either that the pain is significantly reduced or that it does not bother them as much as it used to. When pain behavior is more entrenched (the patient is unresponsive to treatment) early referral to a multidisciplinary pan rehabilitation facility is indicated. Treatment in a pain rehabilitation facility is typically intensive and primarily involves a reduction in pain behaviors and pain perception and an increase in functional activities. The variety of techniques used to increase functional activity include active physical therapy, improved physical tolerances often through occupational therapy, biofeedback, cognitive-behavioral therapy, management of medications, stress management techniques, relaxation training, hypnotherapy, transcutaneous nerve stimulation, vocational counseling, and coping skills training. Treatment is typically offered 6–8 hours/day, 5 days/week, for 3–4 weeks with active follow-up. At the end of treatment patients are usually referred back to their primary care provider with specific recommendations for future treatment or management.

Counseling for treatment of depression, marital therapy for treatment of marital difficulties, and nutritional counseling for dieting in addition to behavioral treatments for pain (Table 30–8) are typically provided in a pain rehabilitation facility but can be useful adjunctive therapies independent of multidisciplinary pain rehabilitation as well.

CHRONIC PROGRESSIVE PAIN: PAIN IN CANCER PATIENTS

 CASE ILLUSTRATION 4

Jorge is a 58-year-old Hispanic man who was diagnosed with colon cancer, Dukes stage C, 18 months before presenting with progressive weight loss and right upper quadrant pain. Chemistries and imaging studies confirmed multiple metastases in his liver. He was increasingly fatigued and was forced to leave his job as an electronics technician. He now reported that

Table 30–8. Behavioral treatment methods for pain.

1. **Biofeedback:** Computer-assisted measurement of physiological changes previously thought to be involuntary, for the purposes of training the patient to bring them into voluntary control. Measurements often include surface electromyelography, temperature, galvanic skin response, respiration, pulse transit time, distal plesmography, and electroencephalograms.
2. **Autogenic training:** A series of mental exercises designed to produce relaxation imagery that may be guided by a practitioner through suggestion or can be coupled with relaxation and exercise.
3. **Progressive muscle relaxation:** A systematic approach to relaxation exercises involving the tensing and relaxing of muscle groups from head to foot.
4. **Hypnosis:** A state of enhanced focus or awareness that can lead to increased levels of suggestibility. This can be helpful in the blocking of painful sensation (hypnoanalgesia).
5. **Cognitive-behavioral therapy:** The approach often involves the monitoring of automatic thoughts that are negative; recognizing the connections between thoughts, affect, and behavior; and altering and replacing dysfunctional thoughts with more reality oriented interpretations.

his pain was expanding to include the entire abdomen, present constantly, but worse in the evening and with any activities. He is married, has five children, and his spouse is employed. A schedule was arranged to allow at least one of his children to be present to help him and his wife each day. Despite this help, he was becoming increasingly incapacitated and complained of pain with minor tasks. His family was concerned that he was "always in pain and losing the will to live."

Cancer pain represents another physical and psychological challenge to both primary care providers and patients. Often pain is an outgrowth of simple tissue destruction by advancing tumor mass. Accompanying this, however, is the progressive loss of "hardiness" (strength, independence, and social identity) that accompanies the cancer. Patients often believe that cancer is a painful condition; for example, it has been shown by verbal report that sciatic pain hurts more and requires more analgesia after a malignant diagnosis is made. In addition, the patient suffers changes in a number of key roles in the face of the disease. As Jorge gives up the roles of parent, spouse, and worker, his pain behavior increases to match his new dependency. Finally, anxiety about both deteriorating health and family responses increases the pain.

CASE ILLUSTRATION 4 (CONT.)

A meeting with the patient and family was scheduled specifically to address the issue of pain. A careful and complete examination to evaluate all pain complaints was performed. The family's concerns were also solicited. Finally, the concepts of cancer pain treatment were reviewed, with an explanation of the importance of identifying and dealing with biological, social, and psychological issues that affect the pain. At the time of this examination, only abdominal pain with radiation to the back was identified as a limiting pain.

Although cancer has a devastating and lasting effect on family function, involving the family in treatment decisions and planning is crucial. In many families it is particularly important to identify the head of the household as well as the primary caregiver. In this case, although Jorge is the head of the household, it is customary that once he becomes sick he is cared for by the family and that he takes on a sick role. It becomes important, therefore, to involve his spouse, who is the primary person in charge of caregiving, in discussions involving treatment decisions and planning.

An early discussion of the effect of the pain on the patient and his family is key to the collaborative treatment of pain. If the patient and family do not understand how the physician needs to integrate treatment as an aspect of daily life, they often feel that reports of pain are being discounted or diminished. Similarly, soliciting and supporting the use of home and cultural remedies can further this communication and collaboration (see Chapter 12). Medications to control cancer pain must be used effectively, regularly, and in adequate doses. Opiates should be used time contingent around the clock in long-acting form rather than on an as needed basis. As needed medications encourage both patient and family to gauge the pain, thus providing an unnecessary focus on the pain. The use of inadequate pain medication also sets up a distrustful resentment between patient and physician. Specific adjunctive medication can be used to afford more relief with less sedation [NSAIDs for bone pain, steroids for pain associated with local inflammation and edema, baclofen (Lioresal) for muscle spasm, and sedatives for insomnia].

Cognitive-behavioral interventions can be tailored to the specific family and cultural circumstances of the patient. In the case of Jorge, his family expects him to yield his traditional roles and to need help as his disease and pain behavior increase. Therapy can thus be directed to both patient and family with the goal of increasing the patient's independence and decreasing the family's tendency to respond to all of his pain behaviors with fear. In addition, Jorge believes that cancer is painful and disabling, neither of which is to be tolerated. This attitude engenders helplessness and suffering. Behavior therapy could address this belief with techniques to provide control over his pain, such as single-symptom autogenic training, relaxation, hypnosis, or cognitive-behavioral therapy. For example, the patient can be trained to interpret sensations as routine rather than threatening. In this way, he and his family can learn to accept rather than potentially distort his disease and pain.

SUMMARY

In this chapter we presented several approaches to the treatment of persons suffering various types of pain that emphasizes the evaluation and treatment of not only the biological, but also the psychological and social implications of the problem.

The primary care physician is encouraged to make good use of the three-function model for interviewing and ongoing communications with his or her patient. The following key factors should be attended to in the treatment of pain:

- **Identifying pain as an issue:** Deal with it in a comprehensive medical, social, and psychological way at onset, instead of when it becomes a problem.
- **Pain behaviors:** Whereas the patient may be quick to understand the pain largely as derived from the precipitating event or factors, the treating physician must always attend to the social causes and consequences of the pain and its implications in the life of the patient at work, at home, and in play.
- **Meaning of the pain:** Cultural influences may dictate differing attitudes and roles in the expression of the pain.
- **Doctor as "change agent":** In addition to providing direct treatment and advice, the doctor, through the patient–doctor relationship, can improve adherence to treatment.
- **Function not dysfunction oriented:** The interests and attention of the doctor influence greatly the thoughts and behaviors of the patient. By commenting on improved functioning as an indicator of heal-

ing, the doctor can redirect the patient's attention away from pain and toward increased functioning.

SUGGESTED READING

Bell G Kidd D, North R: Cost-effectiveness analysis of spinal cord stimulation in treatment of failed back surgery syndrome: J Pain Symptom Manage 1997;13:286.

Bonica T (editor): *The Management of Pain,* Vols. 1 and 2, 2nd ed. Lea & Febiger, 1990.

Cutler R et al: Does nonsurgical pain center treatment of chronic pain return patients to work? Spine 1994:19(6):643.

Fields H, Liebeskind J (editors): *Pharmacological Approaches to the Treatment of Chronic Pain: Concepts and Critical Issues.* IASP Press, 1994.

Fishbain DA et al: Types of pain treatment facilities and referral selection criteria. Arch Family Med 1995;4:58.

Fishman B, Luscalzo M: Cognitive-behavioral intervention in management of cancer pain: principles and applications. Med Clin North Am 1987:71(2):271.

Flor H, Fydrick T, Turk DC: Efficacy of multidisciplinary pain treatment centers: a meta-analytic review. Pain 1992;49:221.

Kobasa SC: Stressful life events, personality and health: an inquiry into hardiness. J Pers Soc Psychol 1979:37:1.

Maddi SR, Kobasa SC (editors): *The Hardy Executive: Health Under Stress.* Dow-Jones-Irwin, 1984.

North RB et al: Failed back surgery syndrome: 5-year follow-up after spinal cord stimulator implantation. Neurosurgery 1991;28:692.

Sullivan MD et al: Chronic pain in primary care. J Family Prac 1991:32(2)193.

Turk DC: Clinician attitudes about prolonged use of opioids and the issue of patient heterogeneity. J Pain Symptom Manage 1996; 11:218.

Turk DC: Treatment of chronic pain: clinical outcomes, cost effectiveness, and cost benefits. Drug Benefit Trends 2001;13(9):36.

Turk DC, Melzack, R (editors): *Handbook of Pain Assessment,* 2nd ed. Guilford Press, 2001.

Turk D, Meichenbaum D, Genest M (editors): *Pain and Behavioral Medicine: A Cognitive Behavioral Perspective.* Guilford Press, 1983.

Turk DC, Okifuji A: Treatment of chronic pain patients: clinical outcomes, cost-effectiveness, and cost-benefits of multidisciplinary pain centers. Crit Rev Phys Med Rehabil Med 1998;10:181.

Turner JA, Loeser JD, Bell KG: Spinal cord stimulation for chronic low back pain: a systematic literature synthesis. Neurosurgery 1995;37:1088.

HIV/AIDS

31

Lisa Capaldini, MD, MPH, Mitchell D. Feldman, MD, MPhil, Jeffrey H. Burack, MD, MPP, BPhil, & Thomas J. Coates, PhD

INTRODUCTION

Infection with the human immunodeficiency virus (HIV) is associated with a range of social, emotional, and neuropsychiatric complications. With the advent of effective antiviral treatment, HIV is now a potentially manageable chronic disease. Living with HIV, however, is a psychospiritual challenge requiring a regime of multiple medications, many of which have side effects, and having to live with a condition that remains stigmatized. Persons at highest risk for HIV [we use the term HIV/acquired immunodeficiency syndrome (AIDS) to designate the entire spectrum of clinical manifestations of HIV disease, from asymptomatic infection through advanced AIDS] are disproportionately likely to suffer behavioral and mood disorders and to be socially disenfranchised and economically disadvantaged. Once infected, they must contend with a widely feared and stigmatized, contagious, and often progressively debilitating medical condition; the loss of capabilities and bodily integrity; multiple bereavements and stressors; and their own suffering and mortality. In addition, many people with HIV may have other significant comorbid conditions, such as chronic hepatitis B or C, psychiatric conditions, and/or substance use that may make coping with HIV more difficult. Although undiagnosed and untreated patients with HIV disease can present with life-threatening neuropsychiatric sequelae of HIV [central nervous system (CNS), opportunistic infections, HIV dementia] most patients' behavioral concerns will be focused on maintaining medication adherence, maximizing quality of life, and managing life-style issues.

EPIDEMIOLOGY & PREVENTION

HIV is primarily transmitted through sexual exposure or shared injection drug paraphernalia (sharing needles). Initially an epidemic concentrated among gay men in cities, new cases of HIV infection now are disproportionately seen in socioeconomically disadvantaged populations, especially women of color. Many patients do not fit "classic" risk factor profiles. For example, a monogamous woman may be infected through her husband who is bisexually active. Although past HIV prevention programs successfully reduced rates of new HIV infections in gay men, the incidence of HIV infection is now rising again. *All* patients are potentially sexually active and should be counseled about HIV prevention and testing, including teens and seniors. HIV positive patients should also be regularly counseled about safer sexual practices.

Harm reduction programs such as needle exchange clearly reduce the spread of HIV infection but have not been implemented in most communities due to political and social concerns about promoting drug use; these concerns are not supported by research. Substance use, including alcohol, is highly correlated with unsafe sex behaviors, and all patients need to be educated about the risk of combining recreational substance use and sexual activity.

Because HIV infection is a major public health problem in the United States, all primary care practitioners must become competent in helping to prevent and treat it.

THE PSYCHOSOCIAL IMPACT OF HIV/AIDS

Overview

Although the course of HIV/AIDS is different for every patient, some common clinical and life events are associated with negative psychological consequences, ranging from mild anxiety and discouragement to feelings of devastation and suicide. Frequent illness and loss of friends and loved ones may allow little time for emotional recovery between episodes of grieving. Persons with HIV/AIDS may be ostracized by family and community and may suffer discrimination in employment, education, housing, and health care.

Later in the course of the illness there may be loss of employment or a reduction in responsibilities, consequent financial hardships compounded by heavy medical expenses, and dislocation or alienation from established social networks. Fatigue, pain, and other symptoms may diminish quality of life. Weight loss and disfiguring body composition changes (eg, lipodystrophy) may lead to loss of pride and bodily integrity as well as privacy concerns (patients who initially chose not to disclose their HIV diagnosis may be forced to do so). Although persons with HIV undergoing treatment are unlikely to suffer from life-threatening opportunistic infections, they may remain or become disabled, often from the side effects of medication or from residual fatigue and cognitive dysfunction. For most patients the challenge is learning to live with the hardships and limitations imposed by chronic HIV disease.

Although with treatment the prognosis of HIV disease has improved, many people still think of HIV disease as a progressive, fatal condition. Patients with HIV infection need validation that although it is challenging to live with HIV, they can still have full and meaningful lives.

Patients with HIV benefit from empathic relationships with their medical providers and from connections with other HIV-positive people. For example, in adherance studies of adult women with HIV, a robust predictor of medication compliance is the patient's perception of her relationship with the clinician. In addition, women who meet other women with HIV (through retreats, support groups, or newsletters) are more likely to adhere to HIV monitoring.

In many urban areas, support groups exist for HIV patients from diverse risk groups (eg, patients in recovery, gay men with HIV, etc). In more rural and underserved areas, public health departments may offer case-management services for people with HIV. In some instances, these case managers may be the only local source of information, clinician referral, and psychosocial support for patients.

Counseling Patients Who Test Positive for HIV

HIV infection is generally diagnosed when an enzyme-linked immunosorbent assay (ELISA) is reactive and confirmed by a Western blot test that is positive for the presence of anti-HIV antibody. Patients tested in the "window period" (up to 6 months after possible exposure) should be offered repeat testing if they are seronegative and possibly direct RNA viral detection testing since treatment during primary infection may be advantageous. By 6 months after exposure, more than 95% of infected patients will test positive. Measurement of viral load allows for earlier diagnosis and intervention.

Patients who test positive for the presence of HIV may experience and express a variety of emotional responses (see Chapter 3). In general, the primary care provider should allow the patient to express his or her feelings, and should actively listen to the expressed emotions in a nonjudgmental manner. Effective use of empathic statements such as "I can understand how difficult this must be for you" and "We can work on this together" can help the patient feel a little less overwhelmed and helpless when presented with a positive test result.

Clinicians should be alert to the potentially wide range of emotional responses expressed by patients and then check their understanding of the response with a reflective statement such as "You seem frightened by this news." Often, the emotion that unexpectedly wells up in the physi-

cian (eg, sadness, anger, panic) is indicative of what the patient also feels. Physicians can use their own emotions as diagnostic information to help gain insight into patients' feelings.

Paradoxically, although many persons seek testing to relieve the uncertainty of not knowing their status, testing positive for HIV can create additional uncertainty. This can be quite unsettling for patients, especially those for whom maintaining tight control over their lives has been highly valued. Suddenly they are confronted with not knowing how long they will remain well, who will care for them if they become ill or debilitated, how they will support themselves, and many other unknowns. The physician can help the patient cope with this sudden uncertainty by providing both information and emotional support. It may be helpful to say: "Many people who test positive for HIV are concerned because they do not know what to expect. Is this true for you?" Some patients are comforted by the physician's acknowledgment that they are the same person they were before the test, but now they possess new information about their health that can be addressed. For example, the clinician can say: "You are the same person today as you were yesterday, only now you *know* that you are HIV positive. It is important that you have this information so that we can now work on keeping you healthy." Patients should be given up-to-date information about treatment, prognosis, and other medical data, especially if they request it. It has been shown that distress can be decreased if patients are informed about their disease and their treatment options.

Physicians should also remember that informing patients of their HIV status is different from informing them of other medical illnesses because of the stigma still associated with AIDS. This may be especially true for gay men who, in addition, have to deal with the social and personal consequences of being gay, such as discrimination, homophobia, and feelings of shame and isolation. It may be important to address these issues of social stigma and shame to help patients cope with their seropositive status. Referral for individual counseling is often helpful.

Other emotions that the seropositive patient may express include anger, fear, denial, and depression. Patients may feel angry for many reasons: about having an incurable illness, about perceived loss of control, and about current or future discrimination. Some patients are angry at themselves for having become infected or at the partner who may have transmitted the virus to them. Allow patients to express their anger and frustration; often the anger dissipates with empathic listening.

Fear is often a less evident emotion and may need to be elicited with questions such as "What are your major fears about HIV?" and "From your experience with other people with HIV, what kinds of things are most frightening for you?" Seropositive persons may fear loss of job, friends, or health insurance or have more global fears of declining health, increasing pain, or becoming a burden on family or friends. These fears should be acknowledged as legitimate, and, when possible, the physician can help the patient to deal concretely with those problems that can be anticipated and ameliorated. It may be helpful to have the patient make two lists, dividing the current or anticipated problems into those that are to some extent controllable and those that are basically uncontrollable. The controllable problems can be addressed through specific **problem-solving** strategies, but the clinician should focus on **emotion-handling skills** for the basically uncontrollable problems and emotions that arise (see Chapters 1 and 2).

Denial is a common response to the news of a positive HIV test. For some patients this may initially be a healthy way of not allowing themselves to be overwhelmed by potentially devastating information. In fact, some people need several months to a year to come to terms with the diagnosis. If, however, denial leads patients to harm themselves (for example, by refusing potentially life-enhancing or life-extending treatment) or to harm others by exposing them to HIV, the physician should challenge the denial. This can be done gently, for example, by saying "I can understand why you would wish that you were not infected, but you are and we need to deal with it." Such statements may need to be repeated at subsequent visits until the patient is ready to accept the fact and consequences of a seropositive status.

Depression and anxiety are also common responses in persons who test positive for HIV. The clinician should assess the severity and duration of these symptoms to determine the appropriate treatment. Some studies have found that the risk of suicide is substantially increased in the 3–6 months following a serological diagnosis, so all patients should be screened for *reactive depression and suicidal ideation.* It is best to use direct, open-ended questions such as "How are you handling your HIV diagnosis?" "What fears or concerns do you have?"

In the weeks and months following a positive test, the clinician can assist patients in coping more effectively by assessing their social support system. This can be done by asking: "Who are you talking to about your concerns and issues?" If patients are isolated, provide them with phone numbers of local AIDS service organizations. Family members can also provide valuable support, but often HIV-infected people avoid seeking their help, or the family has previously rejected them because of their life-style. Clinicians can help patients by offering to have family or significant others attend medical appointments and by integrating supportive others into the treatment team.

Lazarus Phenomenom

Adults diagnosed with HIV prior to 1996 expected to die from it. For those patients who lived long enough to benefit from newly effective HIV antiviral combinations, sur-

viving with HIV can be a paradoxical burden—having planned to die, soon, these patients may have spent their savings, stopped school, left jobs, and made other decisions that make their living with HIV pragmatically and spritually difficult.

In the gay male population, many of these "Lazarus" survivors, in addition to HIV-negative gay men, may feel bewildered, guilty, and angry that they survived while scores of friends and lovers died. These spiritual struggles may result in substance use, HIV medication adherence problems, depression, or unsafe sex. Empathic acknowledgment by the clinician of the paradoxes of living with HIV disease can validate these patients' feelings and struggles. Patients with persistent symptoms should be referred for group and/or individual therapy.

Managing Substance Use

Active substance use is a risk factor for medical nonadherence and for reexposure to HIV through unsafe sex and needle sharing. Many cases of new HIV infection are correlated with unsafe sex during alcohol or drug binges, even in cases in which patients clearly understood the hows and whys of safer sex. Patients in drug and alcohol recovery have been shown to be able to achieve good adherence. All patients with current or past drug or alcohol problems should be screened for comorbid psychiatric disorders.

Methadone has significant interactions with non-nucleoside reverse transcriptase inhibitors (NNRTIs) and protease inhibitors (PIs). These interactions are not always predictable (eg, one agent, nevirapine, can both raise and lower methadone levels). When antiviral drugs are changed, patients should be monitored for both methadone intoxication and withdrawal, and their methadone treatment center should be informed of possible fluctuations in methadone levels.

WORKING WITH ASYMPTOMATIC & SYMPTOMATIC PATIENTS

Without treatment, most persons will remain asymptomatic for 5–10 years after infection with HIV. During this stage, regular preventive medical care includes periodic testing of surrogate markers of disease progression, including CD4 lymphocyte counts and HIV viral load. Waiting for and receiving these results can be intensely stressful for patients. Physicians must counsel patients prior to testing about the day-to-day, even hour-to-hour variability in the test, about the limited clinical significance of a one-time change in counts, and about plans for repeat testing and other follow-up in the event of specific results. Nevertheless, the clinician must anticipate that despite reassurances, any decline in CD4 count may be deeply discouraging. This is particularly true when the CD4 count drops below one of the current staging thresholds, which, although serving only as rules of thumb to experienced HIV clinicians, still represents important clinical benchmarks in the course of HIV/AIDS. These include a CD4 count of 350/mm³, at which many experts recommend initiating antiretroviral therapy and below which symptoms are much more likely; 200/mm³, which presently confers an automatic diagnosis of AIDS and below which the risk of opportunistic infections increases dramatically; and 50/mm³, below which expected survival without antiviral treatment is measured in months and the risks of severe complications and disability are high.

Clinicians use trends in CD4 cells, viral load, and the presence of significant symptoms (fever, weight loss) to determine when antiviral treatment should be initiated. For many patients, especially those familiar with potential medication side effects, needing to start antiviral medication in and of itself may feel like "the beginning of the end" and reduce the patient's sense of health and integrity. Involving patients in the timing and choice of antiviral medications may reduce their anxiety and improve long-term adherence to use of antiviral medications. When patients know what side effects are possible with each medication, and what the demands are of the dosing regimens, they can assist the clinician in selecting the most workable antiviral combination. Adherence to a medication regimen is a challenge for all patients with chronic illness (see Chapter 16). Recent research shows that HIV patients must be 95% adherent (ie, take 19 of every 20 doses) to achieve durable suppression of HIV. Nonadherent patients are at risk for disease progression and for developing viral resistance to antiviral medications.

Clinicians should assess and address adherence initially and on an ongoing basis. Open-ended and supportive questions are useful: "How are you doing with remembering your meds?" "How many doses did you miss yesterday? Last week?" This assessment provides important clinical information and reinforces the critical importance of medication adherence for the patient.

For most patients, linking doses to routine activities (walking the dog, brushing teeth, waking the children) is helpful. Medisets, beepers, and periodic adherence checks by case managers may also be helpful. Risk factors for nonadherence include *active* substance use, change in routine schedules (travel, holiday), medication side effects, and depression. During periods when the patient is at high risk of nonadherance, temporarily suspending antivirals (a structured treatment interruption) may be preferable to poor adherence.

SPECIAL ISSUES & POPULATIONS

Hepatitis B & C Coinfection

All patients with HIV should be offered screening for chronic hepatitis B and C. For some patients learning they have chronic viral hepatitis, in addition to HIV, can be overwhelming. In addition, evaluation for treatment of hepatitis B and C may involve liver biopsy, and currently available treatments (interferon, ribavirin) can cause flu-like symptoms, major depression, and cytopenias.

The clinician should assess each patient's ability to cope with another diagnosis and plan diagnostic studies accordingly. Patients on an interferon-containing regimen should be closely monitored for depression. Noting the high incidence of interferon-associated depression, some investigators have advocated prophylactic antidepressant therapy.

Women

Isolation and stigma are especially common in women with HIV. Irrespective of how they acquired HIV, women fear being judged to be "a whore or an addict." Women may be especially fearful about disclosing their HIV status for fear of domestic abuse, loss of child custody, or loss of employment. Referral to local and national organizations is often helpful (see Web Sites at the end of this chapter).

Pregnant women with HIV benefit from multidisciplinary care teams that can both optimize their HIV care and provide appropriate perinatal care to mother and baby. They should be advised about the risks and appropriate management of perinatal transmission of HIV; many women overestimate the risk and are not aware of the effective treatment options that exist.

Chronic Pain

Chronic pain is a common complication of HIV disease that is commonly underdiagnosed and undertreated. Specific causes of chronic pain include postherpetic neuralgia, peripheral neuropathy, and avascular necrosis (AVN). In 10% of HIV patients with chronic pain a specific etiology is not found.

Untreated pain can cause insomnia, depression, substance use, and medication nonadherence. Patients at high risk of undertreatment are women, minority patients, and patients with prior or active substance use. General pain management principles (see Chapter 30) are used in treating HIV-associated pain: attempt to make a specific diagnosis to target treatment, but do not forego treating pain in the absence of a firm etiological diagnosis.

Many analgesic and adjunctive medications [eg, tricyclic antidepressants (TCAs), carbamazepine, methadone] are metabolized through cytochrome P-450 and may interact with NNRTI and reverse transcriptase inhibitor (RTI) antivirals. Gabapentin (neurontin), nonsteroidal anti-inflammatory drugs (NSAIDs), acetaminophen, and aspirin have no significant interactions, but their use may be complicated by hepatic and renal dysfunction. In patients requiring narcotic therapy, longer acting agents supplemented by fast-acting narcotics as needed for breakthrough are generally most effective.

Fatigue

Many patients with HIV, even those successfully treated with antivirals, suffer from disabling HIV-related fatigue. Typically patients wake with a good deal of energy only to develop severe fatigue with minor activities. Many patients will need to nap and sleep longer than is usual for them. Researchers have speculated that this fatigue may be due to cytokine effects in the brain or be a manifestation of mitochondrial dysfunction.

Before ascribing fatigue to idiopathic HIV-associated fatigue, an extensive differential diagnosis should be considered including depression, anemia, testosterone deficiency, sleep apnea, chronic hepatitis, hypothyroidism, chronic pain, and medication side effects. Idiopathic HIV-related fatigue may respond to bupropion (Wellbutrin) or stimulants. Patients who are otherwise well and wish to resume a full life need validation that their fatigue is real and need to be informed that even with aggressive treatment their activities may remain limited.

NEUROPSYCHIATRIC COMPLICATIONS

Management of Neuropsychiatric Complications of HIV/AIDS

HIV clinicians must be able to identify specific syndromes (eg, depression, psychosis), formulate preliminary differential diagnoses, and make appropriate psychotherapy and psychopharmacological referrals. HIV-related neuropsychiatric syndromes are evaluated and treated with the following guidelines:

1. HIV-associated opportunistic infections, which may present as behavioral disorders, are very uncommon in patients with more than 200 CD4 cells or in patients with fewer than 200 CD4 cells and low or undetectable viral loads.
2. Side effects of prescription medication commonly cause neuropsychiatric symptoms.
3. Drug interactions (both with prescription and recreational drugs) are of special concern in patients receiving potent suppressors of cytochrome P-450 3A4 and 2D6, particularly ritonavir, delavirdine, and lopinavir/ritonavir.
4. Recreational drug use and withdrawal can cause symptoms directly or exacerbate preexisting disorders (eg, bipolar affective disorder).
5. With a few exceptions, HIV-associated neuropsychiatric symptoms are guided by the same treatment principles as used for the general population; most psychiatric medications are used at the same dosages and for the same indications.

Drug Effects

Many of the medications used to treat HIV/AIDS and its complications have common neuropsychiatric side ef-

fects. Side effects may be related to cumulative dose or to peak levels but may be unpredictable and idiosyncratic. Furthermore, the homeostatic mechanisms responsible for maintaining therapeutic drug levels may be disrupted by end-organ involvement, such as decreased renal excretion, hepatic metabolism, or cardiac output; diminished body fat; immunological dysregulation; and a predisposition toward dehydration. Patients with HIV are therefore also more susceptible to side effects from more commonly used medications. The rule of thumb for prescribing to persons with HIV is "say no, start low, and go slow," that is, avoid unnecessary medications, use reduced dosages of those that are necessary, and increase doses slowly and cautiously. Most patients, however, will require conventional doses of medications used to treat psychiatric disorders.

Drug effects and toxicities must always be considered in the initial differential diagnosis of any neuropsychiatric abnormality. Table 31–1 describes the adverse reactions associated with some drugs commonly used in the treatment of HIV/AIDS. A few general principles should be kept in mind. First, use agents with favorable side effect profiles. Second, use caution in the coadministration of medications with similar side effect profiles or those that significantly affect one another's pharmacodynamics. An example of the first situation is the simultaneous use of any combination of antidepressants, antihistamines, neuroleptics, or antimotility agents, all of which have substantial anticholinergic effects.

The second concern arises from the use of agents such as rifampin, which induces the hepatic cytochrome P-450 enzyme system and thereby accelerates the metabolism of many other drugs or, conversely, agents such as ritonavir or delavirdine, which inhibit the P-450 enzyme.

A third concern is that adherence to complex medication regimens is often unreliable. Incorrect dosing may result in undertreatment for some conditions, but confusion may also result in inadvertent overdosing. Always simplify the regimen and use the lowest dose of the fewest drugs likely to be effective. The assistance of a pharmacist is invaluable in addressing these concerns. If possible, the regimens of patients with advanced HIV/AIDS should be periodically reviewed by a pharmacist.

Establishing a drug as the cause of a neuropsychiatric abnormality can be difficult. Look for a temporal relationship between the onset or exacerbation of symptoms and any new medications or dosage increases. In less clear circumstances, the initial strategy might include stopping all nonessential drugs since most drug-induced neuropsychiatric side effects resolve within several days of stopping the agent. If necessary, medications can be added back one by one. Recurrence of symptoms after rechallenge strongly suggests a causal relationship. Finally, there may be other pharmacological causes of neuropsychiatric disturbances, including complementary or nontraditional medical

Table 31–1. Psychiatric side effects of drugs used to treat HIV infection.

Drugs	Adverse Reaction	Comment
Antiretrovirals		
Zidovudine (AZT)	Mania, anxiety, auditory hallucinations, confusion	Idiosyncratic reaction; resolves within 24 h after stopping drug
Didanosine (ddl) Zalcitabine	Anxiety, irritability, insomnia	Idiosyncratic reaction; self-limiting, does not require drug discontinuation
Efavirenz	Confusion, abnormal thinking, impaired concentration, abnormal dreams, insomnia, amnesia, hallucinations, euphoria	Up to 50% of patients experience symptoms that may start on Day 1 and last 2–4 weeks; only 2–5% require discontinuation of the drug
Antivirals		
Acyclovir Ganciclovir (DHPG)	Lethargy, delirium, hallucinations, agitation, paranoia	Dose-related reaction, more common after high-dose oral or parenteral therapy, or in patients with renal impairment. Uncommon with DHPG
Foscarnet	Hallucinations, confusion	Association uncertain. Alterations in calcium and magnesium levels are contributory.
Antimicrobials		
Amphotericin B	Delirium, confusion	Rare reports; might be related to hyperthermia and irreversible leukoencephalopathy
β-Lactam antibiotics	Confusion, paranoia, hallucinations, mania, coma	Dose-related; high doses in patients with renal dysfunction; increased risk with procaine penicillin
Quinolones	Psychosis, delirium, seizures, anxiety, insomnia, depression	Dose-related; high doses in patients with renal dysfunction
Sulfonamides	Psychosis, delirium, confusion, depression, hallucinations	Dose-related; high doses in patients with renal dysfunction and the elderly. Direct neurotoxic effect
Isoniazid (INH)	Paranoia, confusion, anxiety, hallucinations	Doses exceeding 17 mg/kg/day. Intravenous pyridoxine recommended
Dapsone	Mania, psychosis, anxiety	Several reports in patients with overdosages; resolves within 24 h after discontinuation
Anabolic steroids	Mania, psychosis, depression, aggressiveness	Anecdotal reports in patients receiving 10–100 times the recommended doses; abrupt withdrawal after prolonged usage
Dronabinol (Marinol)	Anxiety, confusion, psychosis, mania, depression, hallucinations	Dose-related; self-limited, usually resolves within 12 h after acute usage; abrupt withdrawal produces similar symptoms
Opiates	Delirium, psychosis, depression, nightmares, hallucinations	Dose-related; might be more frequent with tincture of opium and long-acting narcotics; responds to dose reduction
Corticosteroids	Mania, "steroid psychosis," depression, euphoria	Dose-related > 40 mg/daily of prednisone; resolves with dosage reduction
Tricyclic antidepressants, neuroleptics, and other anticholinergics	Confusion, hallucinations, delirium, psychosis, mania, anxiety	Dose-related; resolves within 24–72 h after stopping the drug. Physostigmine 1–2 mg intramuscularly or intravenously can reverse toxicity
Fluoxetine	Anxiety, insomnia, mania	Administer in morning; can inhibit metabolism of TCAs and phenytoin and increase their toxicity
Benzodiazepines	Confusion, disorientation, paradoxical agitation, paranoia and rage; rebound anxiety and insomnia	Related to abuse and abrupt withdrawal after prolonged therapy. Increased risk with short-acting agents

therapies and use of alcohol or substances of abuse. The toxicities of most complementary and alternative therapies have not been well studied, but it is likely, for example, that plant alkaloids present in many herbal or "natural" remedies have psychoactive properties or may interact with HIV medications. For example, St. John's Wort can lower the serum levels of protease inhibitors and other medications.

Persons with HIV/AIDS on average have higher levels of substance abuse, in part because of the association between preexisting drug use and the risk of acquiring HIV, and perhaps because of self-medication for depression or anxiety. Stimulant drugs such as cocaine or amphetamines can cause agitation, psychosis, or delirium, as can withdrawal from sedating drugs such as benzodiazepines and alcohol. Sedatives and narcotics can of course cause somnolence, confusion, and psychomotor slowing, but can also cause paradoxical reactions, including agitation, paranoia, and rage. This may be especially true of the short-acting benzodiazepines, including triazolam (Halcion) and alprazolam (Xanax).

With regards to specific antiviral agents, two points need emphasizing. First, delavirdine or ritonavir-containing regimens, through inhibition of cytochrome P-450 enzymes, *may* dramatically raise the level of many prescribed and recreational drugs. These substrates include many anticonvulsants (eg, carbamazepine, valproic acid, phenytoin), narcotics (meperidine, methadone), recreational drugs (MDMA or Ectasy), and other agents (warfarin, digoxin, estrogen). Patients receiving these cytochrome P-450-inhibiting antivirals should be monitored carefully for these potential interactions (see Table 31–2 for a list of psychotropic medications that interact with the cytochrome P-450 system).

Second, within 2 weeks of starting efavirenz, patients may experience disrupted sleep, depression, agitation, and exacerbation of a previously stable psychiatric disease. Anecdotal reports of delayed or persisting neuropsychiatric symptoms have also been reported. Patients with stable psychiatric disorders may be prescribed efavirenz but should be monitored for drug-associated agitation or depression.

Depression

Major depression is the most common psychiatric disorder in persons with HIV/AIDS. The lifetime incidence is un-

Table 31–2. Clinically important cytochrome P-450 psychotropic interactions in the treatment of patients with HIV/AIDS.

Psychotropic Medication	Key Enzyme	Clinical HIV Implications
Fluoxetine, paroxetine	2D6, 3A4	May raise PI levels, but not to a clinically significant extent; increased TCA levels
Sertraline	2D6, 3A4	Milder effects, not significant
Citalopram	3A4, 2C19	Not clinically significant
Venlafaxine	3A4, 2D6	Few drug–drug interactions
Mirtazapine	3A4, 2D6, 1A2	Not clinically significant
Bupropion	2B6, 3A4	Levels raised with PIs; seizure risk
Nefazodone	3A4	Significant inhibitor; caution with PIs or NNRTIs
Lithium	None	Renally excreted ion
Valproate	2D6	Ritonavir interactions
Alprazolam, triazolam, zolpidem, zaleplon	3A4	Increased sedation with PIs
Risperidone	2D6	Avoid with ritonavir
Olanzapine	1A2, 2D6	Cigarettes will decrease levels
Seroquel	3A4	No reported PI or NNRTI interactions
Ziprasidone	Not significant	Check QTc duration
St. John's wort	3A4	May lower levels of PIs

Reproduced from Levine JM: Psychiatric aspects of HIV care. AIDS Clin Care 2001;13:106.

known but rises dramatically as the disease progresses. As with non-HIV-infected depressed patients, the cardinal symptoms include depressed mood, anhedonia, feelings of worthlessness and hopelessness, disturbances in sleep and appetite, weight loss or gain, fatigue, psychomotor slowing, agitation, and preoccupation with morbid thoughts (see Chapter 21). A family history of an affective disorder or alcoholism may be present. Depression may be more difficult to diagnose in the presence of HIV/AIDS, however, for several reasons. First, its manifestations, and particularly the vegetative symptoms (fatigue, weakness, weight loss, and loss of libido), overlap with the constitutional symptoms commonly attributable to HIV infection or its complications. Second, the multiple losses that many persons with HIV/AIDS often experience may result in a chronic grieving state that shares many of the affective aspects of depression. Third, thoughts of death and suicide may be viewed as appropriate or rational as disease progresses. Fourth, organic impairment due to the HIV-associated dementia complex may have affective manifestations. Fifth, HIV-associated hypogonadism (low testosterone) may cause fatigue, impaired libido, and other depressive symptoms. For some patients, testosterone supplementation has been shown to reverse depressive symptoms. Finally, medication use, and the use of or withdrawal from other psychoactive substances, can have mood-altering effects as described previously. Nevertheless, depressive disorders including major depression and dysthymia are diagnosed by the same criteria for HIV-infected as for non-HIV-infected persons and should never be treated as a normal finding. Indeed, recent surveys have documented that untreated depression is a major correlate of poor quality of life in people with HIV disease.

The clinician should screen for depression with open-ended questions such as "How have things been going for you lately?" or "How are you coping with all of this?" Certain clues may help to distinguish depressive from constitutional symptomatology. For example, progressive fatigue that worsens with exertion and over the course of the day is characteristic of somatic disease (eg, anemia), whereas an inability to get going in the morning, which improves with activity, may suggest depression. Similarly, nondepressed patients may report that nausea or dysgeusia (an abnormal sense of taste) interferes with their appetite, whereas depressed patients often report simply no interest in eating. Nondepressed patients often report their symptoms and limitations with frustration and concern, whereas apathy and resignation are more characteristic of major depression. Anhedonia and a sense of worthlessness are rarely symptoms of a somatic condition, and should therefore be directly investigated as specific indicators of depression. Depressed patients may appear more anxious or preoccupied than sad. Patients with depression and anxiety may self-medicate with recreational drugs or alcohol; patients with substance use should be screened carefully for depression and anxiety disorders.

The treatment of depression in the HIV/AIDS-infected population does not differ from the non-HIV-infected population. Regular, empathic listening and short-term psychotherapeutic techniques may be very effective. Explicit recognition and validation of the patient's losses and fears help to establish a trusting therapeutic relationship and may permit developing joint strategies to cope with them. It is important to emphasize that depression is a common ailment in the setting of HIV/AIDS and is amenable to treatment. All non-monoamine oxidase inhibitor (MAOI) antidepressants can be used to treat depression in patients with HIV disease. As with other patients, choosing among the many available agents should be largely a matter of selecting the most desirable or tolerable side effect profile, and being aware of drug interactions between antivirals and antidepressants.

The clinician must be alert to how the activity and toxicity profile of particular agents may help in simultaneously addressing other concerns of the patient. For example, sedating agents such as mirtazapine may be effective in patients who suffer from insomnia, and doxepin may also relieve pruritus. A tricyclic antidepressant such as nortriptyline may be an ideal choice in a patient with neuropathic pain, who may also benefit from the drug's synergy with other analgesics. The risk of cardiac arrhythmias associated with tricyclic drugs may be increased in persons taking imidazole antifungal agents (such as fluconazole or itraconazole), whereas the selective serotonin reuptake inhibitors (SSRIs) may cause sexual dysfunction. Mirtazapine may be helpful for patients with insomnia and anorexia, as it has antihistamine side effects. Bupropion is especially useful in patients with fatigue and, along with nefazodone and mirtazapine, is unlikely to cause sexual dysfunction.

Stimulants (methylphenidate, dexedrine, modafinil) may be used with other antidepressants in patients with severe refractory fatigue, and can also be used to palliate narcotic-associated fatigue and sedation. Because of their potential for abuse, these agents must be used selectively, and their efficacy varies considerably from patient to patient.

Tearfulness, anhedonia, preoccupation, agitation, and insomnia may characterize an acute grief reaction, which can be expected in the wake of bereavement or at any of the life transition points or disease progression benchmarks mentioned previously. Grieving persons often benefit from emotional and social support and spiritual counseling, and group or individual psychotherapy may be effective in encouraging adaptation. It is appropriate to treat short-term insomnia or agitation with limited courses of benzodiazepines. If vegetative symptoms persist or normal social functioning remains significantly impaired beyond 1 month after the acute loss, treatment for depression should be considered.

Major depression dramatically increases the risk of suicide, which should no more be viewed as the result of a "rational" choice in persons with HIV than it would be in the depressed non-HIV-infected population. Attempting suicide is correlated with a history of psychiatric treatment, substance abuse, persistently high levels of psychological distress, HIV-related interpersonal and occupational problems, poor perceived social support, and recent evidence of disease progression. Physicians should be prepared to intervene under such circumstances with crisis counseling, social support, and psychiatric hospitalization.

Nevertheless, as disability, suffering, and loss of dignity progress, suicide may indeed appear for many to be an attractive and rational alternative to continued deterioration. Perhaps most importantly, the idea that suicide is eventually an option is a comfort to many persons with HIV/AIDS and other chronic degenerative diseases, for whom it represents ultimate control over their condition, and a hedge against the fear of complete dependence and debilitation. Physicians must walk a fine line, detecting and intervening to prevent depression-associated suicide, but remaining careful not to take away the comfort and hope that ultimate control over one's fate confers. Regardless of physicians' own ethical or religious positions on suicide, they must be willing to openly and honestly probe and discuss the patient's suicidal thoughts and, most importantly, the fears and concerns that have led to them. As with requests for assistance in suicide, a discussion of suicide with one's physician is often a disguised cry for help. It may reflect exasperation or exhaustion over symptoms inadequately treated, fear of uncontrollable future pain or suffering, anxiety over burdening caregivers, or the desperate need to be reassured that one will not be abandoned by care providers in one's time of greatest need. What begins as a discussion about suicidal thoughts often ends in the discovery of previously unsuspected or unarticulated fears and needs, a situation that permits physician and patient to work together to chart a clear, practical course to address these (see Chapter 35).

Anxiety

As with some depressive symptoms, anxiety may be a normal response to many of the stressors associated with living with HIV. Symptoms of anxiety may include poor concentration, restlessness, intrusive thoughts, insomnia (particularly trouble falling asleep), and fatigue. Persons with poor coping skills may be particularly prone to periods of uncontrollable anxiety. Withdrawal from nicotine, alcohol, or drugs of abuse, or overuse of caffeine may cause symptoms of anxiety. Some medications used in HIV/AIDS, particularly corticosteroids, decongestants, and nucleoside analogue antiretrovirals, can produce anxiety or agitation and, rarely, anxiety may be the presenting manifestation of underlying CNS disease.

Treatment is indicated if anxiety impairs social or occupational functioning, or is persistently uncomfortable.

Pharmacotherapy generally involves the use of SSRIs and other antidepressants (eg, paroxetine, venlafaxine) or benzodiazepines. For episodic and unpredictable bouts of anxiety, short- to medium-acting benzodiazepines, such as lorazepam (Ativan) or alprazolam (Xanax), are generally more effective, due to their more rapid onset of action. The physician should carefully monitor the frequency of refilling of anxiolytic prescriptions; a pattern of escalating use may suggest that a longer acting agent or antidepressant therapy is preferable. For chronic disabling anxiety, longer acting benzodiazepines such as clonazepam (Klonopin), which maintain more stable blood levels, may be more effective and better tolerated. SSRIs are useful maintenance agents in the treatment of anxiety syndromes such as panic disorder, obsessive-compulsive disorder (OCD), and posttraumatic stress disorder (PTSD).

Patients with anxiety symptoms should be screened for PTSD. PTSD symptoms include easy startling, flashbacks or nightmares, and dissociative symptoms. For some patients, the trauma of living with HIV rekindles memories of prior traumas (abuse, rape, accidents). Studies of incarcerated women with HIV have demonstrated a high rate of PTSD. PTSD is best treated with focused counseling, although SSRIs have been shown to help alleviate some of its symptoms.

Insomnia may complicate depression or anxiety disorders, may be a side effect of medications, including antiretrovirals, or may indicate excessive use of caffeine or stimulants. There are many potential causes of insominia that should be considered. Decreasing levels of daytime activity, due to fatigue, disability, or unemployment, may cause insomnia, particularly if the patient also takes daytime naps, as may the disruption of routine that accompanies hospitalization or a change in living circumstances. Sleeplessness may result from the inability to get comfortable, due to pain or dyspnea, or from fears of fecal incontinence during bouts of diarrhea. A careful history will often reveal the precise nature of the sleep disorder. Nonpharmacological treatment includes limiting evening caffeine, alcohol, and fluid intake; creating a conducive sleeping environment; and learning relaxation techniques. As noted earlier, a sedating antidepressant given at bedtime may be an ideal therapeutic choice for the patient with depression, agitation, and increased sleep latency. For many nondepressed patients, and particularly for those with cognitive impairment who are at risk for adverse reactions to benzodiazepines, moderate bedtime doses of chloral hydrate (500–1000 mg) are safe and effective.

Primary CNS Disease: The HIV-Associated Dementia Complex

HIV-associated dementia is a subcortical dementia characterized initially by cognitive and behavorial dysfunction and in its most advanced stages by motor dysfunction.

Advanced HIV dementia is rarely seen in patients with effectively treated HIV disease. Although antivirals differ in their penetration of cerebrospinal fluid (CSF), all combinations of antivirals that suppress serum viral load are likely to prevent HIV dementia. *Rarely,* genotypic analysis of CSF and blood reveals the presence of different HIV strains. In these rare cases some experts recommend that antiviral medication may need to be adjusted to treat the CSF strains.

All patients with HIV dementia should be evaluated for comorbid depression, as depressive symptoms can easily be misattributed to dementia. A trial of antidepressants may result in gratifying functional improvement in these patients. As in all patients with organic brain disease, sedating agents such as antihistamines and benzodiazapenes should be used with great caution and in general avoided.

Anticholinesterase inhibitors, used to treat Alzheimer's disease, have not been studied in patients with HIV dementia. These agents are unlikely to be useful in HIV dementia, however, as they have shown utility only in cortical dementia, and theoretically could exacerbate a subcortical dementia such as HIV.

HIV-Associated Minor Cognitive Disorders

Although HIV dementia is rare in HIV patients undergoing treatment and in patients with more than 200 CD4 cells, minor cognitive problems can persist and even progress in patients with good surrogate markers (eg, adequate CD4 cells and/or suppressed viral load). HIV-associated minor cognitive disorders are characterized by word-finding problems, difficulty sequencing complex tasks, and immediate memory dysfunction. Patients may note pauses in conversations while searching for words, difficulty performing clerical tasks, and functional forgetfulness (eg, misplacing keys, forgetting medicines).

Minor cognitive disorders may persist or progress in patients who are otherwise responding well to antiviral therapy. While minor cognitive disorders tend not to progress, they are often disabling, despite patients appearing "normal." These cognitive symptoms need to be carefully recorded in patients charts should disability status need to be assessed. Formal neuropsychological testing can document subtle cognitive dysfunction but is rarely more clinically useful than a thorough history.

Delirium

Delirium is an acute confusional state that includes disorientation, inattention, and an altered sensorium or disorganized thinking. It is *never* simply a manifestation of HIV/AIDS and should always be considered to reflect a potentially life-threatening metabolic disruption that has affected the CNS. Patients with cognitive impairment due to the HIV-associated dementia complex or other underlying brain pathology are at particular risk for having delirium precipitated by a metabolic insult, but the dementia itself is never the sole cause of delirium. The list of possible complications of HIV/AIDS that may cause delirium is long and includes disorders of perfusion and gas exchange (hypotension, hypoxia, hypercapnia); fluid and electrolyte abnormalities (dehydration, hyponatremia, hypoglycemia, hyperkalemia, hypercalcemia, uremia); endocrine disorders (adrenal insufficiency, exogenous corticosteroids); CNS injury, infection, or neoplasm; sepsis and other systemic infections; medication side effects (anticholinergics, sedatives, some antimicrobial and antineoplastic agents); and alcohol or drug intoxication or withdrawal. Delirium is generally of abrupt onset and is marked by fluctuating consciousness, poor attention, disorganized thought and speech, and perceptual abnormalities such as visual or auditory hallucinations. It may also be accompanied by either extreme agitation or apathetic withdrawal.

The search for and correction of the underlying abnormalities must be undertaken emergently, in a closely supervised setting such as an intensive care unit. Depending on patients' level of consciousness, frequent attempts may be made to keep them oriented, with careful attention paid to lighting and noise so that sensory stimulation is adequate but not overwhelming. Mechanical restraints should be avoided if possible but are sometimes necessary to prevent patients from injuring themselves or from pulling out lines and catheters. Agitation commonly complicates delirium and can be managed with escalating doses of atypical antipsychotics (eg, olanzapine, risperdal) or haloperidol, and, if necessary, with short-acting parenteral anxiolytics. Delirium should be aggressively treated with these agents while diagnostic studies are in progress.

Mania

Mania can be a terrifying and dangerous complication of HIV/AIDS. As in non-HIV-infected persons, mania is characterized by hyperactivity and psychomotor restlessness, euphoric or irritable mood, insomnia and perceived decreased need for sleep, pressured or rapid speech, grandiosity or paranoia, racing thoughts, distractibility, hypersexuality, and reckless or disinhibited hedonistic behavior. Mania in HIV/AIDS can be due to a preexisting bipolar diathesis precipitated by substance use, stress, or intercurrent illness. Less frequently, mania may be an initial manifestation of HIV-associated organic brain disease such as opportunistic infections or dementia. Medications reported to cause mania include high-dose corticosteroids, antidepressants, zidovudine, efavirenz, and stimulant drugs such as cocaine and amphetamine derivatives.

Treatment involves first discontinuing any potential pharmacological precipitant and ensuring a safe social environment. Pharmacotherapeutic agents effective in treatment of non-HIV-infected patients are also useful here, but their relative usefulness is changed by potential toxicities. Because of their lack of drug interactions with HIV antivirals, gabapentin, valproate, or atypical antipsychotics such as olanzapine are ideal agents in the setting of HIV-associated mania. Patients treated with valproate must be monitored closely for evidence of hepatotoxicity. Lithium, the mainstay of treatment for bipolar affective disorder in non-HIV-infected patients, is risky for patients with advanced AIDS in whom levels appear to fluctuate unpredictably. Dehydration due to diarrhea, fever, or poor intake can quickly result in toxic lithium levels, further complicating management.

Psychosis

As with mania, psychotic symptoms are generally due to underlying psychiatric disease (schizophrenia) or drug side effects. Psychotic symptoms include hallucinations, typically auditory rather than visual; delusions, which tend to be paranoid in content; looseness of association; and flight of ideas. Personal care and hygiene may be neglected, and the risk of violence to self or others is increased. Use of or withdrawal from many drugs of abuse, including amphetamines, phencyclidine, cocaine, alcohol, marijuana, and opiates, may cause a transient psychosis, and psychosis caused by methamphetamine in particular may last for days or weeks. Psychosis may complicate administration of the anticytomegalovirus drugs ganciclovir and foscarnet, anabolic or corticosteroids, zidovudine, efavirenz, opiates, other psychoactive pharmaceuticals including sedatives and antidepressants, and, very rarely, many ordinary antimicrobial agents (Table 31–1). Psychosis is a rare manifestation of underlying secondary CNS infection or neoplasm.

Treatment of HIV/AIDS-associated psychosis involves identification and removal of precipitating drugs and treatment as appropriate of underlying disease. Psychiatric consultation is essential to confirm the diagnosis, identify possible secondary causes, and optimize management. Atypical antipsychotic agents are effective in acute and maintenance treatment of psychosis. These atypical agents are less likely to cause tardive dyskinesia and are less sedating than older agents.

Many patients with schizophrenia and HIV are "triply diagnosed," that is, they also use recreational substances. These patients often benefit from day treatment programs in which medical treatment is integrated with their mental health care, and where adherence to a medication regimen can be facilitated through directly observed therapy.

CONCLUSION

Like all chronic medical disorders, HIV disease can be complicated by a myriad of psychiatric and spiritual challenges, such as isolation from one's family or community, reemergence of previously stable psychiatric disease, and the transition from planning to die of HIV disease to learning to live with it, among many others.

Although accurate psychiatric evaluation is critical, patients also benefit from an ongoing relationship with a clinician they perceive as knowledgeable, caring, and trustworthy. In the authors' experience, no other area of medicine requires such a skillful integration of the science and the art of medicine, nor offers such rewards for doing so.

SUGGESTED READINGS

Boccellari A, Zeifert P: Management of neurobehavioral impairment in HIV-1 infection. Psychiatr Clin North Am 1994;17:183.

Breitbart W: HIV, AIDS, and pain. In: Gatchel R, Turk D (editors): *Psychosocial Factors in Pain.* Guilford Press, 1999.

Breitbart W et al: A randomized, double-blind, placebo-controlled trial of psychostimulants for the treatment of fatigue in ambulatory patients with human immunodeficiency virus disease. Arch Intern Med 2001;161:411.

Capaldini L: HIV disease: psychosocial issues and psychiatric complications. In: Sande M, Volberding PA (editors): *The Medical Management of AIDS,* 6th ed. Saunders, 1999.

Otto-Salaj L, Stevens Y: Influence of psychiatric diagnosis and symptoms on HIV risk behavior in adults with serious mental illness. AIDS Reader 2001;11(4):197.

Treisman GJ, Angelino AF, Hutton HE: Psychiatric issues in the management of patients with HIV infection. JAMA 2001;286:2857.

WEB SITES

ACTIS (AIDS Clinical Trials Information Service) http://www.actis.org/

A central resource for federally and privately funded HIV/AIDS clinical trials information.

HIV Insite
http://hivinsite.ucsf.edu/InSite

Provides comprehensive up-to-date information on HIV/AIDS treatment, prevention, and policy with links for clinicians and patients.

Organizations for People with HIV
http://www.projinf.org

An HIV advocacy organization that issues up-to-date information about HIV research.

WORLD
http://www.womenhiv.org/

A national support group for women with HIV.

Mistakes in Medical Practice

32

Albert W. Wu, MD, MPH, Stephen J. McPhee, MD, & John F. Christensen, PhD

INTRODUCTION

Mistakes are inevitable in the practice of medicine. They result, in part, from individual factors, such as the complexity of medical knowledge, the uncertainty of clinical predictions, the pressures of time, and the need to make treatment decisions in spite of limited or uncertain knowledge. In addition, mistakes are also caused by system factors that influence working conditions. Although much attention has been focused on the effects of errors on patients, it must be understood that medical mistakes are correspondingly distressing for physicians, evoking intense shock and feelings of remorse, guilt, anger, and fear.

If dealt with effectively, mistakes can provide powerful learning experiences for physicians; however, difficulty in dealing with mistakes may impede both learning and efforts to prevent future errors. Professional norms that assume physician infallibility and treat mistakes as anomalies also pose significant barriers to learning. Judgmental institutional responses and fear of litigation are further disincentives to the open discussion of mistakes. Although some individuals may learn from their own mistakes and make subsequent appropriate changes in practice, others are less likely to benefit from these lessons.

Definitions

It is useful to define a number of related terms. A useful set of definitions is maintained by the Australian Safety and Quality Council (http://www.safetyandquality.org/definition/smsequential.htm) and is periodically modified based on comments.

Health care incident: An event or circumstance that could or did lead to unintended and/or unnecessary harm to a person, and/or a complaint, loss, or damage.

Adverse event: An incident in which harm resulted to a person receiving health care.

Medical error or mistake: An action or an omission with potentially negative consequences for the patient that would have been judged wrong by skilled and knowledgeable peers at the time it occurred.

Mistakes differ from negligence or malpractice in that a mistake is not necessarily the proximate cause of harm to a patient. It is clear that not all judgments that precede bad outcomes are necessarily wrong.

Prevalence

Most studies of medical error have focused on the hospital setting and on adverse events rather than mistakes. Although the overall prevalence of medical mistakes is difficult to ascertain, it appears that they are common. One study of hospitalized patients in New York State in 1984 found that injuries occurred in nearly 4% of admissions, with 25% of these events judged to have been due to negligence. A similar study in Colorado and Utah in the 1990s found that adverse events occurred in 3.5% of admissions and a study of 15,000 patients admitted to acute-care hospitals in Australia found that 16.6% were associated with an adverse event. In both of the latter studies, 1.7% of admissions were associated with a major disability and 0.3% with iatrogenic death. Observation of patients hospitalized on a general medical service in a teaching hospital found that the incidence of iatrogenic events was 36%. From the physician's viewpoint, among 254 medical residents, 114 (45%) responded and reported a significant mistake made during the prior year. The prevalence of mistakes in outpatient practice is only beginning to be studied, with one estimate suggesting errors in about 1% of visits.

Types

Mistakes occur in every aspect of medical practice—in diagnosis, in decision making (often because of ignorance of facts), in the pace of evaluation or its timing, in prescribing medications, or in performing procedures (Table 32–1). The Harvard Medical Practice Study found that among 1133 patients with disabling injuries caused by medical treatment, 28% of the injuries were judged to be due to negligence. The most common adverse event involved performance or follow-up of a procedure or operation (35%). Failure to take preventive measures (eg, failure to guard against accidental injury) was the next most common (22%), followed by diagnostic errors (eg, failure to use indicated tests, act on test results, or avoid delays in response) (14%), errors involving drug treatment (9%), and system errors (2%).

A review of malpractice claims in New Jersey from 1977 to 1989, for which payment was made or negligence was determined, found that errors in patient management (eg, diagnostic errors, decision errors, improper management, medication errors, unnecessary treatment, or prob-

Table 32–1. Types of medical mistakes.

Error	Example
Diagnosis or evaluation	Missed diagnosis
Medical decision making	Inappropriate or premature discharge
Treatment	Waiting when treatment is indicated
Medication	Incorrect dosage
Procedural complications	Faulty technique
Faulty communication	Failure to convey information during sign-out
Inadequate supervision	Failure to review treatment plan

Source: Adapted, with permission, from Wu AW et al: Do house officers learn from their mistakes? JAMA 1991;265:2089. © Copyright 1991, American Medical Association.

lems in communication) were more common than errors in technical performance or medical and nursing staff coordination.

Causes

A combination of individual and system-related factors can lead to mistakes. Individual factors include forgetfulness, inattention, poor motivation, carelessness, negligence, and recklessness.

Physicians report a variety of reasons for their mistakes and frequently attribute the mistakes to more than one cause. In one study, house officers most often reported that mistakes were caused in part because they did not possess specific essential knowledge (eg, being unaware of the significance of a prolonged episode of ventricular tachycardia). Almost as often they cited "too many tasks" (one resident neglected to continue a required medication because he was "too busy with other sick patients, and supervising interns and students"). Fatigue was a significant factor (after inadvertently ordering potassium replacement as a bolus, one resident commented, "It was 3:00 AM, and I'm not sure I was completely awake").

A systems-oriented view acknowledges that errors are expected even in the best organizations. Many errors are caused by conditions in the workplace and organizational processes largely independent of clinician attributes. Examples include understaffing, inadequate equipment, long work hours, time pressure, and poor team functioning. There have been few studies of the impact of these factors.

One study of an inpatient medical service found cross-coverage to be a significant predictor of preventable adverse events. Recent studies suggest that staffing ratios tend to be related to patient outcomes. The pressures of prac-

ticing medicine in a managed care setting, especially in capitated systems with higher demands for productivity, may increase the risk that a hurried physician will overlook important diagnostic information or make an error in a prescription. Similarly, the incentives offered by third-party payers to order fewer diagnostic tests and to limit the number of referrals to subspecialists can lead to errors of omission.

Circumstances

Mistakes seem to occur frequently during residency training, possibly because interns and residents are learning new skills, honing their clinical judgment, and accepting new responsibilities. Additionally, they are caring for patients who are acutely ill. Although first-year residents according to one study made the highest proportion of prescription errors (4.25 per 1000 orders), more experienced physicians have also reported making serious medical mistakes.

Many mistakes happen in the inpatient or emergency department setting. Severely ill patients require rapid assessment of a complex clinical picture as well as multiple procedures, evaluations, and decisions, thus affording many opportunities for mistakes to occur. One study found that patients in intensive care units had on average 178 activities performed on them, with 1.7 errors observed per day. Patient characteristics can also increase the risk of mistakes. The risk of iatrogenic events increases with increased age, severity of illness, length of hospital stay, and number of drugs prescribed. Older patients, for example, are likely to have advanced disease and comorbid conditions and are more likely to be taking numerous medications. These factors increase both the risk of errors and the likelihood that complications of treatment will make these errors consequential.

Serious medical mistakes certainly occur in office practice. Some practicing physicians contend that the probability of making a serious error increases with more years in practice and particularly with greater pressures to increase productivity.

THE OUTCOMES OF MEDICAL MISTAKES

Consequences for Patient & Family

Errors, even serious errors if recognized and corrected, may have no major consequences. In such cases, clinicians may not even acknowledge that a mistake has occurred. Often, however, serious errors have significant consequences for the patients involved, such as physical discomfort, emotional distress, the need for additional therapy or procedures, increased and prolonged hospital stay, worsening of disease, permanent disability, or death. Mistakes can also cause distress for family members, including worry, anger, and guilt, particularly if they were involved in making treatment decisions.

Consequences for Physicians & Colleagues

Physicians also experience emotional distress in reaction to a medical mistake, often reporting a variety of emotional responses from remorse, anger, guilt, and feelings of inadequacy to shame and fear—particularly the fear of negative repercussions, such as malpractice suits. After a fatal mistake involving a young patient, one house officer wrote, "This event has been the greatest challenge to me in my training."

Physicians occasionally report persistent negative psychological effects from mistakes. After a mistake caused the death of a patient, one house officer commented, "This case has made me very nervous about clinical medicine. I worry now about all febrile patients, since they may be on the verge of sepsis." For another house officer, a missed diagnosis made him reject a career in subspecialties that would involve "a lot of data collection and uncertainty."

Consequences for the Physician–Patient Relationship

In some cases, depending on the severity of the outcome for the patient and the quality of communication between physician and patient, the physician–patient relationship may be harmed by a mistake. For the physician, feelings of guilt and shame or shaken confidence may lead to avoidance of the patient or to a diminution of open and frank discussion. One physician, for example, reported that his guilt from the death of a patient led him to act like an indentured servant to the patient's family, attempting to expiate his "crime" over a prolonged period of time by spending more time with the family and reducing his fees.

For the patient, learning about a mistake may cause alarm and anxiety, destroying the patient's faith and confidence in the physician's ability to help. There may be anger, an erosion of trust, decreased respect, or feelings of betrayal that diminish openness. Patients may become disillusioned with the medical profession in general, causing them to reduce their adherence to beneficial treatments or habits.

To the extent that doctor and patient can discuss their emotions directly and with mutual understanding and acceptance, the relationship is likely to endure; it may even deepen with time. The negative effect of a mistake on the doctor–patient relationship may also be mitigated if there is a history of shared decision making, which diffuses the responsibility of the physician, especially when there has been uncertainty about treatment.

It should be noted also that mistakes that are nationally—or even locally—reported in the press can damage public trust in the medical profession. Any loss of credibility can be harmful to the public health by creating cynicism about medical care and research and discouraging individuals from seeking care or adopting healthful behaviors.

RESPONDING TO MEDICAL MISTAKES

The way in which physicians respond to mistakes can turn these experiences into powerful opportunities for learning and for personal growth. Figure 32–1 outlines a strategy for responding to a mistake, either made by oneself or made by a colleague.

Individual Responses

After recognizing that a mistake has occurred, the first step is to take any corrective action possible, followed by beginning to cope, disclosure to the patient, disclosure to colleagues and Risk Management (sooner if there is a serious adverse outcome), and attempting to learn from the incident.

COPING WITH MISTAKES

Two major modes of coping are problem focused, in which coping is directed at the problem causing the distress, and emotion focused, in which coping is directed at managing the emotional distress caused by the problem (Table 32–2). Effective coping can prevent unhealthy responses such as denial, cynicism, and excessive concern. The use of effective coping strategies can also play a role in modulating physician stress and increasing physician work satisfaction.

Table 32–2 briefly summarizes some of the many possible strategies for coping with medical mistakes. Among these, accepting responsibility and problem-solving techniques may be those most often used. As an example, "accepting responsibility" would include statements such as "I made a promise to myself that things would be different next time"; "I criticized or lectured myself"; and "I apologized or did something to make it up." Seeking social support and controlling emotions may be somewhat less frequently employed, and escape-avoidance and distancing are used even more rarely.

Accepting responsibility is a prerequisite to an individual learning from a mistake, and physicians who cope by accepting responsibility for their mistakes seem to be more likely to make constructive changes in practice. They may also be more likely to experience emotional distress, however, as in the case of the resident who described persistent feelings of guilt and shame after realizing that inappropriate management of a diabetic patient's foot ulcer led to an amputation.

DISCLOSURE TO PATIENTS AND FAMILIES

It is difficult to disclose mistakes to patients or their families, and several reports suggest that physicians are reluctant to tell patients about mistakes. There are many

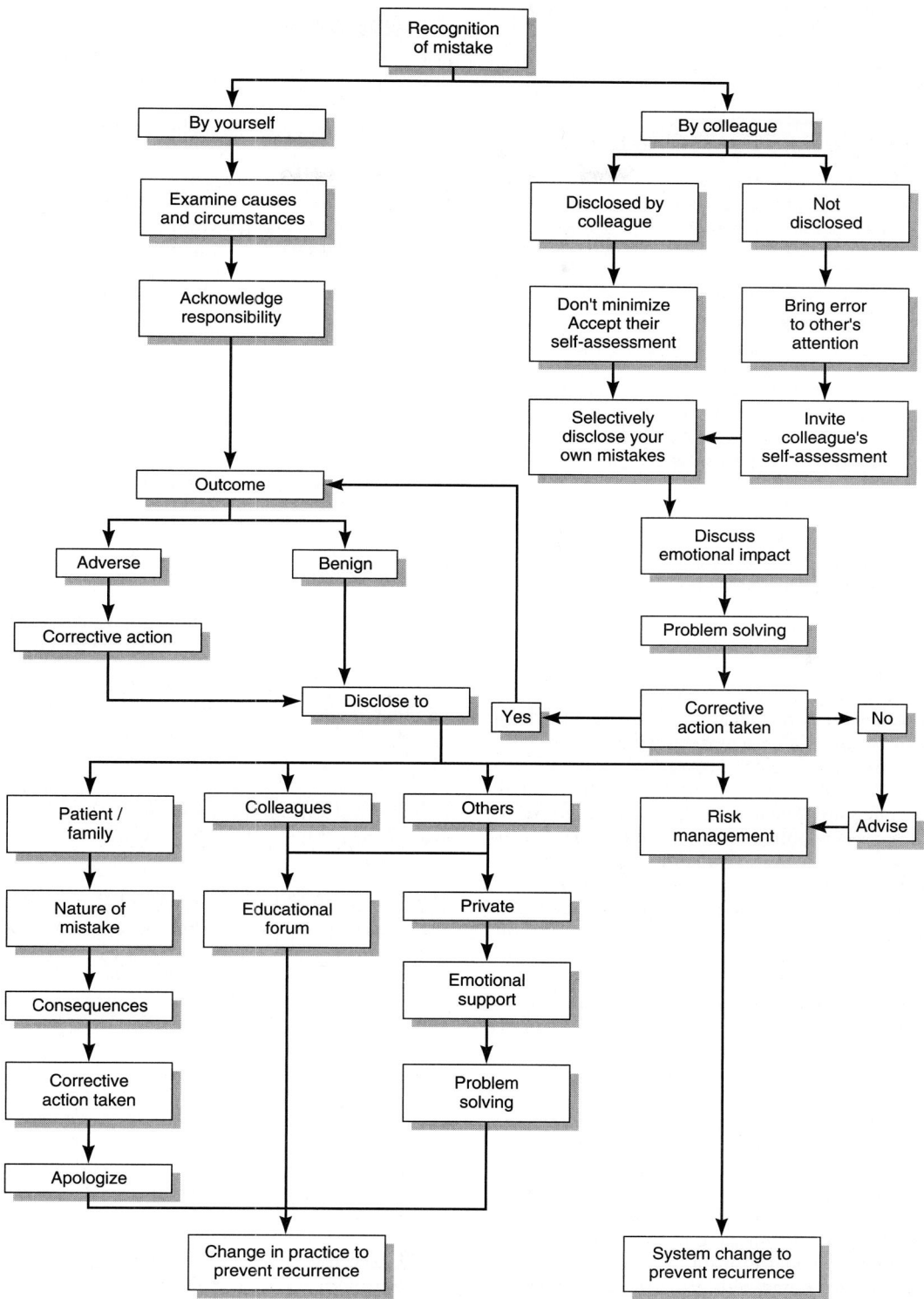

Figure 32–1. Process of responding to a mistake.

Table 32–2. Potential strategies for coping with medical mistakes.

Approach	Strategy
Problem focused	Acceptance of responsibility
	Consultation to understand nature of mistake
	Consultation to correct mistake
	Planned problem solving (eg, obtaining extra training)
Emotion focused	Pursuance of social support
	Disclosure to colleague, friend, or spouse
	Disclosure to patient
	Emotional self-control (eg, repressing one's emotional response)
	Escape-avoidance
	Distancing
	Reframing of mistake (eg, recognizing it as inherent in practicing medicine)

Source: Adapted, with permission, from Wu AW et al: How house officers cope with their mistakes. West J Med 1993; 159:565; and Christensen JF et al: The heart of darkness: The impact of perceived mistakes on physicians. J Gen Intern Med 1992;7:424.

barriers to disclosure include fear for one's reputation, as well as fear of disciplinary action and litigation. Even the National Practitioner Databank, designed to improve quality of care, provokes fear and resentment among physicians. In one study, such disclosure was reported by less than 25% of house officers. Professional societies, including the American Medical Association and American College of Physicians, as well as legal and ethical experts suggest that in general physicians should disclose errors to those involved. In 2001, the Joint Commission on Accreditation of Healthcare Organizations stated that clinicians are obliged to disclose errors to the patient. Disclosure of a mistake also fosters learning by compelling the physician to acknowledge the error truthfully. In addition, when there are serious adverse consequences, disclosing a mistake to the patient may be the only way for the physician to achieve a sense of absolution.

Because there are no guidelines on how to tell a patient about a mistake that has been made, physicians must develop their own approach to each case. Disclosure and discussion of an error with the patient or family can be made easier by several techniques. Physicians should first try to acknowledge their own emotions. Before approaching the patient or family, it may be helpful for physicians to perform a simple relaxation exercise and to remind themselves that the event and present feelings do not define them as either a healer or as a person. Rehearsing a few simple, di-

rect statements ahead of time can provide a road map in this awkward moment. When meeting the patient or family, the physician should make a brief, direct statement, accompanied by a genuine apology. Such directness may help avoid the kind of long and rambling discussion that often increases anxiety for both physician and patient.

The physician who has mistakenly prescribed a medication without checking the patient's allergies, for example, might tell the patient: "Mr. Jones, I've discovered what made you sick last week. I regret to say that I failed to check whether you were allergic to the antibiotic before I prescribed it. You are allergic to it, and that information is clearly written in your chart. I feel awful that my not checking has caused you so much distress. I am truly sorry." It would then be appropriate to pause and allow the patient to respond. Reflecting and accepting the patient's feelings can help to heal the relationship more effectively than overwhelming the patient with information. The doctor–patient relationship can be enhanced by honesty and empathy in this difficult and sensitive moment (see Chapter 3). It is possible that disclosure of an error of which the patient had been unaware may lead to a lawsuit, particularly if there was serious harm. However, it is certain that the risk of a lawsuit is multiplied if there is an attempt at covering the mistake up. Risk may be reduced if disclosure is made promptly, if the patient appreciates the physician's honesty, if it is part of an ongoing dialogue about the patient's care, and if there is a sincere apology. In the event of serious injury, a prompt and fair settlement may be the most helpful measure. There is little research on this topic. However, the favorable experience of the Lexington Kentucky VA Medical Center, which instituted a proactive policy of full disclosure and assistance for the patient in filing claims, suggests that this strategy may decrease the institution's losses.

DISCLOSURE TO COLLEAGUES AND THE INSTITUTION

It may be very important for colleagues to know about a mistake, particularly if they are also participating in the care of the patient as a supervisor or other member of the team. Knowing about a mistake can also benefit the institution, enabling it to provide assistance in handling the mistake, to help individuals appreciate the causes or significance of the incident and learn from the incident, and to prevent future occurrences. However, physicians also seem to be reluctant to tell their colleagues about mistakes. Some physicians report that they find this kind of discussion both threatening, because of the fear of judgment by colleagues, and unhelpful, because of the tendency of colleagues to minimize the event. Most often, discussing mistakes with colleagues serves the purpose of problem-focused coping: correcting the situation that led to the mistake. Sharing mistakes with colleagues can also prevent isolation and start the necessary healing process of remorse and learning.

CHANGES IN PRACTICE

Table 32–3 summarizes changes in practice that often follow medical mistakes. These changes can either be constructive or they can be defensive—and maladaptive—in nature. Constructive changes cited by physicians include paying more attention to detail, confirming clinical data personally, changing protocols for diagnosis and treatment, increasing self-care, changing methods of communication with staff, and being willing to seek advice. Additional constructive action includes attempting to effect institutional change to prevent future incidents.

Physicians also report making defensive changes. These include an unwillingness to discuss the mistake, avoidance of similar patients, and—in some circumstances—ordering additional tests. Defensive changes in practice are more likely to occur if the institutional response to a mistake is punitive or judgmental.

LEARNING FROM MISTAKES

Several factors may determine the extent to which physicians learn from mistakes. When negative emotions such as shame, guilt, or humiliation follow from the mistake, the physician's energy may focus on the emotional aspects of coping. Addressing these negative emotions directly can enhance the physician's ability to learn new information or new approaches to the problem. Failure to appreciate

Table 32–3. Common changes in practice following mistakes.

Constructive Changes	Defensive Changes
Increasing information seeking	Being unwilling to discuss the error
• Asking advice	Avoiding patients with similar problems
• Reading	Ordering additional but unnecessary tests
Increasing vigilance	
• Paying more attention to detail	
• Confirming data personally	
• Changing data organization	
• Ordering additional tests as appropriate	
• Improving screening for disease	
• Improving communication with patients	
Improving self-pacing	
Improving communication with staff	
Supervising others more closely	

these emotions can lead to denial. The cause to which the physician attributes the mistake can also affect learning. Physicians in one study were more likely to report constructive changes if the mistake was caused by inexperience or faulty judgment in a complex case; they were less likely to do so if they believed that the mistake was caused by job overload. Physicians who responded to the mistake with greater acceptance of responsibility and more discussion were also more likely to report constructive changes.

RESPONDING TO COLLEAGUES WHO MAKE MISTAKES

When responding to a colleague who discloses a mistake, it is important to try to elicit or accept the colleague's self-assessment and to not minimize the importance of the mistake. At this point, a selective and discreet disclosure of one's own mistakes can reduce the colleague's sense of isolation and legitimize the discussion. It is then appropriate to inquire about the emotional effect of the mistake and how the colleague is coping with it. An important consideration here is that negative emotions are not necessarily problems to be solved, and they can often be mitigated by acknowledging them. The clinician should return to the content of the mistake and help the colleague to correct it with problem-solving techniques, making the necessary changes in practice and incorporating the new lessons that have been learned.

WITNESSING MISTAKES BY OTHERS

A physician who sees a mistake made by another physician has several options: passively waiting for the physician to disclose the mistake, advising the physician to disclose the mistake, actively telling the patient oneself, or arranging a joint meeting to discuss the mistake. Although some physicians may feel an obligation to report mistakes they have seen, most are reluctant to say anything. Here again, there are many barriers to discussion, including fear of eliciting anger and threatening relationships with colleagues or interference with sources of referrals.

The simplest option, of course, is to wait for the physician who made the mistake to report it. There is no assurance, however, that the patient will actually be informed. Telling the patient directly may be awkward, particularly if the observing physician does not know the patient, and may interfere with the existing doctor–patient relationship. Advising the physician who made the error to tell the patient may fulfill the observing physician's responsibility for disclosure, but the patient may still not be informed. Simultaneously advising the physician and the hospital or clinic quality-assurance or risk-management personnel increases the likelihood that the patient will be told. Arranging a joint conference can satisfy the observer that appropriate disclosure is made while preserving the primacy of the relationship between the patient and the treating physician (Figure 32–1).

Institutional Responses

HOSPITALS

Physicians sometimes feel that the hospital's atmosphere inhibits them from talking about their mistakes and that its administration is judgmental about mistakes. To avoid a vicious circle of blame, denial, and repeated problems, it is crucial for senior leadership in hospitals to assume a blame-free attitude that encourages the reporting and handling of errors. Some institutions have formal settings for discussing mistakes, such as morbidity and mortality conferences. However, important issues such as a discussion of the physician's feelings about the mistake and disclosure by colleagues of how they coped with their own mistakes are commonly avoided in these conferences. The risk-management departments of hospitals could take a leading role in this area—promoting comprehensive, supportive forums for discussing mistakes and using emotion-focused coping to maximize problem-focused learning and to minimize future errors.

GRADUATE MEDICAL EDUCATION

In spite of fears of public disclosure of mistakes, there is growing consensus that patient safety, physician fallibility, and methods of handling medical errors are appropriate topics for medical school, residency, and fellowship training. Although they may experience initial reluctance, physicians sometimes find that discussing a mistake is a positive experience: "Presenting this case at interns' report was difficult—I felt under a lot of scrutiny from my peers. In the end, I felt as though I had gotten more respect from presenting this kind of case rather than one in which I had made a great diagnosis."

Mistakes can be discussed in attending rounds, at morning report, or at morbidity and mortality conferences. When mistakes are discussed in these conferences, it is important to address issues such as overwork, shared responsibility with other physicians (eg, consultants, attending physicians), and appropriate protocols for communicating with staff. In addition, although ensuring that everyone involved learns from the mistake, care should be taken that errors are seen as an unfortunate inevitability in the practice of medicine and that there are appropriate ways of coping with them and of responding to colleagues who make them. A few organizations have begun to organize regular "fallibility rounds," interdisciplinary conferences focused on promoting patient safety that recognize the many factors that contribute to errors.

PRIMARY CARE PRACTICE GROUPS

As group practice becomes the norm in managed care settings, it is important that such groups implement procedures for responding to mistakes. Collegial support should be an explicit rule, providing a safe and confidential setting for discussion of the mistake (see the guidelines discussed earlier for responding to a colleague's mistake). It would also be wise for the practice group to formalize—and thus legitimize—periodic discussions about mistakes; these could broaden the scope of the emotion-focused support, allow members to learn from colleagues' mistakes, and address system flaws that contribute to the mistakes. A bonus of this approach is the gain in personal well-being of the group members—a nonspecific, yet significant, contribution to the practice climate.

PREVENTING MISTAKES

Reducing the frequency and severity of mistakes is the highest priority. There are several ways to help physicians learn from their mistakes and to make constructive changes in practice.

Physician Responsibility

As noted earlier, physicians should be encouraged to accept responsibility for their mistakes. Although those who do so seem more likely than those who do not to make constructive changes in practice, accepting responsibility for mistakes can engender emotional distress. It is therefore important for colleagues and supervising physicians to respond with sensitivity to the distress of practitioners acknowledging their mistakes. The probability of future mistakes can be reduced if the current error can be reviewed in a way that decreases emotional distress, invites disclosure of uncertainty in diagnosis and management, and leads to a discussion of appropriate changes in practice.

Administration & Supervision

Efforts to forestall errors must begin at the highest administrative levels. Leadership acknowledgment of the inevitability of errors and making patient safety an explicit priority are crucial in helping institutions learn from mistakes. Clinically, more active supervision may prevent some mistakes or mitigate their adverse effects. Senior physicians should be more available to their less experienced colleagues for help in making critical decisions about patient care, especially in complex cases that require more mature clinical judgment. Group practice administrators and training-program directors should correct problems in staffing, scheduling, and the nature of work—which may all contribute to mistakes. Serious attention must be paid to the workload. Sleep deprivation during training may be a source of errors; job overload, fatigue, and being expected to perform too many tasks can also lead to mistakes. Working under these conditions may teach house officers to tolerate and rationalize errors; in addition, it may make them less likely to seek the corrective information that could help prevent future mistakes.

Identifying & Reporting Errors

Delineating the cause of a mistake often suggests specific strategies for preventing future mistakes. Routine mechanisms to identify adverse events, such as anonymous reporting by physicians and nurses or computerized feedback about adverse drug reactions, are beginning to prove useful in providing information about the frequency and nature of mistakes. Developing routine methods of conveying information, such as computerized forms that standardize the type and amount of information exchanged between covering physicians, can also reduce errors.

Computerized systems are becoming available that include artificial intelligence to detect and avert medication errors, including overdoses, incorrect routes of administration, drug interactions, and allergies. Computerized order entry systems and bar-coding of medications, blood products, and patients have also been shown to reduce the incidence of adverse events.

Managed Care

The demands of practicing in a managed care setting may increase a busy physician's susceptibility to making mistakes. Fatigue, information overload, and increased pressure to be a more productive member of the practice by seeing more patients for less time can lead the physician to overlook important information. In addition, the role of the physician as the gatekeeper of referrals to specialists in most managed care plans, along with financial incentives for holding down the number of referrals, tests, hospital admissions, and hospital days, has the potential for increasing errors of omission. Ironically, the risk of malpractice litigation may counter this tendency by inducing physicians to practice defensively by ordering more tests. Within the extremes of these incentives and disincentives, there is a need for continuing education of physicians on standards of practice with regard to tests, referrals, and further treatment.

Both physicians and institutions should make whatever changes in practice are warranted to prevent new mistakes and to prevent the recurrence of similar events. Recognizing and dealing with mistakes honestly and directly can improve the quality of patient care and lead to a more rewarding practice.

SUGGESTED READINGS

Anderson RE, Hill RB, Key CR: The sensitivity and specificity of clinical diagnostics during five decades: toward an understanding of necessary fallibility. JAMA 1989;261:1610.

Andrews LB et al: An alternative strategy for studying adverse events in medical care. Lancet 1997;349:309.

Applegate WB: Physician management of patients with adverse outcomes. Arch Intern Med 1986;146:2249.

Bates DW et al: Reducing the frequency of errors in medicine using information technology. J Am Med Inform Assoc 2001;8:299.

Brennan TA et al: Incidence of adverse events and negligence in hospitalized patients: results of the Harvard Medical Practice Study I. N Engl J Med 1991;324:370.

Carmichael DH: Learning medical fallibility. South Med J 1985; 78:1.

Christensen JF, Levinson W, Dunn PM: The heart of darkness: the impact of perceived mistakes on physicians. J Gen Intern Med 1992;7:424.

Classen DC et al: Computerized surveillance of adverse drug events in hospital patients. JAMA 1991;266:2847.

Colford JM, McPhee SJ: The raveled sleeve of care: managing the stresses of residency training. JAMA 1989;261:889.

Donchin Y et al: A look into the nature and causes of human errors in the intensive care unit. Crit Care Med 1995;23:294.

Dubovsky SL, Schrier RW: The mystique of medical training: is teaching perfection in medical house-staff training a reasonable goal or a precursor of low self-esteem? JAMA 1983;250:3057.

Folkman S, Lazarus RS: The Ways of Coping. Consulting Psychologist Press, 1988.

Gander PH et al: Hours of work and fatigue-related error: a survey of New Zealand anaesthetists. Anaesth Intensive Care 2000;28:178.

Hilfiker D: Facing our mistakes. N Engl J Med 1984;310:118.

Institute of Medicine, Committee on Quality of Health Care in America. In: Briere R (editor): Crossing the Quality Chasm. National Academy Press, 2001.

Kraman SS: A risk management program based on full disclosure and trust: does everyone win? Compr Ther 2001;27:253.

Kraman SS, Hamm G: Risk management: extreme honesty may be the best policy. Ann Intern Med 1999;131:963.

Kravitz RL, Rolph JE, McGuigan K: Malpractice claims data as a quality improvement tool, 1. Epidemiology of error in four specialties. JAMA 1991;266:2087.

Laine C et al: The impact of regulations restricting medical house staff working hours on the quality of patient care. JAMA 1993;269:374.

Leape LL: Error in medicine. JAMA 1994;272:1851.

Leape LL et al: The nature of adverse events in hospitalized patients: results of Harvard Medical Practice Study II. N Engl J Med 1991;324:377.

Lesar TS et al: Medication prescribing errors in a teaching hospital. JAMA 1990;263:2329.

Levinson W, Dunn PM: Coping with fallibility. JAMA 1989;261: 2252.

Lo B: Disclosing mistakes. In: Lo B (editor): Problems in Ethics. Williams & Wilkins, 1994.

Meyer BA: A student teaching module: physician errors. Fam Med 1989;21:299.

Mizrahi T: Managing medical mistakes: ideology, insularity and accountability among internists-in-training. Soc Sci Med 1984;196:135.

O'Neil AC et al: Physician reporting compared with medical-record review to identify adverse medical events. Ann Intern Med 1993;119:370.

Petersen LA et al: Does housestaff discontinuity of care increase the risk of preventable adverse events? Ann Intern Med 1994; 121:866.

Pollack C et al: The clinician's role in finding resolution after a medical error. Forthcoming.

Pronovost PJ et al: Organizational characteristics of intensive care units related to outcomes of abdominal aortic surgery. JAMA 1999;281:1310.

Reason JT: *Human Error.* Cambridge University Press, 1990.

Risser DT et al: The potential for improved teamwork to reduce medical errors in the emergency department. The MedTeams Research Consortium. Ann Emerg Med 1999;34:373.

Runciman WB et al: A comparison of iatrogenic injury studies in Australia and America 2: a review of behaviour and quality of care. Int J Qual Health Care 1999;12:379.

Sexton JB et al: Error, stress, and teamwork in medicine and aviation: cross sectional surveys. BMJ 2000;320:745.

Sorensen JR: Biomedical innovation, uncertainty, and the doctor-patient interaction. J Health Soc Behav 1974;15:366.

Steel K et al: Iatrogenic illness on a general medical service at a university hospital. New Engl J Med 1981;304:638.

Thomas EJ et al: Incidence and types of adverse events and negligent care in Utah and Colorado. Med Care 2000;38:261.

Vincent C et al: Framework for analysing risk and safety in clinical medicine. BMJ 1998;316:1154.

Wilson RMcL et al: The Quality in Australian Healthcare Study. Med J Aust 1995;163:458.

Wu AW et al: Do house officers learn from their mistakes? JAMA 1991;265:2089.

Wu AW et al: How house officers cope with their mistakes: doing better but feeling worse? West J Med 1993;159:565.

Wu AW et al: To tell the truth: ethical and practical issues in disclosing medical mistakes to patients. J Gen Intern Med 1997; 12:770.

Domestic Violence

Mitchell D. Feldman, MD, MPhil

INTRODUCTION

Domestic violence is defined as any intentional, controlling behavior consisting of physical, sexual, or psychological assaults in the context of an intimate relationship. The data on domestic violence underscore the magnitude of the problem. In a landmark study, 28% of a random nationwide sample of couples reported violence at some point in their history; almost 4% of the women reported severe violence. If these figures are extrapolated to the general population, it is estimated that 4–8 million women in the United States are subject to battering each year. Women visiting outpatient medical and obstetric/gynecologic clinics as well as the emergency department are often there for complaints directly attributable to domestic violence. Because these complaints are frequently misdiagnosed, they may return time and time again, often with increasingly severe trauma.

Despite its magnitude in society and in medical settings, until recently domestic violence could be described as a "silent epidemic." Considered a private, family problem by the government, and a social problem by the medical establishment, victims of domestic violence often had nowhere to turn. This predicament has gradually improved. Domestic violence is now acknowledged to be an important public health problem, and primary care practitioners now have a variety of diagnostic and treatment guidelines available to them (see Suggested Readings). All primary care practitioners must be knowledgeable about and comfortable with the evaluation and care of patients who are subjected to domestic violence.

EPIDEMIOLOGY

Research conducted in a variety of medical settings has reported on the prevalence of domestic violence. Cross-sectional studies from outpatient primary care clinics and emergency department settings have found the prevalence of domestic violence among women to be from 6% to 28%; lifetime prevalence rates up to 50% have been reported. Similar rates have been reported by studies conducted in obstetric/gynecologic outpatient clinics. In fact, pregnancy may double the risk of domestic violence. Differences in prevalence of domestic violence among different studies can be explained, in part, by their use of different definitions of domestice violence.

Most studies ask about violence exclusively in the context of heterosexual relationships. A similar prevalence of domestic violence appears to exist in gay and lesbian relationships, with the same physical and emotional consequences. Primary care providers should be aware that it may be more difficult for gay and lesbian patients to disclose that they are in an abusive relationship. In addition, the commonly held bias that violence does not occur in these relationships ("women can't hurt women") further lowers detection rates.

Men report being physically abused by their female partners at rates just below those reported by women. The injuries inflicted by women on men, however, are insignificant when compared with same-sex or male-on-female violence, so are not a significant public health or medical problem.

DIAGNOSIS

Many battered women seek medical care both for the direct and indirect sequelae of their battering. Yet only a small percentage of them are diagnosed and treated appropriately. The following case is illustrative of the type of patient commonly seen in the primary care setting.

 CASE ILLUSTRATION

A 40-year-old nurse presents to the general medical clinic with a chief complaint of a headache. She reports having been in a motor vehicle accident 3 days earlier and striking her head on the dashboard. She says that her friends encouraged her to come in, and she is accompanied to the clinic (but not the office) by her partner. On physical examination she appears tense and sad, with bilateral, periorbital ecchymoses.

History

A thorough history is the cornerstone of the diagnosis of domestic violence. Because the presentation is often subtle, with few dramatic injuries, detection requires a high index of suspicion. There are many clues in the medical history, as shown by the case illustration, that should prompt the physician to evaluate the patient for domestic violence (Table 33–1). Clues that should prompt further inquiry include

- Delay in seeking care
- Illogical explanation of injury
- Multiple somatic complaints
- Depression, anxiety, and other mental disorders
- Pregnancy
- Substance use
- Recent diagnosis of human immunodeficiency virus (HIV)
- Family history of domestic violence
- Overbearing partner

DELAY IN SEEKING CARE

Patients who have been assaulted often delay seeking medical attention, in contrast to accident victims who generally seek out medical attention immediately.

ILLOGICAL EXPLANATION OF INJURY

Injuries that are attributed to a mechanism that seems illogical should always raise concern. For example, periorbital ecchymoses ("black eyes") are generally not caused by a motor vehicle accident, a "door knob," or anything other than a fist.

MULTIPLE SOMATIC COMPLAINTS

Some women may present with vague somatic complaints as their only symptom of domestic violence. Fatigue, sleep disturbances, headache, gastrointestinal complaints, abdominal and pelvic pain, genitourinary problems such as frequent urinary tract and genital infections, chest pain, palpitations, and dizziness are just some of the complaints with which women present. Domestic violence should be considered as a sole or contributing cause of these problems.

Table 33–1. When to screen
for domestic violence.

Delay in seeking care
Illogical explanation of injury
Multiple somatic complaints
Depression, anxiety, and other mental disorders
Pregnancy
Substance use
Recent diagnosis of HIV
Family history of domestic violence
Overbearing partner

DEPRESSION, ANXIETY, AND OTHER MENTAL DISORDERS

Depression, eating disorders, and anxiety disorders such as posttraumatic stress disorder and panic disorder are more common among victims of domestic violence than among the general population. If present, the primary care provider should always screen for domestic violence. These emotional disturbances should be thought of as a consequence, not a cause, of the domestic violence. Some patients may feel hopeless and turn toward suicide as a way out. One of every 10 battered women attempts suicide. Of those, 50% try more than once.

PREGNANCY

Many studies have demonstrated that women are at increased risk of physical and sexual abuse during pregnancy. Clues to be alert for include delay in seeking prenatal care, depressed or anxious mood, injuries to breasts or abdomen, frequent spontaneous abortions, and preterm labor. In addition to the physical and emotional trauma to the pregnant woman, these assaults can result in placental separation, fetal fractures, and fetal demise.

SUBSTANCE ABUSE

Although violence and substance abuse often coexist, it is inaccurate and generally not helpful to frame domestic violence as secondary to the substance abuse. Although the perpetrator, and at times the woman herself, often asserts that the violence was a consequence of altered behavior from drugs or alcohol, in fact, the violent behavior must be addressed as a separate issue and is unlikely to end even if the substance abuse does.

Conversely, some studies have found an increased rate of substance use in victims of domestic violence. At times, this may take the form of increased use of pain medications or anxiolytics in an effort to cope with the assaults. It is even more imperative in this instance that physicians not attribute the domestic violence to the substance use; it is precisely this mentality of "blaming the victim" that has often prevented the appropriate evaluation and treatment of domestic violence in all medical settings.

RECENT DIAGNOSIS OF HIV

Some women report an initiation or escalation of domestic violence after informing their partner of their HIV seropositive status. Although every attempt should be made to notify sexual partners of HIV-positive results, practitioners should assess their patient's risk of violence while discussing the issues surrounding notification. Discussion of domestic violence and review of a safety plan should always be part of posttest counseling.

FAMILY HISTORY OF DOMESTIC VIOLENCE

Patients who report a family history of domestic violence, particularly those who witnessed parental violence as a child or adolescent, are at increased risk themselves even if they are not presently in an abusive relationship. Such women should therefore be educated and screened more carefully.

OVERBEARING PARTNER

An overbearing partner who, for example, insists on accompanying the patient into the examining room, acts overly solicitous or concerned (sometimes to the point of knocking on the examining room door to inquire about her well-being), or is hostile to the health care team may be a clue to the presence of domestic violence. Never probe about domestic violence if the perpetrator is in the examining room as this may unintentionally escalate the violence and put the patient in extreme danger.

NOT SOCIOECONOMIC OR ETHNIC STATUS

Many health care providers mistakenly believe that domestic violence disproportionately affects persons in particular ethnic or socioeconomic groups; in fact, it cuts across all ethnic groups and all economic strata. Although some studies have found that women who are uninsured or on medical assistance are at increased risk of domestic violence, this is most likely due to selection bias in the studies. Women from lower socioeconomic status (SES) groups may be overrepresented in some statistics because those from higher SES groups have more resources available to them and the abuse is therefore more likely to remain hidden. Women with fewer resources are forced to take refuge in shelters or county hospital emergency departments, for example, whereas their middle-class counterparts may flee to a hotel or their offices and are therefore underrepresented by some of the surveys.

Physical Examination

The physical examination may provide the first clues of the presence of domestic violence (Table 33–2), including

- Inappropriate behavior
- Multiple injuries
- Central pattern of injury
- Injuries at different stages of healing

INAPPROPRIATE BEHAVIOR

Behavior that appears to be inappropriate at the time of the physical examination may be a sign of domestic violence.

Table 33–2. Physical examination clues to the presence of domestic violence.

Inappropriate behavior
Multiple injuries
Central pattern of injury
Injuries at different stages of healing

Fright, inappropriate embarrassment or laughter, anxiety, passivity, shyness, and avoidance of eye contact may all be clues that the patient has been battered.

MULTIPLE INJURIES

Battered women are more likely to have multiple injuries than are ordinary accident victims. Victims of domestic violence, for example, typically have injuries to the head, neck, abdomen, and chest, whereas accident victims often are able to protect themselves, at least in part, and present with less widespread trauma. The common emotional reactions to assault of denial, confusion, and withdrawal may also lead to more extensive injuries.

CENTRAL PATTERN OF INJURY

Victims of domestic violence often experience injuries such as bruises, lacerations, burns, bites, and more severe injuries secondary to assaults with a deadly weapon or repeated beatings that cause massive internal injuries and fractures. Injuries are most commonly seen in the central areas of the body—the head, neck, chest, abdomen, breasts—and occasionally upper arms from fending off blows.

INJURIES AT DIFFERENT STAGES OF HEALING

As with child abuse, multiple injuries at different stages of healing should always prompt an inquiry about domestic violence.

In summary, primary care providers must be alert to the signs and symptoms of domestic violence. It is important to remember that most domestic violence victims do not present with injuries that require emergency treatment or lead to hospitalization. In fact, for many patients, even in emergency departments, the presenting complaint is often medical or psychological, rather than an actual physical injury. For this reason, detection of domestic violence will increase only if practitioners include it on the differential diagnosis and actively screen for it during the medical encounter.

Screening for Domestic Violence

Questions about domestic violence should be a routine part of the history and physical examination for all female patients. Some practitioners also screen men, particularly men in intimate relationships with other men. This can be done by including questions about abuse on the medical history questionnaire, verbally as a part of the social or past medical history, or (preferably) both. It may help some patients to feel more comfortable revealing domestic violence by screening with the following sorts of questions: "We all fight at home. What happens when you or your partner fight or disagree?" or "Because abuse and violence are so common in women's lives, I've begun to ask about it routinely. At any time, has a partner hit or otherwise hurt or threatened you?" (see Table 33–3 for suggested screening

Table 33–3. Screening questions.

- We all fight at home sometimes. What happens when you or your partner fight or disagree?
- Do you feel safe in your home and in your relationship?
- Do you ever feel afraid of your partner?
- Because abuse and violence are so common in women's lives, I've begun to ask about it routinely. At any time, has a partner hit or otherwise hurt or threatened you?
- Does your partner ever force you to engage in sex that makes you feel uncomfortable?
- Does your partner threaten, hit, or abuse your children?

---

questions). If the answer is vague or evasive, more direct questions must be asked to determine if abuse is taking place. If this is done in a supportive, nonjudgmental manner, the vast majority of patients feel comfortable and respond honestly.

TREATMENT

When domestic violence is detected, five basic tasks must be accomplished (Table 33–4). First, validate the problem by making a clear statement to the patient that violent behavior is unacceptable and illegal, and that nobody has the right to abuse her. The physician's acknowledgment of the domestic violence as a real issue may be the first step in helping to free her from the abuse. Under all circumstances, avoid language that could be interpreted as blaming the victim for the violence.

Because the majority of women are not ready to leave the relationship when the violence is detected, a main task for the primary care provider is to build the relationship with the patient. Statements that express empathy can be an effective way to accomplish this task, for example: "I really respect the way you have been dealing with this" and "we can work on this problem together." It is important to help the patient set short-term goals (eg, to obtain the skills required for a particular job) so that she is not distressed when it takes time to realize her long-term goal of ending the abuse and/or the relationship. Above all, avoid recapit-

Table 33–4. After detection: five tasks to accomplish.

---

1. Validate the problem.
2. Assess the patient's safety, and review an emergency escape plan.
3. Document clearly and completely.
4. Provide information and appropriate referral.
5. Be aware of reporting and other legal requirements.

---

ulating the power and control dynamics that so often characterize the patient's abusive relationship. Never insist that she leave the relationship and always allow her the autonomy to make her own decisions.

Second, it is essential to assess the patient's safety. Is it safe for her to go home? Other options (such as friends, shelters, etc) should be explored and an emergency escape plan reviewed if she chooses to return home. For women not returning home, advise them to inform one or two coworkers about the situation as the perpetrator may attempt to find her at work. It is important to ask if there are children who are potentially at risk. Risk factors for escalating violence such as an increase in the frequency and severity of assaults, an escalation in threats, and the availability of a firearm should be carefully assessed.

Third, it is imperative that practitioners document clearly and completely when they encounter domestic violence. The medical record should include a complete description of the assault with quotes, if possible, from the patient's own account. Include relevant details in the past medical history and social history. Be sure to write legibly; successful prosecution should never be compromised by sloppy recordkeeping. Injuries should be described and visually documented, either with a body chart or with photographs, if the patient consents (include the patient's face in at least one photograph). If the police are called, always include the name of and any actions taken by the investigating police officer.

Fourth, the patient must be provided with information and appropriate referral. Primary care providers should be familiar with the social and legal services available for battered women in their area. Information about shelters should be provided even if the woman intends to return home. All patients should be assessed for the presence of psychiatric or substance abuse problems that would benefit from treatment or referral. Practitioners should have a basic understanding of legal options, such as restraining orders, so that they can help advise women who wish to take immediate action to ensure their safety.

Finally, understand the domestic violence reporting requirements, if any, in your state. For example, in California, health practitioners are required to report to the police all incidents of domestic violence that result in an injury. The usual doctor–patient privileged communication is explicitly preempted by this law.

What to Avoid

Do not insist that the battered woman terminate the relationship, even if you believe that this is the most appropriate action. Only she can make that decision. Trying to control her behavior, albeit subtly, recapitulates the same negative dynamic that is taking place in the battering relationship.

Recommend couple counseling only when the perpetrator acknowledges the problem, wants to change his behavior, and both partners want to preserve the relationship.

Do not use the word *alleged* in the medical record. It implies that you do not believe the woman's story, and you may inadvertently impede her ability to bring her case to court.

Do not ask what the victim did to bring on the violence.

BARRIERS

Physician Barriers to Detection

Many studies have revealed that physicians and other health care practitioners do a poor job of detecting domestic violence, with detection rates rarely exceeding 10%. Several factors are responsible for this dismal record. First, many practitioners lack the appropriate knowledge and training to effectively detect and treat victims of domestic violence. The first step in improving their ability to do so is to disseminate information more widely about its prevalence and consequences and to include domestic violence in medical school, residency, and continuing medical education curricula.

Lack of institutional support is another important barrier. Despite the enormity of the problem and the increasing requirements that all health care institutions have domestic violence protocols in place, most hospitals and clinics have few, if any, adequately trained support staff, accessible guidelines for practitioners, or information for patients. In addition, with growing pressure to see more patients and use fewer resources, issues such as domestic violence may be overlooked. Many of the physicians interviewed in one study identified time constraints as the major deterrent to opening the Pandora's box of domestic violence.

It should be noted, however, that the total annual health care costs from domestic violence exceed $50 million, plus indirect costs such as lost days from paid work. In addition, the diagnostic and treatment strategies outlined here are not particularly time intensive. Inquiry about domestic violence adds less than 1 minute to the typical new patient evaluation; if widely employed, it could yield enormous savings through prevention of injury and decreased health care usage.

The third barrier to detection of domestic violence arises from practitioner discomfort. Many practitioners feel uncomfortable addressing issues that do not fit neatly into the traditional medical model. Numerous studies have shown that many do a poor job discussing issues with their patients having to do with sex, violence, and substance use. Delving into the cause of a suspicious injury may make them uneasy: it is often not amenable to a straightforward solution and may raise embarrassing or uncomfortable feelings. All practitioners must reflect on the feelings that domestic violence raises in them to be effective in caring for these vulnerable patients.

Patient Barriers to Terminating an Abusive Relationship

Primary care providers often have difficulty understanding why more battered women do not terminate their abusive relationship. Why some women remain in these relationships is complex. Some of the reasons include the following:

1. *Fear.* Fear for their own safety or for their children. One-third of women are not at home when the assault takes place, so it is clear that leaving is no guarantee of safety.

2. *Economic.* Many battered women lack employment skills or experience and would find it very difficult to support themselves and/or their children outside of the relationship.

3. Psychological. Some may find it difficult to leave because of the "psychological dependence" the years of repetitive abuse have created. Battered women are told overtly and covertly that they are "worthless"; some eventually internalize this and come to believe that they are incapable of surviving on their own.

4. *Social support—or the lack thereof.* Women are often encouraged by well-meaning friends and family members to "try to work things out," or they are advised to stay "for the children's sake."

5. *Lack of other options.* Shelters are often full, friends and family unavailable, and legal counsel not accessible.

6. Not all women want the relationship to end, just the battering.

CONCLUSION

Along with the criminal justice system, primary care physicians and other health care providers are most likely to come into contact with victims of domestic violence. They have a professional and ethical obligation to recognize domestic violence and intervene appropriately as well as to exert their influence on a broader level. This may be to push for funding of more shelters or to advocate for the teaching about domestic violence at all levels of medical education. Screening for and treating domestic violence should be a routine part of the practice and training of medicine. All primary care practitioners should confront the epidemic of domestic violence and strive to lessen its impact as one of the most important public health issues of our time.

SUGGESTED READINGS

Elliott L et al: Barriers to screening for domestic violence. J Gen Intern Med 2002;17:112.

Family Violence Prevention Fund. *Preventing Domestic Violence: Clinical Guidelines on Routine Screening.* San Francisco, CA, 1999.

McCauley J et al: Inside "Pandora's Box": abused women's experiences with clinicians and health services. J Gen Intern Med 1998;13:549.

Richardson J et al: Identifying domestic violence: cross sectional study in primary care. BMJ 2002;324:1.

Rodriguez M et al: Screening and intervention for intimate partner abuse: practices and attitudes of primary care physicians. JAMA 1999;282:468.

Stark E, Flitcraft A: *Women at Risk: Domestic Violence and Women's Health.* Sage Publications, 1996.

WEB SITES

American Bar Association Commission on Domestic Violence
http://www.abanet.org/domviol/home.html

Family Peace Project
http://www.family.mcw.edu/ahec/ec/medviol.html

Family Violence Prevention Fund
http://www.fvpf.org

Minnesota Center Against Violence and Abuse
http://www.umn.edu/mincava

Same-Sex Domestic Violence
http://www.xq.com/cuav.domviol.html

Chronic Illness

34

Gail F. Brenner, PhD

INTRODUCTION

The incidence of chronic disease in primary care practice is on the rise. Although chronic diseases comprise a diverse group of pathological processes, they share in common long-term and frequent medical intervention with little hope for a cure. Moreover, they can exert a tremendous affect on people's lives, often requiring significant life changes and reevaluation of priorities. The following diseases can be considered chronic include when their presentation is significant enough to cause impairment: diabetes, rheumatoid arthritis and other autoimmune diseases, neuromuscular diseases such as multiple sclerosis, Parkinson's disease, heart disease, stroke, asthma, emphysema, chronic obstructive pulmonary disease (COPD), and acquired immunodeficiency syndrome (AIDS).

The traditional acute-care model of the physician–patient relationship has been shown to be ineffective for patients with chronic illness. In that model, the physician is often in a directive role, informing patients how to treat their illness and expecting them to comply. The result has been a high rate of noncompliance with medical regimens and recommended life-style modifications.

An alternative framework, characterized by a partner relationship between the physician and patient, has been shown to be more effective in treating chronic illness. This chapter will describe how to implement this patient-centered partnership in the context of specific challenges faced by those with chronic illness. The ultimate goal of this approach is to empower patients to develop the skills and attitudes that will help them self-manage the multiple manifestations of their disease.

PATIENT-CENTERED PARTNERSHIP MODEL OF CARE

The role of the physician in the patient-centered partnership is to allow the patient's concerns to guide the medical interview and to consider the patient's concerns, beliefs, and life-style in codesigning an appropriate treatment program. It is useful for the physician to keep in mind that the patient will be making most of the daily treatment decisions. The following methods may be helpful:

1. Provide patient education, not as an intellectualized lecture, but within the context of the patient's life-style and interest about the disease.

2. Elicit and accept the patient's beliefs and views about the illness, symptoms, and treatment. These will guide the patient's treatment behaviors.

3. Elicit the patient's concerns at the beginning of each medical encounter.

4. Collaborate with the patient to address the concerns and design a treatment program that fits within the context of the patient's life. This may be accomplished by asking patients to help discover solutions to their concerns, with the physician giving options and inviting patients to choose.

DIFFERENT WAYS OF COPING

As it is highly effective to promote active participation of the patient in his or her care, the psychological literature on coping suggests more specific guidelines for appropriate coping responses patients can use in different situations. The goal of coping is to respond cognitively or behaviorally to manage, tolerate, or reduce the effect of a stressful event. The two major methods of coping are *problem focused* and *emotion focused*. Problem-focused coping consists of active efforts to change something about oneself or the environment. Emotion-focused coping involves efforts to regulate emotional distress. Most often, people tend to take action to solve problems, but when a stressful experience is uncontrollable, that is, nothing can be done to change it, problem-focused coping can be counterproductive. In these situations, efforts at emotional regulation may more successfully provide relief.

Consider Dan, a 29-year-old attorney recently diagnosed with insulin-dependent diabetes mellitus. With appropriate education he will learn that much of his disease is controllable. He can control his blood sugar levels by engaging in problem-focused coping responses such as frequent blood sugar testing, taking insulin as needed, and complying with diet and exercise recommendations. At times, however, he may be frightened about the possibility of future complications and frustrated with the extent to which his diabetes intrudes on his daily functioning. He may decide to cope with these feelings by distracting himself with an activity he enjoys, by seeking out someone with whom he can talk about his feelings, or by focusing on the present situation and the things he can control. These emotion-focused responses are intended to minimize his emotional distress.

The problem-focused/emotion-focused distinction in coping is useful, not only in understanding people's coping efforts, but in providing guidelines to primary care practitioners about how to facilitate patients' active involvement in their care and adaptation to chronic disease. Asking questions about patients' concerns and helping them to develop coping solutions are integral to developing a patient-centered partnership that will maximize the potential for positive treatment outcomes.

The remainder of this chapter describes the array of challenges that people with chronic disease often encounter and offers suggestions to the primary care practitioner for problem-focused and emotion-focused coping responses.

THE CYCLE OF CHRONIC DISEASE

The experience of living with many chronic illnesses has been described as the interconnection among depression, stress, pain, and the disease process or increased disability (Figure 34–1). Increasing stress in an individual's life, such as greater work demands, might lead to an increase in activity level, greater fatigue, muscle tension, and the psychological experience of feeling stressed and overwhelmed. These may contribute to high levels of pain, which in turn can lead to a decline in daily functioning, immobility, and heightened disease activity. This makes the individual aware of the debilitating aspects of the chronic illness and may negatively affect self-esteem, contributing to depression. Ongoing problems add to this cycle, characterized by poor coping responses and an inability to adapt.

People with chronic illness may benefit from being educated about this cycle. Physicians can empower patients to be alert to the interplay of these factors as they are manifested in their lives. Once aware, patients can make timely and active interventions that interrupt the cycle of chronic disease, leading to decreased stress and pain, increased psychological well-being, and slowing of the disease process.

DIAGNOSIS OF CHRONIC DISEASE

At the Time of Diagnosis

DESCRIPTION

It may take years until the correct diagnosis of a chronic illness becomes evident. From the patient's point of view, knowing a problem exists but being unable to define it is often frightening and frustrating. Physicians can successfully manage this situation by emotion-focused and problem-focused coping techniques (Table 34–1).

INTERVENTION

Patients often worry that their symptoms may not be taken seriously. Physicians can provide emotion-focused support by listening to and reflecting back the patient's concerns and by acknowledging that fear and uncertainty are natural at this time. They can also be reassuring about their commitment to collaborate with the patient to find answers and solutions. Finally, it might be useful for physicians to reflect on their own feelings of frustration or con-

Table 34–1. Physician interventions before diagnosis and at the time of diagnosis.

Before Diagnosis

Emotion-focused interventions

1. Ask about and listen to patient's emotional responses.
2. Acknowledge uncertainty.
3. Reassert your commitment to the patient's care.

Problem-focused interventions

1. Suggest palliative measures for symptom relief.
2. Encourage patient interventions to interrupt the chronic disease cycle.

At the Time of Diagnosis

Emotion-focused interventions

1. Inquire about and reflect back the patient's feelings.
2. Fully attend to the patient, discussing concerns in an unhurried manner.

Problem-focused interventions

1. Schedule a second appointment soon after delivering the diagnosis.
2. Provide patient education in nontechnical language.
3. Discuss the structure of the physician–patient relationship.

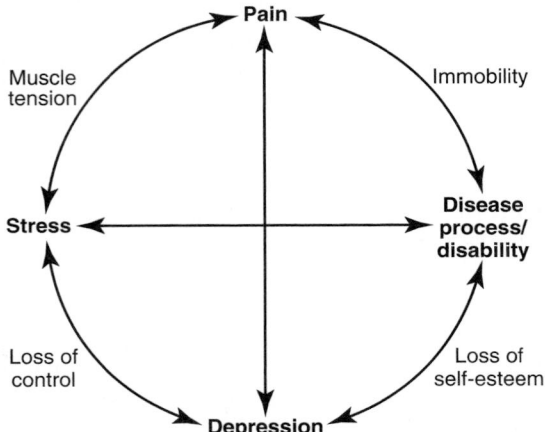

Figure 34–1. The cycle of chronic disease.

cern and acknowledge that these may well be appropriate to the situation.

Problem-focused responses such as palliative measures, including pain medication, physical therapy, occupational therapy, splints, orthotics, adaptive devices, and acupuncture, meditation, and other alternative interventions are likely to be helpful. In addition, patients can be educated about the cycle of chronic disease and pain control techniques so they can make active choices to adapt to their condition.

COMMUNICATING ABOUT THE DIAGNOSIS

Once the diagnosis is clarified, patients are faced with the challenge of adapting to their illness. They may react to the news with shock or disbelief and be unable to absorb information provided at that time. The physician should schedule a second appointment soon after the news is delivered to enable patients to ask questions about the disease and its effect on their life (see Chapter 3).

Some patients are information seekers who need detailed information to reduce uncertainty; others tend to avoid information and cope by distracting themselves from the stressful experience. Physicians should provide as much information as the patient can tolerate, as information is the key to patient empowerment. They should discuss the cause of the disease, treatment options, expected course, and possible complications using nontechnical language. Patients' understanding of the information should be checked by asking them to repeat what they have been told.

Patients may also benefit from a brief discussion of the structure of the physician–patient relationship. The physician might indicate the length of time of the usual appointment and suggest ways the patient can make the best use of that time, for example, by arriving with a list of questions or concerns. Patients may be concerned about physician availability, especially in the event of an acute or urgent medical situation. They are likely to be reassured by discussing in advance ways to deal with these situations.

EMOTIONAL RESPONSES

Many people with a new chronic illness appear to move through a series of stages as they begin to accept their situation. These stages occur as a function of the many losses inherent in adapting to a chronic condition and may include shock, denial, anger, bargaining, sadness, helplessness, and acceptance. It is important to remember that responses to learning about a diagnosis vary greatly, might not occur in any particular order, and are unlikely to adhere to an expected timetable. Moreover, recent evidence suggests that not all people experience grief and depression in response to significant losses; some appear to adapt without substantial emotional distress.

Patients are likely to feel relieved and supported by the physician's willingness to inquire about and show empathy for their emotional experiences in an unhurried manner. This helps to build an effective partnership between physician and patient. Touching may also help communicate caring and concern. The physician might suggest that patients try to manage their feelings with emotion-focused coping such as normalizing the presence of the feelings, seeking support from family and friends, and carrying on with normal daily routines or enjoyable activities as appropriate.

CULTURAL ISSUES

Primary care providers should be aware of patients' culturally based understanding of the disease and its treatment. A patient-centered partnership means that physicians collaborate with patients to design a treatment program that takes into consideration the patient's attitudes, beliefs, and life-style to effect the most positive treatment outcomes.

EFFECT OF CHRONIC DISEASE

Patients with a chronic illness encounter a range of coping challenges that involves nearly every aspect of their lives. The following section details these challenges and offers ways in which physicians can encourage patients to make active treatment and coping decisions (Table 34–2).

 CASE ILLUSTRATION

Jane, a 34-year-old married woman and mother of two young children, recently experienced a severe flare-up of her rheumatoid arthritis (RA). When her arthritis was in remission, she worked full-time, volunteered at her children's school, and was active on the board of a community organization. She considered herself fortunate to be so functional and was pleased with these multiple roles. With the flare-up, however, she needed to take sick leave from work and, with continued deterioration in her condition, she decided to resign from her volunteer positions. Because of pain and fatigue, she became less able to drive her children to different activities, managing only to do the most essential household chores. She found herself relying more on her husband and close friends for assistance and emotional support. Moreover, her arthritis became more apparent to others, as it affected her gait and the appearance of her hands. As her functional abilities became impaired, she began to feel that she was no longer able to contribute to her relationships and her community, and her self-esteem diminished. In addition, she felt less attractive due to changes in her appearance, and she felt disconnected from her body, as it reacted in unfamiliar and unpleasant ways. She became increasingly depressed and isolated from others.

Table 34–2. Physician intervention in areas affected by chronic disease.

Activity Level

Emotion-focused interventions

1. Elicit the patient's reactions to necessary reductions in activity level.
2. Listen to and reflect feelings expressed by the patient.

Problem-focused interventions

1. Suggest planning the day's activities in advance, leaving time for rest and enjoyment.
2. Encourage flexibility about adapting to change.
3. Positively frame changes in activity level.

Activity Choice

Emotion-focused interventions

1. Use active listening and reflection of feelings.
2. Provide hope by encouraging patients to self-manage the effects of the disease.

Problem-focused interventions

1. Suggest connecting with others through disease-specific organizations or by reading about others' experiences with chronic disease.
2. Prescribe physical and occupational therapy as needed.
3. Encourage use of adaptive living devices.
4. Commend patients for their efforts to actively adapt to their disease.

Sexuality

Emotion-focused interventions

1. Raise the topic of sexuality with all chronic disease patients.
2. Normalize and validate the patient's experiences.

Problem-focused interventions

1. Ask questions to pinpoint the problem.
2. Encourage communication with the partner.
3. Suggest planning sex when fatigue and pain are reduced, after use of pain medication, and consider alternative sexual practices.
4. Refer for counseling as needed.

Emotional Response

Emotion-focused interventions

1. Reflect on one's own degree of comfort with experiencing and expressing feelings.
2. Remember that listening, reflecting, and being silent are effective.
3. Suggest focusing on positive or controllable aspects of the situation, using humor, and noticing how having a chronic disease promotes personal growth.
4. If the patient's feelings are intrusive, suggest meditation, relaxation training, refocusing attention, and engaging in enjoyable activities.

Problem-focused interventions

1. Encourage active self-management of the disease.
2. Develop a partnership with patients so they can make decisions about their treatment.
3. Refer for mental health treatment as necessary.

Relationships

Emotion-focused interventions

1. Ask about the effect of the chronic disease on relationships.
2. Validate the difficulty in relationship transitions.
3. Discuss the effectiveness of the physician–patient relationship.

Problem-focused interventions

1. Encourage communication in relationships using effective communication skills.
2. Encourage patients to maintain their usual level of control and decision-making power in their relationships.
3. Refer for individual, couple, or family counseling, as appropriate.

Effect on Activity Level

DESCRIPTION

As a result of pain, fatigue, or physical disability, many people with a chronic disease eventually are unable to maintain their usual level of activity. A common response is to try against all odds to maintain as "normal" a life as possible, sometimes overdoing it. This can result in an increase in disease activity. Others may simply give up and not try to adapt to their new situation. They may feel victimized and controlled by their disease, which leads them to lose their sense of power and become dependent on others. The resulting reduction in activity can be detrimental to their physical condition as well.

 CASE ILLUSTRATION (CONT.)

Jane returned to her busy schedule once her RA was stabilized. She tried desperately to maintain her usual activity level despite pain and overwhelming fatigue. She dropped into bed each night exhausted, waking at 5:00 AM to give her joints time to lose their stiffness. Within a month, she was back in her physician's office, complaining of pain, redness, and swelling in her hands and feet, and asking for a change in medication to enable her to keep going. When her physician commented that she seemed more stressed than usual, she began to cry.

INTERVENTION

Physicians' interventions regarding activity level can help patients adapt to their illness. These interventions are useful both for patients who overdo it and for those who give up. The goal is to achieve a state of maximum functionality by taking as much control as possible. Before providing problem-focused assistance, it is useful for the physician to discuss the patient's feelings about the losses incurred in giving up valued activities. Ask open-ended questions such as, "What do you think about (or feel) when you realize that you can't do it all anymore?" and respond by simply listening or reflecting the emotion expressed: "It seems like you're feeling very sad about your losses."

Using empathic reflection may seem as though nothing is being accomplished, but such communication skills can be highly effective. When patients feel heard and understood, they are more open to discussing problem-focused strategies for addressing their problems (see Chapter 2).

People with chronic disease are likely to benefit from planning each day in advance, making sure to include enjoyable activities and leaving time for a rest or a nap. This process involves making proactive choices to effectively manage the disease. Flexibility is essential to successfully adapting to changes. For example, patients should be encouraged to reevaluate their schedule on days when they wake up feeling poorly. Framing these shifts in activity level in a positive way helps facilitate patients' acceptance of them. Explaining how rest and relaxation can retard the progression of the disease and contribute to life satisfaction can also be helpful. The changes can be viewed in a positive way, for example, an opportunity to spend more quality time with one's children.

Activity Choice

DESCRIPTION

Most people with a chronic disease eventually need to make changes in the kinds of activities in which they participate. These changes can range from giving up a valued hobby or satisfying job to adapting to one's inability to turn a doorknob or climb a flight of stairs. These challenges are significant because they are a constant reminder of the illness and its effects.

 CASE ILLUSTRATION (CONT.)

As Jane's RA progressed, she began having difficulty carrying out her daily activities around the house. She found cooking especially problematic because she could not hold utensils or heavy pots. These problems were caused by her decreased range of motion and flexibility, loss of strength, and pain. She wondered how she could make changes that would enable her to continue to be able to cook for her family.

INTERVENTION

As indicated earlier, physicians should be sensitive to patients' feelings, using active listening and reflection to communicate understanding. Because there are many problem-focused strategies for coping with these changes in activity, patients should be encouraged to adopt an attitude of active self-management and control. The physician can act as a coach, suggesting various coping strategies. Patients might benefit, for example, from connecting with others with similar problems. Local chapters of organizations of people with specific diseases, such as the Arthritis Foundation, are good resources for literature, classes on disease self-management, and support groups.

Patients might also be helped by reading books authored by people with a chronic disease that offer numerous suggestions on how to facilitate activities of daily living.

Adjunctive treatments such as occupational or physical therapy, as well as use of adaptive living devices, may be helpful. The range of possibilities for adaptive change is unlimited, and people with chronic illness can be encouraged by becoming aware of the options. It is also helpful to commend patients for their efforts to actively adapt to their condition.

Sexuality

DESCRIPTION

Sexuality is affected by many chronic illnesses. Interest in sex and the physical ability to engage in sexual activity are reduced as a result of fatigue, pain, loss of strength, altered sense of body image, decreased self-esteem, and relationship stress. Patients concerned about sex may raise the topic with their physicians; others may feel burdened by these concerns but reluctant to discuss them.

 CASE ILLUSTRATION (CONT.)

As Jane's arthritis worsened, she and her husband, Ken, began having sex much less frequently. She was usually exhausted and in pain, and the visible changes in her joints made her feel unattractive. In addition, she was afraid of the pain she would experience with sex. She was also aware, however, of the loss of intimacy and the growing rift with Ken. Ken also felt the lack of closeness and missed the enjoyment of a previously satisfying sex life, yet he was reluctant to burden Jane further by raising a sensitive topic.

INTERVENTION

Primary care physicians should try to discuss sexuality with all patients who have a chronic illness. The physician might say "Sometimes people with RA have concerns about sex. Has this been something you've thought about or worried about?" If patients choose not to discuss it, physicians should make their availability to talk known and follow up at a future appointment. If patients do raise concerns, try to pinpoint the source of the problem, such as "What do you think interferes with your having satisfying sex?" An appropriate emotion-focused response is to listen to patients' concerns and validate their experiences by saying, for example, "It's not unusual for people with RA to have that experience." Suggest that patients communicate with their partner about their concerns, possibly by including the partner in a future appointment. Often couples can work together toward solutions once the problem has been identified and discussed.

Practical problem-focused strategies for helping with sexual difficulties include planning sex at a time when the patient is less tired and experiencing less pain, timing medication so the maximal effect occurs when sex is planned, taking a warm bath prior to sex, and using alternative sexual techniques. Referral to a sex or couple therapist might be useful, particularly when the couple has serious communication problems or obvious sexual dysfunction. This might facilitate communication and help the couple discuss options for sex (see Chapter 27).

Emotional Responses to Chronic Disease

In this section, common emotional responses to chronic disease are described followed by a discussion of emotion-focused and problem-focused coping. The goal is to help primary care providers better understand their patients' internal experiences and outward expression of their emotions and to intervene in ways that promote adaptive coping. Adaptive coping means having available a repertoire of responses that can be used to deal with and modulate the ebb and flow of experience.

Keeping in mind the "chronic" in chronic disease, that is, the longevity of the coping process, no set sequence or intensity of emotions should be expected. For example, the grieving that took place with the initial diagnosis may recur years later with a clear increase in physical disability. In addition, people vary greatly in how they react to their experiences—some may feel their emotions intensely and others may be more modulated or less aware; some may need time to process their feelings and others feel resolved more quickly. Thus, physicians should be attuned to the feelings their patients are experiencing without expecting them to react in a set way.

SADNESS/GRIEF

One of the common emotions experienced by people with a chronic disease is a sense of sadness and loss accompanied by grieving for the loss. Losses are experienced in many areas: health and well-being, body image, the ability to engage in desired activities including work, the core sense of self, independence, important relationships, and future plans. Although grieving is not always necessary to resolve a loss, many patients benefit from an opportunity to discuss their feelings. If they do not, physicians may want to ask about how they are feeling and coping. Some patients may see their physician's office as a place in which they can talk more openly about their feelings, whereas others may be less willing to show their vulnerability. It is often helpful to suggest that discussing feelings is acceptable and often beneficial.

ANGER

Patients may feel angry as they process their feelings about their disease. Although a difficult and uncomfortable emotion for many, anger is a normal part of the grieving process. Anger may be expressed overtly but is often suppressed or displaced. This can lead to increased irritability and conflict in relationships. A patient's irritation at her physician's inability to control her symptoms or at her husband's inefficiency in managing household chores that were once her responsibility may reflect her own underlying anger about the effects of the disease. Repressed anger can show itself in behaviors such as noncompliance or missed appointments. Anger may also be expressed in terms of unfairness, as in the patient asking "Why me?" This question represents a desire to understand events and attribute responsibility for them. People struggle to understand why they developed the disease, wondering whether to blame themselves or others. Eventual acceptance of the disease is facilitated by letting go of the urge to assign blame and focusing attention on the current realities of the disease, including action-oriented coping strategies targeted to aspects of the disease that can be controlled. Patients benefit from acknowledging their anger, understanding that it is to be expected, and communicating it to others in as constructive a way as possible.

Loss of Control/Anxiety

People with chronic disease often experience a sense of loss of control and uncertainty about the future accompanied by anxiety, worry, and fear. Patients worry about future disability, adequacy of financial resources, and ability to maintain significant relationships. As they understand the extent of their loss, they realize that they have diminished choices and no blueprint for the future. A chronic disease imposes on people the need to change without their choosing to do so. They are faced with fear and uncertainty about daily activities that were once taken for granted as well as other issues such as plans for retirement. This uncertainty may manifest itself as anxiety about their medical care.

 CASE ILLUSTRATION (CONT.)

When Jane's physician entered the examining room, she uncharacteristically pointed out that he was 10 minutes late. She pulled a list of complaints from her pocket and stated that she was disturbed about the side effects of her medication and the lack of control over her pain. Rather than responding to her complaints directly, her physician reflected that she seemed upset. When she agreed, her physician invited her to talk about it. She mentioned her constant pain and discomfort, her recent need to reduce her work hours, and her concern that she could end up in a wheelchair. "I just don't feel like I can count on anything anymore," she asserted. Her physician suggested, "It seems like you feel that your whole world is unstable." "It is," she
said sadly, "and sometimes I just don't want to deal with it anymore."

Intervention

To help patients deal with their feelings about their chronic disease, it is useful for physicians to reflect on their own styles of experiencing and expressing feelings. To the extent that practitioners can understand and accept their own feelings, they are likely to be more open to those of their patients. Often, the anxiety physicians experience with patients with a chronic disease has to do with the feeling that they cannot really do anything to help. In this sense, it is useful to remember that patients will benefit from having a supportive place to talk about what they are experiencing and from feeling listened to and understood. Once expressed, feelings are no longer carried around only internally, and the patient is less likely to feel burdened by them. Specific responses the physician might make include reflecting the emotion being expressed ("Sounds like you're angry.") and restating the patient's comment ("So what you're saying is that you're disappointed about not being able to enjoy your retirement the way you had planned."). Simply giving the patient time to talk and feel is often helpful (see Chapters 1 and 2).

Physicians might also suggest that patients reflect on the meaning derived from their current experiences. For example, patients can deal with their feelings by focusing on the positive aspects of the experience, finding humor in the situation, and reflecting on how the situation has helped them to grow as a person (for example, developing patience and greater tolerance). If feelings are overly intrusive, refocusing attention on other thoughts and enjoyable activities may be useful, along with meditation and relaxation training. Moving into problem-focused coping by taking active steps to self-manage the controllable aspects of the problem at hand is also essential.

Practitioners should acknowledge uncertainty and provide information in response to the patient's fears about loss of control. But with some patients, no amount of information can allay all their concerns. Gently setting limits on frequency of phone calls and number and length of appointments may be necessary, or it may be helpful to schedule brief appointments on a regular basis. Patients can be helped by acknowledging their fear and anxiety and by distinguishing between controllable and uncontrollable concerns. When they focus on uncontrollable issues, worry and anxiety increase; recognizing what can be controlled can lead to specific problem-focused coping behaviors that help manage anxiety and decrease their sense of powerlessness.

Physicians can help foster control by engaging patients as partners in their medical care. If appropriate, give patients a choice of treatment options, allowing them to evaluate the pros and cons of each. Some will seek information about their illness and potential treatments from a variety of other sources. Acknowledge that they are attempting to restore a sense of control and seriously consider their proposed remedies.

Effect on Relationships

DESCRIPTION

The toll that a chronic illness can take on close relationships should not be underestimated. Given increasing disability, fatigue, and other changes, roles change and people realize that they cannot be quite the same parent, partner, friend, or co-worker. The experience of loss can be significant. As the role of one person in the relationship changes, the roles of others change as well. The concerns of partners, children, other family members, friends, and other caregivers should not be overlooked. Patients may fear abandonment by those closest to them, including their physician, especially at times of greatest need.

 CASE ILLUSTRATION (CONT.)

As Jane's level of disability increased, she noticed differences in how her two children related to her. Her younger daughter, Molly, aged 7, seemed committed to not further burdening her mother. Her room was always clean and she always helped her mother prepare dinner. When Jane encouraged Molly to spend time with friends in the neighborhood, she declined, saying she preferred to stay home in case she was needed. Jane's other daughter, Lauren, aged 11, reacted quite differently. Lauren stopped having conversations with her mother about the events of the day and spent most of her time in her room listening to music. She often became angry when Jane said she was too tired to drive her to a friend's house. Jane felt guilty and assumed that her children's reactions were due to her illness, but she did not know how to talk to them about so sensitive a topic.

INTERVENTION

Because relationships are often stressed in persons with chronic disease, the primary care provider should inquire about how things are going at home and acknowledge that transitions in relationships as a result of chronic disease can be difficult. Communication is the key to successfully navigating these transitions. Successful communication requires two components: (1) a structure within which people can openly talk about their feelings, for example, a family meeting at home, a session in the physician's office, or counseling with a mental health professional; and (2) use of effective communication skills.

One important issue that often needs to be discussed is the providing or receiving of help. Problems in this area derive from differing perceptions of behaviors that are considered helpful by the people in the relationship as well as from discrepancies in the perceived level of need for help. For example, the wife of a man with multiple sclerosis may encourage him to rest with the intention of helping him feel less fatigued, but he may perceive her efforts as further attempts to control his daily activities. People with chronic disease need to maintain as much control as possible in their relationships. This means, at least in part, continuing to make decisions for themselves. Physicians can be helpful by listening to their patient's concerns about relationships and suggesting possible interventions. Referral to a mental health professional is appropriate, particularly if a problem seems to be escalating to a crisis.

Communication is also important in the physician–patient relationship. The relationship can be supported by periodic assessments of its efficacy ("How is our relationship working for you?") and the understanding that issues can be discussed as needed.

PROBLEMS WITH ADHERENCE

Problems with adherence will be mitigated to the extent that patients with chronic disease are active partners in their medical care. Physicians should try to ascertain the reason for noncompliance in a nonjudgmental fashion, offering to develop patient-centered solutions (Table 34–3). Explanations for nonadherence may include financial problems, lack of information, cultural beliefs, complexity of dosing schedules for multiple medications, adverse side effects, inaccurate expectations about the positive effects of the medication, and the inconvenience of ongoing care.

The physician needs to be flexible regarding the treatment plan, as it will be more successful if it evolves from

Table 34–3. Physician interventions for adherence problems.

1. Collaborate to develop a treatment plan that fits the patient's preferences and life-style.
2. Assess reasons for nonadherence, including financial concerns and cultural beliefs, in a nonjudgmental way.
3. Provide patient education about the expected effects of the medication.
4. Reduce the complexity of medication regimens and dosing frequency.
5. Suggest using a calendar, daily pill box, or diary to keep track of medications.

the patient's preferences, life-style, and beliefs about treatment. Simpler regimens are likely to result in greater adherence. Physicians may feel unappreciated if the patient chooses to resist treatment, but they should not view themselves as having failed, as the ultimate responsibility for carrying out the treatment plan lies with the patient (see Chapter 16).

INDICATIONS FOR REFERRAL

People with a chronic disease can often benefit from a variety of collaborative services, including physical and occupational therapy, counseling, disease self-management programs, social work, nutrition, and employment rehabilitation. Patients should be encouraged to use these services in any way that would be helpful to them. Constraints imposed by managed care, however, may at times limit access to these services. Patients may be helped by referral to community-based resources or by connecting with resources offered by local chapters of national disease-specific organizations.

Referral for mental health services should be offered in the following situations: symptoms of clinical depression or other psychiatric disorder, illness-related concerns that are obstacles to adaptive coping, persistent problems with adherence to medication regimens, and communication problems in close and important relationships. Individual, couple, or family therapy may be appropriate depending on the situation. Cognitive-behavioral therapy may facilitate acceptance of the disease, teach appropriate coping skills, and help the patient to regain a sense of control.

SUMMARY

The effects of chronic disease are broad and potentially severe, affecting physical and psychological well-being, activity level, body image, mood, self-esteem, and important relationships. A patient-centered partnership, in which the physician and patient work together to develop a treatment plan and solve disease-related problems, engenders patient satisfaction and positive treatment outcomes. Patients can learn to self-manage their disease, with the physician's support and assistance, by using intervention strategies that are either emotion focused (aiding in the expression or regulation of emotion) or problem focused (suggesting concrete ways to take action to affect the multiple manifestations of the disease). An effective physician–patient relationship can serve as a vehicle to enable patients with chronic disease to live full, meaningful, and satisfying lives.

SUGGESTED READINGS

Funnell MM: Helping patients take charge of their chronic illnesses. Fam Pract Manage 2000;7:47. PMID 10947289.

Lazarus RS, Folkman S: *Stress, Appraisal, and Coping.* Springer, 1984.

Lorig KR et al: Evidence suggesting that a chronic disease self-management program can improve health status while reducing hospitalization: a randomized trial. Med Care 1999;37:5. PMID 10413387.

Register C: The chronic illness experience: embracing the imperfect life. Hazelden Information Education 1999.

Steyer TE: Complementary and alternative medicine: a primer. Fam Pract Manage 2001;8:37. PMID 11317848.

Wagner EH: The role of patient care teams in chronic disease management. BMJ 2000;320:59. PMID 10688568.

WEB SITES

American Cancer Society
www.cancer.org

American Diabetes Association
www.diabetes.org

American Heart Association
www.americanheart.org

American Lung Association
www.lungusa.org

Arthritis Association
www.arthritis.org

Information and support for chronic illnesses
www.dmoz.org/health/consumer_support_groups

Information on AIDS and HIV
www.thebody.com

List of chat groups and online support for many chronic illnesses
www.noah-health.org/english/support.html

National Center for Chronic Disease Prevention and Health Promotion
www.cdc.gov/nccdphp

Stanford Patient Education Research Center; Information on chronic disease self-management program
www.stanford.edu/group/perc

Death & Dying

Chapter number 35 shown in box.

Michael Eisman, MD, & Timothy E. Quill, MD

INTRODUCTION

Clinicians need to ask themselves how they would want to be treated when they are dying. Answering this question helps them discover and clarify their own beliefs and values concerning the care of dying patients. Although medical practice is usually based on the concepts of healing, cure, and restoration of function, these ideas are called into question when patients are dying. Is death something to be fought at all costs, or is it our responsibility to ease the dying process? Several national initiatives have been undertaken by medical organizations to guide clinicians through the care of dying patients and their families. Despite the fact that about 2 million people die every year in the United States, death's mystery and finality continue to fascinate and terrify us. Death is not a disease, and dying is not an illness that can be cured. Palliation, not cure, and relief of suffering, not restoration of function, are medicine's primary goals in caring for the dying patient.

CASE ILLUSTRATION 1

Ella, a 71-year-old woman, has had pains in her lower chest and upper abdomen for a month before visiting her personal physician. When a chest film shows several nodular masses suggestive of widespread lung cancer, the physician phones Ella and tells her there is a problem, making an office appointment for the next day. At this visit, the doctor discusses the results of the chest film with the patient and her son. Ella, having long suspected she might get lung cancer from smoking heavily, weeps openly. As the diagnosis is not yet certain, bronchoscopy is recommended, and she is referred to a pulmonologist. The bronchoscopy biopsies show a small-cell lung cancer. The pulmonologist refers Ella to an oncologist who recommends chemotherapy and tells the patient that if she doesn't respond to chemotherapy she will have less than a year to live.

The patient and her son return to her primary care doctor to discuss her options. Ella says she would like to proceed with chemotherapy but wants to stop it if she becomes too ill from the treatments. A Roman Catholic, she has discussed with her priest the moral-

ity of refusing extraordinary care, including feeding tubes, if she were to have a terminal condition. She has appointed her son her health-care proxy and discussed with him her desire not to undergo cardiopulmonary resuscitation. The physician gives Ella a living will; she and her son complete it together. Ella undergoes chemotherapy for several months but grows thinner and weaker.

Ella lives alone and does not want to die in her apartment. Neither does she want her son to have to provide home care for her when she becomes too dependent to live alone. She also wants to know whether she could die in the hospital or a nursing home. Her doctor agrees to hospitalize her and find other placement when the need arises.

When she becomes confused and is hospitalized, a brain computed tomography scan shows cerebral metastasis. As Ella loses the capacity to make decisions, her son and her physician decide that based on her previous wishes, she would not want to live under the current conditions. She is moved to a nursing home, with palliative care orders guiding treatment, and dies 6 months after the initial diagnosis.

The psychological and existential step from a seemingly endless life to one in which death appears clearly on the horizon is a momentous one. We usually live in denial about our own mortality. Although we may sometimes abstractly acknowledge that we will die, we do not know when or how. The *when* and *how* of the patient's death become explicit issues when a potentially fatal disorder is diagnosed. Personal, cultural, and spiritual beliefs and experiences shape how we respond to the news about our impending death. After the initial diagnosis, there is often a progressive series of losses in the dying process, each punctuated by the clinician delivering additional bad news. Each step of this process can evoke strong emotional and cognitive reactions. It may elicit overwhelming fear and anxiety, or it may be met with outward equanimity.

NONABANDONMENT OF THE DYING PATIENT

When a patient is informed of a life-threatening illness, a wide spectrum of feelings may emerge: denial, intense anxiety, fear, sadness, and anger. If the practitioner is inexperienced in palliative care or is extremely discomfited by death, there may be a tendency to withdraw from the patient's care. The commitment not to abandon the patient requires that clinicians learn to work through their own feelings, become knowledgeable about palliative care, and recognize that the process of dying can be a unique spiritual and personal experience for both doctor and patient. The goal is to form a partnership that will help the patient face the future with courage and dignity.

The goals of partnership and shared decision making are sometimes limited by strong emotional reactions as well as long-standing personality traits that can isolate the patient from the clinician, friends, and family. In addition, physicians may be unable to commit the time and energy needed to develop close personal contact with the dying patient. Clinicians need to realize that extraordinary effort is sometimes required to be a partner with the patient for a "good" death.

The Difficult Patient

CASE ILLUSTRATION 2

At 68 years old, Albert has severe end-stage emphysema, complicated by mitral regurgitation, congestive heart failure, cardiac arrhythmias, alcoholism, and years of smoking. He lives with his wife, whom he has bullied and dominated throughout their 40-year marriage. He has been on home oxygen and has had multiple hospital admissions for shortness of breath.

Admitted to the emergency room with severe shortness of breath, Albert is found to have pneumonia and heart failure. He had previously decided not to have cardiopulmonary resuscitation and wanted "no part of any of those damned machines." He is admitted to the hospital and treated with aggressive medical means but is not put on a respirator. Albert regularly yells and curses at the respiratory therapists, nursing staff, physicians, and his family for not taking care of him, for making him suffer, and for not being prompt enough with meals, medicines, and treatments. He insists that the only thing wrong with him is that the medicines are making him sick.

Efforts to engage Albert in a dialogue that explores his feelings meet first with an unwillingness to talk and then a life history of feeling abandoned, powerless, betrayed by employers, and subject to bad luck. He describes himself as an "ornery son of a bitch." He fears lingering and suffering in the hospital, and although he hopes he will die quickly, he is also afraid to die. One of Albert's fears is of being buried alive, a phobia fed by a television program he had seen about the difficulty of determining when someone was dead and the pos-

sibility of being sent to the undertaker while still alive. The anxiety of being trapped in a "tight" place is overwhelming to him.

Albert's physicians have resisted placing him on anxiolytic drugs or narcotics out of fear they would compromise his breathing. The issue of palliative care is discussed with him and his wife, and the primary goal of relieving his suffering, rather than prolonging his life, is affirmed. Anxiolytic drugs are started to treat both his sensation of shortness of breath and the associated anxiety. Placed in a room with a large picture window to the outside, he spends long periods of time staring out the window. His complaints diminish and he seems more relaxed, finally telling his wife he has suffered enough and does not want to live any longer. He gradually becomes more confused as a result of the rising carbon dioxide levels and dies several nights later.

It is unusual for a life-long pattern of behavior to be altered by the dying process. Although for some people dying may be a time for personal growth, reflection, and meaning, for others, personal factors and emotional reactions block an acceptance of death. The most frequently encountered of these reactions are denial, anger, depression, fear, and anxiety. These reactions may be present in different degrees and at different times in the dying process. Clinicians need to acknowledge, explore, and eventually understand what function the reaction is serving for the patient. Empathy, rather than withdrawal, is the way to deepen the patient–clinician relationship and create an atmosphere in which personal growth is more likely to occur (see Chapter 2).

The Abandoned Patient

CASE ILLUSTRATION 3

Max, a 63-year-old, recently retired, and previously healthy man, develops abdominal pains and is found to have widely metastasized colon cancer. He goes to a physician and is advised that no treatment would be beneficial and that he has approximately 6–12 months to live. He is given acetaminophen and codeine for pain and told to come back when the combination no longer relieves the discomfort. Max and his wife cannot bear the thought of just waiting for him to die and decide to seek a cure—or at least some kind of treatment. They hear of a cancer-treatment clinic out of the country and go there for a 6-week program of intensive vitamin and herbal treatments, coffee enemas, a variety of teas, and dietary supplements. Max is also given a long list of treatments to follow when he returns home; this keeps him busy trying to "beat" the cancer. The clinic is supposed to provide follow-up by mail or telephone; however, several months go by and there is no contact from the clinic.

Discouraged, Max and his wife go to another physician in their home town when the pains in his liver intensify and ascites and jaundice set in. The physician and the couple discuss the available options and agree on palliative care measures; Max dies 4 weeks later, approximately 9 months from the time of diagnosis. His wife never receives any follow-up information from the overseas clinic, nor does anyone from the original physician's office call to offer condolences on her husband's death.

This patient has been abandoned twice. The first treating physician failed to explore all treatment alternatives and then offered inadequate follow-up. The alternative clinic offered the patient an active treatment approach, which he and his wife needed—but then deserted him by failing to follow through when the treatment did not work (for further discussion, see the section on "Hope & Meaning"). Nonabandonment is a key element in the care of the dying patient.

Dealing with Grief

At times it may be difficult to distinguish normal grief reactions to the dying process from pathological states that may require consultation and special treatment. There is a natural sadness that human beings experience in regard to death. This sadness, which may be a way of preparing for death, has been called **preparatory** or **anticipatory grief.** Grieving over the loss of physical abilities, social position, and contact with pleasurable routines—whether one's own or those of a loved one—is a natural reaction. The absence of grief over these losses may indicate denial and emotional numbing. Sharing and exploring the grief help both patient and clinician enter a relationship that acknowledges one another's humanity. Having the courage to explore these feelings assists the patient in coming to terms with death and may prevent the isolation and subsequent clinical depression to which some patients are prone.

Distinguishing clinical depression from the natural grieving process that accompanies a terminal illness may be difficult, as they share many common symptoms. The vegetative symptoms of depression—fatigue, changes in appetite, sleep disorders, decreased sexual drive—are all common in serious illness. The affective and cognitive signs of depression, such as loss of interest, withdrawal, hope-lessness, shame, guilt, sadness, inability to concentrate, and suicidal ideation, may be realistic assessments in the face of severe suffering, fear of a loss of dignity, and the expectation of death. When the cognitive symptoms, dysphoria, or isolation seem out of proportion to the patient's situation, major depression should be considered and the physician might refer the patient (and the family) to a mental health professional. Psychotherapists who are familiar with the dying process and are experienced with medically ill patients provide an invaluable resource, both diagnostically and therapeutically, in the care of the terminally ill.

TRANSITIONS

Each transition—each diminishment of health—at the end of life includes loss, as well as the potential for personal growth and the acceptance of death. These transitions may initially be treated as another form of bad news, but they provide the opportunity for enhanced meaning and control in the dying process. Physicians caring for terminally ill patients must explore and work through these transitions with their patients. Questions that clinicians can ask their patients in exploring their views on end-of-life issues are listed in Table 35–1. These can be asked as hypothetical questions to explore the patient's beliefs about death and dying. In patients with more advanced illness, the questions and their answers may be highly relevant to immediate treatment decisions.

Education & Information

Clinicians need to provide the patient with information about the disease, the prognosis, the treatment options, and the anticipated course of the illness. Most patients and their families want to know how much time is left when a terminal diagnosis is made. Providing ranges of survival times, allowing for outliers on either end, is better than predicting an exact amount of time. Refusing to give time estimates or withholding other grim information to protect the patient is usually not productive and may not allow the patient and family to prepare for death. The possibility of miracles or rare exceptions to the usual course of the illness allows a glimmer of hope for some patients. In general, the physician should be guided by patients and their families in determining how detailed the information about the course of the illness should be (see Chapter 3).

Advance Directives

Advance directives are formal documents that direct health-care decisions if patients lose the capacity to speak for themselves. There are two types of advance directives: living wills and health-care proxies, or durable powers of attorney.

A living will allows a patient to direct the kinds of treatments wanted at the end of life if the capacity to make decisions is lost. Some living wills focus on general goals,

Table 35–1. End-of-life issues to be discussed with patients.

Life Support

- Do you have an advance directive (a living will or health-care proxy)?
- Do you know what CPR is? If you had a terminal illness would you want to undergo CPR?
- In the event an illness led to your being unable to eat or drink on a permanent basis, would you want to be fed with feeding tubes?
- Do you want your medical care geared to prolonging your life at all costs, or is improving or maintaining your quality of life more important?

Personal Beliefs

- What life experiences have you had around death and dying?
- How have these experiences affected your own attitudes about death?
- What are your worst fears about dying?
- What would be a good death for you?
- What do you believe happens to you when you die?

Long-Term Care and Support Systems

- If you become too ill to take care of yourself, who will take care of you?
- Who would you want to make health-care decisions for you if you became unable to do so?
- If you were dying, would you prefer to be at home or in an institution such as a hospital or nursing home?
- Do you know what hospice care is? Would you want that kind of care if you were terminally ill?
- Who would you want to be present at the time of your dying and death?
- Is there anything you need to get done before you die?

whereas others specify exact treatments and explicit circumstances. Living wills become operative only when patients are unable to communicate for themselves.

A **health-care proxy,** or **durable power of attorney,** allows patients to designate a person to make decisions on their behalf should they become unable to do so. These directives allow more flexibility than do living wills, an important point, as it is difficult to anticipate all possible medical conditions and treatment options.

Many people complete both documents: a living will to present an overarching philosophy and a health-care proxy to designate a person to help interpret that philosophy when the patient can no longer do so. For healthy persons, discussing a living will or a health-care proxy may be the first time they have had to face their own mortality. For those with terminal illness, completing an advance directive may be seen as another indication of their inevitable deterioration.

Involving family members in the discussions of advance directives is useful. A proxy who is uninformed about the values and wishes of the patient has an arduous job when difficult care decisions must be made. Although they cannot cover every situation, living wills with clear statements about goals, values, and directions help the clinician and the designated proxy formulate a care plan. In addition, having a form to fill out helps many patients and their families discuss death-related issues. For severely ill patients, the ad-

vance directive decisions can provide a starting point for discussions about the limits of care and the burdens of suffering as well as orders not to resuscitate.

DO NOT RESUSCITATE

The "do not resuscitate" (DNR) order refers to the withholding of cardiopulmonary resuscitation (CPR), specifically closed-chest cardiac massage, defibrillation, and artificially supplied respiratory support. For most patients with a terminal disease, CPR is at best ineffective and at worst a cruel and expensive technological death ritual. Many studies have shown that CPR provides no increase in out-of-hospital survival for patients with multisystem disease, particularly patients with advanced cancers and renal failure.

Unfortunately many patients and their families interpret a DNR order as an abandonment, or giving up, and agonize over its issuance. This is in part due to the way medical personnel emphasize what will be withheld rather than what will be done. When alternative treatment strategies are not explained, patients and families think that a DNR order means nothing will be done to treat potentially reversible conditions or to relieve uncomfortable symptoms. They sense that second-class treatment will be given—which may indeed happen if clinicians and the institutions they work in are not knowledgeable about the narrow focus on a DNR directive. It should be understood that agreement to a DNR order in no way limits other treatment options.

DNR orders do, however, signal that things are different. The notion that being resuscitated from cardiopulmonary arrest will not add appreciably to the quality and or quantity of life is an open acknowledgment that death is near—and that reversing the dying process is not within the power of medicine. Although some patients are initially frightened by this discussion, many feel relieved and appreciate the opportunity to avoid treatment they do not want.

Emergency rescue crews are obligated to attempt resuscitation unless they have specific instructions not to proceed. DNR orders that are valid in the inpatient setting may not be valid in the outpatient setting unless special forms, which vary by locality, are completed. These issues should be addressed with terminally ill patients who want to remain at home, as resuscitation may be carried out in times of crisis if the proper documentation is not on hand.

PALLIATIVE CARE

The goal of palliative care is to provide the best possible quality of life for the patient and family. Palliative care addresses the biological, psychosocial, and spiritual dimensions of suffering of seriously ill patients, emphasizing state-of-the-art pain and symptom management, and a fresh look at goals and prognosis. Unlike Medicare-sponsored hospice programs, palliative care does not require a patient to give up on aggressive treatment of his underlying disease, to accept a prognosis of 6 months or less, and accept palliation as the central goal of therapy. Thus, it allows "hospice-like" treatments to be made available to those seriously ill patients who want to continue some or all disease-directed treatments. Thus, a patient who is highly likely to die, but wants to try improbable experimental therapy in hopes that it might prolong his or her life, could receive palliative care but would not qualify for a Medicare-sponsored hospice program. Similarly, a patient with advanced emphysema or Alzheimer's disease who has a 50 percent chance of dying in the next 6 months, but might live several years, could receive palliative care but would not qualify for hospice even if their goals were palliation and comfort. Thus palliative care allows better pain and symptom management, careful attention to quality of life, an examination of the goals of treatment, and an opportunity to consider issues of life closure to be provided to a much broader range of patients.

Patients confronting a severe potentially terminal illness may opt for all-out, aggressive, disease-oriented medical treatment, or a trial of aggressive medical care with set limits (such as a DNR order). Of course, palliative care should also be initiated simultaneously with this more disease-oriented care. When limited trials of aggressive care are undertaken, the patient has the opportunity to gauge whether the suffering engendered by the treatment, given the odds of success, is worth it. When treatments begin to fail, or if supposedly curative treatments become too burdensome, the patient can stop at any time and consider a transition to an approach that emphasizes pure palliation. Relieving symptoms and alleviating suffering then take precedence over attempts to treat the underlying disease.

HOSPICE

Hospice programs provide comprehensive care to dying patients, with a multidisciplinary team of nurses, physicians, social workers, volunteers, and clergy. These programs accept only patients who have a life expectancy of less than 6 months and are willing to forgo disease-directed therapies and hospitalizations. In the United States, only about 50,000 deaths annually (out of almost 2 million) occur in hospice programs. Unfortunately, many patients are referred to a hospice too late in the course of their illness to take full advantage of the resources and supports available. The palliative care philosophy underlying hospice can be applied in a range of settings from acute-care hospitals to nursing homes to the patient's home. The advantage of hospice programs is the expertise brought to techniques of palliative care by the multidisciplinary staff. In most outpatient programs, the primary care physician and the hospice team form a partnership to care for the patient. The primary care provider, with whom the patient may have a long-term relationship, should be intimately involved in both the decision for hospice referral and the patient's ongoing care. Once distressing symptoms are controlled, the hospice team may then help the patient find avenues to hope, meaning, and ways of saying good-bye.

CASE ILLUSTRATION 4

Carlos, a 70-year-old man, has been diagnosed with a hepatocellular carcinoma. In exploring the treatment options with his physician, he is clear about wanting only palliative measures, and referral to a home hospice program is initiated. Carlos is not a verbal man, and discussions about death and dying meet with little response.

At first, periodic nursing visits are all that is needed. He has an antique tool collection and spends countless hours labeling and ordering the tools. His nurse talks to him about this process, which has come to symbolize his anticipatory grief. As he deteriorates, nursing visits become more frequent, and home health aides come to help with his personal care. Carlos gradually becomes bed bound. Although his family initially feels uncomfortable with his dying at home, a family meeting with the physician and hospice nurse sets up a rotation of visits to provide for both company and supervision. Children who had been estranged are in the rotation, and it becomes a time of family healing. Although little is explicitly said about his approaching death, the presence of family and talk about the tools provide a vehicle for saying good-bye. Carlos dies quietly at home with his family present.

Hospice care, with its supportive team of physicians, nurses, and other caregivers, eases the patient's way to death by providing quality palliative care.

PAIN AND SYMPTOM RELIEF

An important goal in palliative care is to keep patients as pain free as they choose. Long-acting opioid preparations, when given in sufficient quantity in a regular dosing schedule around the clock, with proportionate supplemental doses as needed, are effective in alleviating chronic pain without significantly compromising quality of life. Knowing that they can control their own pain is reassuring to patients, especially those who have seen painful deaths. Unrealistic concerns about addiction from patients, families, and caregivers should be anticipated and addressed, as these worries often present a major obstacle to adequate pain relief. Withholding narcotics in the terminally ill because of fears about addiction is unwarranted and cruel.

Delirium & Coma

Many patients die in profoundly altered states of sensorium. There is also an increasing number of patients with dementing illnesses in whom cognitive and affective life may have diminished significantly prior to the terminal episode. Terminally ill patients with delirium present the physician and the patient's family with a dilemma. Delirium may be due to reversible factors that, if treated, could extend life. The extent to which reversible causes of delirium are searched for and treated depends on the patient's current goals, previous directives, and concurrent discussions with the family. The prior degree of suffering and the patient's wishes should largely determine what should be done.

The internal, subjective experience of a person dying with altered mental status may vary significantly from the outside perception. Patients who recover from delirium and coma sometimes report nightmarish, terrifying visions, out-of-body travel, or visions of light and angelic beings, or they may not be able to remember anything about the experience. Occasionally the disorientation becomes profound and the sense of the world is lost.

 CASE ILLUSTRATION 5

Caleb, a 101-year-old rugged dairy farmer, has become partly deaf and then blind in the last 5 years of his life but remains alert and communicative. He develops a cough and fever, and despite treatment for pneumonia, becomes progressively more dyspneic. He tells his physician that he does not wish to be resuscitated. Because his elderly wife cannot care for him at home, Caleb is hospitalized. He becomes progressively more confused and withdrawn, and his deafness and blindness further confound communication. He lies still in bed for long periods of time. Efforts by physicians and nurses to engage him in conversation are usually met with short responses such as yes, no, or okay. His physician asks him one morning what experiences he is having, and he replies that he is flying over fields of golden wheat on a sunny day. Then, in a voice of wonderment, he asks if he is still alive or if he has died. His physician replies that he is still alive. Caleb dies later that day.*

Patients who experience altered states at the end of life need supportive treatment. Once this stage has been reached, decisions about artificial hydration and feeding should have already been made and formalized through advance directives. If they have not (as is frequently the case) the designated health care agent or the family, taking into consideration the patient's condition and prognosis, must make a substituted judgment as to what the patient would want. If this cannot be determined, the physician's decision should be based on a consensus among family and providers about what is in the best interest of the patient.

There is growing evidence that terminal dehydration and inanition may ease the dying process. Providing nutrition and hydration through feeding tubes and intravenous lines when the dying patient can no longer eat or drink may appear compassionate, but such practices may inadvertently prolong dying and aggravate suffering. The person with terminal illness is dying; our acceptance of this should guide all treatments in the direction of decreasing the suffering, enhancing the quality of life left, and respecting the patient's dignity.

The Wish to Die

Sometimes, even with the best methods of palliative care, suffering cannot be alleviated to the patient's satisfaction. If this occurs, the patient may feel that dying is the only way out. The patient may no longer be able to tolerate the pain, humiliation, loss of control, increased dependency, or burden the illness places on the family. Such patients often actively begin to contemplate ending their life.

 CASE ILLUSTRATION 6

Marvin is 63 years old; he has amyotrophic lateral sclerosis and has been on a respirator at home for a year.

He has lost the ability to use his arms and legs and requires total care. He increasingly resents his life on the respirator and finally requests that it be removed and he be permitted to die. He makes this request repeatedly over the course of a month. His primary care physician sees him several times on home visits and discusses the request with Marvin's family. They agree that the respirator should be stopped. A psychiatrist visits the patient and indicates that he finds Marvin competent, not depressed; he concurs with the patient, family, and primary care physician on removing the respirator. An attempt to remove the respirator without the sedative effects of morphine leads to air hunger and feelings of suffocation. A morphine drip is instituted and the respirator is turned off. The patient dies comfortably several minutes later, attended by his family and physician.

The ***double effect*** of providing medications intended to relieve suffering and yet could inadvertently shorten the patient's life is an accepted part of medical practice and palliative care provided the patient's suffering is proportionately severe. Withdrawing life-sustaining but burdensome treatments, even though the withdrawal leads to death, is also an accepted part of practice. These practices have widespread legal, ethical, and medical acceptance and should not be confused with the controversy surrounding assisted suicide and voluntary euthanasia. In this case, the patient's wish to die can be acceded to, as a treatment that is life-sustaining but very burdensome could be removed in conjunction with the provision of a high-dose narcotic that is intended to lessen panic and suffering (Table 35–2). Patients, however, may ask the clinician, sometimes in an off-hand way, as if testing the water, about help in dying (either assisted suicide or euthanasia). This subject has both ethical and legal repercussions, and patients are often as reluctant as their physicians to discuss it.

If the patient has terrible suffering but does not have a life-sustaining treatment that can be withdrawn (eg, respirator, dialysis) or the kind of pain that can justify high doses of narcotics, the request for help in dying would put

Table 35–2. Euthanasia and assisted death: definitions.

Term	Definition	Legal Status in the United States
Double effect	Administering drugs that are intended to relieve suffering but may unintentionally shorten life. The risk of shortening life must be proportionate to the degree of suffering.	Legal
Withholding or withdrawing life-sustaining treatment (also called passive euthanasia)	Withholding or withdrawing life-sustaining care that results in the patient's death with the consent of the patient or surrogate.	Legal with the proper consent
Palliative sedation (also called terminal sedation)	With consent from the patient or surrogate, the patient is sedated to unconsciousness to relieve otherwise intractable suffering, and then food and fluids are withdrawn. Generally viewed as a combination of double effect and withdrawal of treatment, but not without moral controversy if viewed in aggregate.	Legal with the proper consent
Physician aid-in-dying (also called physician-assisted suicide)	Physician provides, at the patient's request, the means for the patient to end his or her own life. The patient then takes or does not take the overdose at a future time.	Illegal in most states except for Oregon, but difficult to prosecute
Active euthanasia	Intentionally intervening to cause the patient's death with the competent patient's informed consent. The physician is the direct agent causing death at the patient's request.	Illegal, and likely to be successfully prosecuted if discovered

the clinician in a more difficult position legally and ethically. Voluntary active euthanasia is the act of intentionally intervening to cause the patient's death, at the explicit request of, and with the full informed consent of, the competent patient. The physician administers a lethal agent, with the intent of both alleviating suffering and causing death. Voluntary active euthanasia is illegal in the United States and would lead to prosecution if discovered. In assisted suicide, the physician provides the means (such as a prescription for barbiturates) at the request of the patient, but the patient administers the lethal intervention. Assisted suicide is illegal in many states, but its legal status is currently in flux. A referendum legalizing assisted suicide at the request of a terminally ill patient was passed in Oregon in 1997, and now there are several years of data about the legalized practice.

CASE ILLUSTRATION 7

Sara, a bedridden 84-year-old woman with end-stage congestive heart failure, is seen on rounds. She is on multiple medications, including morphine, to relieve her dyspnea and pulmonary edema. Despite intensive treatment, even eating causes her to be dyspneic. She looks up from her bed and asks to be given a lethal dose of medicine so that she can die. When asked why she wants to die now, Sara replies that she has lived long enough—through the deaths of her husband, two of her children, three of her brothers, and both her sisters. Her one remaining son is dying of leukemia and has only weeks to live. She wants to die before him so she won't have to grieve his death. Her request for lethal medication is not granted. Sara leaves the hospital with public health nurses and family to look after her. Her physician agrees to make home visits as Sara is too weak to travel to the office. A few days later, Sara is found dead in bed by the visiting nurse. The physician, called to the house to pronounce the patient dead, notices several empty pill bottles, including those from the morphine, at the bedside. The physician thinks that this may have been a suicide, but decides not to pursue it and simply completes the death certificate as for a natural death.

The patient's request to hasten death should be explored in detail. It may represent the wish to escape from depression, anxiety, uncontrolled physical pain, shame of dependency, and other psychosocial issues. Once the purpose of the request is understood, the problem can usually be ameliorated through appropriate techniques of palliative care, and the request is frequently withdrawn. If the request is ignored or belittled, the patient is left to deal with these feelings alone, and may, in fact, commit suicide because of suffering that might have been dealt with by other means.

There are times, however, as in our example, when protracted pain and other debilitating symptoms make choosing death a desirable alternative to continued suffering. The relationship between the physician, patient, and family as well as the physician's own values determine the response to such requests. Clinicians who refuse to participate in assisted suicide, because of their own moral positions, should make this clear to the patient. In this event, they have an obligation to seek common ground with the patient and to continue to search for other avenues to relieve suffering. Usually such intractable suffering can be addressed with symptom management, withdrawal of all potentially life-sustaining therapies, and terminal sedation if all else fails. Those who are considering these last-resort options should fully explore the potential personal, professional, and legal consequences. Guidelines for assisted suicide have been published, and clinicians confronted with a reasonable request to end life should refer to these, as well as to colleagues experienced in terminal care, for help.

HOPE & MEANING

Throughout the dying process, the search for hope and meaning is always in the background. Hopelessness and despair are disturbing emotions. Hope helps patients and their loved ones endure suffering when faced with a terminal illness. It comes in many forms, not simply through cure or recovery. To hope for a peaceful death, to have a little more time to finish business, to find new meaning and the possibility of personal growth in our dying, or to become emotionally closer to loved ones or to God are all hopes and wishes not dependent on cure of the body.

CASE ILLUSTRATION 8

Rhea, a 64-year-old woman with metastatic breast cancer, is on high-dose long-acting morphine because of bone pain. She has fractures of the clavicle and both femurs and has requested no resuscitation in the event of cardiac or pulmonary arrest. She hopes to be able to die at home, where she has very close family support, without more painful episodes or fractures.

Rhea now shows signs of increasing confusion and dehydration but wants to avoid hospitalization. She expresses the strong wish not to die yet because her children and their families are arriving in 2 weeks.

She wants not only to see them, but to be as alert and pain free as possible while they visit. Hypercalcemia is found on evaluation and hospitalization is advised. Because she wishes to die at home with only palliative measures taken, she remains at home for another day. She knows that she could let herself die from the effects of the calcium, but that she then would not get to see her daughters. Despite attempts at oral treatment she becomes progressively less alert and is brought to the hospital by her family when her oral intake stops.

Treatment is initiated with intravenous fluids and diuretics and the hypercalcemia is corrected; her confusion clears, and she is able to go home after a week. By the time her children arrive, Rhea is alert and able to communicate coherently. She is quite elated that she can have last words with them and her grandchildren. Despite the need for increased doses of morphine and multiple other medications to control her symptoms, she is not hospitalized again and dies at home several months later.

The hope for more time may be reasonable. Relatively invasive interventions that exceed the boundaries of hospice care but that extend meaningful life and are consistent with the patient's goals are sometimes appropriate. Remaining flexible in the face of changing, difficult situations and letting the patient's goals guide the treatment permit the clinician to hope, along with the patient, for a death with as little meaningless suffering as possible. When no hope is offered or found, the patient is left alone and isolated.

Case illustration 3 (the case of the patient who had been abandoned twice) is also germane here. The hopelessness engendered by the first clinician, who prescribed acetaminophen and codeine for metastatic cancer, led to feelings of despair. These were alleviated when the patient looked elsewhere for treatment and was given a complicated regimen to follow. By providing an activity on which to focus, the alternative clinic offered him hope, however false. In sum, the lack of continuity with the primary practitioner resulted in a desperate search for help and left the patient and his wife open to exploitation.

Alternative healing methods often offer hope to some patients when traditional methods are not working, have proven too burdensome, or are not consistent with the patient's preferences or beliefs about illness and healing. Patients who are interested in pursuing alternative methods of treatment should be encouraged to do so, particularly if those treatments are noninvasive, and are therefore unlikely to harm. There is nothing to systematically preclude combining nontraditional treatments with traditional treatments as part of an individually tailored treatment plan. Some may be turning to alternative treatment because they have been told their case is hopeless and there is nothing left to be done. However, selecting such therapies because of a sense of futility, desperation, and abandonment is very different from choosing them because they are consistent with a person's goals and values. Aggressive if unconventional therapeutic alternatives often offer the patient some degree of hope. However, the validity of this type of hope needs to be explored by the clinician and patient together. Examining the risks and benefits of the therapy is frequently enough to begin the dialogue, which can then continue by exploring the possibilities and probabilities of improvement and by distinguishing false hope from a meaningful alternative (see Chapter 28).

Trying to find and maintain hope when it becomes evident that recovery is hopeless calls for personal and spiritual exploration. The patient's feeling of hopelessness may need to be probed in depth before possible new avenues for hope and meaning can be examined. It is important not to provide false hope through simple or formulaic solutions to complex problems; hopeful solutions are often uniquely personal and may be discovered through continuing exploration by the patient with family, friends, health care providers, and clergy.

Some patients are not afraid of dying and come to accept death as a natural step in completing the life cycle. Such persons die with grace and ease, demonstrating that death does not always have to be feared or denied. Furthermore, some patients experience profound personal growth in the process of dying. For some highly independent persons, this becomes a time to be more accepting and appreciative of the love and care of others.

 CASE ILLUSTRATION 9

A 64-year-old veterinarian, Richard, develops headaches so severe that he can no longer carry on his surgical practice. Within 3 months, he is diagnosed with an inoperable brain tumor. Over the ensuing 6 months, he loses the ability to walk and swallow. Because of recurrent aspiration, he is placed on a home ventilator and fed through a gastrostomy tube. In the face of his overwhelming losses, he decides he wants to tape a description of his life and journey to the point at which he is now. Relatives, friends, colleagues, and members of his church come to his home, and joint recollections and reflections are taped. When this process is complete Richard says good-bye to his wife and family and requests that the respirator and fluids be withdrawn. With his physician's consent and instructions to family members, he is given regular doses of morphine and the respirator is turned off. He dies with his loved ones in attendance. His life and death leave a legacy of courage and an acquiescence to fate that touches the hearts of those he knew.

The search for love, a connection to others, and a sense of meaning are essential in helping patients through the dying process. The ability to experience love and meaning can ameliorate considerable suffering. If love and purpose can be found, then fears usually lessen, and dying may be accepted as an adventure and entry into the next phase of existence.

CARE OF THE FAMILY

Terminal illness can help resolve or intensify family conflict. Issues of power, money, allegiances, previous losses, and grief may surface along with unforeseen courage and the noblest sacrifices that family members may ever have made on behalf of one another. Paradoxical feelings of anger and love, fear and bravery, anxiety and compassion, depression and transcendence never seem to be far removed on the part of the dying patient and his or her caregivers.

The physician can be a healing presence in this volatile mix by including the patient's family and other caregivers as part of the treatment team. Such collaboration broadens the patient's network of support, enlisting new allies and more widely distributing the burden of care.

The clinician needs to communicate clearly with family members regarding plans for care, prognosis, complications, and who will make decisions if the patient cannot. Establishing advance directives with the patient and the proxy is essential when it is likely the patient will lose capacity during the illness. The selection of a proxy forces the patient to choose among family members and may trigger old family wounds over who was favored and who has more power. The patient's wishes and choices should take precedence over what family members may want, although in actual practice this is sometimes difficult to achieve. When the patient loses mental capacity, the family becomes the focus of decision making, and processes are brought into play that may create conflict. Family pressures may influence even what the competent patient does. The clinician may need to remind family members that whether the patient is competent or not, the patient's values, beliefs, and preferences need to be honored.

When a family has many members, the clinician may want to meet regularly with a small group and at special times with more members. The family can be asked to designate representatives who can stay in close touch with the physician. If patients have lost the capacity to express their wishes and family members are in conflict about a certain plan, it is best to focus on what the patient would have wanted, applying the ethical principle of substituted judgment. If the patient's wishes are unknown, what is in the patient's best interest must be discussed. Views on what is truly in the patient's best interest may vary widely between family members and clinicians (see Chapter 8).

Unexpected Death

An unexpected death puts a particular strain on the family and the clinician. Sudden or traumatic death sends a shock through the family and, when it occurs in a medical facility, may elicit strong doubt about competence in clinicians. Meeting with the family, expressing sympathy, and answering questions in as straightforward a way as possible may be helpful. Family members should be allowed to view and stay with the deceased; when possible, the eyes and mouth should be closed and the limbs arranged peacefully. Strong emotional reactions should be anticipated and the tears of grief welcomed.

The clinician should recognize each family member present and solicit each person's reaction. Cultural norms may vary widely in the emotional behaviors displayed. The normal reactions to grief in some cultures (screaming, yelling, falling to the ground) may seem inappropriate or embarrassing to a clinician from another, less demonstrative background. Only through experience with various manifestations of grief can the clinician judge what "normal" grief should look like. Physicians and nurses may want to call in clergy and social workers; each may have something to offer a family that is trying to integrate the shock and loss.

When an unexpected death occurs in the context of ongoing medical care, the practitioner should critically examine what, if anything, could have been done to prevent its occurrence. Self-recrimination and blame may initially be part of this process for the clinician, especially if a medical misjudgment is involved. Learning from the experience, discussing it with trusted colleagues, and, if necessary, disclosing it to the family are often appropriate. It is important that clinicians not bear the burdens of these experiences alone (see Chapter 32).

Unresolved Grief

Of all the causes of unremitting grief, one of the most overwhelmingly difficult for families and practitioners is the death of a child, especially when the death is unexpected. The parents' grief must be followed closely for signs of becoming pathological. The physician should not try to ameliorate the pain of the loss prematurely. Supportive listening, acknowledging and legitimizing the suffering, and expressing empathy may be the best initial approach. Follow-up visits to elicit stories and memories give the parents a chance to talk about the deceased if they choose. Discussing and expressing anger, guilt, and sadness can help the bereavement process. In many other cases, survivors are unable to deal with the loss of a parent, a sibling, a spouse or partner, or a long-time friend. Grief that is unresolved may lead to clinical depression, social isolation, and emotional numbing as well as multiple physical symptoms. Social problems such as drug abuse, marital and work conflicts, and feelings of hopelessness and abandonment may also appear. If the clinician cannot help the family resolve the grief, referral should be made to an appropriate support group or a therapist for counseling.

SELF-CARE

How health-care workers take care of themselves when involved in work related to death and dying has not received a great deal of attention. Burnout is common among physicians and nurses who work with patients who are suffering a terminal illness. Having responsibility for dying patients' care and management, in a society that denies death, exacerbates the problem. From the initial delivery of bad news to decisions about whether to attend the funeral, clinicians are confronted with thoughts and feelings that enmesh them with the patient and the family. How closely the patient's family resembles their own may determine how emotionally involved they become. The grief that follows the death of a close patient may be quite profound and requires time and reflection to heal. Unfortunately, most institutions do not have an organized way for caregivers to get and give support during these times. The feelings of loss need to be recognized and discussed. Support or bereavement groups may help in this process. Hospital morbidity and mortality committees review the decedent's medical care, but they rarely reflect on how caregivers felt about the death, or what effect it has on the staff. Setting aside time to review the death from this perspective is likely to be helpful for staff morale, cohesiveness, and healing (see Chapter 7).

Taking care of the dying patient enables clinicians to view death at very close range. Feelings of compassion and love as well as loneliness and vulnerability are frequently stirred up in providers. Healing responses may include turning to music, art, religion, literature, nature, humor, or psychotherapy for solace and understanding. Spiritual questions of purpose and meaning in life become more immediate in the face of impending death. Not only do workers in the realm of death and dying midwife patients through the dying process, but the dying patient midwifes us into a fuller experience of life.

SUGGESTED READINGS

American Board of Internal Medicine, End of Life Care Project Committee: Caring for the dying: identification and promotion of physician competency, 1996.

American Medical Association: Good care of the dying patient. JAMA 1996;275:474.

Clinical practice guideline: Management of cancer pain. Agency for Health Care Policy and Research. Publication No. 94-0592. Available through the National Cancer Institute.

Ebell MH: Prearrest predictors of survival following in-hospital cardiopulmonary resuscitation. J Fam Pract 1992;34:551.

Field MJ, Cassel CK for the Committee on Care at the End of Life, Institute of Medicine: *Approaching Death: Improving Care at the End of Life.* National Academy Press, 1997.

Quill TE: *Caring for Patients at the End of Life: Facing an Uncertain Future Together.* Oxford University Press, 2001.

Snyder L, Quill TE (editors): *Physician Guide to End-of-Life Care.* ACP-ASIM Publishing, 2001.

Waisel DB, Truog RD: The cardiopulmonary-resuscitation-not-indicated order: futility revisited. Ann Intern Med 1995; 122:304.

WEB SITES

American Academy of Hospice and Palliative Medicine
www.aahpm.org
Americans Academy on Physician and Patient
www.physicianpatient.org
American for Better Care of the Dying
www.abcd-caring.org
American Hospice Foundation
www.americanhospice.org
American Medical Association: Education for Physicians in End-of-Life Care
www.ama-assn.org/ethic
Compassion in Dying
www.compassionindying.org
Last Acts
www.lastacts.org

Index

Note: Page numbers followed by the letter "*t*" indicates tables, those followed by the letter "*f*" indicate figure.

Q

Quinolones, psychiatric side effects of, 326*t*

R

Rape, 291
Rapid ejaculation, 288–289
RBD (REM-behavior disorder), 270
Reactance, 136
Reactive depression, 188
screening in HIV-positive patients, 323
Reassurance and hope, offering, 20–21
Reductionism, 55, 56*t*
Reflection, 13
Reframing, 71*t*
Rehabilitation, older patients, 100
Relapse stage, 135, 136*t*, 147–148
Relational model, 56
Relationship-centered care, 57, 173
Relaxation techniques
anxiety disorders, 218*t*
hypnosis, 49
REM (rapid eye movement) sleep, 263
REM-behavior disorder (RBD), 270
Remeron. *See* Mirtazapine
Renal failure, depression and, 192*t*
Reproductive system, stress and, 305
Resistance, "rolling with," 178, 178*t*
Respect, 14
Respiratory problems, hypnosis for, 50
Resting metabolic expenditure (RME), 163
Restless legs syndrome (RLS), 266
Reverse transcriptase inhibitors (RTIs), interaction with pain medications, 323
Risperidone, cytochrome P-450 psychotropic interactions in HIV/AIDS patients, 327*t*
Rivastigmine, for Alzheimer's disease, 261*t*
RLS (restless legs syndrome), 266
RME (resting metabolic expenditure), 163
Rollnick, Stephen, 135–136
Runaway adolescents, 91–92

S

Sadness , in reaction to chronic disease, 352
Schizoid personality disorder. *See also* Personality disorders
case illustration, 239
differential diagnosis, 239
doctor–patient relationship, 239
illness experience and behavior, 239
management, 234*t*, 239
symptoms and signs, 233*t*, 238–239, 238*t*
Schizotypal personality disorder. *See also* Personality disorders
case illustration, 240–241
differential diagnosis, 240
doctor–patient relationship, 240
illness experience and behavior, 240
management, 234*t*, 240
symptoms and signs, 233*t*, 239–240, 240*t*
School age children. *See also* Children
attention deficit disorders, 84–85, 84*t*-85*t*
primary nocturnal enuresis, 83–84
SCL-90 (Hopkins Symptom Checklist 90 Revised), 208
SCOFF questionnaire for eating disorders, 125
Selective serotonin reuptake inhibitors. *See* SSRIs
Self-awareness as physician skill, 21
Self-care, physicians and health-care workers, 57. *See also* Physician well-being
working with dying patients, 366
Self-efficacy model, 135–137
Self-hypnosis, 51, 52*t*
Seroquel, cytochrome P-450 psychotropic interactions in HIV/AIDS patients, 327*t*
Sertraline (Zoloft), 197–198
adverse effects, 198, 198*t*
cytochrome P-450 psychotropic interactions in HIV/AIDS patients, 327*t*
for obsessive-compulsive disorder (OCD), 214, 217*t*
for panic disorder, 217*t*

pharmacodynamics, 197*t*
for posttraumatic stress disorder (PTSD), 215
sexual dysfunction and, 279
for weight loss, 166
Serzone. *See* Nefazodone
Sexual activity
assessment in adolescent medical interview, 90
chronic illness, effects on, 352
Sexual addiction, 291
Sexual aversion disorder, 283, 284*t*, 285–286
Sexual issues and professional development
ambiguity, 34–35
awareness, 37–38
boundaries, 33–34, 42–43
colleagues, relationships with, 39, 43
connectedness, 35
developmental experiences, 36–37, 41
historical perspective, 33
identity, 35
intensity and physical intimacy, 35–36
mentoring, 43–44
overview, 33, 41, 44
power differences, 39–40
progression to termination of relationship, 38–39
recommendations, 44
sexuality, 33, 42–43
shame and humiliation, 40–42
training programs, 42
workshop experience, 34
Sexual problems
challenge for primary care providers, 274
common issues, 275–276
common sexual disorders
female sexual arousal disorder, 286
hypoactive sexual desire, 283, 285–286
male erectile disorder, 286–288
orgasmic disorder, 289–290
rapid ejaculation, 288–289
sexual aversion disorder, 283, 285–286
sexual pain, 290–291